AF761670

RESEARCH ON MELANOMA – A GLIMPSE INTO CURRENT DIRECTIONS AND FUTURE TRENDS

Edited by **Mandi Murph**

INTECHWEB.ORG

Research on Melanoma – A Glimpse into Current Directions and Future Trends
Edited by Mandi Murph

Published by InTech
Janeza Trdine 9, 51000 Rijeka, Croatia

Copyright © 2011 InTech
All chapters are Open Access articles distributed under the Creative Commons Non Commercial Share Alike Attribution 3.0 license, which permits to copy, distribute, transmit, and adapt the work in any medium, so long as the original work is properly cited. After this work has been published by InTech, authors have the right to republish it, in whole or part, in any publication of which they are the author, and to make other personal use of the work. Any republication, referencing or personal use of the work must explicitly identify the original source.

Statements and opinions expressed in the chapters are these of the individual contributors and not necessarily those of the editors or publisher. No responsibility is accepted for the accuracy of information contained in the published articles. The publisher assumes no responsibility for any damage or injury to persons or property arising out of the use of any materials, instructions, methods or ideas contained in the book.

Publishing Process Manager Petra Nenadic
Technical Editor Teodora Smiljanic
Cover Designer Jan Hyrat
Image Copyright dean bertoncelj, 2011. Used under license from Shutterstock.com

First published August, 2011
Printed in Croatia

A free online edition of this book is available at www.intechopen.com
Additional hard copies can be obtained from orders@intechweb.org

Research on Melanoma – A Glimpse into Current Directions and Future Trends,
Edited by Mandi Murph
p. cm.
ISBN 978-953-307-293-7

INTECH OPEN ACCESS PUBLISHER

INTECH open

free online editions of InTech
Books and Journals can be found at
www.intechopen.com

Contents

Preface

This is an exciting time for the field of melanoma research. So far in 2011 the FDA has approved two new immunotherapies against this malignancy and is likely to vote on a targeted therapeutic soon. The clinical trials evaluating BRAF inhibitors are being discussed at major symposia and appearing in popular news media. There hasn't been this much activity on melanoma therapeutics since 1998. For researchers it is particularly exciting to see years of studying aberrant molecular mechanisms in the laboratory translate into the clinic. The goal of scientists who tirelessly study mechanisms of disease is this – to contribute to developing lifesaving interventions. Now is the time when this dream is coming to fruition. Although the ability to cure every melanoma patient may still be elusive, exploiting melanoma's molecular weaknesses and observing dramatic effects provides hope and confidence to researchers that it can be done.

Thus, this book on melanoma research provides a glimpse of many diverse scientific aspects that are currently underway in melanoma research laboratories around the world. Although the topics are different they all have the same goals, to develop better understandings of malignancy and treatment methods. The sections of this book are organized to reflect emerging trends in research, starting with epigenetics. The role of epigenetics is under investigation in melanoma as well as other types of cancers. There is much progress to be made in this complex area to help explain the etiology of disease, a topic that patients always ask when attempting to pinpoint the source of their cancer. In addition, a subsequent section contains work discussing emerging, promising and much-needed therapeutics. Although newer drugs have an enhanced ability for treatment, they also suffer from chemoresistance development, a huge clinical problem among other cancer types. Thus, there is still much work to be done in the area of melanoma therapeutics.

In the section on Molecular Signaling, the manuscripts cover a broad range of areas. The classical pathways are discussed, including BRAF, along with some emerging proteins that are likely highly relevant to melanoma. This theme is continued with the final section on Tumor Progression and the Microenvironment. Manuscripts organized in this section are focused on angiogenesis, the tumor microenvironment and metastasis. All of these reflect clinical problems in need of additional research, whereby contributions aimed towards melanoma are likely to be translatable to numerous cancer types.

This book would not have been possible without the help of several wonderful people. These include Ana Pantar, Petra Nenadic, Juliet Eneh and Molly Altman. I would also like to thank my spouse, Gary Rollie, who has always been incredibly supportive of my career and dealt with me this past year as I worked on this project. I think he knew when I said, "This will only take a few more minutes", that it wasn't true, but he patiently understood that at some point I would finish.

Sincerely,

Mandi Murph, Ph.D.
Assistant Professor Department of Pharmaceutical and
Biomedical Sciences University of Georgia College of Pharmacy
Athens, GA,
USA

Part 1

Epigenetics

1

Predictive Capacity and Functional Significance of MicroRNA in Human Melanoma

Xiaobo Li and Yaguang Xi
Mitchell Cancer Institute, University of South Alabama, USA

1. Introduction

Melanoma is one of the most serious forms of cutaneous malignancies with an incidence of over two million people worldwide[1]. During 2010, an estimated 68,130 new patients were diagnosed with melanoma, and 8,700 deaths were attributed to the development of metastatic disease in the United States[2]. Compared to earlier stages of melanoma, the prognosis for patients with metastatic (stage IV) melanoma is very poor with six out of every seven skin cancer-related deaths being attributed to melanoma. However, our diagnostic and prognostic methods for melanoma are primarily histologic, such as Breslow's depth of invasion, falling far short of being able to accurately predict the overall survival, recurrence risk, or clinical outcomes for patients[3]. There are several methods of treatment for metastatic melanoma, including radiation therapy, immunotherapy, chemotherapy, and palliative surgery[2, 4, 5]. However, there exists a clear and unfortunate understanding that these therapies are only minimally effective in treating patients with advanced disease[6].

MicroRNAs(miRNAs) are a set of small, average 22 nt in length, single-stranded, non-protein-coding RNA molecules that can recognize and bind 3'-untranslated regions (UTR) of mRNA, blocking translation of the gene or inducing cleavage of the mRNA[7, 8]. To date, a total of 15,172 miRNAs (Version 16.0), including 1,049 human miRNAs, have been registered in the miRbase database. The biogenesis of miRNA is similar to the other RNA starting from DNA transcription. A primary miRNA (pri-miRNA) is an independent transcript processed by RNA polymerase II (Pol II), which are bound in the nucleus by the microprocessor complex consisting of the RNase III-type endonuclease, Drosha, and its co-factor, Pasha (DGCR8). These enzymes can crop the pri-miRNA into a hairpin loop, cleaving off 3' and 5' regions of excess mRNA to give precursor miRNA (pre-miRNA) ~70 nt in length. Pre-miRNA is then actively transported to the cytoplasm by exportin-5 where it is bound by the RNAse III-type endonuclease, Dicer, which removes the loop, resulting in a duplex of complementary, mature miRNA sequences. One strand is bound by the RNA-induced silencing (RISC) complex, which guides mature miRNA to target mRNA for subsequent silencing. The remaining strand is usually degraded, but it may be bound by RISC and target its own mRNAs, which are denoted with an asterisk (i.e., miR-10b and miR-10b*)[9, 10].

In both plants and animals, miRNAs are capable of mediating gene expression by influencing the RNA's stability and/or translational resspression[11, 12]. Impressively, a single miRNA can potentially bind hundreds to thousands of its cognate mRNA 3'UTR sequences. It is predicted that miRNAs may regulate upwards of 30% of all mammalian genes' expression, due to their critical function in gene regulation and expression[8]. Thus, it is meaningful to understand their roles and significance in the essential cellular events, such as development, differentiation, proliferation, and apoptosis, which account for carcinogenesis, tumor progression, and metastasis[13-16]. MiRNA synthesis and function is summarized in Figure 1.

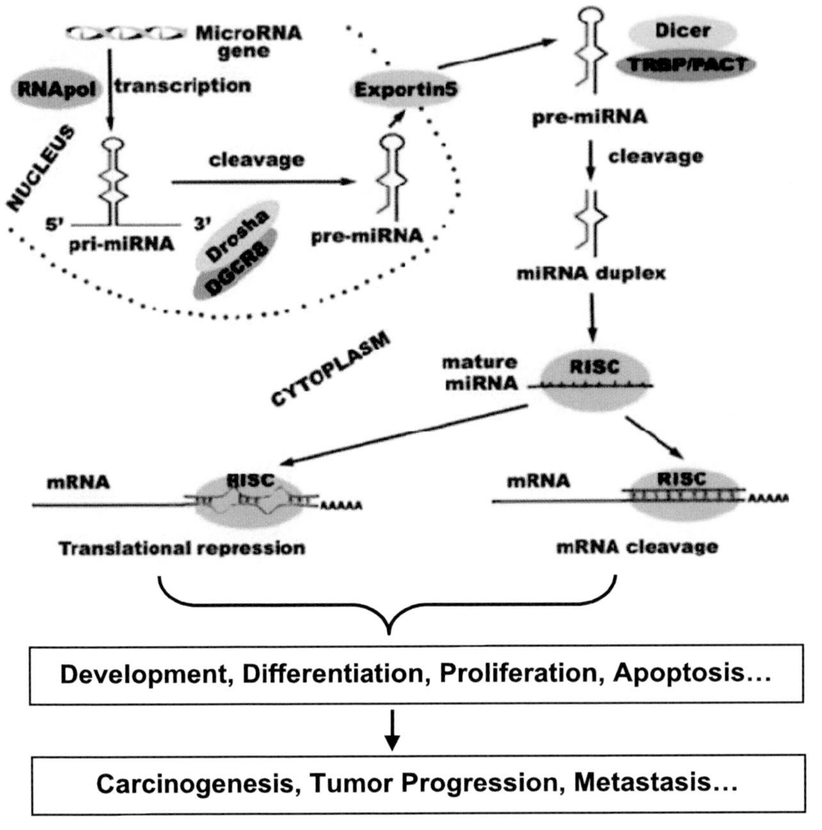

Fig. 1. MicroRNA biogenesis and biological functions

Following a pilot study connecting B-cell chronic lymphocytic leukemia (CLL) and deregulated expression of miR-15a and miR-16-1[17], it has been demonstrated that more than 50% of miRNA genes are located in cancer-associated genomic regions or within fragile sites[18], and more and more miRNAs have been identified to play a central role in the pathogenesis of human cancers. Although it was in 2006 that the first study on miRNA in melanoma has reported that 86% of primary melanoma cell lines had DNA copy number alterations in genomic loci containing miRNA genes[19], studies focusing on the roles of miRNA in the pathogenesis and development of melanoma have bloomed since 2008. Figure 2 illustrates the miRNAs reported by more than two studies or confirmed by functional studies in the progression of melanoma[20-26], suggesting that miRNAs play an important role in melanocyte and melanoma biology. To date, there are 77 publications that can be retrieved in PUBMED when using keywords "melanoma and miRNA"; more than 99% of them were published in the latest three years, and half of them were published from 2010 to 2011, which is evidence that this research field is rapidly expanding. However, a few knowledge and understanding gaps need to be filled before taking full advantage of miRNA signatures in melanoma research. In 2010, we were invited to author a review summarizing the accomplishments on the research of miRNA and melanoma[27]. Here, based on the previous review, we will highlight the latest progress in this field.

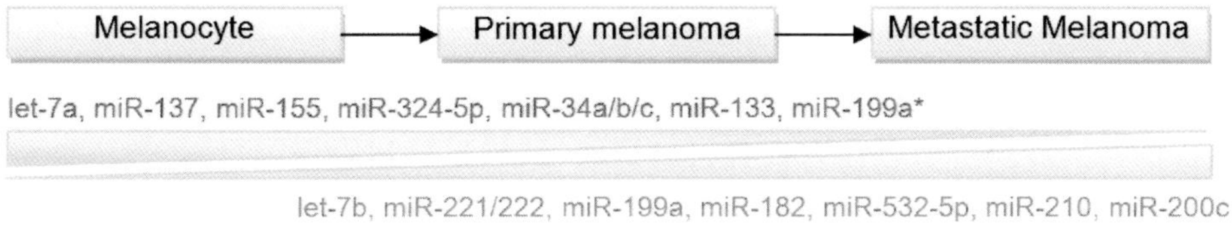

Fig. 2. Representative miRNAs involved in the progression of melanoma

2. Oncogenic miRNAs in melanoma

The role of miRNAs in tumorigenesis depends on their target genes' classification and abundance. When targeting tumor suppressor genes, these over-expressed miRNAs will play the promoting tumor roles as oncogenes; likewise, when targeting oncogenes, these miRNAs will have the characteristics of tumor suppressors. Kitago et al. reported that miR-532-5p directly targeted the runt-related transcription factor 3 (RUNX3) tumor suppressor during the progression from melanocyte to metastatic melanoma[28]. MiR-532-5p was shown to be significantly up-regulated in melanoma cells compared to normal melanocytes and in metastatic melanoma tissue compared to primary melanoma tissue. The transfection of anti-miR-532-5p molecules to the melanoma cells rescued the expression of RUNX3. Methylation analysis of the RUNX3 promoter region showed that transcriptional regulation was not a major regulatory mechanism for the down-regulation of RUNX3 expression in melanoma, suggesting miR-532-5p induced post-transcriptional regulation played an important role in melanoma progression.

Zhang et al. demonstrated that the expression of miR-210, the most prominent miRNA up-regulated by hypoxia and a direct transcriptional target of hypoxia inducible factors (HIFs), was elevated in multiple cancer types and correlated with breast cancer and melanoma metastases, respectively. MiR-210 over-expression in cancer cells bypassed hypoxia-induced cell-cycle arrest by directly targeting the expression of MNT, which is a gene known as one of the Myc antagonists. The miR-210-mediated abolishment of hypoxia-induced cell-cycle arrest was restored by the loss of Myc[5]. This finding indicated that miR-210 influenced the hypoxia response in tumor cells by triggering a Myc-like response by targeting MNT expression.

The miR-200 family has received much attention for suppressing epithelial-mesenchymal transition (EMT) as well as their down-regulation in some tumors promotes invasion and metastasis. Interestingly, Elson et al. showed that levels of miR-200 are increased in melanoma cell lines compared to normal melanocytes. In melanoma cell lines, the expression of miR-200 members has no significant effect on suppressing invasion but instead leads to a switch between modes of invasion. For example, miR-200c results in a higher proportion of cells thus adopting the rounded, amoeboid-like mode of invasion by reduced expression of myristoylated alanine-rich protein kinase C substrate (MARCKS); meanwhile, miR-200a results in a protrusion-associated elongated mode of invasion by reduced actomyosin contractility. This study improved our understanding of the impacts of the miR-200 family on suppressing invasion and metastasis, and implied a novel insight of these miRNAs in melanoma[29].

3. Tumor suppressor miRNAs in melanoma

Recently, miR-34 was identified as a target and a potential key responder of the tumor suppressor gene product, p53. Ectopic expression of miR-34a induced a G1 cell-cycle arrest, senescence, and apoptosis, which suggested that miR-34 was a potential tumor suppressor[12]. The altered expression of miR-34 was also found in melanoma progression[22, 24, 30]. Lodygin et al. reported that miR-34a expression is silenced in several types of cancer due to the aberrant CpG methylation of its promoter. Reportedly, 43.2% of melanoma cell lines and 62.5% of primary melanoma samples displayed CpG methylation of the miR-34a promoter and loss of miR-34a expression, whereas the two samples of normal melanocytes included in the study did not show promoter methylation[30]. Migliore et al. identified three miRNAs, miR-34b, miR-34c, and miR-199a*, in melanoma cells that negatively regulate the expression of MET, which is an oncogene that encodes the tyrosine kinase receptor for hepatocyte growth factor[24]. MET is frequently over-expressed in many human tumors and promotes the 'invasive growth' that results from the stimulation of cell motility and protection from apoptosis. Exogenous expression of these miRNAs in primary melanoma cells led to a decreased MET protein expression and resulted in the impairment of MET-mediated motility in these cells[24]. Recently, Yan et al. detected the expression level of miR-34a in uveal melanoma cells and melanocytes and found that miR-34a had been actively expressed in melanocytes but not in uveal melanoma cells. Additionally, the transfection of miR-34a into melanoma cells led to a significant repression of their growth and migration by down-regulating the expression of c-Met directly and the expression of phosphorylated Akt (p-Akt) and other cell-cycle-related proteins indirectly [22].

Mazar et al. found the levels of miR-211 were reduced in melanoma cell lines compared with expression levels in melanocytes. Ectopically expressing miR-211 in different melanoma cell lines caused significant growth inhibition and reduced invasiveness by cleaving the mRNA and inhibiting the translation of KCNMA1, a highly expressed protein in metastasizing melanoma, prostate cancer, and glioma[31]. Another research study resulted in a similar but more interesting conclusion. MiR-211 is encoded within the sixth intron of TRPM1, which is known as melastatin and is greatly down-regulated in metastatic melanomas; it is widely believed to function as a melanoma tumor suppressor. Levy et al. reported that the tumor suppressive activity of TRPM1 in melanoma is not mediated by this gene itself but instead by miR-211 hosted within an intron of TRPM1 because of the increasing expression of miR-211 but not a TRPM1 reduced migration and invasion of invasive human melanomas cells. This result implicates miR-211 as a suppressor of melanoma invasion whose expression is silenced or selected against via the suppression of the entire TRPM1 locus during human melanoma progression. Additionally, they also identified three central node genes, IGF2R, TGFBR2, and NFAT5, as the target of miR-211[32]. Notably, the micropthalmia-associated transcription factor (MITF), which is important for melanocyte development and function, is needed for high TRPM1 expression[31], and thus, MITF contributes to miR-211 expression, suggesting that the tumor-suppressor activities of MITF may at least be partially executed through miR-211's tumor suppressing effect.

MiR-196a is another documented tumor suppressor in melanoma by Dr.Bosserhoff's group [33, 34]. First, they found that miR-196a was significantly down-regulated in malignant melanoma cell lines and tissue samples when screening differential miRNAs. Re-expressing miR-196a *in vitro* can dramatically reduce the invasive behavior of melanoma cells, which is partially believed to account for the negative regulating expression of the transcription factor HOX-C8, which is a member belonging to the homeobox genes family. By investigating a potential "miR-196a → HOX-C8 → target gene" model, they further identified cadherin-11, calponin-1, and osteopontin as the downstream targets of miR-196a[34]. Additionally, they elucidated that down-regulated miR-196a in melanoma cells leads to enhanced HOX-B7 mRNA and protein levels, another member of the homeobox genes family, which subsequently raise Ets-1 activity, another transcription factor, by inducing basic fibroblast growth factor (bFGF). Ets-1 eventually up-regulates bone morphogenetic protein 4 (BMP-4) playing an important role in melanoma progression[33].

Chen et al. reported that the over-expression of miR-193b in melanoma cell lines repressed cell proliferation by down-regulating cyclin D1 (CCND1). They identified 31 miRNAs that are differentially expressed (13 up-regulated and 18 down-regulated) in metastatic melanomas relative to benign nevi by profile-analyzing tissue samples from benign nevi and metastatic melanomas. Notably, miR-193b was significantly down-regulated in the melanoma tissues examined. Functional studies revealed miR-193b is a tumor suppressor in melanoma. Their study indicates that miR-193b is able to repress cell proliferation and regulate CCND1 expression, suggesting that the deregulation of miR-193b may play an important role in melanoma development[35].

4. Molecular mechanism of microRNA associated with melanoma

The development of rational treatments for melanoma will depend on our taking advantage of its clinical features' molecular basis. The necessary understanding of the molecular genetics underlying melanoma is gradually emerging[36]. Many key genes and signaling pathways have been characterized for their functions associated with melanoma. For example, the micropthalmia-associated transcription factor (MITF) is one of the most recognizable oncogenes in melanoma, which regulates cell proliferation and apoptosis, and is over-expressed in 10-20% of human melanoma[32]. Also, it is a member in Myc supergene family of basic helix-loop-leucine-zipper transcription factors, which are necessary for functional melanocyte formation[37]. Because MITF's critical role in melanoma progression, several recent studies have explored miRNAs' impact on melanoma through MITF mediated pathways.

4.1 MicroRNAs targeting MITF

MicroRNA.org, an online database for miRNA targets prediction, provides more than 300 miRNA candidates that putatively target MITF. However, only few of them have been verified.

MiR-137 is located in the chromosomal region, 1p22, which is known to harbor an allele for melanoma susceptibility. The bioinformatics and *in vitro* analyses verified that miR-137 had targeted MITF in melanoma cells[20]. Most recently, Chen et al. reported the down-regulation of MITF by miR-137 in uveal melanoma cells[38]. Additionally, the over-expression of miR-137 in uveal melanoma cells can lead to a significant decrease in cell growth through inducing G1 cell cycle arrest, which might be due to its suppression on oncogenic tyrosine kinase protein receptor c-Met, cell cycle-related protein CDK6, and MITF[38].

Segura et al. described miR-182 also as a negative regulator of MITF expression[25]. MiR-182 is located in 7q31-34, a chromosomal region frequently altered in melanoma. MiR-182 was demonstrated to increase the invasive potentials of melanoma cells by repressing MITF and FOXO3, a Forkhead family transcription factor. Importantly, 7q31-34 also harbors c-Met (encodes hepatocyte growth factor receptor with tyrosine-kinase activity) and BRAF (member of the raf/mil family of serine/threonine protein kinases), two important regulators in the MAPK/ERK signaling pathway[39]. They found that miR-182 was over-expressed not only in human melanoma cell lines but also in tissue specimens. These results were inversely correlated with MITF and FOXO3 expression in the prediction of melanoma progression and development. Moreover, miR-182 ectopic expression in melanoma cells stimulated the anchorage-independent growth and invasion using an *in vitro* extracellular matrix assay, and promoted melanoma lung metastasis in a mouse model, whereas miR-182 down-regulation impeded invasion and triggered apoptosis of melanoma cells.

MiR-340 is capable of causing mRNA degradation by interacting with its 3'-UTR of MTIF. Interestingly, the RNA-binding protein coding region determinant-binding protein (CRD-BP) is highly expressed in melanoma and can directly bind the 3'-UTR of MITF mRNA thus preventing miR-340 access, resulting in the stabilization of the MITF transcript and the elevation the transcription of MITF[40].

4.2 MiRNAs regulated by MITF in transcription

As described earlier, miRNA has a similar transcription and regulatory process to other RNA molecules. MITF has been demonstrated as a transcriptional factor[37]. Ozsolak et al. identified a number of miRNAs that were regulated by MITF in melanoma cells using nucleosome mapping and linker sequence analyses[41]. These miRNAs included some members of let-7 family (let-7a-1, -7d, -7f-1 and -7i), miR-221/222, miR-17-92 cluster, miR-106-363 cluster, miR-29, miR-146a, miR-148b and miR-125b[41]. A few of them, such as let-7, miR-17-92, miR-221/222, and miR-148, have been documented for their abilities to connect many key genes and to signal pathways to melanoma. Here, we will illustrate a MITF-centered regulatory loop with the involvement of multiple miRNAs/mRNAs/pathways (Figure 3).

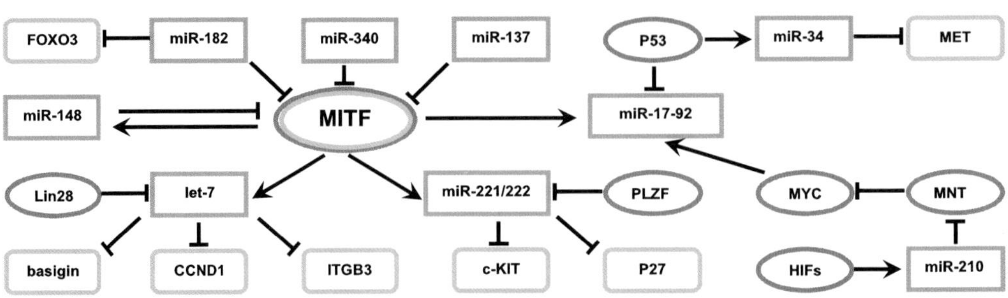

Fig. 3. Molecular mechanism of microRNA regulation in melanoma ▬ miRNA ▬ target gene ▬ transcription factor

The Let-7 family is highly conserved across species in sequence and function, which were first validated to be involved in tumorigenesis[42]. Schultz et al. revealed five members of the let-7 family (let-7a, -7b, -7d, -7e, and -7g) as being significantly down-regulated in primary melanoma when compared with benign nevi, which suggested that the let-7 family might be tumor suppressors in melanoma[43]. The ectopic over-expression of let-7b diminished the anchorage-independent growth ability of melanoma cells and inhibited the cell-cycle progression. The over-expression of let-7b eventually repressed cyclins (D1, D3 and A) and cyclin-dependent kinase (CDK4) all of which had been described to play a role in melanoma development. Most recently, another study showed that the over-expression of let-7b in the melanoma cell line B16-F10 exhibited an inhibition of both cellular proliferation and colony formation. Let-7b can reduce lung metastasis by repressing the expression of basigin, which is a stimulator for tumor cells producing matrix metalloproteinases (mmps) and is highly expressed on the surface of tumor cells[44].

Let-7a is considered lost in melanoma when one is comparing primary melanocytes to malignant melanoma cell lines. Sequencing analysis suggested Let-7a had an interaction with the 3'UTR of integrin β3 mRNA[26]. Integrin β3 is highly related to melanoma progression and leads to an enhanced migratory and an enhanced invasive potential of melanoma cells[45]. The transfection of melanoma cells with let-7a pre-miR molecules resulted in the down-regulation of integrin β3 mRNA and protein expression, which suggested that the loss of let-7a expression might be one of the essential regulatory mechanisms leading to an increase integrin β3 expression in melanoma cells[26]. Muller et al. also proved that the over-expression of let-7a in melanoma cells reduced their invasive potential by approximately 75%; meanwhile transfection with let-7a anti-miRs and anti-sense oligonucleotides that directly binds and inhibits the actions of miRNAs, resulted in the induction of the integrin β3 expression and induced the migration of anti-let-7a-transfected melanocytes. These findings revealed let-7a to be an important integrin β3 regulator, and the loss of let-7a is thus involved in the development and progression of malignant melanoma.

The miR-17-92 cluster locates to chromosome 13 and contains 6 members (miR-17, -18a, -19a, -20a, -19b-1 and -92a-1), while another miRNA cluster, miR-106-363that shares many similarities with the miR-17-92 cluster locates to the X chromosome; it also consists of 6 members (miR-106a, -18b, -20b, -19b-2, -92a-2 and -363). Both miRNA clusters are described as being oncogenic and found to be highly expressed in a variety of cancers[46, 47]. Muller et al. compared the miRnomes of normal human melanocytes and well characterized melanoma cell lines derived from primary tumors and melanoma metastases and showed that all members of the miR-17-92 cluster were up-regulated in primary tumor cell lines compared with normal melanocytes. The expression of the miR-17-92 cluster was even higher in metastatic cell lines with an approximately two-fold up-regulation as compared to primary melanoma cell lines. The expression of the miR-106-363 cluster was similar to the expression of the miR-17-92 cluster in melanocytes and melanoma cells. They detected a strong up-regulation of miR-106a expression in primary tumor cells and a further increase in expression levels in metastatic melanoma cells[48]. In addition to finding miR-17-5p, miR-18a, miR-20a, and miR-92a over-expressed and miR-146a, miR-146b, and miR-155 down-regulated in the majority of melanoma cell lines with respect to melanocytes, Levati et al. found that ectopic expression of miR-155 in melanoma cells inhibits the proliferation[49]. These results imply that the miR-17-92 cluster would be involved in melanoma progression.

Both miR-221 and miR-222 are regulated by MITF at the transcription level[21]. These two miRNAs are clustered on the X chromosome, are transcribed as a common precursor, and are over-expressed in a variety of cancers with the function of repressing the c-Kit receptor. In normal melanocytes, stem cell factor (SCF)-dependent c-Kit-mediated signaling supports proliferation, migration, and differentiation of cells[50]. Constitutive activation of c-Kit receptor tyrosine kinase (RTK) alone does not induce a tumorigenic transformation of the melanocytes in neither *in vitro* nor *in vivo*[51]; however, cutaneous melanoma are often characterized with a loss of c-Kit expression[52]. The inhibition of c-Kit RTK in c-Kit-positive melanoma showed an increased apoptosis and G1 phase cell-cycle arrest[52], while the re-expression of c-Kit in the c-Kit-negative melanoma cells restored c-Kit-mediated apoptosis and resulted in a loss of tumorigenic potential[53]. In accordance with these observations, Felicetti et al. found that up-regulated miR-221/222 repressed the expression of the c-Kit receptor and p27Kip1 (cyclin-dependent kinase inhibitor 1B, CDKN1B) tumor suppressor during melanoma progression from a weakly invasive primary tumor to a more invasive phenotype[21]. The over-expression of miR-221/222 in melanoma cells led to an increase in their proliferation and invasion *in vitro* and accelerated tumor growth in a mouse melanoma model. Conversely, treatment with anti-miRs against both miRNAs resulted in a reduced proliferation rate and migration of melanoma cells with a high level of miR-221/222 abilities. They also found that the elevated expression of miR-221/222 in melanoma cells was caused by the loss of a transcription factor, promyelocytic leukemia zinc finger (PLZF). PLZF binds to the miR-221/222 promoter and inhibits their transcription in normal melanocytes.

Cyclin-dependent kinase 2 (CDK2) has been reported to phosphorylate PLZF, triggering its ubiquitination and subsequent degradation[54]. Furthermore, p27Kip1 is important for the efficient induction of G1 cell-cycle arrest by PTEN and is necessary for PTEN-induced down-regulation of CDK2 [55, 56]. Additionally, PTEN is an inhibitor for Ha-ras-mediated astrocyte elevated gene-1 (AEG-1) transactivation [57]. AEG-1 directly binds PLZF, preventing it from binding its target promoters[58], including those of miR-221/222. Therefore, PTEN may be an important negative regulator of miR-221/222 in melanoma as it is capable to maintain PLZF levels to bind the miR-221/222 promoters, preventing their transcription. Although there are no miRNAs currently described to target PTEN in melanoma, recent reports highlighted miR-221/222 in aggressive non-small cell lung cancer (NSCLC) and hepatocarcinoma as oncomirs capable of directly targeting and inhibiting the expression of the tumor suppressor, PTEN [59, 60]. As a result, there may be a positive feedback loop for miR-221/222 expression, promoting melanoma progression through the joint inhibition of PTEN and p27Kip1 and blocking PTEN/AEG-1/PLZF and/or p27Kip1/CDK2/PLZF-mediated repression of miR-221/222.

Additionally, Igoucheva et al. confirmed that c-Kit was down-regulated by miR-221/222 and revealed that c-Kit regulation was mainly based on miRNA-dependent post-transcriptional mechanisms instead of an AP-2-dependent transcriptional mechanism[50]. Recently, mutations have been identified in both miRNAs and target genes that disrupt regulatory relationships. Godshalk et al. described a genetic variant in the 3' UTR of the KIT; this KIT variant results in a mismatch in the seed region of a miR-221 complementary site and thus leads to an increased expression of the KIT oncogene [61].

Haflidadóttir et al. suggested that miR-148 affects MITF mRNA expression in melanoma cells through a conserved binding site in the 3'UTR sequence of mouse and human MITF[37]. Interestingly, it seemed that MITF transcriptionally regulated the expression of miR-148b in melanoma cells[41], which showed that there was a negative feedback regulation between miR-148 and MITF to control their balance.

5. Clinical applications of miRNA in melanoma

5.1 Diagnostic miRNAs

Several years ago, we and other groups independently demonstrated that miRNAs were relatively more stable and tolerate RNAases better than mRNAs in both archived tissue samples and in blood samples[27, 41, 62], which suggests that miRNAs have the potential to be valuable, practical, and reliable biomarkers for disease states.

Recently, several groups employed a high through-put microarray technique to discover miRNA biomarkers from formalin-fixed and paraffin-embedded (FFPE) melanoma samples[9, 63, 64]. A number of miRNAs have shown the potential to become diagnostic markers for melanoma based on data from clinical samples and array analysis[9, 63, 64].Radhakrishnan et al. examined the presence of oncogenic miRNA (oncomirs) in uveal melanoma using FFPE specimens by comparing miRNA expression profiles between non-invasive tumor and melanoma metastatic to the liver. They revealed 19 miRNAs that were expressed in non-metastatic melanoma but were absent in metastatic melanoma, and they revealed 11 miRNAs with the opposite expression pattern[65].

In addition to FFPE samples, blood samples have been used to identify the melanoma tumor biomarkers[66]. Leidinger et al screened almost 900 human miRNAs, 55 blood samples, including 20 samples of healthy individuals, 24 samples of melanoma patients as test set, and 11 samples of melanoma patients as independent validation set. They identified 51 altered miRNAs (21 down-regulated miRNAs and 30 up-regulated miRNAs) that can potentially distinguish melanoma patients from healthy controls. More excitingly, the panel consisting of 16 deregulated miRNAs can reach a classification accuracy of 97.4%, a specificity of 95%, and a sensitivity of 98.9%. Therefore, this study again demonstrates that signatures of miRNA expression can act as useful biomarkers for melanoma[66]

Kanemaru et al, in particular, indentified the serum level of miR-221 as a new tumor marker in patients with malignant melanoma[67]. MiR-221 is usually up-regulated in malignant melanoma cells as we discussed earlier. By measuring the miR-221 levels in serum from 94 malignant melanoma patients and 20 healthy controls, they found that the circulating miR-221 was detectable and could be quantified in serum samples; the serum levels of miR-221 were significantly increased in malignant melanoma patients when compared to healthy controls. Among the malignant melanoma patients, the miR-221 levels were significantly increased in patients with advanced melanoma compared to those with melanoma in situ, and the levels were correlated with tumor thickness. Moreover, they also revealed a decreasing tendency for the miR-221 levels along with the surgical removal of the primary tumor, but miR-221 was found to increase again at recurrence, which strongly suggested that circulating miR-221 may be useful not only for diagnosing malignant melanoma and for differentiating melanoma with different stages, but it could also be useful as a prognostic marker for patients with malignant melanoma[67].

5.2 Prognostic miRNAs

Like miR-221, some other miRNAs have been reported for their prognostic signatures in melanoma. Worley et al. were the first to use a genome-wide, microarray-based approach to investigate the value of miRNA expression patterns in predicting metastatic risk in uveal melanoma. They found the most significant discriminator to classify low and high metastatic risk was let-7b and miR-199a expression. A classifier system that included the top six miRNA discriminators accurately distinguished melanoma patient tissues with high metastatic propensity with 100% sensitivity and specificity[23]. Satzger et al. found that miR-15b and miR-210 were significantly up-regulated in parallel with the down-regulation of miR-34a in melanoma compared to nevi. These three miRNAs were then analyzed in 128 primary melanoma patients, including detailed clinical follow-up information; only the high expression of miR-15b was significantly correlated with the poor recurrence-free survival and overall survival by the univariate Kaplan-Meier and the multivariate Cox analyses. Furthermore, the transfection of anti-miR-15b into melanoma cells led to a reduced tumor cell proliferation and an increased apoptosis. Their results showed that miR-15b might be a novel melanoma biomarker contributing to poor prognosis and tumorigenesis[68]. Segura et al. identified the signature of a panel of miRNAs for predicting post-recurrence survival in metastatic melanoma by analyzing 59 formalin-fixed paraffin-embedded melanoma metastasis samples. Eighteen over-expressed miRNAs are significantly correlated with longer survival (>18 months). The signature of a six-miRNA panel (miR-150, miR342-3p, miR-455-3p, miR-145, miR-155, and miR-497) can have a better advantage to classify stage III patients into different prognostic categories because it is an independent predictor of survival[69]. Additionally, the down-regulation of miR-191 and the up-regulation of miR-193b were reported to be associated with poor melanoma-specific survival[70].

5.3 Therapeutic miRNAs

Since miRNAs are critical in regulating many cellular events and are highly deregulated in various cancers, including melanoma, it is likely that miRNAs could be effective targets for treatment. The basic strategies of miRNA-based therapeutics are: first, delivering highly expressed miRNAs that are tolerated in normal tissues but are lost in diseased cells , which may provide a general strategy for miRNA replacement therapies[71]; and second, using specific compounds targets aberrant oncogenic miRNAs, especially for over-expressed miRNAs.

Sun et al. recently found that genistein, an isoflavone isolated from soybeans, inhibited human uveal melanoma cells growth in vitro and in vivo and altered the expression of miR-27a and its target gene zinc finger and BTB domain containing 10 (ZBTB10), hinting at the contributions of miR-27a to genistein's inhibitory effect on melanoma growth[72]. Das et al. found that human polynucleotide phosphorylase (hPNPase(old-35)), a type I IFN-inducible 3'-5' exoribonuclease, can specifically down-regulate the expression of miR-221, a regulator of p27(kip1) and usually over-expressed in melanoma, as stated previously. This study implied that targeting over-expression of hPNPase(old-35) might provide an effective therapeutic strategy for miR-221-overexpressing and IFN-resistant tumors, such as melanoma[73]. MiR-137 acted as a tumor suppressor and usually decreased in uveal melanoma as previously described. Chen et al described one avenue to increase the expression levels of miR-137 through treatment with a DNA hypomethylating agent, 5-aza-2'-deoxycytidine, or a histone deacetylase inhibitor, trichostatin A, for down-regulating its cognate target genes MITF and CDK6[38]. MiR-182 is a pro-metastatic miRNA frequently over-expressed in melanoma. Huynh et al. assessed the effect of anti-miR-182 oligonucleotides in a mouse model with melanoma liver metastasis and confirmed that miR-182 levels were effectively down-regulated in the tumors of anti-miR-treated mice. This study implies that anti-miR may be a promising therapeutic strategy for metastatic melanoma[74]. Targeted delivery of RNA-based therapeutics for cancer therapy remains a challenge. By developing an improved liposome-polycation-hyaluronic acid (LPH) nanoparticle vehicle, Chen et al. reported that miR-34a was successfully delivered to B16-F10 melanoma lung metastasis-bearing mice, and it could specifically suppress the surviving expression in the metastatic tumor and reduced tumor load in the lung[75].

Progression		miRNA	Target(s)	Regulatory Factor	Associations
		let-7a	ITGB3		↓ Migration, invasion
		let-7b	CCND1		↓ Proliferation, differentiation
		miR-137	MITF		↓ Cell migration, invasion and survival
	↓	miR-155			↑ Proliferation
		miR-324-5p			
Melanocyte		miR-34a	MET	Promoter methylation	↓Proliferation
↓		miR-106a			
		miR-126			
Primary Melanoma		miR-133a			
		miR-141			
	↑	miR-145			
		miR-15b			↑ Proliferation, survival
		miR-200c			Migration style transition
		miR-27b			
		miR-210	MNT		↑ Proliferation
		miR-126			
		miR-200c			
		miR-141			
	↓	miR-133a			
		miR-34a			
Primary Melanoma		miR-199a*	c-Met		↓ Cell migration, invasion and survival
		miR-34b/c	c-Met		↓ Cell migration, invasion and survival
↓		miR-106a			
		miR-133a			
Metastasis		miR-199a*			
	↑	miR-182	MITF, FOXO3		↑ Migration, invasion and survival
		let-7b			
		miR-133a			
		miR-155			↓ Proliferation, survival
	↓	miR-193b			
		miR-196a	HOX-C8 HOX-B7		↓Invasion
Melanocyte		miR-133a			
↓		miR-17-5p			
		miR-18a			
Metastasis		miR-19a/b			
	↑	miR-221/222	c-Kit, p27	PLZF	↑ Proliferation, invasion; ↓ differentiation
		miR-532-5p	RUNX3		↑Invasion
		miR-20a			
		miR-92a			

Table 1. MicroRNAs in melanoma progression

6. Summary

There were approximately 40 publications from the past year and a half that reported the involvement of miRNA in melanoma research from both laboratory and clinical settings, which evidences the perspective of miRNA as one of the most valuable biomarkers and therapeutic targets in current melanoma research. We are pleased to find the that research trend of miRNA and melanoma has changed from solely searching altered specific miRNAs to exploring molecular networks and connections between miRNAs and signaling pathways involved in the progression of melanoma (Table 1). Certainly, a better understanding of the biological machinery of miRNA function will allow us to visibly observe the genetic impacts on carcinogenesis and to explore effective therapeutic strategies for conquering melanoma in the near future.

7. Acknowledgement

We specifically acknowledge the Ochsner Journal for giving us a permission to represent partial contents from our pervious publication "MicroRNA in melanoma". We also appreciate Ms. Amy Brown for her editorial assistance.

8. References

[1] Melanoma FAQ. World Health Organization, 2008.
[2] Jemal A, Siegel R, Xu J, Ward E. Cancer statistics, 2010. CA Cancer J Clin 2010;60:277-300.
[3] Sekulic A, Haluska P, Jr., Miller AJ, Genebriera De Lamo J, Ejadi S, Pulido JS, Salomao DR, Thorland EC, Vile RG, Swanson DL, Pockaj BA, Laman SD, et al. Malignant melanoma in the 21st century: the emerging molecular landscape. Mayo Clin Proc 2008;83:825-46.
[4] Bapat SA, Jin V, Berry N, Balch C, Sharma N, Kurrey N, Zhang S, Fang F, Lan X, Li M, Kennedy B, Bigsby RM, et al. Multivalent epigenetic marks confer microenvironment-responsive epigenetic plasticity to ovarian cancer cells. Epigenetics 2010;5:716-29.
[5] Zhang Z, Sun H, Dai H, Walsh RM, Imakura M, Schelter J, Burchard J, Dai X, Chang AN, Diaz RL, Marszalek JR, Bartz SR, et al. MicroRNA miR-210 modulates cellular response to hypoxia through the MYC antagonist MNT. Cell Cycle 2009;8:2756-68.
[6] Tarhini AA, Agarwala SS. Cutaneous melanoma: available therapy for metastatic disease. Dermatol Ther 2006;19:19-25.
[7] Friedman RC, Farh KK, Burge CB, Bartel DP. Most mammalian mRNAs are conserved targets of microRNAs. Genome Res 2009;19:92-105.
[8] Lewis BP, Burge CB, Bartel DP. Conserved seed pairing, often flanked by adenosines, indicates that thousands of human genes are microRNA targets. Cell 2005;120:15-20.
[9] Glud M, Klausen M, Gniadecki R, Rossing M, Hastrup N, Nielsen FC, Drzewiecki KT. MicroRNA expression in melanocytic nevi: the usefulness of formalin-fixed, paraffin-embedded material for miRNA microarray profiling. J Invest Dermatol 2009;129:1219-24.
[10] Okamura K, Phillips MD, Tyler DM, Duan H, Chou YT, Lai EC. The regulatory activity of microRNA* species has substantial influence on microRNA and 3' UTR evolution. Nat Struct Mol Biol 2008;15:354-63.
[11] Bartel DP. MicroRNAs: genomics, biogenesis, mechanism, and function. Cell 2004;116:281-97.

[12] Gaur A, Jewell DA, Liang Y, Ridzon D, Moore JH, Chen C, Ambros VR, Israel MA. Characterization of microRNA expression levels and their biological correlates in human cancer cell lines. Cancer Res 2007;67:2456-68.

[13] Lee HC, Park IC, Park MJ, An S, Woo SH, Jin HO, Chung HY, Lee SJ, Gwak HS, Hong YJ, Yoo DH, Rhee CH, et al. Sulindac and its metabolites inhibit invasion of glioblastoma cells via down-regulation of Akt/PKB and MMP-2. J Cell Biochem 2005;94:597-610.

[14] Takamizawa J, Konishi H, Yanagisawa K, Tomida S, Osada H, Endoh H, Harano T, Yatabe Y, Nagino M, Nimura Y, Mitsudomi T, Takahashi T. Reduced expression of the let-7 microRNAs in human lung cancers in association with shortened postoperative survival. Cancer Res 2004;64:3753-6.

[15] Carmell MA, Xuan Z, Zhang MQ, Hannon GJ. The Argonaute family: tentacles that reach into RNAi, developmental control, stem cell maintenance, and tumorigenesis. Genes Dev 2002;16:2733-42.

[16] Karube Y, Tanaka H, Osada H, Tomida S, Tatematsu Y, Yanagisawa K, Yatabe Y, Takamizawa J, Miyoshi S, Mitsudomi T, Takahashi T. Reduced expression of Dicer associated with poor prognosis in lung cancer patients. Cancer Sci 2005;96:111-5.

[17] Calin GA, Dumitru CD, Shimizu M, Bichi R, Zupo S, Noch E, Aldler H, Rattan S, Keating M, Rai K, Rassenti L, Kipps T, et al. Frequent deletions and down-regulation of micro- RNA genes miR15 and miR16 at 13q14 in chronic lymphocytic leukemia. Proc Natl Acad Sci U S A 2002;99:15524-9.

[18] Calin GA, Sevignani C, Dumitru CD, Hyslop T, Noch E, Yendamuri S, Shimizu M, Rattan S, Bullrich F, Negrini M, Croce CM. Human microRNA genes are frequently located at fragile sites and genomic regions involved in cancers. Proc Natl Acad Sci U S A 2004;101:2999-3004.

[19] Zhang L, Huang J, Yang N, Greshock J, Megraw MS, Giannakakis A, Liang S, Naylor TL, Barchetti A, Ward MR, Yao G, Medina A, et al. microRNAs exhibit high frequency genomic alterations in human cancer. Proc Natl Acad Sci U S A 2006;103:9136-41.

[20] Bemis LT, Chen R, Amato CM, Classen EH, Robinson SE, Coffey DG, Erickson PF, Shellman YG, Robinson WA. MicroRNA-137 targets microphthalmia-associated transcription factor in melanoma cell lines. Cancer Res 2008;68:1362-8.

[21] Felicetti F, Errico MC, Segnalini P, Mattia G, Care A. MicroRNA-221 and -222 pathway controls melanoma progression. Expert Rev Anticancer Ther 2008;8:1759-65.

[22] Yan D, Zhou X, Chen X, Hu DN, Dong XD, Wang J, Lu F, Tu L, Qu J. MicroRNA-34a inhibits uveal melanoma cell proliferation and migration through downregulation of c-Met. Invest Ophthalmol Vis Sci 2009;50:1559-65.

[23] Worley LA, Long MD, Onken MD, Harbour JW. Micro-RNAs associated with metastasis in uveal melanoma identified by multiplexed microarray profiling. Melanoma Res 2008;18:184-90.

[24] Migliore C, Petrelli A, Ghiso E, Corso S, Capparuccia L, Eramo A, Comoglio PM, Giordano S. MicroRNAs impair MET-mediated invasive growth. Cancer Res 2008;68:10128-36.

[25] Segura MF, Hanniford D, Menendez S, Reavie L, Zou X, Alvarez-Diaz S, Zakrzewski J, Blochin E, Rose A, Bogunovic D, Polsky D, Wei J, et al. Aberrant miR-182 expression promotes melanoma metastasis by repressing FOXO3 and microphthalmia-associated transcription factor. Proc Natl Acad Sci U S A 2009;106:1814-9.

[26] Muller DW, Bosserhoff AK. Integrin beta 3 expression is regulated by let-7a miRNA in malignant melanoma. Oncogene 2008;27:6698-706.

[27] Howell P, Li X, Riker A, Xi Y. MicroRNA in Melanoma. The Ochsner Journal 2010;10:83-92.

[28] Kitago M, Martinez SR, Nakamura T, Sim MS, Hoon DS. Regulation of RUNX3 tumor suppressor gene expression in cutaneous melanoma. Clin Cancer Res 2009;15:2988-94.

[29] Elson-Schwab I, Lorentzen A, Marshall CJ. MicroRNA-200 family members differentially regulate morphological plasticity and mode of melanoma cell invasion. PLoS One 2010;5.

[30] Lodygin D, Tarasov V, Epanchintsev A, Berking C, Knyazeva T, Korner H, Knyazev P, Diebold J, Hermeking H. Inactivation of miR-34a by aberrant CpG methylation in multiple types of cancer. Cell Cycle 2008;7:2591-600.

[31] Mazar J, DeYoung K, Khaitan D, Meister E, Almodovar A, Goydos J, Ray A, Perera RJ. The regulation of miRNA-211 expression and its role in melanoma cell invasiveness. PLoS One 2010;5:e13779.

[32] Levy C, Khaled M, Iliopoulos D, Janas MM, Schubert S, Pinner S, Chen PH, Li S, Fletcher AL, Yokoyama S, Scott KL, Garraway LA, et al. Intronic miR-211 assumes the tumor suppressive function of its host gene in melanoma. Mol Cell 2010;40:841-9.

[33] Braig S, Mueller DW, Rothhammer T, Bosserhoff AK. MicroRNA miR-196a is a central regulator of HOX-B7 and BMP4 expression in malignant melanoma. Cell Mol Life Sci 2010;67:3535-48.

[34] Mueller DW, Bosserhoff AK. MicroRNA miR-196a controls melanoma-associated genes by regulating HOX-C8 expression. Int J Cancer 2010.

[35] Chen J, Feilotter HE, Pare GC, Zhang X, Pemberton JG, Garady C, Lai D, Yang X, Tron VA. MicroRNA-193b represses cell proliferation and regulates cyclin D1 in melanoma. Am J Pathol 2010;176:2520-9.

[36] Haluska FG, Tsao H, Wu H, Haluska FS, Lazar A, Goel V. Genetic alterations in signaling pathways in melanoma. Clin Cancer Res 2006;12:2301s-7s.

[37] Haflidadottir BS, Bergsteinsdottir K, Praetorius C, Steingrimsson E. miR-148 regulates Mitf in melanoma cells. PLoS One 2010;5:e11574.

[38] Chen X, Wang J, Shen H, Lu J, Li C, Hu DN, Dong XD, Yan D, Tu L. Epigenetics, MicroRNAs, and Carcinogenesis: Functional Role of MicroRNA-137 in Uveal Melanoma. Invest Ophthalmol Vis Sci 2011;52:1193-9.

[39] Dhomen N, Marais R. BRAF signaling and targeted therapies in melanoma. Hematol Oncol Clin North Am 2009;23:529-45.

[40] Goswami S, Tarapore RS, Teslaa JJ, Grinblat Y, Setaluri V, Spiegelman VS. MicroRNA-340-mediated degradation of microphthalmia-associated transcription factor mRNA is inhibited by the coding region determinant-binding protein. J Biol Chem 2010;285:20532-40.

[41] Ozsolak F, Poling LL, Wang Z, Liu H, Liu XS, Roeder RG, Zhang X, Song JS, Fisher DE. Chromatin structure analyses identify miRNA promoters. Genes Dev 2008;22:3172-83.

[42] Roush S, Slack FJ. The let-7 family of microRNAs. Trends Cell Biol 2008;18:505-16.

[43] Schultz J, Lorenz P, Gross G, Ibrahim S, Kunz M. MicroRNA let-7b targets important cell cycle molecules in malignant melanoma cells and interferes with anchorage-independent growth. Cell Res 2008;18:549-57.

[44] Fu TY, Chang CC, Lin CT, Lai CH, Peng SY, Ko YJ, Tang PC. Let-7b-mediated suppression of basigin expression and metastasis in mouse melanoma cells. Exp Cell Res 2011;317:445-51.

[45] Haass NK, Smalley KS, Li L, Herlyn M. Adhesion, migration and communication in melanocytes and melanoma. Pigment Cell Res 2005;18:150-9.

[46] He L, Thomson JM, Hemann MT, Hernando-Monge E, Mu D, Goodson S, Powers S, Cordon-Cardo C, Lowe SW, Hannon GJ, Hammond SM. A microRNA polycistron as a potential human oncogene. Nature 2005;435:828-33.
[47] Landais S, Landry S, Legault P, Rassart E. Oncogenic potential of the miR-106-363 cluster and its implication in human T-cell leukemia. Cancer Res 2007;67:5699-707.
[48] Mueller DW, Rehli M, Bosserhoff AK. miRNA expression profiling in melanocytes and melanoma cell lines reveals miRNAs associated with formation and progression of malignant melanoma. J Invest Dermatol 2009;129:1740-51.
[49] Levati L, Alvino E, Pagani E, Arcelli D, Caporaso P, Bondanza S, Di Leva G, Ferracin M, Volinia S, Bonmassar E, Croce CM, D'Atri S. Altered expression of selected microRNAs in melanoma: antiproliferative and proapoptotic activity of miRNA-155. Int J Oncol 2009;35:393-400.
[50] Igoucheva O, Alexeev V. MicroRNA-dependent regulation of cKit in cutaneous melanoma. Biochem Biophys Res Commun 2009;379:790-4.
[51] Curtin JA, Busam K, Pinkel D, Bastian BC. Somatic activation of KIT in distinct subtypes of melanoma. J Clin Oncol 2006;24:4340-6.
[52] Smalley KS, Contractor R, Nguyen TK, Xiao M, Edwards R, Muthusamy V, King AJ, Flaherty KT, Bosenberg M, Herlyn M, Nathanson KL. Identification of a novel subgroup of melanomas with KIT/cyclin-dependent kinase-4 overexpression. Cancer Res 2008;68:5743-52.
[53] Huang S, Luca M, Gutman M, McConkey DJ, Langley KE, Lyman SD, Bar-Eli M. Enforced c-KIT expression renders highly metastatic human melanoma cells susceptible to stem cell factor-induced apoptosis and inhibits their tumorigenic and metastatic potential. Oncogene 1996;13:2339-47.
[54] Costoya JA, Hobbs RM, Pandolfi PP. Cyclin-dependent kinase antagonizes promyelocytic leukemia zinc-finger through phosphorylation. Oncogene 2008;27:3789-96.
[55] Gottschalk AR, Basila D, Wong M, Dean NM, Brandts CH, Stokoe D, Haas-Kogan DA. p27Kip1 is required for PTEN-induced G1 growth arrest. Cancer Res 2001;61:2105-11.
[56] Mamillapalli R, Gavrilova N, Mihaylova VT, Tsvetkov LM, Wu H, Zhang H, Sun H. PTEN regulates the ubiquitin-dependent degradation of the CDK inhibitor p27(KIP1) through the ubiquitin E3 ligase SCF(SKP2). Curr Biol 2001;11:263-7.
[57] Lee SG, Su ZZ, Emdad L, Sarkar D, Fisher PB. Astrocyte elevated gene-1 (AEG-1) is a target gene of oncogenic Ha-ras requiring phosphatidylinositol 3-kinase and c-Myc. Proc Natl Acad Sci U S A 2006;103:17390-5.
[58] Thirkettle HJ, Mills IG, Whitaker HC, Neal DE. Nuclear LYRIC/AEG-1 interacts with PLZF and relieves PLZF-mediated repression. Oncogene 2009;28:3663-70.
[59] Zhang L, Deng T, Li X, Liu H, Zhou H, Ma J, Wu M, Zhou M, Shen S, Li X, Niu Z, Zhang W, et al. microRNA-141 is involved in a nasopharyngeal carcinoma-related genes network. Carcinogenesis 2010;31:559-66.
[60] Garofalo M, Di Leva G, Romano G, Nuovo G, Suh SS, Ngankeu A, Taccioli C, Pichiorri F, Alder H, Secchiero P, Gasparini P, Gonelli A, et al. miR-221&222 regulate TRAIL resistance and enhance tumorigenicity through PTEN and TIMP3 downregulation. Cancer Cell 2009;16:498-509.
[61] Godshalk SE, Paranjape T, Nallur S, Speed W, Chan E, Molinaro AM, Bacchiocchi A, Hoyt K, Tworkoski K, Stern DF, Sznol M, Ariyan S, et al. A Variant in a MicroRNA complementary site in the 3' UTR of the KIT oncogene increases risk of acral melanoma. Oncogene 2010.

[62] Cortez MA, Calin GA. MicroRNA identification in plasma and serum: a new tool to diagnose and monitor diseases. Expert Opin Biol Ther 2009;9:703-11.
[63] Liu A, Tetzlaff MT, Vanbelle P, Elder D, Feldman M, Tobias JW, Sepulveda AR, Xu X. MicroRNA expression profiling outperforms mRNA expression profiling in formalin-fixed paraffin-embedded tissues. Int J Clin Exp Pathol 2009;2:519-27.
[64] Ma Z, Lui WO, Fire A, Dadras SS. Profiling and discovery of novel miRNAs from formalin-fixed, paraffin-embedded melanoma and nodal specimens. J Mol Diagn 2009;11:420-9.
[65] Radhakrishnan A, Badhrinarayanan N, Biswas J, Krishnakumar S. Analysis of chromosomal aberration (1, 3, and 8) and association of microRNAs in uveal melanoma. Mol Vis 2009;15:2146-54.
[66] Leidinger P, Keller A, Borries A, Reichrath J, Rass K, Jager SU, Lenhof HP, Meese E. High-throughput miRNA profiling of human melanoma blood samples. BMC Cancer 2010;10:262.
[67] Kanemaru H, Fukushima S, Yamashita J, Honda N, Oyama R, Kakimoto A, Masuguchi S, Ishihara T, Inoue Y, Jinnin M, Ihn H. The circulating microRNA-221 level in patients with malignant melanoma as a new tumor marker. J Dermatol Sci 2011;61:187-93.
[68] Satzger I, Mattern A, Kuettler U, Weinspach D, Voelker B, Kapp A, Gutzmer R. MicroRNA-15b represents an independent prognostic parameter and is correlated with tumor cell proliferation and apoptosis in malignant melanoma. Int J Cancer 2010;126:2553-62.
[69] Segura MF, Belitskaya-Levy I, Rose AE, Zakrzewski J, Gaziel A, Hanniford D, Darvishian F, Berman RS, Shapiro RL, Pavlick AC, Osman I, Hernando E. Melanoma MicroRNA signature predicts post-recurrence survival. Clin Cancer Res 2010;16:1577-86.
[70] Caramuta S, Egyhazi S, Rodolfo M, Witten D, Hansson J, Larsson C, Lui WO. MicroRNA expression profiles associated with mutational status and survival in malignant melanoma. J Invest Dermatol 2010;130:2062-70.
[71] Kota J, Chivukula RR, O'Donnell KA, Wentzel EA, Montgomery CL, Hwang HW, Chang TC, Vivekanandan P, Torbenson M, Clark KR, Mendell JR, Mendell JT. Therapeutic microRNA delivery suppresses tumorigenesis in a murine liver cancer model. Cell 2009;137:1005-17.
[72] Sun Q, Cong R, Yan H, Gu H, Zeng Y, Liu N, Chen J, Wang B. Genistein inhibits growth of human uveal melanoma cells and affects microRNA-27a and target gene expression. Oncol Rep 2009;22:563-7.
[73] Das SK, Sokhi UK, Bhutia SK, Azab B, Su ZZ, Sarkar D, Fisher PB. Human polynucleotide phosphorylase selectively and preferentially degrades microRNA-221 in human melanoma cells. Proc Natl Acad Sci U S A 2010;107:11948-53.
[74] Huynh C, Segura MF, Gaziel-Sovran A, Menendez S, Darvishian F, Chiriboga L, Levin B, Meruelo D, Osman I, Zavadil J, Marcusson EG, Hernando E. Efficient in vivo microRNA targeting of liver metastasis. Oncogene 2010.
[75] Chen Y, Zhu X, Zhang X, Liu B, Huang L. Nanoparticles modified with tumor-targeting scFv deliver siRNA and miRNA for cancer therapy. Mol Ther 2010;18:1650-6.
[76] Molnar V, Tamasi V, Bakos B, Wiener Z, Falus A. Changes in miRNA expression in solid tumors: an miRNA profiling in melanomas. Semin Cancer Biol 2008;18:111-22.

2

Epigenetic Changes in Melanoma and the Development of Epigenetic Therapy for Melanoma

Duc P. Do[1] and Syed A.A. Rizvi[2]
[1]*Department of Pharmaceutical Sciences*
College of Pharmacy, Chicago State University
[2]*Department of Pharmaceutical Sciences*
College of Pharmacy, Nova Southeastern University
USA

1. Introduction

Melanoma is responsible for 80% of all skin cancer deaths (Miller & Mihm, 2006), and it is the most common cause of cancer deaths between the age of 20 and 35 years old (Houghton & Polsky, 2002). Melanoma is a highly heterogeneous cancer that is caused by the accumulation of genetic and epigenetic defects allowing the cell to escape normal cellular controls. Genetic changes are caused by irreversible alterations in the DNA sequence, including chromosomal amplification or deletions and gene mutations that culminate in aberrant cellular functions, such as activation of oncogenes and inactivation of tumor suppressors. However, recent progress in cancer research has shown that epigenetic events may play a major role in establishing the correct program of gene expression. Epigenetics is defined as heritable changes in gene expression that are not due to any changes in the DNA sequence. Currently, four epigenetic drugs, vorinostat (Marks & Breslow, 2007), romidepsin (Campas-Moya, 2009), azacitidine (Mani & Herceg, 2010; Wijermans et al., 2005), and decitabine (Mani & Herceg, 2010), have been approved for the treatment of hematologic malignancies in the United States by the Food and Drug Administration (U.S. FDA).

In a human cell, there are approximately two meters of diploid DNA that are packaged inside the nucleus with a volume of about 1000 μm^3 (Kamakaka & Biggins, 2005). This packaging of DNA is facilitated by histones. Histones are a group of highly conserved, basic (positively-charged) proteins that are rich in arginine and lysine residues. This DNA-protein complex is called the chromatin. In chromatin, proteins account for more than half of the weight, from which, histone proteins being the most abundant. There are five distinct families of histones, each with numerous variants or individual genes. DNA is packaged into nucleomes comprising a histone octamer of two copies of each core histones (H2A, H2B, H3, and H4) (Luger et al., 1997). The core histones interact in pairs. Two H3:H4 dimers interact together forming a tetramer, and two H2A:H2B dimers associate with the H3:H4 tetramer to form a nucleosome. About 146 bp of DNA is wrapped around a histone octamer. One molecule of histone H1 associates at the position where the DNA enters and exits the nucleosome core, thus sealing the two turns of DNA (Luger et al., 1997).

These core histones contain a conserved C-terminal histone fold domain and unique N-terminal tails. The histone N-terminal tails protrude from the nucleosome core and provide sites for posttranslational modifications, including acetylation, methylation, phosphorylation, and ubiquitination (Jenuwein & Allis, 2001). These distinct patterns of posttranslational modifications make up the histone code that is read by multiprotein chromatin remodelling complexes to determine the transcriptional status of the target gene (Strahl & Allis, 2000).

2. Histone acetylation and histone deacetylases

Epigenetic phenomena can be viewed as changes in the packaging and modifications of the DNA. In the case of DNA, it is modified only by methylation. Changes in the packaging of DNA include both histone modifications and chromatin remodeling. Histones can be modified by methylation, acetylation, phosphorylation, biotinylation, ubiquitination, sumoylation, and ADP-ribosylation. Lysine residues in the histone tails can be acetylated or methylated. Arginine residues can be methylated (Howell et al., 2009).

Among all of the posttranslational modifications on histone tails, histone acetylation is among the most extensively studied. In normal cells, acetylation and deacetylation exist in equilibrium. Acetylation is a reaction that is catalyzed by histone acetyltransferases (HATs), and the deacetylation reaction is catalyzed by histone deacetylases (HDACs). These two families of enzymes regulate the delicate balance needed for maintaining the states of chromatin and chromatin dynamics (Figure 1).

Acetylation is a reversible reaction occurring on lysine residues within the N-terminal tails of core histones H3 and H4. For histone acetylation, one of the hydrogens in the free amino group of internal lysine is substituted with an acetyl (CH_3CO) group. The addition of an acetyl group removes the positive charge from the NH_3^+ group on lysine, thus neutralizing the basic charge of the histone tails. This modification is suggested to reduce the affinity between histones and DNA, which, in turn, correlates with active gene expression. Acetylated histone is usually associated with transcriptionally active chromatin (Hebbes et al., 1992; Kouzarides, 2007; Turner, 1993). In addition, it is involved in many processes, such as replication, nucleosome assembly, higher-order chromatin packing and interactions of nonhistone proteins (Grant & Berger, 1999). Lysine at amino acid positions 9, 14, 18, and 23 for histone H3 and at amino acid positions 5, 8, 12, 16 for histone H4 are frequent targets for acetylation. These histone modifications facilitate access and binding of transcription factors.

Histone deacetylation is associated with an inactive (closed) state of chromatin and transcriptional repression (Kouzarides, 2007; Strahl & Allis, 2000). Deacetylation is catalyzed by histone deacetylases (HDAC). HDACs catalyze the removal of acetyl groups from lysine residues. HDACs and HATs are either part of a multiprotein transcriptional complex or interact with DNA binding proteins (Haberland et al., 2009; Jenuwein & Allis, 2001). Deregulation in the activity of HDACs and HATs may lead to alterations in gene expression and has been linked to diseases, particularly cancers. Fraga et al (2005) found that the loss of acetylation of histone H4 at K16 and K20 is a common hallmark of human cancer. Recently, Kondo et al. (2008) found, 5% of the genes are silenced by trimethylation of H3K27 independent of DNA methylation.

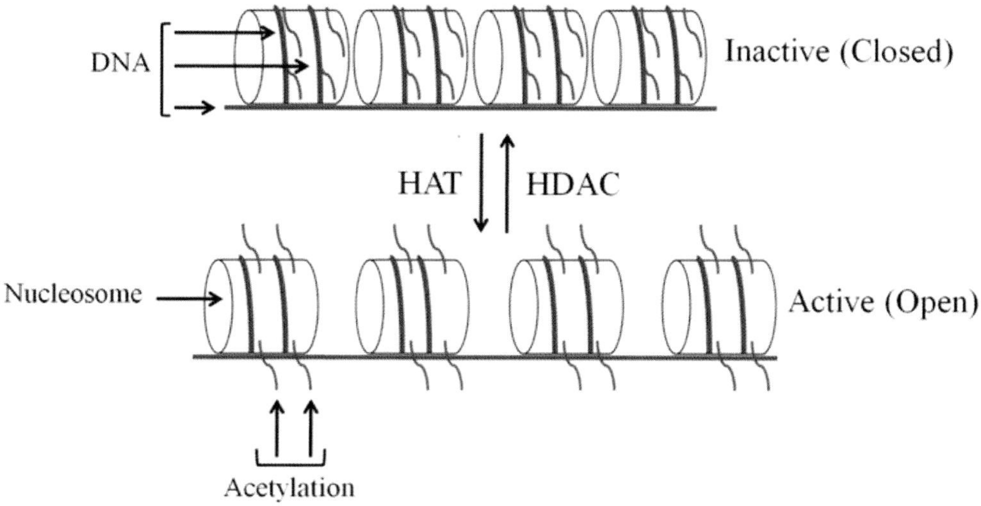

Fig. 1. The states of chromatin and regulation of gene expression. HAT: Histone acetyltransferase; HDAC: Histone deacetylase.

To date, 18 HDACs have been identified in humans. They are divided into four classes based on their homology to yeast HDACs (Table 1). Class I enzymes, which included HDACs 1, 2, 3, and 8, are related to the yeast RPD3 (de Ruijter et al., 2003; Paris et al., 2008). Class I HDACs 1, 2, and 3 are ubiquitously expressed and are almost exclusively found in the nuclei of cells in various cell lines and tissues (de Ruijter et al., 2003; Paris et al., 2008). Unlike HDACs 1-3, HDAC 8 is found only in cells with smooth muscle/myoepithelial differentiation. HDAC8 expression was found in smooth muscle cells where its expression is suggested to play a role in regulating the dynamics of smooth muscle cytoskeleton (Waltregny et al., 2004). These class I HDACs are involved in the regulation of proliferation, apoptosis, cardiac morphogenesis, and interferon (INF) expression through regulating gene expressions (Bernstein et al., 2000; Foglietti et al., 2006; Zupkovitz et al., 2006). Class II proteins, which included HDACs 4, 5, 6, 7, 9, and 10, share domains with the yeast HDAC-1 (de Ruijter et al., 2003; Paris et al., 2008). Class II HDACs can shuttle between the nucleus and the cytoplasm (Paris et al., 2008). Class II HDAC 6 is not seen in lymphocytes, stromal cells, and vascular endothelial cells (Yoshida et al., 2004; Zhang et al., 2004). It is localized mainly in the cytoplasm. This HDAC6 enzyme is also found on the perinuclear and leading-edge subcellular regions of cells. It is a microtubule-associated deacetylase (Hubbert et al., 2002). HDAC 7 inhibits the expression of Nur77, which is involved in the regulation of apoptosis and negative selection during developing thymocytes (Dequiedt et al., 2005). Unlike class I HDACs, class II HDACs are found only in some tissues. The recently described class IV, comprised solely of HDAC 11 enzyme, shares features of classes I and II HDACs, such as the dependence on zinc for their enzymatic activity. Classes I, II and IV are zinc dependent proteases (de Ruijter et al., 2003; Gao et al., 2002; Glozak & Seto, 2007). Class III HDACs (sirtuins) have been identified based on sequence homology with the yeast transcription repressor Sir2. To date, seven different sirtuins have been identified, and all of the enzymes of class III require NAD^+ for their activity. This class of enzymes is localized in the nucleus (de Ruijter et al., 2003; Glozak & Seto, 2007). HDACs can deacetylase non-histone proteins, such as tumor suppressors (e.g., p53), and signaling molecules (e.g., STAT1 and STAT3) (Minucci & Pelicci, 2006).

HDAC		Example of Biological Functions	Tissue Distribution	Localization	Reference
Class I	HDAC1	essential in cell survival and proliferation	ubiquitous	nucleus	(Bernstein et al., 2000; Paris et al., 2008; Sun & Hampsey, 1999)
	HDAC2				(Foglietti et al., 2006; Paris et al., 2008)
	HDAC3				(Lagger et al., 2002; Paris et al., 2008; Zupkovitz et al., 2006)
	HDAC8				(Montgomery et al., 2007; Paris et al., 2008)
Class IIa	HDAC4	mediator of neuronal death	heart; brain; skeletal muscle	nucleus/ cytoplasm	(Paris et al., 2008; Waltregny et al., 2004; Waltregny et al., 2005)
	HDAC5	cardiac development	heart; brain; skeletal muscle		(Bolger & Yao, 2005; Paris et al., 2008)
	HDAC7	regulation of apoptosis in developing thymocytes	heart; skeletal muscle; pancreas; spleen		(Paris et al., 2008; Vega et al., 2004)
	HDAC9	cardiac development	brain; skeletal muscle		(Bolger & Yao, 2005; Paris et al., 2008)
Class IIb	HDAC6	regulation of tubulin and Hsp90 acetylation	heart; liver; kidney; pancreas	mainly cytoplasm	(Chang et al., 2004; Dequiedt et al., 2003; Paris et al., 2008; Zhang et al., 2002)
	HDAC10	regulation of thioredoxin-interacting protein expression	spleen; liver; kidney		(Lee et al., 2010)
Class V	HDAC11	regulation of immune function	heart; brain; skeletal muscle; kidney	nucleus/ cytoplasm	(Villagra et al., 2009)

Table 1. Histone deacetylases.

2.1 Clinical applications of histone modifications

Given the association between HDAC enzymes and cancers, there is growing interest in using HDAC inhibitors (HDACI) as antitumor agents. Inhibition of HDAC activity should lead to chromatin decondensation and an increase in gene transcription (Figure 1) (Karagiannis & El-Osta, 2006). HDACIs have been shown to have pleiotropic effects, including cell cycle arrest, growth inhibition and chromatin decondensation. They interfere directly with the mitotic spindle checkpoint, differentiation, and apoptosis in cancer cell types (Choi et al., 2007; Marchion & Munster, 2007; Stearns et al., 2007; Xu et al., 2005). Imre et al. (2006) showed that HDACIs reduce the responsiveness of tumor cells to the tumor necrosis factor-α (TNF-α) mediated activation of the nuclear factor-kappa B (NF-kappa B). All HDACIs upregulate p21, an important mediator of growth arrest (Richon et al., 2000). Studies in clinical trials have attempted to use HDACIs in combination therapy with some successes (Johnstone, 2002). This combined strategy has shown promise in some malignancies (Bishton et al., 2007).

To date, more than 18 HDACIs have been tested in clinical trials for cancer therapy (Carew et al., 2008; Paris et al., 2008). In the United States, two histone deacetylase inhibitors, namely vorinostat (Zolinza) and romidepsin (Istodax), have been approved for the treatment of cutaneous T-cell lymphoma. HDACIs are usually classified into various groups based on their structures, including hydroxamic acids, cyclic peptides, short chain fatty acids, and benzamides. Hydroxamic acid derived compounds (trichostatin A, oxamflatin) have been used in clinical trials for treating both hematologic malignancies and solid tumors. These compounds contain an acid moiety that can fit into the catalytic site and bind to the zinc atom, thus inhibiting the HDAC enzyme (Marchion & Munster, 2007; Marks et al., 2000). For cyclic peptide group (depsipeptide, trapoxin), HDACIs are effective in nanomolar range. On the other hand, short chain fatty acid compounds (butyrate, trybutyrin) require relatively high concentrations for their action. A member of this group, valproic acid has been used in antiepileptic treatment. The use of valproic acid as an anti-epileptic underlines the wide functional distribution of HDACs, contributing to problems targeting the cancer treatments using histone deacetylase inhibitors. The benzamide group molecules (MS-275, CI-994) exert their action at micromolar concentrations. Since the enzymatic pocket is highly conserved in nature, most HDACIs do not selectively inhibit individual HDAC enzymes. Rather, HDACIs inhibit several HDAC enzymes simultaneously. They target mainly classes I and II HDACs (Marks & Xu, 2009; Paris et al., 2008). Table 2 shows the histone deacetylase inhibitors.

Histone deacetylase inhibitors have been investigated in clinical trials for melanoma (Table 3). A multicenter, phase II clinical trial was conducted to evaluate the efficacy, safety, and pharmacokinetics of the histone deacetylase inhibitor, pyridylmethyl-N-{4-[(2-aminophenyl)-carbamoyl]-benzyl}-carbamate (MS-275) in 28 patients with pretreated metastatic melanoma. MS-275 is an oral benzamide HDACI. In the study, patients with unresectable American Joint Committee on Cancer (AJCC) stage IV melanoma, refractory to at least one earlier systemic therapy, were randomized to receive MS-275 3 mg bi-weekly or 7 mg weekly on a 28-day cycle. The primary endpoint of the study was objective tumor response, and the secondary study endpoints were safety and time-to-progression. No objective responses were observed in pretreated metastatic melanoma patients. The median time-to-progession was comparable in both arms of the study. MS-275 was well tolearted, with nausea, diarrhea, and hypophosphatemia as the most frequently reported adverse events (Hauschild et al., 2008).

Compound	Chemical Group	[Range]	HDAC Specificity	*In Vitro* Effect	Reference
Sodium butyrate	Short-chain fatty acid	mM	Class I, IIa	Apoptosis Cell-cycle arrest	(Bhalla, 2005; Bolden et al., 2006; Johnstone, 2002; Schwabe & Lubbert, 2007)
Valproic acid (VPA)	Short-chain fatty acid	mM	Class I, IIa	Apoptosis Differentiation	(Bhalla, 2005; Bolden et al., 2006; Johnstone, 2002; Schwabe & Lubbert, 2007)
Trichostatin A (TSA)	Hydroxamic acid	nM	Class I, IIa	Apoptosis Cell-cycle arrest Differentiation	(Bhalla, 2005; Bolden et al., 2006; Johnstone, 2002; Schwabe & Lubbert, 2007)
Suberoylanilide hydroxamic acid (SAHA) or vorinostat	Hydroxamic acid	µM	Class I, II	Apoptosis Cell-cycle arrest	(Bhalla, 2005; Bolden et al., 2006; Johnstone, 2002; Schwabe & Lubbert, 2007)
Depsipeptide (FK 228)	Cyclic tetrapeptide	nM	Class I	Apoptosis Cell-cycle arrest	(Bhalla, 2005; Bolden et al., 2006; Johnstone, 2002; Schwabe & Lubbert, 2007)
Apicidin	Cyclic tetrapeptide	nM	HDACs 1 and 3	Apoptosis Cell-cycle arrest	(Bolden et al., 2006; Johnstone, 2002; Schwabe & Lubbert, 2007; Vannini et al., 2004)
MS-275	Benzamide	µM	Class I	Cell-cycle arrest	(Bolden et al., 2006; Hu et al., 2003; Johnstone, 2002; Schwabe & Lubbert, 2007)

Table 2. Histone deacetylase inhibitors

Due to the low response rates of HDACIs as single-agent therapies, HDACIs have also been investigated in combination with other therapeutic agents (Table 3). In a phase I/II clinical trial for patients with stage IV melanoma, the combination of valproic acid and the topoisomerase I inhibitor karenitecin associated with disease stabilization in 47% of patients. The median overall survival and time-to-progression were 32.8 and 10.2 weeks, respectively. In addition, histone hyperacetylation was observed in peripheral blood mononuclear cells (Daud et al., 2009).

HDACIs have also been investigated in combination with other treatment modalities. A phase I/II study of HDACI valproic acid with standard chemoimmunotherapy in patients with advanced melanoma was conducted to evaluate its clinical activity and to assess toxicity. In the study, patients were treated initialy with valproic acid alone for 6 weeks. After the treatment with valproic acid alone, dacarbazine plus interferon-α therapy was started in combination with the valproic acid. However, the results showed that the combination of valproic acid and chemoimmunotherapy did not produce superior results as compared to standard therapy (Rocca et al., 2009).

Epigenetic Agent	Combination	Malignancy	Phase	Reference
Histone Deacetylase Inhibitors (HDACIs)				
Valproic acid	Karenitecin (topoisomerase I inhibitor)	Melanoma	I, II	(Cang et al., 2009; Howell et al., 2009; Sigalotti et al., 2010)
Vorinostat (Zolinza)	NPI-0052 (proteasome inhibitor)	Melanoma	I	(Cang et al., 2009; Howell et al., 2009; Sigalotti et al., 2010)
Vorinostat (Zolinza)		Unresectable Metastatic Melanoma (Stage IV)	II	(Cang et al., 2009; Howell et al., 2009; Sigalotti et al., 2010)
MS-275		Melanoma	II	(Cang et al., 2009; Howell et al., 2009; Sigalotti et al., 2010)
Romidepsin		Nonresectable Intraocular Melanoma or Unresectable Stage III or Stage IV Melanoma	II	(Cang et al., 2009; Howell et al., 2009; Sigalotti et al., 2010)
DNA Methyltransferase Inhibitors (DNA Hypomethylating Agents) (DNMTIs)				
5-azacytidine (Vidaza)	Recombinant Interferon α-2b	Melanoma	I	(Cang et al., 2009; Howell et al., 2009; Sigalotti et al., 2010)
5-aza-2-deoxycytidine (Dacogen)	Temozolomide	Melanoma	I, II	(Cang et al., 2009; Howell et al., 2009; Sigalotti et al., 2010)
	Pegylated Interferon α-2b	Melanoma	I, II	(Cang et al., 2009; Howell et al., 2009; Sigalotti et al., 2010)
	Panobinostat, Temozolomide	Melanoma	I, II	(Cang et al., 2009; Howell et al., 2009; Sigalotti et al., 2010)

Table 3. Current epigenetic agents used in clinical trials for melanoma patients

3. DNA methylation

DNA methylation is carried out by different DNA methyltransferases (DNMT). DNMT1 involves in the maintenance of established methylation patterns. DNMT3a and DNMT3b are implicated in *de novo* DNA methylation (Bestor, 2000; Okano et al., 1999; Rothhammer & Bosserhoff, 2007). This epigenetic event takes place at the C5 position of cytosine on the CpG dinucleotide rich regions (CpG islands) that are distributed throughout the genome. Proper DNA methylation patterns are essential for human development and normal functioning. In normal cells, CpG islands located in the promoter regions are mainly unmethylated; however, in melanoma cancer cells, aberrant hypermethylation occur. In addition, genome-wide hypomethylation occurs in melanoma cancer cells (Jones & Baylin, 2007). This epigenetic modification results in silencing the transcription of selected tumor suppressor genes (Robertson, 2005; Rothhammer & Bosserhoff, 2007). Aberrant DNA hypermethylation of promoter regions has been shown to result in the silencing of at least 50 genes (Fulda et al., 2001; Gallagher et al., 2005; Mori et al., 2005; Muthusamy et al., 2006; Paz et al., 2003; Rothhammer & Bosserhoff, 2007; Soengas et al., 2001; van der Velden et al., 2003). Table 4 shows some genes affected by promoter DNA hypermethylation in melanoma. For example, *CDKN2A* is a major gene involved in the pathogenesis of melanoma. It is the most frequently mutated gene inherited in familial cutaneous melanoma (Palmieri et al., 2009; Sigalotti et al., 2010). Freedberg et al (2008) showed that aberrant promoter DNA hypermethylation at CDKN2A locus independently affects the tumor suppressors $p16^{INK4A}$ and $p14^{ARF}$, which function in the pRB and p53 pathways, respectively. In human melanoma, $p16^{INK4A}$ and $p14^{ARF}$ are methylated.

Gene	Pathway	Reference
APAF1(apoptotic protease activating factor 1)	Apoptosis	(Soengas et al., 2001)
MT2A (methallothionein 2A)	Apoptosis	(Gallagher et al., 2005)
HSPB1 (heat shock 27 kDa protein)	Apoptosis	(Gallagher et al., 2005)
MAGE-A1(melanoma antigen, family A1)	Immune recognition	(De Smet et al., 1996; Karpf et al., 2004; Sigalotti et al., 2010)
ER-α (estrogen receptor alpha)	Signaling	(Mori et al., 2006)
WFDC1 (wap 4-disulfide core domain 1)	Proliferation	(Muthusamy et al., 2006)
CDKN1B (cyclin-dependent kinase inhibitor 1B	Cell cycle	(Worm et al., 2000)
CDKN1C (cyclin-dependent kinase inhibitor 1C)	Cell cycle	(Shen et al., 2007)
APC (adenomatous polyposis coli gene)	Cell fate determination	(Worm et al., 2004)
GDF15 (growth/differentiation factor 15)	Differentiation	(Muthusamy et al., 2006)
TPM1 (tropomyosin 1)	Anchorage-independent growth	(Liu et al., 2008)
MIB2 (skeletrophin)	Cell fate determination	(Takeuchi et al., 2006)
MGMT (0^6-methylguanine-DNA-methyltransferase)	DNA repair	(Hoon et al., 2004)
CDH1 (E-cadherin)	Invasion/metastasis	(Liu et al., 2008)
CDH8 (cadherin 8)	Invasion/metastasis	(Muthusamy et al., 2006)

Table 4. Genes with an altered DNA methylation status in melanoma

3.1 Clinical applications of DNA methylation

DNA methylation is a reversible epigenetic event and can be nullified by specific DNA demethylating agents (DNA methyltransferase inhibitors). Several ongoing clinical trials are conducted to investigate their clinical effectiveness and safety in melanoma patients (Table 3). In these studies, DNA demethylating agents 5-azacytidine (Vidaza) and 5-aza-2-deoxycytidine (decitabine, Dacogen) are the most intensively studied. Azacytidine is a pyrimidine nucleoside analog of cytidine, and decitabine is a cytosine nucleoside (cytidine) analog. These epigenetic agents were approved by the FDA for the treatment of myelodysplastic syndromes and acute myeloid leukemia. Agents that inhibit DNA methyltransferases can reactivate silenced genes and induce apoptosis of cancerous cells (Howell et al., 2009). Since epigenetic modifications affect cellular pathways, epigenetic agents also display pleiotropic activities (Howell et al., 2009). In a phase I trial, Gollob et al. (2006) found that a low dose of 5-aza-2'-deoxycytidine (decitabine) can be safely administered with high-dose interleukin to cancer patients and has antitumor activity in melanoma. The inclusion of decitabine resulted in DNA hypomethylation. In addition, Appleton et al. (2007) showed that decitabine reduces DNA methylation and can be combined safely with carboplatin for the treatment of melanoma.

In addition to therapeutic applications, modifications of DNA methylation may serve as biomarkers in clinical use for melanoma (Howell et al., 2009). Mori et al. (2006) showed that methylated ER-α can be detected in paraffin-embedded primary and metastatic melanoma tumors. In addition, methylated ER-α DNA was detected in the serum of melanoma patients with AJCC stage I to IV disease. Methylated ER-α was detected in 42% of stage III and 86% of stage IV metastatic melanomas. Serum methylated ER-α is an unfavorable prognostic factor. Liu et al (2008) found that SOCS1, SOCS2, RARβ2, DcR1, and DcR2 genes were the most frequently methylated genes in melanoma. The investigators also found that RECK, IRF7, PAWR, DR5, and Rb were not methylated in melanoma although these genes were found to be highly methylated in other cancers (Howell et al., 2009; Liu et al., 2008), suggesting that different cancers have distinct methylated genes. This is important since biomarkers must be specific and be able to differentiate between different forms of malignancies.

4. Conclusions and future perspectives

Melanoma is a complex disease that is caused by aberrant genetic and epigenetic events.
Epigenetic modifications play a significant role in the biology of melanoma, and epigenetic therapy emerges as a promising treatment modality for melanoma as well as for dignostic developments for the malignancy. A major difference between the two events is that epigenetic changes can be reversed by chemical and/or environmental modalities. Histone modifications and DNA methylation are extensively studied epigenetic events that affect the expression of genes. Currently, four epigentic agents have been approved by the U.S. FDA for hematologic malignancies and many HDACIs and DNMTIs are being investigated in clinical trials for solid tumors, such as melanoma. However, there have not been any FDA-approved epigenetic agents for solid tumors. Consequently, further investigations are required to find successful treatment strategies or protocols involving epigenetic agents. Future developments would address the issues of systemic toxicities, nonspecific epigenetic effect, and low bioavailability. In addition, a promising strategy is combination therapy. In tumors, DNA methylation and histone acetylation can act synergistically to silence tumor

suppressor genes. This approach could potentially enhance the reversal of epigenetic silencing. Although in its infancy, epigenetic therapy has been shown to be an effective treatment modality for cancers, as evident by the approval of 4 epigenetic drugs by the U.S. FDA. Encouraging results from preclinical and clinical trials prompts further investigations into designing new drugs or strategy that are more suitable for epigenetic therapies for melanoma patients, with the goal of improving patient outcomes.

5. References

Appleton, K., Mackay, H. J., Judson, I., Plumb, J. A., McCormick, C., Strathdee, G., Lee, C., Barrett, S., Reade, S., Jadayel, D., Tang, A., Bellenger, K., Mackay, L., Setanoians, A., Schatzlein, A., Twelves, C., Kaye, S. B. & Brown, R. (2007). Phase I and pharmacodynamic trial of the DNA methyltransferase inhibitor decitabine and carboplatin in solid tumors. *J Clin Oncol,* Vol.25, No.29, pp. 4603-4609

Bernstein, B. E., Tong, J. K. & Schreiber, S. L. (2000). Genomewide studies of histone deacetylase function in yeast. *Proc Natl Acad Sci U S A,* Vol.97, No.25, pp. 13708-13713

Bestor, T. H. (2000). The DNA methyltransferases of mammals. *Hum Mol Genet,* Vol.9, No.16, pp. 2395-2402

Bhalla, K. N. (2005). Epigenetic and chromatin modifiers as targeted therapy of hematologic malignancies. *J Clin Oncol,* Vol.23, No.17, pp. 3971-3993

Bishton, M., Kenealy, M., Johnstone, R., Rasheed, W. & Prince, H. M. (2007). Epigenetic targets in hematological malignancies: combination therapies with HDACis and demethylating agents. *Expert Rev Anticancer Ther,* Vol.7, No.10, pp. 1439-1449

Bolden, J. E., Peart, M. J. & Johnstone, R. W. (2006). Anticancer activities of histone deacetylase inhibitors. *Nat Rev Drug Discov,* Vol.5, No.9, pp. 769-784

Bolger, T. A. & Yao, T. P. (2005). Intracellular trafficking of histone deacetylase 4 regulates neuronal cell death. *J Neurosci,* Vol.25, No.41, pp. 9544-9553

Campas-Moya, C. (2009). Romidepsin for the treatment of cutaneous T-cell lymphoma. *Drugs Today (Barc),* Vol.45, No.11, pp. 787-795

Cang, S., Ma, Y. & Liu, D. (2009). New clinical developments in histone deacetylase inhibitors for epigenetic therapy of cancer. *J Hematol Oncol,* Vol.2, pp. 22

Carew, J. S., Giles, F. J. & Nawrocki, S. T. (2008). Histone deacetylase inhibitors: mechanisms of cell death and promise in combination cancer therapy. *Cancer Lett,* Vol.269, No.1, pp. 7-17

Chang, S., McKinsey, T. A., Zhang, C. L., Richardson, J. A., Hill, J. A. & Olson, E. N. (2004). Histone deacetylases 5 and 9 govern responsiveness of the heart to a subset of stress signals and play redundant roles in heart development. *Mol Cell Biol,* Vol.24, No.19, pp. 8467-8476

Choi, S., Lew, K. L., Xiao, H., Herman-Antosiewicz, A., Xiao, D., Brown, C. K. & Singh, S. V. (2007). D,L-Sulforaphane-induced cell death in human prostate cancer cells is regulated by inhibitor of apoptosis family proteins and Apaf-1. *Carcinogenesis,* Vol.28, No.1, pp. 151-162

Daud, A. I., Dawson, J., DeConti, R. C., Bicaku, E., Marchion, D., Bastien, S., Hausheer, F. A., 3rd, Lush, R., Neuger, A., Sullivan, D. M. & Munster, P. N. (2009). Potentiation of a topoisomerase I inhibitor, karenitecin, by the histone deacetylase inhibitor valproic acid in melanoma: translational and phase I/II clinical trial. *Clin Cancer Res,* Vol.15, No.7, pp. 2479-2487

de Ruijter, A. J., van Gennip, A. H., Caron, H. N., Kemp, S. & van Kuilenburg, A. B. (2003). Histone deacetylases (HDACs): characterization of the classical HDAC family. *Biochem J,* Vol.370, No.Pt 3, pp. 737-749

De Smet, C., De Backer, O., Faraoni, I., Lurquin, C., Brasseur, F. & Boon, T. (1996). The activation of human gene MAGE-1 in tumor cells is correlated with genome-wide demethylation. *Proc Natl Acad Sci U S A,* Vol.93, No.14, pp. 7149-7153

Dequiedt, F., Kasler, H., Fischle, W., Kiermer, V., Weinstein, M., Herndier, B. G. & Verdin, E. (2003). HDAC7, a thymus-specific class II histone deacetylase, regulates Nur77 transcription and TCR-mediated apoptosis. *Immunity,* Vol.18, No.5, pp. 687-698

Dequiedt, F., Van Lint, J., Lecomte, E., Van Duppen, V., Seufferlein, T., Vandenheede, J. R., Wattiez, R. & Kettmann, R. (2005). Phosphorylation of histone deacetylase 7 by protein kinase D mediates T cell receptor-induced Nur77 expression and apoptosis. *J Exp Med,* Vol.201, No.5, pp. 793-804

Foglietti, C., Filocamo, G., Cundari, E., De Rinaldis, E., Lahm, A., Cortese, R. & Steinkuhler, C. (2006). Dissecting the biological functions of Drosophila histone deacetylases by RNA interference and transcriptional profiling. *J Biol Chem,* Vol.281, No.26, pp. 17968-17976

Fraga, M. F., Ballestar, E., Villar-Garea, A., Boix-Chornet, M., Espada, J., Schotta, G., Bonaldi, T., Haydon, C., Ropero, S., Petrie, K., Iyer, N. G., Perez-Rosado, A., Calvo, E., Lopez, J. A., Cano, A., Calasanz, M. J., Colomer, D., Piris, M. A., Ahn, N., Imhof, A., Caldas, C., Jenuwein, T. & Esteller, M. (2005). Loss of acetylation at Lys16 and trimethylation at Lys20 of histone H4 is a common hallmark of human cancer. *Nat Genet,* Vol.37, No.4, pp. 391-400

Freedberg, D. E., Rigas, S. H., Russak, J., Gai, W., Kaplow, M., Osman, I., Turner, F., Randerson-Moor, J. A., Houghton, A., Busam, K., Timothy Bishop, D., Bastian, B. C., Newton-Bishop, J. A. & Polsky, D. (2008). Frequent p16-independent inactivation of p14ARF in human melanoma. *J Natl Cancer Inst,* Vol.100, No.11, pp. 784-795

Fulda, S., Kufer, M. U., Meyer, E., van Valen, F., Dockhorn-Dworniczak, B. & Debatin, K. M. (2001). Sensitization for death receptor- or drug-induced apoptosis by re-expression of caspase-8 through demethylation or gene transfer. *Oncogene,* Vol.20, No.41, pp. 5865-5877

Gallagher, W. M., Bergin, O. E., Rafferty, M., Kelly, Z. D., Nolan, I. M., Fox, E. J., Culhane, A. C., McArdle, L., Fraga, M. F., Hughes, L., Currid, C. A., O'Mahony, F., Byrne, A., Murphy, A. A., Moss, C., McDonnell, S., Stallings, R. L., Plumb, J. A., Esteller, M., Brown, R., Dervan, P. A. & Easty, D. J. (2005). Multiple markers for melanoma progression regulated by DNA methylation: insights from transcriptomic studies. *Carcinogenesis,* Vol.26, No.11, pp. 1856-1867

Gao, L., Cueto, M. A., Asselbergs, F. & Atadja, P. (2002). Cloning and functional characterization of HDAC11, a novel member of the human histone deacetylase family. *J Biol Chem,* Vol.277, No.28, pp. 25748-25755

Glozak, M. A. & Seto, E. (2007). Histone deacetylases and cancer. *Oncogene,* Vol.26, No.37, pp. 5420-5432

Gollob, J. A., Sciambi, C. J., Peterson, B. L., Richmond, T., Thoreson, M., Moran, K., Dressman, H. K., Jelinek, J. & Issa, J. P. (2006). Phase I trial of sequential low-dose 5-aza-2'-deoxycytidine plus high-dose intravenous bolus interleukin-2 in patients with melanoma or renal cell carcinoma. *Clin Cancer Res,* Vol.12, No.15, pp. 4619-4627

Grant, P. A. & Berger, S. L. (1999). Histone acetyltransferase complexes. *Semin Cell Dev Biol,* Vol.10, No.2, pp. 169-177

Haberland, M., Montgomery, R. L. & Olson, E. N. (2009). The many roles of histone deacetylases in development and physiology: implications for disease and therapy. *Nat Rev Genet,* Vol.10, No.1, pp. 32-42

Hauschild, A., Trefzer, U., Garbe, C., Kaehler, K. C., Ugurel, S., Kiecker, F., Eigentler, T., Krissel, H., Schott, A. & Schadendorf, D. (2008). Multicenter phase II trial of the histone deacetylase inhibitor pyridylmethyl-N-{4-[(2-aminophenyl)-carbamoyl]-benzyl}-carbamate in pretreated metastatic melanoma. *Melanoma Res,* Vol.18, No.4, pp. 274-278

Hebbes, T. R., Thorne, A. W., Clayton, A. L. & Crane-Robinson, C. (1992). Histone acetylation and globin gene switching. *Nucleic Acids Res,* Vol.20, No.5, pp. 1017-1022

Hoon, D. S., Spugnardi, M., Kuo, C., Huang, S. K., Morton, D. L. & Taback, B. (2004). Profiling epigenetic inactivation of tumor suppressor genes in tumors and plasma from cutaneous melanoma patients. *Oncogene,* Vol.23, No.22, pp. 4014-4022

Houghton, A. N. & Polsky, D. (2002). Focus on melanoma. *Cancer Cell,* Vol.2, No.4, pp. 275-278

Howell, P. M., Jr., Liu, S., Ren, S., Behlen, C., Fodstad, O. & Riker, A. I. (2009). Epigenetics in human melanoma. *Cancer Control,* Vol.16, No.3, pp. 200-218

Hu, E., Dul, E., Sung, C. M., Chen, Z., Kirkpatrick, R., Zhang, G. F., Johanson, K., Liu, R., Lago, A., Hofmann, G., Macarron, R., de los Frailes, M., Perez, P., Krawiec, J., Winkler, J. & Jaye, M. (2003). Identification of novel isoform-selective inhibitors within class I histone deacetylases. *J Pharmacol Exp Ther,* Vol.307, No.2, pp. 720-728

Hubbert, C., Guardiola, A., Shao, R., Kawaguchi, Y., Ito, A., Nixon, A., Yoshida, M., Wang, X. F. & Yao, T. P. (2002). HDAC6 is a microtubule-associated deacetylase. *Nature,* Vol.417, No.6887, pp. 455-458

Imre, G., Gekeler, V., Leja, A., Beckers, T. & Boehm, M. (2006). Histone deacetylase inhibitors suppress the inducibility of nuclear factor-kappaB by tumor necrosis factor-alpha receptor-1 down-regulation. *Cancer Res,* Vol.66, No.10, pp. 5409-5418

Jenuwein, T. & Allis, C. D. (2001). Translating the histone code. *Science,* Vol.293, No.5532, pp. 1074-1080

Johnstone, R. W. (2002). Histone-deacetylase inhibitors: novel drugs for the treatment of cancer. *Nat Rev Drug Discov,* Vol.1, No.4, pp. 287-299

Jones, P. A. & Baylin, S. B. (2007). The epigenomics of cancer. *Cell,* Vol.128, No.4, pp. 683-692

Kamakaka, R.T. & Biggins, S. (2005). Histone variants: deviants? *Genes Dev,* Vol.19, No.3, pp. 295-310

Karagiannis, T. C. & El-Osta, A. (2006). Clinical potential of histone deacetylase inhibitors as stand alone therapeutics and in combination with other chemotherapeutics or radiotherapy for cancer. *Epigenetics,* Vol.1, No.3, pp. 121-126

Karpf, A. R., Lasek, A. W., Ririe, T. O., Hanks, A. N., Grossman, D. & Jones, D. A. (2004). Limited gene activation in tumor and normal epithelial cells treated with the DNA methyltransferase inhibitor 5-aza-2'-deoxycytidine. *Mol Pharmacol,* Vol.65, No.1, pp. 18-27

Kondo, Y., Shen, L., Cheng, A. S., Ahmed, S., Boumber, Y., Charo, C., Yamochi, T., Urano, T., Furukawa, K., Kwabi-Addo, B., Gold, D. L., Sekido, Y., Huang, T. H. & Issa, J. P. (2008). Gene silencing in cancer by histone H3 lysine 27 trimethylation independent of promoter DNA methylation. *Nat Genet,* Vol.40, No.6, pp. 741-750

Kouzarides, T. (2007). Chromatin modifications and their function. *Cell,* Vol.128, No.4, pp. 693-705

Lagger, G., O'Carroll, D., Rembold, M., Khier, H., Tischler, J., Weitzer, G., Schuettengruber, B., Hauser, C., Brunmeir, R., Jenuwein, T. & Seiser, C. (2002). Essential function of histone deacetylase 1 in proliferation control and CDK inhibitor repression. *EMBO J,* Vol.21, No.11, pp. 2672-2681

Lee, J. H., Jeong, E. G., Choi, M. C., Kim, S. H., Park, J. H., Song, S. H., Park, J., Bang, Y. J. & Kim, T. Y. (2010). Inhibition of histone deacetylase 10 induces thioredoxin-interacting protein and causes accumulation of reactive oxygen species in SNU-620 human gastric cancer cells. *Mol Cells,* Vol.30, No.2, pp. 107-112

Liu, S., Ren, S., Howell, P., Fodstad, O. & Riker, A. I. (2008). Identification of novel epigenetically modified genes in human melanoma via promoter methylation gene profiling. *Pigment Cell Melanoma Res,* Vol.21, No.5, pp. 545-558

Luger, K., Mader, A. W., Richmond, R. K., Sargent, D. F. & Richmond, T. J. (1997). Crystal structure of the nucleosome core particle at 2.8 A resolution. *Nature,* Vol.389, No.6648, pp. 251-260

Mani, S. & Herceg, Z. (2010). DNA demethylating agents and epigenetic therapy of cancer. *Adv Genet,* Vol.70, pp. 327-340

Marchion, D. & Munster, P. (2007). Development of histone deacetylase inhibitors for cancer treatment. *Expert Rev Anticancer Ther,* Vol.7, No.4, pp. 583-598

Marks, P. A. & Breslow, R. (2007). Dimethyl sulfoxide to vorinostat: development of this histone deacetylase inhibitor as an anticancer drug. *Nat Biotechnol,* Vol.25, No.1, pp. 84-90

Marks, P. A., Richon, V. M. & Rifkind, R. A. (2000). Histone deacetylase inhibitors: inducers of differentiation or apoptosis of transformed cells. *J Natl Cancer Inst,* Vol.92, No.15, pp. 1210-1216

Marks, P. A. & Xu, W. S. (2009). Histone deacetylase inhibitors: Potential in cancer therapy. *J Cell Biochem,* Vol.107, No.4, pp. 600-608

Miller, A. J. & Mihm, M. C., Jr. (2006). Melanoma. *N Engl J Med,* Vol.355, No.1, pp. 51-65

Minucci, S. & Pelicci, P. G. (2006). Histone deacetylase inhibitors and the promise of epigenetic (and more) treatments for cancer. *Nat Rev Cancer,* Vol.6, No.1, pp. 38-51

Montgomery, R. L., Davis, C. A., Potthoff, M. J., Haberland, M., Fielitz, J., Qi, X., Hill, J. A., Richardson, J. A. & Olson, E. N. (2007). Histone deacetylases 1 and 2 redundantly regulate cardiac morphogenesis, growth, and contractility. *Genes Dev,* Vol.21, No.14, pp. 1790-1802

Mori, T., Martinez, S. R., O'Day, S. J., Morton, D. L., Umetani, N., Kitago, M., Tanemura, A., Nguyen, S. L., Tran, A. N., Wang, H. J. & Hoon, D. S. (2006). Estrogen receptor-alpha methylation predicts melanoma progression. *Cancer Res,* Vol.66, No.13, pp. 6692-6698

Mori, T., O'Day, S. J., Umetani, N., Martinez, S. R., Kitago, M., Koyanagi, K., Kuo, C., Takeshima, T. L., Milford, R., Wang, H. J., Vu, V. D., Nguyen, S. L. & Hoon, D. S. (2005). Predictive utility of circulating methylated DNA in serum of melanoma patients receiving biochemotherapy. *J Clin Oncol,* Vol.23, No.36, pp. 9351-9358

Muthusamy, V., Duraisamy, S., Bradbury, C. M., Hobbs, C., Curley, D. P., Nelson, B. & Bosenberg, M. (2006). Epigenetic silencing of novel tumor suppressors in malignant melanoma. *Cancer Res,* Vol.66, No.23, pp. 11187-11193

Okano, M., Bell, D. W., Haber, D. A. & Li, E. (1999). DNA methyltransferases Dnmt3a and Dnmt3b are essential for de novo methylation and mammalian development. *Cell,* Vol.99, No.3, pp. 247-257

Palmieri, G., Capone, M., Ascierto, M. L., Gentilcore, G., Stroncek, D. F., Casula, M., Sini, M. C., Palla, M., Mozzillo, N. & Ascierto, P. A. (2009). Main roads to melanoma. *J Transl Med,* Vol.7, pp. 86

Paris, M., Porcelloni, M., Binaschi, M. & Fattori, D. (2008). Histone deacetylase inhibitors: from bench to clinic. *J Med Chem,* Vol.51, No.6, pp. 1505-1529

Paz, M. F., Fraga, M. F., Avila, S., Guo, M., Pollan, M., Herman, J. G. & Esteller, M. (2003). A systematic profile of DNA methylation in human cancer cell lines. *Cancer Res,* Vol.63, No.5, pp. 1114-1121

Richon, V. M., Sandhoff, T. W., Rifkind, R. A. & Marks, P. A. (2000). Histone deacetylase inhibitor selectively induces p21WAF1 expression and gene-associated histone acetylation. *Proc Natl Acad Sci U S A,* Vol.97, No.18, pp. 10014-10019

Robertson, K. D. (2005). DNA methylation and human disease. *Nat Rev Genet,* Vol.6, No.8, pp. 597-610

Rocca, A., Minucci, S., Tosti, G., Croci, D., Contegno, F., Ballarini, M., Nole, F., Munzone, E., Salmaggi, A., Goldhirsch, A., Pelicci, P. G. & Testori, A. (2009). A phase I-II study of the histone deacetylase inhibitor valproic acid plus chemoimmunotherapy in patients with advanced melanoma. *Br J Cancer,* Vol.100, No.1, pp. 28-36

Rothhammer, T. & Bosserhoff, A. K. (2007). Epigenetic events in malignant melanoma. *Pigment Cell Res,* Vol.20, No.2, pp. 92-111

Schwabe, M. & Lubbert, M. (2007). Epigenetic lesions in malignant melanoma. *Curr Pharm Biotechnol,* Vol.8, No.6, pp. 382-387

Shen, L., Kondo, Y., Guo, Y., Zhang, J., Zhang, L., Ahmed, S., Shu, J., Chen, X., Waterland, R. A. & Issa, J. P. (2007). Genome-wide profiling of DNA methylation reveals a class of normally methylated CpG island promoters. *PLoS Genet,* Vol.3, No.10, pp. 2023-2036

Sigalotti, L., Covre, A., Fratta, E., Parisi, G., Colizzi, F., Rizzo, A., Danielli, R., Nicolay, H. J., Coral, S. & Maio, M. (2010). Epigenetics of human cutaneous melanoma: setting the stage for new therapeutic strategies. *J Transl Med,* Vol.8, pp. 56

Soengas, M. S., Capodieci, P., Polsky, D., Mora, J., Esteller, M., Opitz-Araya, X., McCombie, R., Herman, J. G., Gerald, W. L., Lazebnik, Y. A., Cordon-Cardo, C. & Lowe, S. W. (2001). Inactivation of the apoptosis effector Apaf-1 in malignant melanoma. *Nature,* Vol.409, No.6817, pp. 207-211

Stearns, V., Zhou, Q. & Davidson, N. E. (2007). Epigenetic regulation as a new target for breast cancer therapy. *Cancer Invest,* Vol.25, No.8, pp. 659-665

Strahl, B. D. & Allis, C. D. (2000). The language of covalent histone modifications. *Nature,* Vol.403, No.6765, pp. 41-45

Sun, Z. W. & Hampsey, M. (1999). A general requirement for the Sin3-Rpd3 histone deacetylase complex in regulating silencing in Saccharomyces cerevisiae. *Genetics,* Vol.152, No.3, pp. 921-932

Takeuchi, T., Adachi, Y., Sonobe, H., Furihata, M. & Ohtsuki, Y. (2006). A ubiquitin ligase, skeletrophin, is a negative regulator of melanoma invasion. *Oncogene,* Vol.25, No.53, pp. 7059-7069

Turner, B. M. (1993). Decoding the nucleosome. *Cell,* Vol.75, No.1, pp. 5-8

van der Velden, P. A., Zuidervaart, W., Hurks, M. H., Pavey, S., Ksander, B. R., Krijgsman, E., Frants, R. R., Tensen, C. P., Willemze, R., Jager, M. J. & Gruis, N. A. (2003). Expression profiling reveals that methylation of TIMP3 is involved in uveal melanoma development. *Int J Cancer,* Vol.106, No.4, pp. 472-479

Vannini, A., Volpari, C., Filocamo, G., Casavola, E. C., Brunetti, M., Renzoni, D., Chakravarty, P., Paolini, C., De Francesco, R., Gallinari, P., Steinkuhler, C. & Di Marco, S. (2004). Crystal structure of a eukaryotic zinc-dependent histone deacetylase, human HDAC8, complexed with a hydroxamic acid inhibitor. *Proc Natl Acad Sci U S A,* Vol.101, No.42, pp. 15064-15069

Vega, R. B., Matsuda, K., Oh, J., Barbosa, A. C., Yang, X., Meadows, E., McAnally, J., Pomajzl, C., Shelton, J. M., Richardson, J. A., Karsenty, G. & Olson, E. N. (2004). Histone deacetylase 4 controls chondrocyte hypertrophy during skeletogenesis. *Cell,* Vol.119, No.4, pp. 555-566

Villagra, A., Cheng, F., Wang, H. W., Suarez, I., Glozak, M., Maurin, M., Nguyen, D., Wright, K. L., Atadja, P. W., Bhalla, K., Pinilla-Ibarz, J., Seto, E. & Sotomayor, E. M. (2009). The histone deacetylase HDAC11 regulates the expression of interleukin 10 and immune tolerance. *Nat Immunol,* Vol.10, No.1, pp. 92-100

Waltregny, D., De Leval, L., Glenisson, W., Ly Tran, S., North, B. J., Bellahcene, A., Weidle, U., Verdin, E. & Castronovo, V. (2004). Expression of histone deacetylase 8, a class I histone deacetylase, is restricted to cells showing smooth muscle differentiation in normal human tissues. *Am J Pathol,* Vol.165, No.2, pp. 553-564

Waltregny, D., Glenisson, W., Tran, S. L., North, B. J., Verdin, E., Colige, A. & Castronovo, V. (2005). Histone deacetylase HDAC8 associates with smooth muscle alpha-actin and is essential for smooth muscle cell contractility. *FASEB J,* Vol.19, No.8, pp. 966-968

Wijermans, P. W., Lubbert, M., Verhoef, G., Klimek, V. & Bosly, A. (2005). An epigenetic approach to the treatment of advanced MDS; the experience with the DNA demethylating agent 5-aza-2'-deoxycytidine (decitabine) in 177 patients. *Ann Hematol,* Vol.84 Suppl 1, pp. 9-17

Worm, J., Bartkova, J., Kirkin, A. F., Straten, P., Zeuthen, J., Bartek, J. & Guldberg, P. (2000). Aberrant p27Kip1 promoter methylation in malignant melanoma. *Oncogene,* Vol.19, No.44, pp. 5111-5115

Worm, J., Christensen, C., Gronbaek, K., Tulchinsky, E. & Guldberg, P. (2004). Genetic and epigenetic alterations of the APC gene in malignant melanoma. *Oncogene,* Vol.23, No.30, pp. 5215-5226

Xu, C., Shen, G., Chen, C., Gelinas, C. & Kong, A. N. (2005). Suppression of NF-kappaB and NF-kappaB-regulated gene expression by sulforaphane and PEITC through

IkappaBalpha, IKK pathway in human prostate cancer PC-3 cells. *Oncogene,* Vol.24, No.28, pp. 4486-4495

Yoshida, N., Omoto, Y., Inoue, A., Eguchi, H., Kobayashi, Y., Kurosumi, M., Saji, S., Suemasu, K., Okazaki, T., Nakachi, K., Fujita, T. & Hayashi, S. (2004). Prediction of prognosis of estrogen receptor-positive breast cancer with combination of selected estrogen-regulated genes. *Cancer Sci,* Vol.95, No.6, pp. 496-502

Zhang, C. L., McKinsey, T. A., Chang, S., Antos, C. L., Hill, J. A. & Olson, E. N. (2002). Class II histone deacetylases act as signal-responsive repressors of cardiac hypertrophy. *Cell,* Vol.110, No.4, pp. 479-488

Zhang, Z., Yamashita, H., Toyama, T., Sugiura, H., Omoto, Y., Ando, Y., Mita, K., Hamaguchi, M., Hayashi, S. & Iwase, H. (2004). HDAC6 expression is correlated with better survival in breast cancer. *Clin Cancer Res,* Vol.10, No.20, pp. 6962-6968

Zupkovitz, G., Tischler, J., Posch, M., Sadzak, I., Ramsauer, K., Egger, G., Grausenburger, R., Schweifer, N., Chiocca, S., Decker, T. & Seiser, C. (2006). Negative and positive regulation of gene expression by mouse histone deacetylase 1. *Mol Cell Biol,* Vol.26, No.21, pp. 7913-7928

3

Genetic, Epigenetic and Molecular Changes in Melanoma: A New Paradigm for Biological Classification

Stefania Staibano, Massimo Mascolo, Maria Siano, Gennaro Ilardi and Gaetano De Rosa
University Federico II of Naples/Department of Biomorphological and Functional Sciences – Pathology Section/School of Medicine
Italy

1. Introduction

The last two decades have registered a progressive decline of both the incidence and mortality rates for some human cancers, worldwide (Jemal et al., 2010). However, in the same time interval, the incidence of cutaneous melanoma (CM), has progressively increased (Gallagher et al., 2005; Jemal et al., 2010), up to an epidemic level in Western countries and Australia (Beddingfield et al., 2003; Cancer facts & Figures, 2009). To date, the average lifetime risk for developing melanoma ranges from 1/50 in the United States (men and women) (Meyle & Guldberg, 2009; Horner et al. 2011) up to 1/25 for Australian men (Hocker et al., 2008). CM is an extremely aggressive skin cancer, and constitutes one of the most lethal human malignancies, notwithstanding the progressive increase of early diagnosis and surgical excision registered from 1990s. This poor prognosis may be due, at least in part, to the possible occurrence of metastasis even in early phases of melanoma progression, as well as to the very low response to current systemic therapy. The 5 year-survival rate for patients with disseminated disease is about 10%, with death for disease ultimately occurring within 2 years from metastases (Balch et al., 2000; Chin et al., 2006; Zbytek et al., 2008; Ugurel et al., 2009; Cancer facts & Figures, 2009). This underscores the need to uncover the mechanisms underlying melanoma biology, with the aim to identify reliable early markers of response and to select patients eligible for new rational avenues for therapy (Siena et al., 2009). The formidable aggressive potential of CM is thought to represent the result of multiple intersecting molecular alterations of the control pathways governing cell proliferation, cell death, DNA-repair, and tumor-stromal interaction. These molecular alterations are thought to be involved also in the peculiar histomorphological features and different biological behavior of the four "classical" types of CM. Three of them (superficial spreading melanoma, SSM; malignant lentigo melanoma, LM; acral melanoma, AM) are characterized by the sequential progression from junctional (radial) and pagetoid (intraepithelial) growth phase, to invasive (vertical) growth. The radial growth phase (RGP) is characterized by lateral melanocyte growth at the dermo-epidermal interface (junctional area), whereas the vertical growth phase (VGP) shows the spreading of melanoma cells into the dermis and subcutis, this being correlated with the occurrence of metastasis. The fourth type of CM, the "nodular" melanoma (NM), shows an *ab initio* invasive growth, and a more aggressive clinical course. Considerable insights have recently been made with respect to these topics. An impressive number of putative biomarkers of CM progression and drug response are being increasingly proposed, and new hypotheses concerning the interrelationship between histopathological features and clinical behavior are in progress. To date, however, we have to face with an "overload" of research data, which has already had a great impact on our understanding of melanoma progression, but is only beginning to unravel the real complexity of CM biology. Further work is required before we definitively know how we can use correctly these data to fight melanoma. We here review the more recent advances in molecular events involved in melanoma progression, drawing on a limited set of examples focused on the seminal findings of several research groups that have provided insight on melanoma biology. We discuss also the surprising interactions between some of these molecular pathways, both at genetic and epigenetic level, with particular attention to their role in defining potential markers for prognosis and therapeutic management of melanoma patients.

2. Genetics

Since the announcement of the completion of the Human Genome Project in 2003 (Noble, 2003), the first comprehensive analysis of cancer genomes has been completed: the entire genome of cutaneous melanoma and lung cancer has been sequenced. This formidable amount of information concerning the specific mutations of these cancer types will be of paramount importance in our understanding of the key molecular events that determine cancer evolution in every single patient. In tumors, most mutations are "passengers", meaning that they do not contribute to oncogenesis. Still, they provide information about the various steps leading to the oncogenic transformation of cells, as occurs, for example, for UV-exposure in skin cancer. This kinds of mutation, then, are very useful to study the pathogenesis of cancer. Only a small subset of somatic mutations is made of "driver mutations", which confer the oncogenic stigmata to cancer cells, being thus eligible for diagnosis and molecular therapy (Stratton et al, 2009). To date, more than 300 "driver" genes have been identified across all human cancers. Not surprisingly, they all converge over the few key cellular pathways which regulate cell life and differentiation (Vogelstein, 2010). The development and progression of melanoma is characterized by the acquisition of chromosomal deletions, amplification and gene mutations (Chin et al., 2006). The many gene expression profile studies performed up to now have evidenced that melanomas show significant genetic heterogeneity (Fecher et al., 2007; Ryu et al., 2007). Overall, large regions of the genome exhibiting DNA copy number changes and genes relevant for melanoma progression (Lin et al., 2008) as the Wnt5a, which misregulation results in increased motility in melanoma, have been identified (Lin et al., 2008). This also occurs for genes fundamental for basic melanocyte biology, such as Rab38, involved in melanosomal protein trafficking. We here refer to several genetic changes specifically linked to particular aspects of melanoma biology.

2.1 UVR

The dominant mutational signature emerging from sequencing the entire genome of cutaneous melanoma (Stratton et al, 2009) reflects DNA damage due to ultraviolet light exposure. Ultra-Violet Radiation (UVR) exerts direct or indirect damaging effects on nucleic acids and proteins (Kyrgidis et al., 2010). UVA mutate DNA indirectly, via absorption by non-DNA endogenous sensitizers which generate Reactive Oxygen Species (ROS) responsible for DNA damage (Lund & Timmins, 2007). UVB directly cause two types of DNA lesions: cyclobutane pyrimidine dimers (CPDs), arising between adjacent thymine(T) or cytosine(C) residues, and -pyrimidine 4-pyrimidone photoproducts (6-4PP) . The "UVB signature mutations" are characterized by CT→T and CC→TT transitions. Variants in MC1R, ASIP, TYR and TYRP1 have been identified as independent low-penetrance susceptibility genes for UV-induced melanomagenesis. These genes seem to contribute to the interrelation between pigmentation, cutaneous phototypes and exposure to UV light in affecting predisposition to melanoma (Thompson et al., 2009). Moreover, in melanomas of photoexposed skin, we have found defective expression of the mismatch-repair genes MHS2, which constitutes the phototype of mismatch-repair genes. It is actually thought that this may trigger microsatellite instability, thus contributing to the development of UV related skin tumors. In a previous study, we have shown also in oral melanomas that a deregulating expression of both hMSH2 and hMLH1 (mut L homologue 1) occurs. hMLH1 is frequently silenced in tumors with microsatellite instability. Both these genes can actually predispose to mutational events during tumor progression. We hypothesized that the altered expression of both HMSH2 and hMLH1 contributes to the mutagenic effect of UVR on melanocytes and, in turn, may be also involved in melanoma resistance to DNA damaging agents (Lo Muzio et al., 2000; Staibano et al., 2001).

2.2 BRAF

Alteration of the RAF/MEK/ERK pathway influences proliferation, invasion and survival of melanoma cells in vitro. For this reason it emerges then that B-Raf mutation has a pivotal role in determining melanoma biology, even if its exact function in melanoma progression remains still controversial. BRAF is a serine/threonine kinase that signals downstream of RTKs and RAS protein. Point mutations of B-Raf alter its auto-regulatory activation (Rother & Jones, 2009). The frequency of B-Raf mutations in melanoma and nevi is really impressive, being detectable in 30 to 80% of cases. Very interestingly, melanomas have a BRAF mutational spectrum different from other tumours, this probably reflecting the UVR environmental exposure (Thomas et al., 2006). This idea is further supported by the frequent occurrence of these mutations in SSM or NM of intermittently sun-exposed skin and in younger patients, whereas they are rare in AM (5-10%) and non-cutaneous melanomas (Platz et al., 2008). Over 30 distinct BRAF mutations, varying in biological activity, have been found and may be predictive of clinically relevant tumour differences (Thomas et al., 2006). The most common is constituted by a glutamic acid (glu) for valine (val) substitution at residue 599 (V600E) in the activation segment. At present, in spite of all these technical information, we are far away to the understanding of the real meaning of BRAF mutation in melanoma. It seems to correlate with distinct histopathologic features, such as intraepidermal "pagetoid" spreading of cohesive nests of malignant melanocytes, and "pushing" rather than infiltrative border of the tumor, as well as with the younger age and lymph node metastasis at diagnosis (Rother & Jones, 2009). However, these hypotheses show considerable inconsistencies, if we consider that benign nevi show even higher rates of V600E BRAF mutation and cell line or transgenic mouse models of melanoma have failed to unequivocally demonstrate the transforming ability of this mutation (Rother J et al, 2009). Recently, Dhomen N et al. have developed a mouse model of BRAFv600E-driven melanoma, showing that V600E BRAF mutation alone stimulates proliferation of melanocytes but cannot induce full transformation, which presumably requires the acquisition of additional mutations (Dhomen N, et al., 2009). Nevertheless, the $BRAF^{V600E}$ has evolved into the most important target in melanoma. First-generation non-selective RAF inhibitor (Sorafenib) as a single therapy or in combination with carboplatin and paclitaxel (Hauschild et al., 2009), iinhibitors of the MAPK pathways with activity for either BRAF or MEK (as PLX4032, Flaherty et al., 2010), induction of specific cellular immunity against $BRAF^{V600E}$, $BRAF^{V600E}$ inhibitors based on the crystal structure of $BRAF^{V600E}$ complexes, are providing conflicting results in patients with metastatic melanoma. New potent small molecule inhibitors of mutant BRAF, combined to the immunotherapy agent ipilimumab have demonstrated promising clinical activity. However, despite initial high response rates, in most cases these results persist for a short time and melanomas recur after a few months, showing resistance to the previously effective B-RAFv600E inhibitors (Nazarian et al., 2010; Villanueva et al., 2010). One invoked mechanism which can influence the clinical response to antineoplastic therapy could be the pharmacogenomic variation in both the tumor and the patient's genome (Wang et al., 2011). Recently, high-throughput screening methods have been proposed to uncover the mechanisms of resistance in these tumors (Garraway, 2010). However, further studies on B-RAF mutant melanomas are needed before definitive results will be reached. A recent genome-wide RNA-interference screening targeting 28,000 genes, identified 17 genes able to block uncontrolled proliferation of melanocytes in the presence of BRAFV600E, among them a relevant role seems to be played by IGFBP7 (insulin-like growth factor binding protein 7), which is often epigenetically silenced in primary melanomas. The functional relevance of these genes in human melanoma remains unclear. Overall, it seems evident that several mechanisms act together during malignant transformation and progression of melanoma. Activating or inactivating mutations of members of the Akt signalling pathway (phosphatidylinositol 3-kinase CA, PI3KCA and Akt kinase) and mutations of tumor suppressor phosphatase and tensin homolog (PTEN) are frequently found in melanomas. Hopefully, targeting these molecular pathways will change the standard of care of metastatic melanoma in the future, but further studies focused on identifying predictors of chemotherapeutic response are needed.

2.3 PTEN/AKT

PTEN is a phosphatase that acts as a tumor suppressor gene, regulating the activation of the global regulators of cell proliferation serine/theronine kinases AKT1/2-3. Complete PTEN loss (usually due to genomic deletion) is found in 20-25% of melanomas, sometimes in combination with BRAF mutation, and leads to high-level AKT activation (Rother & Jones, 2009). Rare activating mutations of the AKT1 or AKT3 isoforms have been found in sun-exposed melanoma subtypes. Moreover, AKT overexpression may be associated with melanoma growth in situ.

2.4 Timing of melanoma progression

The central theme of melanoma research actually focuses on changes in gene expression occurring at the RGP/VGP shifting. We are now in a conceptual transition phase, in which the Clark model of neoplastic progression of melanocytes is being questioned. Basing upon the growing body of molecular data and considering the finding that many melanomas arise de novo on normal skin instead of from pre-exsisting melanocytic nevi, the biology of melanocytic lineage could be examined from a point-of-view alternative to the postulated classical Clark model. This latter postulated that melanoma derives from (Takata et al., 2009) benign melanocytic nevus, which usually temporarily undergoes proliferation via oncogenic BRAF signalling, followed by growth arrest due to senescence induced by p16INK4/Rb. When a disruption of p16INK4a-retinoblastoma (Rb) pathway occurs, mostly by the inactivation of CDKN2A, the nevus become "dysplastic" and progressively more atypical, up to the RGP melanoma. At this stage, melanoma cells are dependent on growth factors secreted from keratinocytes, such as endothelin-1 (Murata et al., 2007), and are immortal, due to the activation of human telomerase reverse transcriptase (hTERT). In the vertical growth phase (VGP), mutations repressing apoptosis and favouring invasion (as PTEN loss, RAS activation, b-catenin activation) allow neoplastic melanocytes to survive in the absence of keratinocytes (Bennett 2003).

According to this theory, the interaction between melanoma cells and stromal fibroblasts further promotes tumor growth, migration, and angiogenesis (Li et al. 2003), but recently it has been proposed to revise this model of neoplastic progression of melanocytes, basing on the same evidences. Firstly, melanocytic nevi often consist of polyclonal population of either wild-type BRAF and BRAF mutated-nevus cells; moreover as before mentioned, many melanomas arise de novo (Takata et al., 2009). The p16INK4a-Rb inactivation (by deletion, mutation or promoter methylation of the CDKN2A gene, amplification of CCND1 or CDK4, or Rb mutation) (Bennett, 2008) has been demonstrated in early RGP melanomas (Takata et al., 2009), which in turn acquire a proliferative mutation, such as BRAFV600E, and clonally proliferate, maintaining a minimum telomere length through activation of hTERT. The full oncogenic transformation to VGP melanoma requires additional genetic or epigenetic changes, suppressing apoptosis, altering cell-cell adhesion, and leading to hyperproliferation and stromal invasion, for example via up-regulation of genes coding for cell surface and secreted proteins, as Neuropilin-2 (NRP2), which plays a critical role in mediating melanoma-endothelial interactions (Stine et al., 2011).

2.5 HIF1/ROS and melanoma-microenvironment

ROS are mutagenic molecules. Most of apoptosis regulators are known to be potentially mutated or functionally altered by ROS: BRAF (RAS, MEK, and ERK within the MAPK pathway), PTEN, Rb and AKT (Wittgen & van Kempen, 2007; Fruehauf & Trapp, 2008).

Melanoma cells generate large intracellular amounts of ROS (Sander et al., 2003) and excrete them into the extra cellular space. An upgraded ROS production has also been observed in dysplastic nevi (Pavel et al., 2004). ROS emerging as bio product during physiological melanin synthesis are neutralized within melanosomes by the anti-oxidant melanin. Melanosomes of malignant melanocytes produce excessive amounts of ROS (Gidanian et al., 2008; Josse et al., 2010) and in addition produce, instead of the regular eumelanin, pheomelanin, which is associated with more oxidative stress. In view of these unique melanoma properties, elevated production of ROS seems to be a melanoma- specific defect (Fruehauf and Trapp, 2008). Other factors may contribute to elevate ROS levels around the primary tumor: the skin is a hypoxic tissue, leading to ROS production (Wittgen & van Kempen, 2007) and exogenous attacks (e.g. UV-radiation) further increase oxidative stress. In addition, tumor-associated immune cells also excrete ROS (Nishikawa, 2008). Reactive oxygen species derived from immune cells have been proposed to exert a 'selective pressure' on MM cells to develop ROS-resistance (Wittgen & van Kempen, 2007). Following this hypothesis, the entire 'ROS-saturated environment' in and around the primary tumor may exert a selective pressure on MM cells, causing the selection of those with the highest ROS resistance, whereas unfit cells die of ROS-induced apoptosis. After acquiring ROS resistance to block apoptosis, MM cells can also use high ROS levels to further stimulate their metastatic potential (Nishikawa and Hashida, 2006) through an impressive variety of pathways; from induction of DNA changes and activation of cell proliferation, to destruction of surrounding tissue, induction of adhesion molecules, activation of metastatic processes and escaping immune surveillance. In summary, ROS act as pro-metastatic agents through a wide range of pathways (Josse et al., 2010), which in melanoma cells accumulates early in tumor progression due to the alteration of melanin produced by characteristically abnormal melanosomes (Fruehauf & Trapp, 2008; Meyskens, 2001; Gidanian et al., 2008). HIF-1 activity is highly regulated by hydroxyl radicals and other reactive oxygen species (ROS) (Kietzmann & Gorlach, 2005; Wittgen & van Kempen, 2007, Kuphal et al., 2010) HIF-1 molecular complex is the major transcriptional regulator of the cellular and systemic response to a hypoxic environment, and is involved in cancerogenesis, regulating the expression of factors fundamental for angiogenesis (VEGF) and tumour invasion (glycolytic enzymes) (Forsythe et al., 1996; Wenger, 2002; Wiesener & Maxwell, 2003; Erler et al., 2006). HIF-1 contributes also to the induction of vasculogenic mimicry (Sun et al., 2007). In melanoma cells HIF-1 expression is also regulated both at the translational and transcriptional level by various other molecular ways, comprising the AKT/phosphatidylinositol 3-kinase (PI3K) pathway, (Jiang et al., 2001) enhanced by the hypoxic skin environment, and by V600E BRAF (Minet et al., 2000; Galabova-Kovacs et al., 2006) and the transcription factor NFkappaB (Bonello et al., 2007, Rius et al., 2008). This latter, in turn, is constitutively upregulated in melanoma cell lines (Kuphal et al., 2004) and, in addition, may be regulated by ROS and/or JNK, either induced by UVR or directly triggered by the activation of the RAS/RAF/MEK pathway (Tobar et al., 2008; Bonello et al., 2007; Li & Karin, 1999; Kuphal et al., 2010). HIF-1 activity is modulated also by mTOR. In particular, it has been shown that downregulation of HIF-1 by the mTOR inhibitor rapamycin prevents transformation under hypoxia, this suggesting that Rapamycin may be proposed as a therapeutic approach in melanoma treatment (Bedogni et al., 2005; Michaylira & Nakagawa, 2006). This is of particular interest, considering that Rapamicin has been shown to stimulate apoptosis in melanoma cell lines through the specific inhibition of FK506-binding protein 51 (FKBP51) isomerase activity (Romano et al., 2004).This protein belongs to a family of immunophilins physiologically expressed in lymphocytes, involved in the regulation of several fundamental biological processes and over-expressed in cancers and premalignant lesions. FKBP51 has been associated to the apoptosis resistance of malignant melanoma. In a recent study, we demonstrated that the expression of FKBP51 is markedly increased in vertical growth phase of melanomas and in metastatic lesions, providing evidence that FKBP51 is a marker of melanocyte malignancy (Romano et al., 2010a, 2010b). In addition we found that FKBP51 is a factor of resistance to genotoxic agents, including anthracyclins and ionizing radiations, through NF-kB activation.

2.6 cKIT

KIT encodes a receptor tyrosine kinase (RTK), which is recognized as a ligand for a stem cell factor (SCF) (Takata et al., 2009). Dysregulation of KIT plays a role in systemic mastocytosis, acute myelogenous leukaemia, gastrointestinal stromal cell tumors (GISTs) and germ cell tumors (Patnaik et al., 2007). A critical role for c-Kit for normal neural crest and normal melanocyte development, (Rother & Jones, 2009) differentiation, proliferation, survival and migration (Wehrle-Haller, 2003) has been recognized, but its function in melanoma remains somewhat unclear. As a rule, c-Kit expression is lost during melanoma progression, but a subset of melanomas has been found to overexpress it and mutations activating c-Kit, mostly constituted by L576P (up to 50% of mutations), have recently been identified in some mucosal and AL melanoma subtypes (5-20% of cases), but not in cases arising from chronic sun-damaged skin (Rother & Jones, 2009; Monsel et al., 2010). KIT is expressed at maximum level at the invading edge of tumors, this suggesting a role for dynamic RTK activation in metastasis (Handolias et al., 2010). Monsel et al (Monsel et al., 2010) demonstrated that c-Kit mutated melanocytes require a specific epigenetic environment to be transformed in melanoma cells. c-Kit mutants cause in fact a strong activation of the phosphatidyl-inositol-3 kinase (PI3K) pathway, which, *per se*, is not sufficient to promote transformation of melanocytes. However, in the chronic hypoxic skin microenvironment, and/or when a constitutively active form of hypoxia-inducible factor 1alpha (HIF-1alpha) is coexpressed, c-Kit mutants activate also the Ras/Raf/Mek/Erk pathway, transforming the melanocytes, (Monsel et al., 2010). This scenario is extremely interesting, considering that KIT mutations are mutually exclusive with BRAF and NRAS, to identify a subset of melanomas arising from a distinct molecular mechanism of transformation, which may be specifically targeted by KIT inhibitors, such as imatinib or sorafenib (Monsel et al., 2010).

2.7 Plexin B1

Plexin B1 interacts with small G proteins to regulate cell proliferation, migration, and apoptosis, and is repressed by oncogenic B-RAF signalling; its loss of expression *in vivo* has been documented in breast cancer and renal cell carcinoma (Stevens et al., 2010). Plexin B1 functions as a tumor suppressor in melanoma cells, as it has been recently shown in a mouse model (Stevens et al., 2010; Argast et al., 2009). Introduction of plexin B1 into melanoma cell lines suppresses tumor formation in mice (Rody et al., 2009; Gomez Roman et al., 2008; Argast et al., 2009), this being thought to be due, at least in part, to suppression of c-Met signalling and c-Met-dependent migration. Recently, it has been evidenced that plexin B1 is lost in metastatic and deeply invasive melanoma in patient samples in vivo (Stevens et al., 2010), whereas it is generally hyperexpressed in benign nevi and thin melanomas. This finding suggests that the loss of plexin B1 contributes to late stages of melanoma progression, including invasion and metastasis. Recent evidences indicate that plexin B1 can also activates the PI3-kinase-Akt pathway, thus functioning as a tumor promoter and inhibitor of apoptosis in melanomas not driven by c-Met activation (Stevens et al., 2010). These results require further investigation. If confirmed, they could indicate that the final action of plexin B1 on melanoma progression may depend on the balance between c-Met receptor blockade and the interaction of plexin B1 receptor to downstream targets independent of c-Met signalling, such as Akt.

2.8 Tumor-stromal interactions

Mutant BRAF melanomas show high levels of constitutively activated Erk 1,2 (Houben et al., 2004). Consequences of Erk 1,2 pathway activation include induction of cell proliferation, expression of melanoma transcription factors, matrix metalloproteinases, specific integrin subunits, and resistance to apoptosis (Rubinstein et al., 2010). Melanoma chondroitin sulfate proteoglycan (MCSP) is a plasma membrane-associated proteoglycan which interacts with distinct Erk-binding sites (Yang et al., 2009). As for Erk 1,2, its functions range from remodelling tumor microenvironments, facilitating the growth, invasion and motility of tumor cells to modify the organization of the cytoskeleton by modulating the activity of Rho family. Normal melanocytes express little or no MCSP, while the protein expression increases from benign and dysplastic nevi (Campoli et al., 2004) to melanoma. In RGP melanoma, MCSP expression enhances integrin function and constitutive activation of Erk 1,2. As already shown in acral lentiginous melanoma (such as in acute lymphoblastic leukaemia) MCSP expression is thought to be associated with a poor prognosis (Kageshita et al., 1991). These evidences indicate that MCSP, as a member of the Erk 1,2 pathway, may be considered as a promising therapeutic target in the treatment of melanoma.

3. Epigenetics

Epigenetics refers to changes in phenotype or gene expression without alterations of the DNA sequence. These changes occur at a much higher frequency compared to gene mutation, and may persist for the entire cell life and even for multiple generations (Kyrgidis et al., 2010). These "epimutations"allow the cell to modulate the transcriptional activity of a given gene, from high-level expression to complete silencing. Transcription results from the activity of the RNA polymerase machinery and depends on the ability of transcription activators and repressors to access chromatin at specific promoters (Santos-Rosa & Caldas, 2005). Chromatin is the dynamic scenario in which all the genomic functions take place; its structure is governed by the interplay of complex regulatory systems, which guarantee the maintenance of higher order chromosomal organization. Our understanding of how modulation of chromatin influences cell fate in normal as in neoplastic cells has been greatly improved during the last two decades. DNA replication, repair and transcription are achieved through the interplay of DNA modification and alteration in DNA packaging (Rountree et al., 2001). These mechanisms cooperate to establish the pattern of gene expression (Hashimshony et al., 2003) concerning every fundamental cell function, from cell growth and differentiation, to DNA repair and apoptosis. They operate through the induction of changes in chromatin architecture induced by histones (Dong & Bode, 2006) and "chromatin modifiers" (Kyrgidis et al., 2010). Histones are the main protein components of chromatin. Covalent post-translational modifications of the amino termini of the core histones in nucleosomes consist of methylation, acetylation, phosphorylation, ubiquitination and SUMOylation, and determine the "histone code" (Berger, 2002).

3.1 DNA methylation

DNA methylation occurs on lysine and arginine residues on histone tails. One preferred site of methylation is the C5 position of cytosine in the context of CpG dinucleotides. The latter may be found throughout the genome but are frequently clustered in short regions of 0.5–4kb, known as CpG islands (Bird, 2002), mostly located at the promoter regions of genes and unmethylated in normal cells. Hypermethylation of these regions causes the "silencing" of the target gene. DNA methylation is carried out by different DNA methyltransferases (DNMT) that use s-adenosyl-methionine as a methyl donor to replace a hydrogen atom with a methyl group (Board et al., 2008) and have distinct substrate specificities: DNMT1 (Pradhan et al., 1999), DNMT3a and 3b (Okano et al., 1999). All these DNMTs cooperate in establishing and maintaining DNA methylation patterns (Rhee et al., 2000; Kim et al., 2002).

In normal cells, methylation of CpG sites within promoter regions is used for controlling gene expression (Klose & Bird, 2006). In cancer cells, hypermethylation of the promoter regions of growth-regulatory genes leads to transcriptional silencing (Eden et al., 2003; Bonazzi et al., 2009), whereas hypo/demethylation results in de-repression of proto-oncogenes and genome wide hypomethylation leads to increased mutation rates and chromosome instability, which constitutes an early hallmark of tumour cells (Feinberg et al. 2002; Robertson, 2005; Martinez et al., 2009). The peculiar changes in DNA methylation patterns of human cancers are commonly constituted by reduced levels of DNA methylation and aberrantly hypermethylated CpG islands (Bird, 2002), which has been termed "the CpG island methylator phenotype" (CIMP) (Board et al., 2008). In cancer, epigenetic silencing through methylation occurs at even greater frequency than mutations or deletions and may be a more frequent cause of loss of function of tumor-suppressor genes than genetic defects (Jones & Baylin, 2002; Herman, 1999), suggesting that epigenetic changes have a major role in every step of tumor progression (Baylin, 2005). The genes that are known to be frequently hypermethylated and silenced in cancers frequently reside in chromosome regions that commonly show loss of heterozygosity, and their loss-of-function provides a selective growth advantage to neoplastic cells, and/or are implicated in tumor metastasis and angiogenesis (Baylin, 2005). Among these genes, we found most of them frequently mutated in cancers, as: ATM, ataxia telangiectasia mutated; APC, adenomatosis polyposis coli; BRCA1/2, breast cancer1/2; CDKN2A/B, cyclin-dependent kinase inhibitor 2A/B; GSTP1, glutathione S-transferase pi; MLH1, mutL homologue 1, colon cancer, non-polyposis type 2; MSH2, mutS homologue 2, colon cancer, non-polyposis type 1; NF12PTCHPTEN, phosphatase and tensin homologue; RB1, retinoblastoma 1; SWI/SNF-related, matrix-associated, actin-dependent regulator of chromatin, subfamily A, member 3/subfamily B, member 1; TIMP3, tissue inhibitor of metalloproteinase 3; TP53/73, tumour protein p53/p73.

3.2 Histone acetylation

In an opposite manner respect to methylation, acetylation of histones reduces the positive charge, relaxing chromatin and making DNA in a transcriptionally active state, mediated mainly by the binding of transcriptional factors and histone acetylates. By a simplified point-of-view, we can assume that hyper acetylated histones are mostly associated with activated genomic regions, whereas deacetylation/hypoacetylation results in repression/silencing. In addition, histone acetylation allows also the binding of some regulatory transcriptional co-activators (Baylin, 2005), as the SWI/SNF adenosine triphosphatase (ATP)-dependent chromatin remodelling complex. Chromatin remodelling complex ("chromatin modifiers") is large protein complexes with enzymatic activity able to modify the structure and transcriptional activity of the chromatin. In an indirect manner, then, histone acetylation cooperates also to the regulation of gene expression mediated by the modification of higher-order chromatin folding (Verdone et al., 2006).

3.3 Phosphorylation

Other chromatin modifications, in concert with DNA methylation and acetylation, regulate gene transcription, in normal as in cancer cells, by affecting local chromatin structure. One of these modifications is constituted by phosphorylation of serines and threonines (Dong & Bode, 2006). Berger (Berger, 2002) showed that phosphorylation of histone (Ser10) is fundamental for neoplastic cell transformation.

3.4 Ubiquitination and SUMOylation

The other histone post-translational modifications include ubiquitination and SUMOylation. Ubiquitin is a highly conserved protein associated with most of fundamental cellular processes and its deregulated activity is thought to contribute to cancer onset or progression. SUMOylation directly affects nucleosomal structure, but the exact molecular mechanism is still not clear (Gill, 2004). Recently it has been shown that histone H4 is modified by SUMO, and SUMO-modification of histones has been suggested to contribute to transcriptional repression (Shiio & Eisenman, 2003), regulation of protein–protein interactions and activity of many factors involved in maintenance of the genome stability. Many factors and enzymes associated with DNA replication and repair including PCNA, and Topoisomerases I and II, are post-translationally modified by SUMO (Muller et al., 2004). The activity and/or localization of several tumor supressors and oncogenes are regulated by SUMO modification, and this has been hypothesized to provide new chances for new target therapy for cancer (Gill, 2004).

3.5 Interplay between different post-translational modifications

It has to be pointed out that single histone modifications may have distinct biological effects depending on their context. Methylation of H3 on K9, for example, is largely associated with silencing and repression. Methylation of lysine 9 on histone H3 is associated with epigenetically silenced chromatin, and loss of the H3K9me3 mark results in genomic instability (Cloos et al., 2006). Methylation of H3 on K4, by reverse, is most often associated with active or permissive chromatin regions. Moreover, demethylation of H3-K4 occurs at both inactive and active euchromatic genes, whereas tri-methylation is present exclusively at active genes. Similarly, the phosphorylation of H3 at S10 has been implicated not only in transcriptional activation, but also in mitotic chromosome condensation. This led to the suggestion that multiple readouts of a certain covalent mark could be obtained by various combinations of different modifications in the same chromatin region. Particular sets of modifications might occur concomitantly on the same histone tail. Mounting evidence suggests that different histone modifications can influence or 'communicate' with each other at several levels (Fischle et al., 2003). Moreover, as a rule, histone acetylation/deacetylation and methylation operate synergistically in cancer cells (Rountree et al., 2001), but competition for lysines may create crosstalk between SUMO and other modifiers. Acetylation may enhance SUMOylation of histone H4 (Gill, 2004); HATs and HDACs (that respectively add and remove acetyl groups) are post-translationally modified by SUMO, which regulates also their localization and/or activity (Girdwood et al., 2003). Cross-talk between the SUMOylation, ubiquitination, and acetylation occurs during signal-dependent regulation of several proteins (Hoege et al., 2002; Ross et al., 2002). From these data it emerges that the epigenetic framework which regulates gene expression is an extremely complex process, constituted by a multitude of intersecting molecular factors converging on chromatin.

3.6 miRNA

MicroRNAs (miRNAs) are recently discovered endogenous non-coding RNAs, about 22 nucleotide long (Guil & Esteller, 2009; Sigalotti et al., 2010). They play a role as mediators of epigenetic gene regulation, by interacting with mRNA, either by inhibiting mRNA translation or causing mRNA degradation (Sood et al., 2006). Their regulatory nature, as well as the large number of presumptive target genes, candidate them as regulators of several fundamental cellular processes, in normal as in cancer cells.

3.7 Melanoma epigenetics

3.7.1 Methylation

At present, it is not clear if UVR can initiate melanomagenesis through an epigenetic mechanism. Nevertheless, epigenetic changes, as mutations, increase after ultraviolet radiation (UVR) (Kyrgidis et al., 2010). This is of a great interest, considering that intermittent, intense exposure to UVR, especially during childhood, is major environmental risk factor in the etiology of melanoma (Maddodi & Setaluri, 2008). Deregulation of gene expression in melanoma progression requires epigenetic mechanisms which are currently uncompletely characterized, but have a potential great impact on the process of melanoma tumorigenesis and metastatic potential (Howell et al., 2009; Schinke et al., 2010). To date, more than 50 genes have been shown to be silenced through epigenetic changes during melanoma development, progression, and metastasis, mainly by promoter CpG island hypermethylation (Rothhammer & Bosserhoff, 2007; Howell et al., 2009), as it has been reported for MAGEA1 (Karpf et al.,2004). Most of these genes are not specific for melanoma, being involved in the control of cell cycle, cell signalling, immune recognition, angiogenesis, apoptosis, tumor cell invasion and metastasis in almost all cancer types (Rothhammer & Bosserhoff, 2007). Among these, there are CDKN2A, PTEN, APAF-1, TPM1 and TIMP3, several human leukocyte class I antigens and CASP8. Recently, have been found methylated in melanoma other genes linked to apoptosis (DAPKb, HSPB6, HSPB8, TMS1, TP53INP1, TRAILR1, XAF1), anchorage-independent growth (TPM1; cell cycle: CDKN1B, CDKN1C, CDKN2A, TSPY); chromatin remodeling (NPM2); differentiation (HOXB13, ENC1, GDF15); DNA repair (MGMT); invasion/metastasis (CCR7, CXCR4, SERPINB5); signaling (PGRbeta); transcription (RUNX3) (Sigalotti et al., 2010). In several cases, these aberrant hyper-methylations are recognizable in an high percentage of melanomas, as for Suppressors of cytokine signaling SOCS-1 (75%), SOCS-2 (75%), SOCS-3 (60%) (Liu et al., 2008), ER-α Estrogen receptor alpha (42%-86%) (Mori et al., 2006), p101(PIK3R5) Phosphoinositide-3-kinase, regulatory subunit 5 (88%), TNFRSF10C (DcR1) Tumor necrosis factor receptor superfamily, member 10c (55%) and TNFRSF10D (8 5%) (Liu et al., 2008), THBS4 Thrombospondin 4 (63%), RASSF1A RAS association domain family protein 1A (involved in apoptosis: its expression negatively correlates with lymph node metastasis, 55%), (Yi et al., 2010), HSP11, Heat shock protein H11 (60%), and RARβ2, Retinoic acid receptor, beta isoform 2 (70%, linked to the low retinoid sensitivity of melanoma) (Hoon et al., 2004). Up to 100% of melanoma cases show hyper-methylated CYP1B1 (Cytochrome P450, subfamily 1, polypeptide 1, linked to drug metabolism) and QPCT (Glutaminyl-peptide cyclotransferase) (Muthusamy et al., 2006). Recently, in cutaneous melanoma the loss of expression/methylation of gene promoter for Tumor suppressor in lung cancer 1 (TSLC1), encoding a member of the immunoglobulin superfamily, has been described (You et al., 2010). In some cancer types, this phenomenon leads to poor prognosis, and in melanoma it is significantly associated with advanced tumor stage and shorter disease-related survival, thus appearing as an important event in the pathogenesis of CM and a marker of poor prognosis (You et al., 2010). Similarly, recent findings indicated that a frequently aberrant methylated region in CM resides within the Zygote arrest 1 (ZAR1) gene, demonstrating a distinct methylation pattern between melanoma and nevus, thus hypothesizing that the aberrant methylation of ZAR1 may be a useful tumor biomarker to distinguish nevus from melanoma for early diagnosis (Shinojima et al., 2010). As well, there is an increasing body of evidence that, indicating the inactivation of the dimeric 14-3-3σ proteins member of the oncogene RAS/RAF/MEK/Erk pathway, involved in DNA damage repair or arrest of cell cycle after severe damage, plays an important role in primary melanoma development. This has been reported for several malignant tumors (Schultz et al., 2009). Moreover, enhanced 14-3-3σ gene methylation in lymph node and cutaneous melanoma metastases compared with primary tumors was associated with significant 14-3-3σ downregulation. Treatment of melanoma cells with methylation and histone deacetylase inhibitors has led to the increase of 14-3-3σ expression, inhibition of cell proliferation, and induction of melanoma cell senescence. Epigenetic profiling showed, in addition, that multiple metastases after a single primary melanoma either share similar methylation patterns for many genes, or show differences in methylation between the lesions for several genes, as for PTEN, TFAP2C, and RARB (Harbst et al., 2010). Less is known on the presence and role of demethylation in CM, this reflecting the state-of-the art of the research on genome-wide demethylation in cancer, which has been overshadowed, to date, by studies of gene-specific hypermethylation events. It is generally thought that global demethylation early in tumorigenesis might predispose cells to genomic instability and further genetic changes, whereas gene-specific demethylation frequently constitutes a later event that favours the establishment of metastasis (Robertson, 2005). Recent study report that MAGE-A1, A2, A3, A4, which are involved in immune recognition and belong to the melanoma antigen family of cancer–testis genes, encoding tumour antigens of mostly unknown function, are frequently demethylated and re-expressed in cancer (Robertson, 2005) and hypomethylated in 44% of CM (MAGEA1) (Sigalotti et al., 2010; Tellez et al., 2009). This is very interesting, if we consider that the same family of genes, as before reported, may be found frequently hypermethylated in melanoma. This is also the case for the Testis-specific protein, Y-encoded (TSPY) (Oram et al., 2006; Howell et al., 2009), and maspin, a mammary serine protease inhibitor, acting as a TSG in breast cancer (Wada et al., 2004) that is repressed in normal melanocytes.

3.7.2 Phosphorylation

Phosphorylation of histone H3 at serine 28 and 10 is strongly induced by UV irradiation (Dong et al., 2006), and is mediated by the MAP kinase cascades (Zhong SP et al., 2000). UVA and UVB differentially induce the MAP kinase pathways at different levels (Bode & Dong, 2003): ERKs and p38 kinase mediate UVB-induced H3 (Ser10) phosphorylation in mouse epidermal skin cells and in vitro. It has been hypothesized that the p53 protein may directly regulate this phosphorylation by serving as a link or a bridge between these kinases and histone H3. Moreover, it has been found that also (He Z et al., 2005). Fyn, a member of the Src kinase family, and Aurora B kinase overexpression are involved in the UVB-induced phosphorylation of histone H3 (Ser10) (Ota et al., 2002). Recent data suggest that H3 histone phosphorylation plays a role in UV-mediated carcinogenesis.

3.7.3 Acetylation

Three members of the HATs family, the transcriptional coactivators, GNAT (general control non-depressible 5 (Gcn5)-related *N*-acetyltransferase), MYST (family members: MOZ, Ybf2-Sas3, Sas2, and Tip60) and p300/CBP-adenoviral E1A-associated protein, 300 kDa, (CREB-binding protein), have been recently found linked to melanoma progression. Members of the GNAT family (including GCN5, HAT1) and PCAF (p300/CREB-binding associated factor) acetylate histones H3 and H4 and non-histone transcriptional activators. P300 and CBP are global transcription coactivators that acetylate core histones and non-histone proteins such as p53, Rb, and E2F, involved in regulation of cellular proliferation, differentiation and apoptosis

(Shiama et al., 1997). Both CBP and p300 have been also shown to associate with microphthalmia-associated transcription factor (MITF), a melanocyte lineage survival oncogene (Garraway et al., 2005), which regulates melanoma proliferation, apoptosis and invasiveness (Dynek et al., 2008), and is mostly upregulated in metastatic melanomas (Lomas et al., 2008) being associated with decreased survival of patients (Ugurel et al., 2007).

3.7.4 Ubiquitination/SUMOylation

Accumulating evidence confirms the involvement of ubiquitin and ubiquitin-related pathways in melanomagenesis. Transcription factors such as MiTF, beta-catenin and IkB, which regulate the proliferation and differentiation of melanocytes, are subjected to this process (Wu et al., 2000). In normal melanocytes, MITF may be in turn subjected to ubiquitination or SUMOylation. In melanoma, ubiquitination leads to the corresponding elevated activity of MITF (Nakayama, 2010). In addition, melanoma cells show an alterated ubiquitination-dependent degradation of IKB, with consequent high rate of nuclear translocation of free NF-kB and activation of its target genes (Nakayama, 2010). Notably, also B-catenin is a target of the ubiquitin–proteasome pathway in melanoma. Several beta-catenin mutants lack sites of ubiquitination and, consequently, become stabilized because of the inhibition of proteasome-mediated proteolysis; thus promoting proliferation and survival of melanoma cells (Aberle et al., 2007; Rubinfeld et al., 1997; Widlund et al., 2002).

3.7.5 Chromatin texture

The neoplastic growth-induced modification of composition and distribution of histone and non-histone nuclear proteins provokes alterations of the distribution of heterochromatin in the nucleus. This reflects on the characteristics of the nuclear architecture, as seen on routinely stained histopathological sections, and has suggested as prognostic markers in cancer (Montironi et al., 2007). The determination of fractality characterizes the complexity of a structure not revealed by classical morphometry. The fractal nature of nuclear chromatin and of the surrounding nucleoplasmic space (Lieberman-Aiden et al., 2009; Bancaud A et al., 2009) are of prognostic importance in neoplasias (Goutzanis et al., 2008; Mashiah et al., 2008). Unstable, aggressive tumors with a high number of genetic or epigenetic changes, are characterized by a complex chromatin rearrangement, with an increased number of darker and lighter areas. The increased nuclear fractal dimension found in the most aggressive melanomas is the mathematical equivalent of this complex chromatin architecture, constituting a new and promising variable in prognostic models (Bedin et al., 2010), able to provide prognostic information independent from the invasion level of melanomas.

3.7.6 Chromatin assembly

Nuclear structure and function interact reciprocally at all the three hierarchical nuclear levels (coordination of nuclear processes, higher-order chromatin fiber organization, and spatial arrangement of genome) (Misteli, 2007). The chromatin template undergoes structural reorganizations during DNA replication and cell cycle progression (Fischle et al., 2003). Nucleosomes, made of 146 base pairs of DNA wrapped around a histone octamer core comprising two copies each of histones H2A, H2B, H3 and H4, represent the basic functional units of chromatin. Each histone contains flexible N-terminal tails protruding from the nucleosomes, which are extensively targeted by post-translational modifications, including acetylation and methylation (Sigalotti et al., 2010). When in open configuration, they allow access of transcription factors. By converse, when they are in a hyper-compacted state, as in heterochromatin, inhibit transcription (Jones & Baylin, 2002; Jenuwein & Allis, 2001; Noma et al., 2001). Nucleosome structure and histone acetylation/methylation equally affect chromatin structure, regulating gene transcription (Baylin, 2005). Among molecules responsible of the chromatin assembly, a pivotal role is exerted by the Chromatin Assembly Factor-1 (CAF-1), a protein complex, formed of three subunits with different molecular weight: p48, p60 and p150. CAF-1 deliveres histones H3 and H4 to DNA during DNA replication and DNA repair, and CAF-1/p60 has been found overexpressed in a series of human malignancies, including breast, prostate, oral squamous and salivary glands cancers, in close association with their biological aggressiveness. We have evaluated by immunohistochemistry the expression of CAF-1/p60 in a selected series of cutaneous melanomas paraffinized tissue (Mascolo et al., 2010), comparing results with the clinical and pathological features of each tumor and with patient's outcome. We found a significant association between hyperexpression of CAF-1/p60 and the occurrence of node and/or distant metastases in SM patients. These findings indicate that CAF-1 may have a role as novel, sensible proliferation and prognostic marker for CM. CAF-1 overexpression can be easily evaluated by immunohistochemistry on formalin-fixed, paraffin-embedded tissue, and may constitute a potential useful adjunctive tool for pathologists for predicting the individual prognosis of melanoma patients.

3.7.7 Remodeling proteins

Recent studies have shown that SWI/SNF ATP dependent chromatin remodeling enzymes are involved in the molecular alterations occurring in melanoma (Saladi et al., 2010) and regulate the expression of genes important for tumor metastasis. SWI/SNF enzymes promote neural crest migration and differentiation and interact with Microphthalmia - Associated Transcription Factor (MITF), a known lineage survival oncogene in melanoma (de la Serna et al., 2006; Matsumoto et al., 2006; Saladi et al., 2010). SWI/SNF are multisubunit complexes that contain either BRG1 or BRM as the catalytic subunit (Li B et al., 2007) regulating important aspects of melanoma phenotype. While BRM expression is variable in melanoma (cell lines), BRG1 expression is increased at the protein levels in primary melanoma tumors compared to dysplastic nevi, and in most melanoma cell lines (Keenen et al., 2010; Vachtenheim et al., 2010). A BRG1 expression increases during melanoma progression and is thought to play an important role in melanoma metastasis, as it promotes melanoma invasive ability in vitro. This is supported by the ability of BRG1 to modulate the expression of a subset of cell surface receptors, adhesion proteins, and extracellular matrix remodeling enzymes in normal as in cancer cells, interacting with a transcriptional regulator of MMP2, the SP1 transcription factor, being also recruited to the matrix metalloproteinase (MMP2) promoter. However, up to date there was found no significant difference in BRG1 levels between primary and metastatic melanoma samples, but there has been evidenced a tendency for negative to weak BRG1 expression in the cases with a better patient survival (Lin et al., 2010).

3.7.8 miRNA

As before outlined, microRNAs (miRNAs) may act as either oncogenes or tumor suppressor genes. Recently, it has been shown that miRNAs act as tumor suppressors in uveal melanoma cells through downregulation of MITF and CDK6, and, particularly, that miR-137 is frequently silenced in this tumor (Chen et al., 2011). Up to now, limited data are available on miRNA deregulation in CM, almost all relative to small series of cases (Mueller et al., 2009; Sigalotti et al., 2010). However, a recent specific miRNA profiling study reports extensive modifications of miRNA patterns in CM as compared to normal melanocytes, and identifyies modifications of miRNA expression potentially associated to the different phases of CM progression (Mueller et al., 2009). Another study reports that miR-17-5p, miR-18a, miR-20a and miR-92a are over-expressed, while miR-146a, miR-146b, and miR155 are down-regulated in the majority of the examined CM cell lines as compared to normal melanocytes (Levati et al., 2009). Of particular interest, the master regulator of melanocytes biology, transcription factor MITF, has been found to be regulated by at least 2 different miRNAs, miR-137 and miR-182, which showed opposite alterations (Bemis et al., 2008). Other miRNAs have been found overexpressed in CM cell lines and tissues. Among them, miR-182 appeared to be involved in CM progression, being increasingly over-expressed from primary to metastatic disease. Its action has been related to the repression of MITF and FOXO3 (Segura. et al., 2009). The overexpression of miR-29c has been recently reported to be inversely correlated to DNMT3A and DNMT3B protein expression (Nguyen et al., 2011) and predictive of overall survival in AJCC stage III melanoma patients by multivariate analysis. On the contrary, members of the let-7 family of miRNAs are significantly downregulated in primary melanomas compared with benign nevi (Schultz et al., 2008). As in normal cells let-7 miRNAs exhert a regulatory activity on the expression of cyclins D1, D3, and A, as well as cyclin-dependent kinase (Cdk) 4, all of which have been described to play a role in melanoma development, (Müller & Bosserhoff, 2008). It appears evident that the loss of let-7a expression may contribute in the development and progression of melanoma.

3.7.9 Epigenetic drugs

DNA methylation inhibitors (as azacitidine and decitabine), along with inhibitors of histone deacetylation, have improved the therapeutic options of some cancer types, and particularly of several hematologic malignancies, where gene hypermethylation typically occurs (Baylin, 2005). The potential reversibility of epigenetic changes via pharmacologic manipulation, confers to this area of research particular relevance for the alternative therapeutic treatment of patients with advanced melanoma. New agents affecting epigenetic alterations in melanoma are thus being increasingly produced. The treatment of CM with these "epigenetic drugs" generally produce multiple effects, due to the reactivation and/or suppression of many of intersecting pathways that became altered during melanoma progression (Sigalotti et al., 2007). There is a tendency to combine epigenetic intervention with conventional and/or innovative therapeutic approaches that would take specific advantages from the epigenetically-restored pathways. As an example, strategies to restore the loss of expression of spindle checkpoint proteins, such as RASSF1A, by use of demethylating agents may be of utility in reversing genetic instability associated with melanoma progression (Rother & Jones, 2009). Indeed, in advanced stage melanoma, RASSF1A appears to correlate at some degree with response to chemotherapy. As a result, profiling of the activation state or degree of mitotic spindle dysfunction using these markers, shows promise in identifying those patients who would benefit from spindle toxins. The drugs typically used as multi-agent chemotherapy regimens to treat melanoma include carboplatin and cisplatin, alkylating agents, and mitotic spindle poisons such as vinblastine and paclitaxel. Since therapeutic activity of alkylating agents and DNA-damaging agents requires tumor cell division, melanomas with high proliferative rate or those with genetic alterations in checkpoint function may be more likely to respond (Rother & Jones, 2009). Similarly, a particular clinical benefit might be expected from the synergistic effect of the pharmacologic inhibition of DNA methyltransferases and/or of histone deacetylases with chemo-, radio-, and immuno-therapeutic approaches in melanoma patients (Sigalotti, 2010). The introduction of new epigenetic drugs in this context is

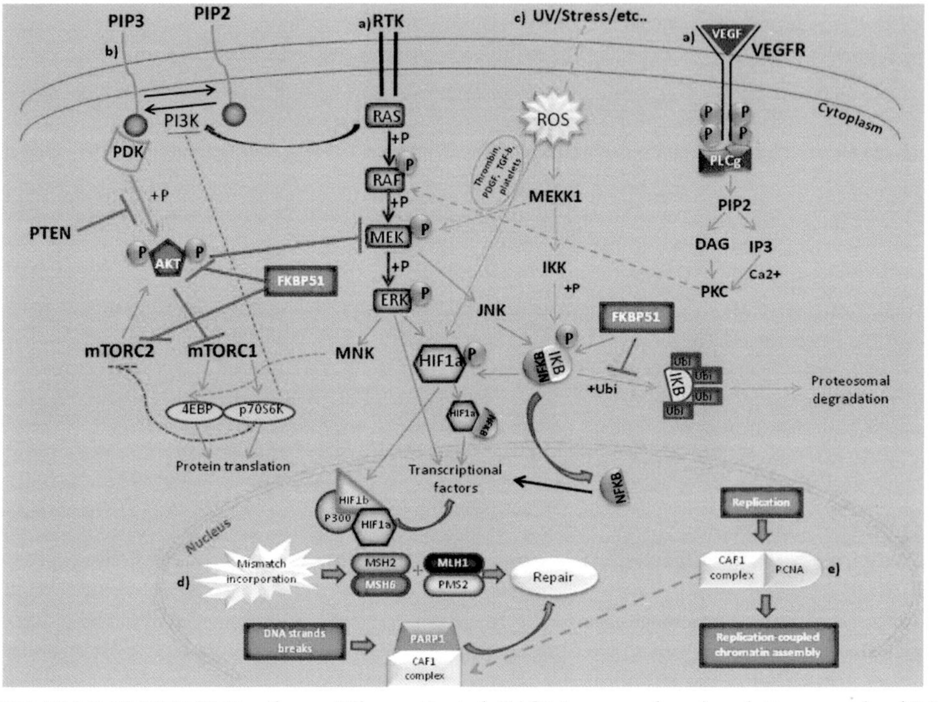

a) RTK-RAS-RAF-MEK-ERK pathway. When activated, RAS triggers a phosphorylation cascade of RAF, MEK and ERK. MEK, when phosphorylated, activates Jun N-terminal kinase (JNK) cascade; ERK translocates to the nucleus, where it activates transcription factors for cell proliferation. VEGFR is a RTK and, therefore, when activated, leads to activation of this pathway. b) PI3K-AKT pathway. Activation of RTKs leads to activation of PI3K and, subsequently, of PDK1 that phosphorylates and activates AKT. AKT regulates several proteins affecting cell growth and survival. c) ROS signaling pathway. ROS production can induce HIF-1a (hypoxia-inducible transcription factors 1) under normoxia in response to some factors. Intracellular ROS activates also the NFkB (nuclear factor-kappa route B). d) DNA-repair pathways. PARP1 (Poly [ADP-ribose] polymerase 1) has a role in repair of single-stranded DNA (ssDNA) breaks, modifying nuclear proteins by polyADP-ribosylation. Component of the post-replicative DNA mismatch repair system (hMSH2 and hMLH) binds to DNA mismatches thereby initiating DNA repair. e) The Chromatin Assembly Factor-1 (CAF-1) promotes also the first step of nucleosome assembly during DNA replication, driving the incorporation of different histones into DNA to the sites where chromatin has to be newly formed or remodeled. CAF-1 promotes chromosome assembly during resetting of the chromatin structure after DNA repair (d).

Fig. 1. Crosstalks between signaling pathways involved in melanomagenesis and progression

GENETIC CHANGES	
Mutations	ASIP, β-catenin, BRAF, CCND1, CDKN2A, CDK4, Rb, cKIT, HIF1/ROS, IGFBP7, MC1R, NEUROPILIN2, NFkB, NRAS, PI3KCA, p16INK4, PLEXIN B1, PTEN/AKT, Rab38, TYR, TYRP1, WNT5A
EPIGENETIC ALTERATIONS	
Hypermethylation	ATM, APAF-1, APC, BRCA1, BRCA2, CASP8, CCR7, CXCR4, CDKN1B, CDKN1C, CDKN2A, CDKN2B, CYP1B1, DAPKb, ENC1, ER-α, GDF15, GSTP, H3, HLA class I, HOXB13, HSPB6, HSPB8, HSP11, MAGE-A1, MGMT, MLH1, MSH2, NF12PTCHPTEN, NPM2, p101(PIK3R5), PGRbeta, PTEN, QPCT, RARβ2, RASSF1A, RB1, RUNX3, SERPINB5, SOCS1, SOCS2, SOCS3, Stratifin (14-3-3sigma), SWI/SNF, TFAP2C, THBS4, TIMP3, TMS1, TNFRSF10C (DcR1), TNFRSF10D, TP53INP1, TP53/73, TPM1, TRAILR1, TSCL1, TSPY, XAF1, ZAR1
Hypomethylation	MAGE-A1, MAGE-A2, MAGE-A3, MAGE-A4, Maspin, TSPY,
Phosphorylation	H3 (ser 28), H3 (ser 10)
Acethylation	E2F, H3, H4, MITF, p53, Rb, SWI/SNF (ATP)-dependent chromatin remodelling complex,
Ubiquitination/SUMOylation	H4, PCNA, Topoisomerase 1, Topoisomerase 2, MiTF, IkB, β-catenin
Chromatin assembly	Chromatin Assembly Factor-1 (CAF-1)
Remodelling proteins	SWI/SNF chromatin remodelling enzymes
miRNA overexpressed	miR-29c, miR-17-5p, miR-18a, miR-20a, miR-92a, miR-182
miRNA downregulated	miR137, miR-146a, miR-146b, miR155, miRNA let-7a
Tumor-stromal interactions	MCSP/NG2

Table 1. Summary of major genetic and epigenetic alterations in melanoma.

expected to reduce systemic toxicities of traditional therapies. Histone deacetylase (HDAC) inhibitors represent a promising therapeutic option for melanoma treatment (Facchetti F et al., 2004) and are particularly interesting with this regard. It has been shown, in fact, that HDAC inhibitors enhance the response of human tumor cells to ionizing radiation (Munshi et al., 2006) and synergize with radiation, reducing the clonogenic survival of CM cells. This beneficial effect seems to be related to their ability to sensitize CM cells to radiation-induced apoptosis, impairing also the ability of CM cells to repair DNA damages through the down-regulation of the repair proteins Ku70, Ku80, Ku86 and Rad50) (Munshi et al., 2006). These exciting results support the idea that combined epigenetic chemo/radiotherapies might overcome the resistance of CM to traditional therapies. In addition, HDAC inhibitors have been shown to sensitize melanoma cells to retinoid treatment, leading to the increase of tsg p16INK4A, either mutated or with homozygous deletion in most of late-stage melanoma cells, thus correlating with their increased senescence. A further interesting example of possible integration between "old" and "new, epigenetic" therapies, is offered by the major polyphenolic constituent of green tea, the epigallocatechin-3-gallate (EGCG), which has anti-proliferative, pro-apoptotic and chemopreventive effects against cancer cells, including melanoma (Nihal et al., 2010), mediated through its demethylating activity. EGCG sensitizes melanoma cells to interferon in mouse models of human melanoma, by down-regulating NF-κB promoter activity, induced by reactive oxygen species (Fried & Arbiser, 2008). EGCG synergizes with the HDAC inhibitory action of vorinostat to help de-repress silenced tumor-suppressor genes regulating key functions, such as proliferation and survival. Lastly, it has to be outlined the potential beneficial effect of therapeutically restoring miRNA activity in CM.

4. Conclusions

Cross-talk between different signaling cascades has emerged as a paradigm of cell biology, in that they direct the local and global cell functions (Fischle et al., 2003). The epigenetic code is made of post-translational marks which correlate with specific transcriptional states and may influence one another (Berger, 2002), their combinations ultimately directing downstream functions. We are beginning to unravel the complexities of gene expression, which is conditioned by a myriad of diverse stimuli, acting in a multidimensional fashion (Dong & Bode, 2006), with histone modification and ATP-dependent chromatin remodeling being functionally connected for gene regulation. DNA methylation is controlled at several different levels in normal and tumor cells, directly by DNA methyltransferases (DNMTs), and indirectly by nucleosome spacing and histone deacetylases (HDACs) (Baylin, 2005; Bird A, 2002; Bird & Wolffe, 1999). Synergism/antagonism of adjacent modifications in the same histone tail is the rule ('cis' effects), but modifications on different histones affect each other ('trans' effects) (Fischle et al., 2003). Overall, it is now clear that each specific genetic or epigenetic alteration may impact the biology of CM cells by concurrently affecting multiple proteins/pathways. Further study will determine which panels of genes are most effective as biomarkers for prediction of response to therapy and prognosis and may be translated into clinically applicable tests. The different methylation or acetylation patterns may indicate important differences in tumorigenesis and may help identify subsets of patients with different clinical behaviour. The reported correlation of alterations in tumour DNA with circulating tumour DNA allows the basis for the development of biomarker blood tests for early detection of melanoma metastasis and prediction of response to therapy. Being a relatively rare event in normal melanocytes, specific hypermethylations of CpG islands are ideal candidate as biomarkers for early melanoma metastasis detection in body fluids (Howell et al., 2009). In line with this hypothesis, it has been recently reported that estrogen receptor A (ER-A) methylation can predicts melanoma progression, and serum methylated ER-A constitutes an unfavorable prognostic factor and negative predictor of progression-free survival in patients treated with biochemotherapy (Mori et al., 2006; Satzger I, 2009). Many studies are investigating the methylation status of several genes in sera of CM patients (Satzger I, 2009). We have now summarized only a selection of the hot topics concerning the genetic and epigenetic alterations that contribute to the development and progression of melanoma. Many questions remain unanswered. Cancer research is moving away from an histology-based view of cancer toward a genomic concept of the neoplastic disease (Garraway, 2010), and therapy is shifting toward pharmacogenomics, engineered to hit the specific genetic and epigenetic profile (the "genomic grade") of the single tumor in each single patient, (Kim et al., 2010; Piccart-Gebhart, 2010). These goals are necessary for ultimately improve melanoma patient outcomes and increase drug efficacy against this lethal cancer. Further work is required to improve our understanding of the precise role of interlinked modifications that dictate specific genomic states, such as gene activation, repression, DNA repair in melanoma progression. Bioinformatics-based tools are being currently used to generate complex fingerprints based on a combination of genetic and epigenetic markers. Recent mathematical modeling of the dynamics of transcriptional control of gene expression will be relevant to a full understanding of MITF, SOX10, and PAX3 functions (Ben-Tabou de-Leon & Davidson, 2009). An unconditioned approach to the importance of the yet known key molecules involved in melanocyte development and function, under the light of the growing body of newly discovered interrelationships between new and old members of the most relevant pathways involved in melanoma progression, will be fundamental to improve the chances of the pigment research community to fight melanoma. The shift occurring towards personalized therapy in cancer is also beginning to be seen in melanoma, and new generation epigenetic drugs are be expected to reduce systemic toxicities with more specific effects (Sigalotti et al., 2010), even if additional pre-clinical studies are required to define even more precisely their consequences on normal cells and to predict their safety when used on patients. Convincing evidence that we are on the right way to truly understand melanoma biology already exists. A comprehensive point-of-view, considering simultaneously the phenotype, genotype and epigenotype of melanoma cells with respect to the differences in clinical behavior (Shackleton & Quintana, 2010) will help us to guide treatment and target those patients with specific, personalized therapies.

5. Acknowledgment

We thank Ms. Amanda Tedeschi for the editing of the English style. We also acknowledge the many colleagues and collaborators with whom we have worked or discussed ideas. We apologize for all the authors we have not mentioned, due to space restriction.

6. References

Aberle, H., Bauer, A., Stappert, J., Kispert, A., & Kemler, R. (1997). beta-catenin is a target for the ubiquitin-proteasome pathway. *EMBO J*, Vol. 16, No. 13, (Jul 1997), pp. 3797-3804, ISSN 0261-4189

Argast, G.M., Croy, C.H., Couts, K.L., Zhang, Z., Litman, E., Chan, D.C., & Ahn, N.G. (2009). Plexin B1 is repressed by oncogenic B-Raf signaling and functions as a tumor suppressor in melanoma cells. *Oncogene*, Vol. 28, No. 30, (Jul 2009), pp. 2697-2709, ISSN 0950-9232

Balch, C.M., Buzaid, A.C., Atkins, M.B., Cascinelli, N., Coit, D.G., Fleming, I.D., Houghton, A. Jr, Kirkwood, J.M., Mihm, M.F., Morton, D.L., Reintgen, D., Ross, M.I., Sober, A., Soong, S.J., Thompson, J.A., Thompson, J.F., Gershenwald, J.E., & McMasters, K.M. (2000). A new American Joint Committee on Cancer staging system for cutaneous melanoma. *Cancer*, Vol. 88, No. 6, (Mar 2000), pp. 1484-1491, ISSN 1097-0142

Bancaud, A., Huet, S., Daigle, N., Mozziconacci, J., Beaudouin, J., & Ellenberg, J. (2009). Molecular crowding affects diffusion and binding of nuclear proteins in heterochromatin and reveals the fractal organization of chromatin. *EMBO J*, Vol. 28, No. 24, (Dec 2009), pp. 3785-3798, ISSN 0261-4189

Bauer, J., & Bastian B.C. (2006). Distinguishing melanocytic nevi from melanoma by DNA copy number changes: comparative genomic hybridization as a research and diagnostic tool. *Dermatol Ther*, Vol. 19, No. 1, (Jan-Feb 2006), pp. 40-49, ISSN 1529-8019

Baylin, S.B. (2005). DNA methylation and gene silencing in cancer. *Nat Clin Pract Oncol*, Vol. 2, Suppl 1, (Dec 2005), pp. S4-11, ISSN 1743-4262

Beddingfield, F.C. 3rd. (2003). The melanoma epidemic: res ipsa loquitur. *Oncologist*, Vol. 8, No. 5, (2003), pp. 459-465, ISSN 1083-7159

Bedin, V., Adam, R.L., de Sá, B.C., Landman, G., & Metze, K. (2010). Fractal dimension of chromatin is an independent prognostic factor for survival in melanoma. *BMC Cancer*, Vol. 10, (Jun 2010), pp. 260, ISSN 1471-2407

Bedogni, B., Welford, S.M., Cassarino, D.S., Nickoloff, B.J., Giaccia, A.J., & Powell, MB. (2005). The hypoxic microenvironment of the skin contributes to Akt-mediated melanocyte transformation. *Cancer Cell*, Vol. 8, No. 6, (Dec 2005), pp. 443-454, ISSN 1535-6108

Bemis, L.T., Chen, R., Amato, C.M., Classen, E.H., Robinson, S.E., Coffey, D.G., Erickson, P.F., Shellman, Y.G., & Robinson, W.A. (2008). MicroRNA-137 targets microphthalmia-associated transcription factor in melanoma cell lines. *Cancer Res*, Vol. 68, No. 5, (Mar 2008), pp. 1362-1368, ISSN 0008-5472.

Ben-Tabou de-Leon, S., & Davidson, E.H. (2009). Modeling the dynamics of transcriptional gene regulatory networks for animal development. *Dev Biol*, Vol. 325, No. 2, (Jan 2009), pp. 317-328, ISSN 0012-1606

Bennett, DC. (2003). Human melanocyte senescence and melanoma susceptibility genes. *Oncogene*, Vol. 22, No. 20, (May 2003), pp. 3063-3069, ISSN 0950-9232

Bennett, D.C. (2008). How to make a melanoma: what do we know of the primary clonal events? *Pigment Cell Melanoma Res*, Vol. 21, No. 1, (Feb 2008), pp. 27-38, ISSN 1755-1471

Berger, S.L. (2002) Histone modifications in transcriptional regulation. *Curr Opin Genet Dev*, Vol. 12, No. 2, (Apr 2002), pp.142-148, ISSN 0959-437X

Bird, A. (2002). DNA methylation patterns and epigenetic memory. *Genes Dev*, Vol. 16, No. 1, (Jan 2002), pp. 6-21, ISSN 0890-9369

Bird, A.P., & Wolffe, A.P. (1999). Methylation-induced repression--belts, braces, and chromatin. *Cell*, Vol. 99, No. 5, (Nov 1999), pp. 451-454, ISSN 0092-8674

Bittner, M., Meltzer, P., Chen, Y., Jiang, Y., Seftor, E., Hendrix, M., Radmacher, M., Simon, R., Yakhini, Z., Ben-Dor, A., Sampas, N., Dougherty, E., Wang, E., Marincola, F., Gooden, C., Lueders, J., Glatfelter, A., Pollock, P., Carpten, J., Gillanders, E., Leja, D., Dietrich, K., Beaudry, C., Berens, M., Alberts, D., & Sondak, V. (2000). Molecular classification of cutaneous malignant melanoma by gene expression profiling. *Nature*, Vol. 406, No. 6795, (Aug 2000), pp 536-540, ISSN 0028-0836

Board, R.E., Knight, L., Greystoke, A., Blackhall, FH., Hughes, A., Dive, C., & Ranson M. (2008). DNA methylation in circulating tumour DNA as a biomarker for cancer. *Biomark Insights*, Vol. 2. (Jan 2008), pp. 307-319, ISSN 1177-2719

Bode, A.M., & Dong, Z. (2003). Mitogen-activated protein kinase activation in UV-induced signal transduction. *Sci STKE*, Vol. 2003, No. 167, (Jan 2003), pp. RE2, ISSN 1945-0877

Bonazzi, V.F., Irwin, D., & Hayward, N.K. (2009). Identification of candidate tumor suppressor genes inactivated by promoter methylation in melanoma. *Genes Chromosomes Cancer*, Vol. 48, No. 1, (Jan 2009), pp 10-21, ISSN 1045-2257

Bonello, S., Zähringer, C., BelAiba, R.S., Djordjevic, T., Hess, J., Michiels, C., Kietzmann, T., & Görlach, A. (2007). Reactive oxygen species activate the HIF-1alpha promoter via a functional NFkappaB site. *Arterioscler Thromb Vasc Biol*, Vol. 27, No. 4 (Apr 2007), pp. 755-761, ISSN 1049-8834

Campoli, M.R., Chang, C.C., Kageshita, T., Wang, X., McCarthy, J.B., & Ferrone, S. (2004). Human high molecular weight-melanoma-associated antigen (HMW-MAA): a melanoma cell surface chondroitin sulfate proteoglycan (MSCP) with biological and clinical significance. *Crit Rev Immunol*, Vol. 24, No. 4, (2004), pp. 267-296, ISSN 1040-8401

Cancer facts and figures; 2009. Atlanta Cancer Society, Available from: http://www.cancer.org/acs/groups/content/@nho/documents/document/f861009final90809pdf.pdf

Chen, X., Wang, J., Shen, H., Lu, J., Li, C., Hu, D.N., Dong, X.D., Yan, D., & Tu, L. (2011). Epigenetics, MicroRNAs, and Carcinogenesis: Functional Role of MicroRNA-137 in Uveal Melanoma. *Invest Ophthalmol Vis Sci*, Vol. 52, No. 3, (Mar 2011), pp. 1193-1199, ISSN 0146-0404

Chin, L., Merlino, G., & DePinho, R.A. (1998) Malignant melanoma: modern black plague and genetic black box. *Genes Dev*, Vol. 12, No. 22, (Nov 1998), pp 3467-3481, ISSN 0890-936

Chin, L., Garraway, L.A., & Fisher, D.E. (2006). Malignant melanoma: genetics and therapeutics in the genomic era. *Genes Dev*, Vol. 20, No. 16, (Aug 2006), pp. 2149-2182, ISSN 0890-9369

Cloos, P.A., Christensen, J., Agger, K., Maiolica, A., Rappsilber, J., Antal, T., Hansen, K.H., & Helin, K. (2006). The putative oncogene GASC1 demethylates tri- and dimethylated lysine 9 on histone H3. *Nature*, Vol. 442, No. 7100, (Jul 2006), pp. 307-311, ISSN 0028-0836

de la Serna, I.L., Ohkawa, Y., Higashi, C., Dutta, C., Osias, J., Kommajosyula, N., Tachibana, T., & Imbalzano, A.N. (2006). The microphthalmia-associated transcription factor requires SWI/SNF enzymes to activate melanocyte-specific genes. *J Biol Chem*, Vol. 281, No. 29, (Jul 2006), pp. 20233-20241, ISSN 0021-9258

Dhomen, N., Reis-Filho, J.S., da Rocha Dias, S., Hayward, R., Savage, K., Delmas, V., Larue, L., Pritchard, C., & Marais, R. (2009). Oncogenic Braf induces melanocyte senescence and melanoma in mice. *Cancer Cell*, Vol. 15, No. 4, (Apr 2009), pp. 294-303, ISSN 1535-6108

Dong, Z., & Bode, A.M. (2006). The role of histone H3 phosphorylation (Ser10 and Ser28) in cell growth and cell transformation. *Mol Carcinog*, Vol. 45, No. 6, (Jun 2006), pp. 416-421, ISSN 0899-1987

Dynek, J.N., Chan, S.M., Liu, J., Zha, J., Fairbrother, W.J., & Vucic, D. (2008). Microphthalmia-associated transcription factor is a critical transcriptional regulator of melanoma inhibitor of apoptosis in melanomas. *Cancer Res*, Vol. 68, No. 9, (May 2008), pp. 3124-3132, ISSN 0008-5472

Eden, A., Gaudet, F., Waghmare, A., & Jaenisch, R. (2003). Chromosomal instability and tumors promoted by DNA hypomethylation. *Science*, Vol. 300, No. 5618, (Apr 2003), pp. 455, ISSN 0036-8075

Erler, J.T., Bennewith, K.L., Nicolau, M., Dornhöfer, N., Kong, C., Le, Q.T., Chi, J.T., Jeffrey, S.S., & Giaccia, A.J. (2006). Lysyl oxidase is essential for hypoxia-induced metastasis. *Nature*, Vol. 440, No. 7088, (Apr 2006), pp. 1222-1226, ISSN 0028-0836

Facchetti, F., Previdi, S., Ballarini, M., Minucci, S., Perego, P., & La Porta, C.A. (2004). Modulation of pro- and anti-apoptotic factors in human melanoma cells exposed to histone deacetylase inhibitors. *Apoptosis*, Vol. 9, No. 5, (Sep 2004), pp. 573-582, ISSN 1360-8185

Fecher, L.A., Cummings, S.D., Keefe, M.J., & Alani, R.M. (2007). Toward a molecular classification of melanoma. *J Clin Oncol*, Vo. 25, No 12, (Apr 2007), pp. 1606-1620, ISSN 0732-183X

Feinberg, A.P., Cui, H., & Ohlsson, R. (2002). DNA methylation and genomic imprinting: insights from cancer into epigenetic mechanisms. *Semin Cancer Biol*, Vol. 12, No. 5, (Oct 2002), pp. 389-398, ISSN 0008-5472

Fischle, W., Wang, Y., & Allis, C.D. (2003). Histone and chromatin cross-talk. *Curr Opin Cell Biol*, Vol. 15, No. 2, (Apr 2003), pp. 172-183, ISSN 1369-5266.

Flaherty, K.T., Puzanov, I., Kim, K.B., Ribas, A., McArthur, G.A., Sosman, J.A., O'Dwyer, P.J., Lee, R.J., Grippo, J.F., Nolop, K., & Chapman, P.B. (2010). Inhibition of mutated, activated BRAF in metastatic melanoma. *N Engl J Med*, Vol. 363, No. 9, (Aug 2010), pp. 809-819, ISSN 0028-4793

Forsythe, J.A., Jiang, B.H., Iyer, N.V., Agani, F., Leung, S.W., Koos, R.D., & Semenza, G.L. (1996). Activation of vascular endothelial growth factor gene transcription by hypoxia-inducible factor 1. *Mol Cell Biol*, Vol. 16, No. 9, (Sep 1996), pp. 4604-4613, ISSN 0270-7306

Fried, L., & Arbiser, J.L. (2008). The reactive oxygen-driven tumor: relevance to melanoma. *Pigment Cell Melanoma Res*, Vol. 21, No. 2, (Apr 2008), pp. 117-122, ISSN 1755-148X

Fruehauf, J.P., & Trapp, V. (2008). Reactive oxygen species: an Achilles' heel of melanoma? *Expert Rev Anticancer Ther*, Vol. 8, No. 11, (Nov 2008), pp. 1751-1757, ISSN 1473-7140

Galabova-Kovacs, G., Matzen, D., Piazzolla, D., Meissl, K., Plyushch, T., Chen, A.P., Silva, A., & Baccarini, M. (2006). Essential role of B-Raf in ERK activation during extraembryonic development. *Proc Natl Acad Sci U S A*, Vol. 103, No. 5, (Jan 2006), pp. 1325-1330, ISSN 0027-8424

Gallagher, W.M., Bergin, O.E., Rafferty, M., Kelly, Z.D., Nolan, I.M., Fox, E.J., Culhane, A.C., McArdle, L., Fraga, M.F., Hughes, L., Currid, C.A., O'Mahony, F., Byrne, A., Murphy, A.A., Moss, C., McDonnell, S., Stallings, R.L., Plumb, J.A., Esteller, M., Brown, R., Dervan, P.A., & Easty, D.J. (2005). Multiple markers for melanoma progression regulated by DNA methylation: insights from transcriptomic studies. *Carcinogenesis*, Vol. 26, No. 11, (Nov 2005), pp.1856-1867, 0143-3334

Garraway, L.A., Widlund, H.R., Rubin, M.A., Getz, G., Berger, A.J., Ramaswamy, S., Beroukhim, R., Milner, D.A., Granter, S.R., Du, J., Lee, C., Wagner, S.N., Li, C., Golub, T.R., Rimm, D.L., Meyerson, M.L., Fisher, D.E., & Sellers, W.R. (2005). Integrative genomic analyses identify MITF as a lineage survival oncogene amplified in malignant melanoma. *Nature*, Vol. 436, No. 7047, (Jul 2005), pp. 117-122, ISSN 0028-0836

Garraway, L.A. (2010). From cancer genomics to personalized oncology. *Program and abstracts of the American Association for Cancer Research 101st Annual Meeting*, Plenary PL02, Washington, DC, USA, April 17-21, 2010

Gidanian, S., Mentelle, M., Meyskens, F.L. Jr, & Farmer, P.J. (2008). Melanosomal damage in normal human melanocytes induced by UVB and metal uptake--a basis for the pro-oxidant state of melanoma. *Photochem Photobiol*, Vol. 84, No. 3, (May-Jun 2008), pp. 556-564, ISSN 1751-1097

Gill, G. (2004). SUMO and ubiquitin in the nucleus: different functions, similar mechanisms? *Genes Dev*, Vol. 18, No. 17, (Sep 2004), pp. 2046-2059, ISSN 0890-9369

Girdwood, D., Bumpass, D., Vaughan, O.A., Thain, A., Anderson, L.A., Snowden, A.W., Garcia-Wilson, E., Perkins, N.D., & Hay, R.T. P300 transcriptional repression is mediated by SUMO modification. *Mol Cell*, Vol. 11, No. 4, (Apr 2003), pp. 1043-1054, ISSN 1097-2765.

Gómez Román, J.J., Garay, G.O., Saenz, P., Escuredo, K., Sanz Ibayondo, C., Gutkind, S., Junquera, C., Simón, L., Martínez, A., Fernández Luna, J.L., & Val-Bernal, J.F. (2008). Plexin B1 is downregulated in renal cell carcinomas and modulates cell growth. *Transl Res*, Vol. 151, No. 3, (Mar 2008), pp. 134-140, ISSN 1931-5244

Goutzanis, L., Papadogeorgakis, N., Pavlopoulos, P.M., Katti, K., Petsinis, V., Plochoras, I., Pantelidaki, C., Kavantzas, N., Patsouris, E., & Alexandridis, C. (2008). Nuclear fractal dimension as a prognostic factor in oral squamous cell carcinoma. *Oral Oncol*, Vol. 44, No. 4, (Apr 2008), pp. 345-353, ISSN 1368-8375

Guil, S., & Esteller, M. (2009). DNA methylomes, histone codes and miRNAs: tying it all together. *Int J Biochem Cell Biol*, Vol. 41, No. 1, (Jan 2009), pp. 87-95, ISSN 1357-2725

Handolias, D., Hamilton, A.L., Salemi, R., Tan, A., Moodie, K., Kerr, L., Dobrovic, A., & McArthur, G.A. (2010). Clinical responses observed with imatinib or sorafenib in melanoma patients expressing mutations in KIT. *Br J Cancer*, Vol. 102, No. 8, (Apr 2010), pp. 1219-1223, ISSN 0007-0920

Harbst, K., Staaf, J., Måsbäck, A., Olsson, H., Ingvar, C., Vallon-Christersson, J., Ringnér, M., Borg, A., & Jönsson, G. (2010). Multiple metastases from cutaneous malignant melanoma patients may display heterogeneous genomic and epigenomic patterns. *Melanoma Res*, Vol. 20, No. 5, (Oct 2010), pp. 381-391, ISSN 1473-5636

Hashimshony, T., Zhang, J., Keshet, I., Bustin, M., & Cedar, H. (2003). The role of DNA methylation in setting up chromatin structure during development. *Nat Genet*, Vol. 34, No. 2, (Jun 2003), pp 187-92, ISSN 1061-4036

Hauschild, A., Agarwala, S.S., Trefzer, U., Hogg, D., Robert, C., Hersey, P., Eggermont, A., Grabbe, S., Gonzalez, R., Gille, J., Peschel, C., Schadendorf, D., Garbe, C., O'Day, S., Daud,A., White, J.M., Xia, C., Patel, K., Kirkwood, J.M., & Keilholz, U. (2009). Results of a phase III, randomized, placebo-controlled study of sorafenib in combination with carboplatin and paclitaxel as second-line treatment in patients with unresectable stage III or stage IV melanoma. *J Clin Oncol*, Vol. 27, No. 17, (Jun 2009), pp. 2823-2830, ISSN 0732-183X

He, Z., Cho, Y.Y., Ma, W.Y., Choi, H.S., Bode, A.M., & Dong, Z. (2004). Regulation of ultraviolet B-induced phosphorylation of histone H3 at serine 10 by Fyn kinase. *J Biol Chem*, Vol. 280, No. 4, (Jan 2005), pp. 2446-2454, ISSN 0021-9258

Herman, J.G. (1999). Hypermethylation of tumor suppressor genes in cancer. *Semin Cancer Biol*, Vol. 9, No. 5, (Oct 1999), pp. 359-367, ISSN 1044-579X

Hocker, T.L., Singh, M.K., & Tsao, H. (2008). Melanoma genetics and therapeutic approaches in the 21st century: moving from the benchside to the bedside. *J Invest Dermatol*, Vol. 128, No. 11, (Nov 2008), pp. 2575-2595, ISSN 0022-202X

Hoege, C., Pfander, B., Moldovan, G.L., Pyrowolakis, G., & Jentsch, S. (2002). RAD6-dependent DNA repair is linked to modification of PCNA by ubiquitin and SUMO. *Nature*, Vol. 419, No. 6903, (Sep 2002), pp. 135-141, ISSN 0028-0836

Hoek, K.S., Schlegel, N.C., Brafford, P., Sucker, A., Ugurel, S, Kumar, R., Weber, B.L., Nathanson, K.L., Phillips, D.J., Herlyn, M., Schadendorf, D., & Dummer, R. (2006). Metastatic potential of melanomas defined by specific gene expression profiles with no BRAF signature. *Pigment Cell Res*, Vol. 19, No. 4, (Aug 2006), pp. 290-302, ISSN 0893-5785

Hoon, D.S., Spugnardi, M., Kuo, C., Huang, SK., Morton, D.L., & Taback, B. (2004). Profiling epigenetic inactivation of tumor suppressor genes in tumors and plasma from cutaneous melanoma patients. *Oncogene*, Vol. 23, No. 22, (May 2004), pp. 4014-4022, ISSN 0950-9232

Horner, M.J., Ries, L.A.G., Krapcho, M., Neyman, N., Aminou, R., Howlader, N., Altekruse, S.F., Feuer, E.J., Huang, L., Mariotto, A., Miller, B.A., Lewis, D.R., Eisner, M.P., Stinchcomb, D.G., & Edwards, B.K. (January, 7, 2011). In: *SEER Cancer Statistics Review, 1975-2006. Bethesda, MD: National Cancer Institute*, Available from: http://www.seer.cancer.gov/csr/1975_2007/index.html

Houben, R., Becker, J.C., Kappel, A., Terheyden, P., Bröcker, E.B., Goetz, R., & Rapp, U.R. (2004). Constitutive activation of the Ras-Raf signaling pathway in metastatic melanoma is associated with poor prognosis. *J Carcinog*, Vol. 3, No. 1, (Mar 2004). pp. 6, ISSN 0974-6773

Howell, P.M. Jr, Liu, S., Ren, S., Behlen, C., Fodstad, O., & Riker, A.I. (2009). Epigenetics in human melanoma. *Cancer Control*, Vol. 16, No. 3, (Jul 2009), pp. 200-218, ISSN 1073-2748

Jenuwein, T., & Allis, C.D. (2001). Translating the histone code. *Science*, Vol. 293, No. 5532, (Aug 2001), pp. 1074-1080, ISSN 0036-8075

Jiang B.H., Jiang G., Zheng J.Z., Lu Z., Hunter T., & Vogt, P.K. (2001). Phosphatidylinositol 3-kinase signaling controls levels of hypoxia-inducible factor 1. *Cell Growth Differ*, Vol. 12, No. 7, (Jul 2001), pp. 363-369, ISSN 1044-9523

Jones, P.A., & Baylin, S.B. (2002). The fundamental role of epigenetic events in cancer. *Nat Rev Genet*, Vol. 3, No. 6, (Jun 2002), pp. 415-428, ISSN 1471-0056

Joosse, A., De Vries, E., van Eijck, C.H., Eggermont, A.M., Nijsten, T., & Coebergh, J.W. (2010). Reactive oxygen species and melanoma: an explanation for gender differences in survival? *Pigment Cell Melanoma Res*, Vol. 23, No. 3, (Jun 2010), pp. 352-364, ISSN 1755-1471

Kageshita, T., Nakamura, T., Yamada, M., Kuriya, N., Arao, T., & Ferrone, S. (1991). Differential expression of melanoma associated antigens in acral lentiginous melanoma and in nodular melanoma lesions. *Cancer Res*, Vol. 51, No. 6, (Mar 1991), pp. 1726-1732, ISSN 0008-5472

Karpf, A.R., Lasek, A.W., Ririe, T.O., Hanks, A.N., Grossman, D., & Jones, D.A. (2004). Limited gene activation in tumor and normal epithelial cells treated with the DNA methyltransferase inhibitor 5-aza-2'-deoxycytidine. *Mol Pharmacol*, 65, No. 1 (Jan 2004), pp. 18-27, ISSN 0026-895X

Keenen, B., Qi, H., Saladi, S.V., Yeung, M., & de la Serna, I.L. (2010). Heterogeneous SWI/SNF chromatin remodeling complexes promote expression of microphthalmia-associated transcription factor target genes in melanoma. *Oncogene*, Vol. 29, NO. 1, (Jan 2010), pp. 81-92, ISSN 0950-9232

Kietzmann, T., & Görlach, A. (2005). Reactive oxygen species in the control of hypoxia-inducible factor-mediated gene expression. *Semin Cell Dev Biol*, Vol. 16, No. 4-5, (Aug-Oct 2005), pp. 474-486, ISSN 1084-9521

Kim, E.S., Herbst, R.S., Lee, J.J., Blumenschein, G.R. Jr, Tsao, A., Alden, C.M., Tang, X., Liu, S., Stewart, D.J., Heymach, J.V., Tran, H.T., Hicks, M.E., Erasmus, J. Jr, Gupta, S., Powis, G., Lippman, S.M., Wistuba, I.I., & Hong, W.K. (2010). The BATTLE trial (Biomarker-integrated Approaches of Targeted Therapy for Lung Cancer Elimination): personalizing therapy for lung cancer. *Program and abstracts of the American Association for Cancer Research 101st Annual Meeting*, LB-01, Washington, DC, USA, April 17-21, 2010

Kim, G.D., Ni, J., Kelesoglu, N., Roberts, R.J., & Pradhan, S. (2002). Co-operation and communication between the human maintenance and de novo DNA (cytosine-5) methyltransferases. *EMBO J*, Vol. 21, NO. 15, (Aug 2002), pp. 4183-4195, ISSN 0261-4189

Kietzmann, T.,& Görlach, A. (2005). Reactive oxygen species in the control of hypoxia-inducible factor-mediated gene expression. *Semin Cell Dev Biol*, Vol. 16, No. 4-5, (Aug-Ott 2005, pp. 474-486, ISSN 1084-9521

Klose, R.J., & Bird, A.P. (2000). Genomic DNA methylation: the mark and its mediators. *Trends Biochem Sci*, Vol. 31, No, 2, (Feb 2006), pp. 89-97, ISSN 0968-0004

Kuphal, S., Poser, I., Jobin, C., Hellerbrand, C., & Bosserhoff, A.K. (2004). Loss of E-cadherin leads to upregulation of NFkappaB activity in malignant melanoma. *Oncogene*, Vol. 23, No. 52, (Nov 2004), pp. 8509-8519, ISSN 0950-9232

Kyrgidis, A., Tzellos, T.G., & Triaridis, S. (2010). Melanoma: Stem cells, sun exposure and hallmarks for carcinogenesis, molecular concepts and future clinical implications. *J Carcinog*, Vol. 9, (Apr 2010), pp. 3, ISSN 0143-3334

Kuphal, S., Winklmeier, A., Warnecke, C., & Bosserhoff, A.K. (2010). Constitutive HIF-1 activity in malignant melanoma. *Eur J Cancer*, Vol. 46, No. 6, (Apr 2010), pp. 1159-1169, ISSN 0959-8049

La Vecchia, C., Bosetti, C., Lucchini, F., Bertuccio, P., Negri, E., Boyle, P., & Levi, F. (2010). Cancer mortality in Europe, 2000-2004, and an overview of trends since 1975. *Ann Oncol*, Vol. 21, No. 6, (Jun 2010), pp. 1323-1360, ISSN 0923-7534

Levati, L., Alvino, E., Pagani, E., Arcelli, D., Caporaso, P., Bondanza, S., Di Leva, G., Ferracin, M., Volinia, S., Bonmassar, E., Croce, C.M., & D'Atri, S. (2009). Altered expression of selected microRNAs in melanoma: antiproliferative and proapoptotic activity of miRNA-155. *Int J Oncol*, Vol. 35, No. 2, (Aug 2009), pp. 393-400, ISSN 1019-6439

Li, B., Carey, M., & Workman, J.L. (2007). The role of chromatin during transcription. *Cell*, Vol. 128, No. 4, (Feb 2007), pp. 707-719, ISSN 0092-8674

Li, G., Kalabis, J., Xu, X., Meier, F., Oka, M., Bogenrieder, T., & Herlyn, M. (2003). Reciprocal regulation of MelCAM and AKT in human melanoma. *Oncogene*, Vol. 22, No. 44, (Oct 2003), pp. 6891-6899, ISSN 0950-9232

Li, N., & Karin, M. (1999). Is NF-kappaB the sensor of oxidative stress? *FASEB J*, Vol. 13, No. 10, (Jul 1999), pp. 1137-1143, ISSN 0892-6638

Lieberman-Aiden, E., van Berkum, N.L., Williams, L., Imakaev, M., Ragoczy, T., Telling, A., Amit, I., Lajoie, B.R., Sabo, P.J., Dorschner, M.O., Sandstrom, R., Bernstein, B., Bender, M.A., Groudine, M., Gnirke, A., Stamatoyannopoulos, J., Mirny, L.A., Lander, E.S., & Dekker, J. (2009). Comprehensive mapping of long-range interactions reveals folding principles of the human genome. *Science*, Vol. 326, No. 5950, (Oct 2009), pp 289-293, ISSN 0036-8075

Lin, H., Wong, R.P., Martinka, M., & Li, G. (2010). BRG1 expression is increased in human cutaneous melanoma. *Br J Dermatol*, Vol. 163, No. 3, (Sep 2010), pp. 502-510, ISSN 0007-0963

Lin, W.M., Baker, A.C., Beroukhim, R., Winckler, W., Feng, W., Marmion, J.M., Laine, E., Greulich, H., Tseng, H., Gates, C., Hodi, F.S., Dranoff, G., Sellers, W.R., Thomas, R.K., Meyerson, M., Golub, T.R., Dummer, R., Herlyn, M., Getz, G., & Garraway, L.A. (2008). Modeling genomic diversity and tumor dependency in malignant melanoma. *Cancer Res*, Vol. 68, No. 3, (Feb 2008), pp. 664-673, ISSN 0008-5472

Liu, S., Ren, S., Howell, P., Fodstad, O., & Riker, A.I. (2008). Identification of novel epigenetically modified genes in human melanoma via promoter methylation gene profiling. *Pigment Cell Melanoma Res*, Vol 21., No. 5, (Oct 2008), pp. 545-558, ISSN 1755-148X

Lomas, J., Martin-Duque, P., Pons, M., & Quintanilla, M. (2008). The genetics of malignant melanoma. *Front Biosci*, Vol. 13, (May 2008), pp. 5071-5093, ISSN 1093-9946

Lo Muzio, L., Nocini, P., Mignogna, M.D., Pannone, G., Staibano, S., Procaccini, M., Rubini, C., Fioroni, M., Fanali, S., & Piattelli, A. (2000). Immunocytochemical detection of hMSH2 and hMLH1 expression in oral melanoma. *Anticancer Res*, Vol. 20, No. 2, (Mar-Apr 2000), pp. 741-748, ISSN 0250-7005

Lund, L.P., & Timmins, G.S. (2007). Melanoma, long wavelength ultraviolet and sunscreens: controversies and potential resolutions. *Pharmacol Ther*, Vol. 114, No. 2, (May 2007), pp. 198-207, ISSN 0163-7258

Maddodi, N., & Setaluri, V. (2008). Role of UV in cutaneous melanoma. *Photochem Photobiol*, Vol. 84, No. 2, (Mar-Apr 2008), pp. 528-536, ISSN 0031-8655

Martinez, R., Martin-Subero, J.I., Rohde, V., Kirsch, M., Alaminos, M., Fernandez, A.F., Ropero, S., Schackert, G., & Esteller, M. (2009). A microarray-based DNA methylation study of glioblastoma multiforme. *Epigenetics*, Vol. 4, No. 4, (May 2009), pp. 255-264, ISSN 1559-2294

Mascolo, M., Vecchione, M.L., Ilardi, G., Scalvenzi, M., Molea, G., Di Benedetto, M., Nugnes, L., Siano, M., De Rosa, G., & Staibano, S. (2010). Overexpression of Chromatin Assembly Factor-1/p60 helps to predict the prognosis of melanoma patients. *BMC Cancer*, Vol. 10, (Feb 2010), pp 63, ISSN 1471-2407

Mashiah, A., Wolach, O., Sandbank, J., Uziel, O., Raanani, P., & Lahav, M. (2008). Lymphoma and leukemia cells possess fractal dimensions that correlate with their biological features. *Acta Haematol*, Vol. 199, No. 3, (Apr 2008), pp. 142-150, ISSN 0001-5792

Matsumoto, S., Banine, F., Struve, J., Xing, R., Adams, C., Liu, Y., Metzger, D., Chambon, P., Rao, M.S., & Sherman, L.S. (2005). Brg1 is required for murine neural stem cell maintenance and gliogenesis. *Dev Biol*, Vol. 289, No. 2, (Jan 2006), pp. 372-383, ISSN 0012-1606

Meyle, K.D., & Guldberg, P. (2009). Genetic risk factors for melanoma. *Hum Genet*, Vol. 126, No. 4, (Oct 2009), pp. 499-510, ISSN 0340-6717

Meyskens, F.L. Jr, Farmer, P., & Fruehauf, J.P. (2001). Redox regulation in human melanocytes and melanoma. *Pigment Cell Res*, Vol. 14, No. 3, (Jun 2001), pp. 148-154, ISSN 0893-5785

Michaylira, C.Z., & Nakagawa, H. (2006). Hypoxic microenvironment as a cradle for melanoma development and progression. *Cancer Biol Ther*, Vol. 5, No. 5, (May 2006), pp. 476-479, ISSN 1538-4047

Minet, E., Arnould, T., Michel, G., Roland, I., Mottet, D., Raes, M., Remacle, J., & Michiels, C. (2000). ERK activation upon hypoxia: involvement in HIF-1 activation. *FEBS Lett*, Vol. 468, No. 1, (Feb 2000), pp. 53-58, ISSN 0014-5793

Misteli, T. (2007). Beyond the sequence: cellular organization of genome function. *Cell*, Vol. 128, No. 4, (Feb 2007), pp. 787-800, ISSN 0092-8674

Monsel, G., Ortonne, N., Bagot, M., Bensussan, A., & Dumaz, N. (2010). c-Kit mutants require hypoxia-inducible factor 1alpha to transform melanocytes. *Oncogene*, Vol. 29, No. 2, (Jan 2010), pp. 227-236, ISSN 0950-9232

Montironi, R., Scarpelli, M., Lopez-Beltran, A., Mazzucchelli, R., Alberts, D., Ranger-Moore, J., Bartels, H.G., Hamilton, P.W., Einspahr, J., & Bartels, P.H. (2007). Chromatin phenotype karyometry can predict recurrence in papillary urothelial neoplasms of low malignant potential. *Cell Oncol*, Vol. 29, No. 1, (2007) pp. 47-58, ISSN 1570-5870

Mori, T., Martinez, S.R., O'Day, S.J., Morton, D.L., Umetani, N., Kitago, M., Tanemura, A., Nguyen, S.L., Tran, A.N., Wang, H.J., & Hoon, D.S. (2006). Estrogen receptor-alpha methylation predicts melanoma progression. *Cancer Res*, Vol. 66, No. 13, (Jul 2006), pp. 6692-6698, ISSN 0008-5472

Mueller, D.W., Rehli, M., & Bosserhoff, A.K. (2009). miRNA expression profiling in melanocytes and melanoma cell lines reveals miRNAs associated with formation and progression of malignant melanoma. *J Invest Dermatol*, Vol. 129, No. 7, (Jul 2009), pp. 1740-1751, ISSN 0022-202X

Müller, S., Ledl, A., & Schmidt, D. (2004). SUMO: a regulator of gene expression and genome integrity. *Oncogene*, Vol. 23, No. 11, (Mar 2004), pp. 1998-2008, ISSN 0950-9232

Müller, D.W., & Bosserhoff, A.K. (2008). Integrin beta 3 expression is regulated by let-7a miRNA in malignant melanoma. *Oncogene*, Vol. 27, No. 52, (Nov 2008), pp. 6698-6706, ISSN 0950-9232

Munshi, A., Tanaka, T., Hobbs, M.L., Tucker, S.L., Richon, V.M., & Meyn, R.E. (2006). Vorinostat, a histone deacetylase inhibitor, enhances the response of human tumor cells to ionizing radiation through prolongation of gamma-H2AX foci. *Mol Cancer Ther*, Vol. 5, No. 8, (Aug 2006), pp. 1967-1974, ISSN 1535-7163

Murata, H., Ashida, A., Takata, M., Yamaura, M., Bastian, B.C., & Saida, T. (2007) Establishment of a novel melanoma cell line SMYM-PRGP showing cytogenetic and biological characteristics of the radial growth phase of acral melanomas. *Cancer Sci*, Vol. 98, No. 7, (Jul 2007), pp. 958-963, ISSN 1349-7006

Muthusamy,V., Duraisamy, S., Bradbury, C.M., Hobbs, C., Curley, D.P., Nelson, B., & Bosenberg, M. (2006). Epigenetic silencing of novel tumor suppressors in malignant melanoma. *Cancer Res*, Vol. 66, No. 33, (Dec 2006), pp. 11187-11193, ISSN 0008-5472

Nakayama, K. (2010). Growth and progression of melanoma and non-melanoma skin cancers regulated by ubiquitination. *Pigment Cell Melanoma Res*, Vol. 23, No. 3, (Jun 2010), pp. 338-351, ISSN 1755-1471

Nazarian, R., Shi, H., Wang, Q., Kong, X., Koya, R.C., Lee, H., Chen, Z., Lee, M.K., Attar, N., Sazegar, H., Chodon, T., Nelson. S.F., McArthur, G., Sosman, J.A., Ribas, A., & Lo, R.S. (2010). Melanomas acquire resistance to B-RAF(V600E) inhibition by RTK or N-RAS upregulation. *Nature*, Vol. 468, No. 7326, (Dec 2010), pp. 973-977, ISSN 0028-0836

Nguyen, T., Kuo, C., Nicholl, M.B., Sim, M.S., Turner, R.R., Morton, D.L., & Hoon, D.S. (2011). Downregulation of microRNA-29c is associated with hypermethylation of tumor-related genes and disease outcome in cutaneous melanoma. *Epigenetics*, Vol. 6, No. 3, (Mar 2011), pp. 388-394, ISSN 1559-2294

Nihal, M., Roelke, C.T., & Wood, G.S. Anti-melanoma effects of vorinostat in combination with polyphenolic antioxidant (-)-epigallocatechin-3-gallate (EGCG). *Pharm Res*, Vol. 27, No. 6, (Jun 2010), pp. 1103-1114, ISSN 0724-8741

Nishikawa, M., & Hashida, M. (2006). Inhibition of tumour metastasis by targeted delivery of antioxidant enzymes. *Expert Opin Drug Deliv*, Vol. 3, No. 3, (May 2006), pp. 355-369, ISSN 1742-5247

Nishikawa, M. (2008). Reactive oxygen species in tumor metastasis. *Cancer Lett*, Vol. 266, No. 1, (Jul 2008), pp. 53-9, ISSN 0304-3835

Noble, I. (2003-04-14). "Human genome finally complete". *BBC News*. *http://news.bbc.co.uk/1/hi/sci/tech/2940601.stm*. Retrieved 2006-07-22.

Noma, K., Allis, C.D., & Grewal, S.I. (2001). Transitions in distinct histone H3 methylation patterns at the heterochromatin domain boundaries. *Science*, Vol. 293, No. 5532, (Aug 2001), pp. 1150-1155, ISSN 0036-8075

Okano, M., Bell, D.W., Haber, D.A, & Li, E. (1999). DNA methyltransferases Dnmt3a and Dnmt3b are essential for de novo methylation and mammalian development. *Cell*, Vol. 99, No. 3, pp. 247-257, ISSN 0092-8674

Oram, S.W., Liu, X.X., Lee, T.L., Chan, W.Y., & Lau, Y.F. (2006). TSPY potentiates cell proliferation and tumorigenesis by promoting cell cycle progression in HeLa and NIH3T3 cells. *BMC Cancer*, Vol. 6, (Jun 2006), pp. 154, ISSN 1471-2407

Ota, T., Suto, S., Katayama, H., Han, Z.B., Suzuki, F., Maeda, M., Tanino, M., Terada, Y., & Tatsuka, M. (2002). Increased mitotic phosphorylation of histone H3 attributable to AIM-1/Aurora-B overexpression contributes to chromosome number instability. *Cancer Res*, Vol. 62, No. 18, (Sep 2002), pp. 5168-5177, ISSN 0008-5472

Patnaik, M.M., Tefferi, A., & Pardanani, A. (2007). Kit: molecule of interest for the diagnosis and treatment of mastocytosis and other neoplastic disorders. *Curr Cancer Drug Targets*,Vol. 7, No. 5, (Aug 2007), pp. 492-503, ISSN 1568-0096

Pavel, S., van Nieuwpoort, F., van der Meulen, H., Out, C., Pizinger, K., Cetkovská, P., Smit, N.P., & Koerten, H.K. (2004). Disturbed melanin synthesis and chronic oxidative stress in dysplastic naevi. *Eur J Cancer*, Vol. 40, No. 9, (Jun 2004), pp. 1423-1430, ISSN 1359-6349

Piccart-Gebhart, M.J.(2010). The Breast International Group (BIG): building on an accelerated path to tailored adjuvant cancer therapy. *Program and abstracts of the American Association for Cancer Research 101st Annual Meeting*, Plenary PL01, Washington, DC, USA, April 17-21, 2010

Platz, A., Egyhazi, S., Ringborg, U., & Hansson, J. (2008). Human cutaneous melanoma; a review of NRAS and BRAF mutation frequencies in relation to histogenetic subclass and body site. *Mol Oncol*, Vol. 1, No. 4, (Apr 2008), pp. 395-405, ISSN 1574-7891

Pradhan, S., Bacolla, A., Wells, R.D., & Roberts, R.J. (1999). Recombinant human DNA (cytosine-5) methyltransferase. I. Expression, purification, and comparison of de novo and maintenance methylation. *J Biol Chem*, Vol. 274, No. 46, (Nov 1999), pp. 33002-33010, ISSN 0021-9258

Rhee, I., Jair, K.W., Yen, R.W., Lengauer, C., Herman, J.G., Kinzler, K.W., Vogelstein, B., Baylin, S.B., & Schuebel, K.E. (2000). CpG methylation is maintained in human cancer cells lacking DNMT1. *Nature*, Vol. 404, No. 6781, (Apr 2000), pp. 1003-1007, ISSN 0028-0836

Rius, J., Guma, M., Schachtrup, C., Akassoglou, K., Zinkernagel, A.S., Nizet, V., Johnson, R.S., Haddad, G.G., & Karin, M. (2008). NF-kappaB links innate immunity to the hypoxic response through transcriptional regulation of HIF-1alpha. *Nature*, Vol. 453, No. 7196, (Jun 2008), pp. 807-811, ISSN 0028-0836

Robertson, K.D. (2005). DNA methylation and human disease. *Nat Rev Genet*, Vol. 6, No. 8, (Aug 2005), pp. 597-610, ISSN 1471-0056

Rody, A., Karn, T., Ruckhäberle, E., Hanker, L., Metzler, D., Müller, V., Solbach, C., Ahr, A., Gätje, R., Holtrich, U., & Kaufmann, M. (2009). Loss of Plexin B1 is highly prognostic in low proliferating ER positive breast cancers--results of a large scale microarray analysis. *Eur J Cancer*, Vol. 45, No. 3, (Feb 2009), pp. 405-413, ISSN 0959-8049

Romano, M.F., Avellino, R., Petrella, A., Bisogni, R., Romano, S., & Venuta, S. (2004). Rapamycin inhibits doxorubicin-induced NF-kappaB/Rel nuclear activity and enhances the apoptosis of melanoma cells. *Eur J Cancer*, Vol. 40, No. 18, (Dec 2004), pp.2829-2836, ISSN 0014-2964

Romano, S., D'Angelillo, A., Pacelli, R., Staibano, S., De Luna, E., Bisogni, R., Eskelinen, E.L., Mascolo, M., Calì, G., Arra, C., & Romano, M.F. (2010). Role of FK506-binding protein 51 in the control of apoptosis of irradiated melanoma cells. *Cell Death Differ*, Vol. 17, No. 1; (Jan 2010), pp. 145-157, ISSN 1350-9047

Romano, S., D'Angelillo, A., Staibano, S., Ilardi, G., & Romano, M.F. (2010) FK506-binding protein 51 is a possible novel tumoral marker. *Cell Death Dis*, Vol. 1, No. 7, (Jul 2010), pp. e55, ISSN: 2041-4889Ross, S., Best, J.L., Zon, L.I., & Gill, G. (2002). SUMO-1 modification represses Sp3 transcriptional activation and modulates its subnuclear localization. *Mol Cell*, Vol. 10, No.4, (Oct 2002), pp 831-842, ISSN 1097-2765

Rothhammer, T., & Bosserhoff, A.K. (2007). Epigenetic events in malignant melanoma. *Pigment Cell Res*, Vol. 20, No. 2, (Apr 2007), pp. 92-111, ISSN 0893-5785

Rother, J., & Jones, D. (2009). Molecular markers of tumor progression in melanoma. *Curr Genomics*, Vol. 10, No. 4, (Jun 2009), pp. 231-239, ISSN 1389-2029

Rountree, M.R., Bachman, K.E., Herman, J.G., & Baylin, S.B. (2001). DNA methylation, chromatin inheritance, and cancer. *Oncogene*, Vol. 20, No. 24, (May 2001), pg 3156-3165, ISSN 0950-9232

Rubinfeld, B., Robbins, P., El-Gamil, M., Albert, I., Porfiri, E., & Polakis, P. (1997). Stabilization of beta-catenin by genetic defects in melanoma cell lines. *Science*, Vol. 275, No. 5307, (Mar 1997), pp. 1790-1792, ISSN 0036-8075

Rubinstein, J.C., Sznol, M., Pavlick, A.C., Ariyan, S., Cheng, E., Bacchiocchi, A., Kluger, H.M., Narayan, D., & Halaban, R. (2010).Incidence of the V600K mutation among melanoma patients with BRAF mutations, and potential therapeutic response to the specific BRAF inhibitor PLX4032. *J Transl Med*, Vol. 14, No. 8, (Jul 2010), pp. 67, ISSN 1479-5876

Ryu, B., Kim, D.S., Deluca, A.M., & Alani, R.M. (2007). Comprehensive expression profiling of tumor cell lines identifies molecular signatures of melanoma progression. PLoS One, Vol. 2, No. 7, (Jul 2007), e594, ISSN 1932-6203

Saladi, S.V., Keenen, B., Marathe, H.G., Qi, H., Chin, K.V., & de la Serna, I.L. (2010). Modulation of extracellular matrix/adhesion molecule expression by BRG1 is associated with increased melanoma invasiveness. *Mol Cancer*, Vol. 9, (Oct 2010), pp. 280; ISSN 1476-4598

Sander, C.S., Hamm, F., Elsner, P., & Thiele, J.J. (2003). Oxidative stress in malignant melanoma and non-melanoma skin cancer. *Br J Dermatol*, Vol. 148, No. 5, (May 2003), pp. 913-922, ISSN 0007-0963

Santos-Rosa, H., & Caldas, C. (2005). Chromatin modifier enzymes, the histone code and cancer. *Eur J Cancer*, Vol. 41, No. 16, (Nov 2005), pp. 2381-2402, ISSN 1359-6349

Satzger, I., Mattern, A., Kuettler, U., Weinspach, D., Voelker, B., Kapp, A., & Gutzmer, R. (2010). MicroRNA-15b represents an independent prognostic parameter and is correlated with tumor cell proliferation and apoptosis in malignant melanoma. *Int J Cancer*, Vol. 126, No. 11, (Jun 2010), pp 2553-2562, ISSN 0020-7136

Schinke, C., Mo, Y., Yu, Y., Amiri, K., Sosman, J., Greally, J., & Verma, A. (2010). Aberrant DNA methylation in malignant melanoma. *Melanoma Res*, Vol. 20, No. 4, (Aug 2010), pp. 253-265, ISSN 0960-8931

Schultz, J., Lorenz, P., Gross, G., Ibrahim, S., & Kunz M. (2008). MicroRNA let-7b targets important cell cycle molecules in malignant melanoma cells and interferes with anchorage-independent growth. *Cell Res*, Vol. 18, No. 5, (May 2008), pp. 549-557, ISSN 1001-0602

Schultz, J., Ibrahim, S.M., Vera, J., & Kunz, M. (2009). 14-3-3sigma gene silencing during melanoma progression and its role in cell cycle control and cellular senescence. *Mol Cancer*, Vol.8, (Jul 2009), pp. 53, ISSN 14764598

Segura, M.F., Hanniford, D., Menendez, S., Reavie, L., Zou, X., Alvarez-Diaz, S., Zakrzewski, J., Blochin, E., Rose, A., Bogunovic, D., Polsky, D., Wei, J., Lee, P., Belitskaya-Levy, I., Bhardwaj, N., Osman, I., & Hernando, E. (2009). Aberrant miR-182 expression promotes melanoma metastasis by repressing FOXO3 and microphthalmia-associated transcription factor. *Proc Natl Acad Sci U S A*, Vol. 106, No. 6, (Feb 2009), pp. 1814-1819, ISSN 0027-8424

Shackleton, M., & Quintana, E. (2010). Progress in understanding melanoma propagation. *Mol Oncol*, Vol. 4, No. 5, (Oct 2010), pp. 451-457, ISSN 1574-7891

Shen, L., Kondo, Y., Guo, Y., Zhang, J., Zhang, L., Ahmed, S., Shu, J., Chen, X., Waterland, R.A., & Issa, J.P. (2007). Genome-wide profiling of DNA methylation reveals a class of normally methylated CpG island promoters. *PLoS Genet*, Vol. 3, No. 10, (Oct 2007), pp 2023-2036, ISSN 1553-7390

Shiama, N. (1997). The p300/CBP family: integrating signals with transcription factors and chromatin. *Trends Cell Biol*, Vol. 7, No. 6, (Jun 1997), pp. 230-236, ISSN 0962-8924

Shiio, Y., & Eisenman, R.N. (2003). Histone sumoylation is associated with transcriptional repression. *Proc Natl Acad Sci U S A*, Vol. 100, No. 23, (Nov 2003), pp. 13225-13230, ISSN 0027-8424

Shinojima, Y., Terui, T., Hara, H., Kimura, M., Igarashi, J., Wang, X., Kawashima, H., Kobayashi, Y., Muroi, S., Hayakawa, S., Esumi, M., Fujiwara, K., Ghosh, S., Yamamoto, T., Held, W., & Nagase, H. (2010). Identification and analysis of an early diagnostic marker for malignant melanoma: ZAR1 intra-genic differential methylation. *J Dermatol Sci*, Vol. 59, No. 2, (Aug 2010), pp. 98-106, ISSN 0923-1811

Siena, S., Sartore-Bianchi, A., Di Nicolantonio, F., Balfour, J., & Bardelli, A. (2009). Biomarkers predicting clinical outcome of epidermal growth factor receptor-targeted therapy in metastatic colorectal cancer. *J Natl Cancer Inst*, Vol. 101, No. 19, (Oct 2009), pp. 1308-1324, ISSN 0027-8874

Sigalotti, L., Fratta, E., Coral, S., Cortini, E., Covre, A., Nicolay, H.J., Anzalone, L., Pezzani, L., Di Giacomo, A.M., Fonsatti, E., Colizzi, F., Altomonte, M., Calabrò, L., & Maio, M. (2007). Epigenetic drugs as pleiotropic agents in cancer treatment: biomolecular aspects and clinical applications. *J Cell Physiol*, Vol. 212, No. 2, (Aug 2007), pp. 330-344, ISSN 0021-9541

Sigalotti, L., Covre, A., Fratta, E., Parisi, G., Colizzi, F., Rizzo, A., Danielli, R., Nicolay, H.J., Coral, S., & Maio, M. (2010). Epigenetics of human cutaneous melanoma: setting the stage for new therapeutic strategies. *J Transl Med*, Vol. 8, (Jun 2010), pp. 56, ISSN 1479-5876

Sood, P., Krek, A., Zavolan, M., Macino, G., & Rajewsky, N. (2006). Cell-type-specific signatures of microRNAs on target mRNA expression. *Proc Natl Acad Sci U S A*, Vol. 103, No. 8, (Feb 2006), pp 2746-2751, ISSN 0027-8424

Staibano, S., Lo Muzio, L., Pannone, G., Somma, P., Farronato, G., Franco, R., Bambini, F., Serpico, R., & De Rosa, G. (2001). P53 and hMSH2 expression in basal cell carcinomas and malignant melanomas from photoexposed areas of head and neck region. *Int J Oncol*, Vol. 19, No. 3, (Sep 2001), pp. 551-559, ISSN 1019-6439

Stevens, L., McClelland, L., Fricke, A., Williamson, M., Kuo, I., & Scott, G. (2010). Plexin B1 suppresses c-Met in melanoma: a role for plexin B1 as a tumor-suppressor protein through regulation of c-Met. *J Invest Dermatol*, Vol. 130, No. 6, (Jun 2010), pp. 1636-1645, ISSN 0022-202X

Stine, M.J., Wang, C.J., Moriarty, W.F., Ryu, B., Cheong, R., Westra, W.H., Levchenko, A., & Alani, R.M. (2011). Integration of Genotypic and Phenotypic Screening Reveals Molecular Mediators of Melanoma-Stromal Interaction. *Cancer Res*, Vol. 71, No. 7, (Apr 2011), pp 2433-2444, ISSN 0008-5472

Stratton, M.R., Campbell, P.J., & Futreal, P.A. (2009). The cancer genome. *Nature*, Vol. 458, No. 7239, (Apr 2009), pp. 719-724, ISSN 0028-0836

Sun B., Zhang D., Zhang S., Zhang W., Guo H., & Zhao, X. (2007). Hypoxia influences vasculogenic mimicry channel formation and tumor invasion-related protein expression in melanoma. *Cancer Lett*, Vol. 249, No. 2, (May 2007), pp. 188-197, ISSN 0304-3835

Takata, M., Murata, H., & Saida, T. (2010). Molecular pathogenesis of malignant melanoma: a different perspective from the studies of melanocytic nevus and acral melanoma. *Pigment Cell Melanoma Res*, Vol. 23, No. 1, (Feb 2010), pp. 64-71, ISSN 1755-1471

Tellez, C.S., Shen, L., Estécio, M.R., Jelinek, J., Gershenwald, J.E., & Issa, J.P. (2009). CpG island methylation profiling in human melanoma cell lines. *Melanoma Res*, Vol. 19, No. 3, (Jun 2009), 146-155, ISSN 1473-5636

Thomas, N.E., Berwick, M., & Cordeiro-Stone, M. (2006) Could BRAF mutations in melanocytic lesions arise from DNA damage induced by ultraviolet radiation? *J Invest Dermatol*, Vol. 126, No. 8, (Aug 2006), pp. 1693-1696, ISSN 0022-202X

Thompson, J.F., Scolyer, R.A., & Kefford, R.F. (2009). Cutaneous melanoma in the era of molecular profiling. *Lancet*, Vol. 374, No. 9687, (Aug 2009), pp 362-365, ISSN 0140-6736

Tobar, N., Cáceres, M., Santibáñez, J.F., Smith, P.C., & Martínez, J. (2008). RAC1 activity and intracellular ROS modulate the migratory potential of MCF-7 cells through a NADPH oxidase and NFkappaB-dependent mechanism. *Cancer Lett*, Vol. 267, No. 1, (Aug 2008), pp. 125-132, ISSN 0304-3835

Ugurel, S., Houben, R., Schrama, D., Voigt, H., Zapatka, M., Schadendorf, D., Bröcker, E.B., & Becker, J.C. (2007). Microphthalmia-associated transcription factor gene amplification in metastatic melanoma is a prognostic marker for patient survival, but not a predictive marker for chemosensitivity and chemotherapy response. *Clin Cancer Res*, Vol. 13, No. 21, (Nov 2007), pp. 6344-6350, ISSN 1078-0432

Ugurel, S., Utikal, J., & Becker, J.C. Tumor biomarkers in melanoma. *Cancer Control*, Vol. 16, No. 3, (Jul 2009), pp. 219-224, ISSN 1073-2748

Vachtenheim, J., Ondrusová, L., & Borovanský, J. (2010). SWI/SNF chromatin remodeling complex is critical for the expression of microphthalmia-associated transcription factor in melanoma cells. *Biochem Biophys Res Commun*, Vol. 392, No. 3, (Feb 2010), pp. 454-459, ISSN 0006-291X

Verdone, L., Agricola, E., Caserta, M., & Di Mauro, E. (2006). Histone acetylation in gene regulation. *Brief Funct Genomic Proteomic*, Vol. 5, No. 3, (Sep 2006), pp. 209-221, ISSN 2041-2649

Villanueva, J., Vultur, A., Lee, J.T., Somasundaram, R., Fukunaga-Kalabis, M., Cipolla, A.K., Wubbenhorst, B., Xu, X., Gimotty, P.A., Kee, D., Santiago-Walker, A.E., Letrero, R., D'Andrea, K., Pushparajan, A., Hayden, J.E., Brown, K.D., Laquerre, S., McArthur, G.A., Sosman, J.A., Nathanson, K.L., & Herlyn, M. (2010). Acquired resistance to BRAF inhibitors mediated by a RAF kinase switch in melanoma can be overcome by cotargeting MEK and IGF-1R/PI3K. *Cancer Cell*, Vol. 18, No. 6, (Dec 2010), pp. 683-695, ISSN 1535-6108

Wada, K., Maesawa, C., Akasaka, T., & Masuda, T. (2004). Aberrant expression of the maspin gene associated with epigenetic modification in melanoma cells. *J Invest Dermatol*, 2004, Vol. 122, No. 3, (Mar 2004), pp. 805-811, ISSN 0022-202X

Wang, L., McLeod, H.L., & Weinshilboum, R.M. (2011). Genomics and drug response. *N Engl J Med*, Vol. 364, No. 12, (Mar 2011), pp. 1144-1153, ISSN 0028-4793

Wehrle-Haller, B. (2003). The role of Kit-ligand in melanocyte development and epidermal homeostasis. *Pigment Cell Res*, Vol. 16, No. 3, (Jun 2003), pp. 287-296, ISSN 0893-5785

Wenger, R.H. (2002). Cellular adaptation to hypoxia: O2-sensing protein hydroxylases, hypoxia-inducible transcription factors, and O2-regulated gene expression. *FASEB J*, Vol. 16, No. 10 (Aug 2002), pp. 1151-1162, ISSN 0892-6638

Wiesener, M.S., & Maxwell, P.H. (2003). HIF and oxygen sensing; as important to life as the air we breathe? *Ann Med*, Vol. 35, No. 3, (2003), pp. 183-190, ISSN 0785-3890

Wittgen, H.G., & van Kempen, L.C. (2007). Reactive oxygen species in melanoma and its therapeutic implications. *Melanoma Res*, Vol. 17, No. 6, (Dec 2007), pp. 400-409, ISSN 0960-8931

Wu, K., Fuchs, S.Y., Chen, A., Tan, P., Gomez, C., Ronai, Z., & Pan, Z.Q. (2000). The SCF(HOS/beta-TRCP)-ROC1 E3 ubiquitin ligase utilizes two distinct domains within CUL1 for substrate targeting and ubiquitin ligation. *Mol Cell Biol*, Vol.20, No. 4, (Feb 2000), pp.1382-1393, ISSN 0270-7306

Yang, J., Price, M.A., Li, G.Y., Bar-Eli, M., Salgia, R., Jagedeeswaran, R., Carlson, J.H., Ferrone, S., Turley, E.A., & McCarthy, J.B. (2009). Melanoma proteoglycan modifies gene expression to stimulate tumor cell motility, growth, and epithelial-to-mesenchymal transition. *Cancer Res*, Vol. 69, No. 19, (Oct 2009), pp. 7538-7547, ISSN 0008-5472

Yi, M., Yang, J., Chen, X., Li, J., Li, X., Wang, L., Tan, Y., Xiong, W., Zhou, M., McCarthy, J.B., Li, G., Xiang, B., & Xie, H. (2010). RASSF1A Suppresses melanoma development by modulating apoptosis and cell cycle progression. *J Cell Physiol*, (Dec 2010), ISSN 0021-9541

You, Y., Ma, L., You, M., Li, X., Wang, S., Li, H., Wu, D., Yang, H., & Li, Z.Y. (2010). TSLC1 gene silencing in cutaneous melanoma. *Melanoma Res*, Vol. 20, No.3, (Jun 2010), pp. 179-183, ISSN 1473-5636

Zbytek, B., Carlson, J.A., Granese, J., Ross, J., Mihm, M.C., & Slominski, A. (2008).Current concepts of metastasis in melanoma. *Expert Rev Dermatol*, Vol. 3, No. 5, (Oct 2008), pp. 569-585, ISSN 1746-9872

Zhong, S.P., Ma, W.Y., & Dong, Z. (2000). ERKs and p38 kinases mediate ultraviolet B-induced phosphorylation of histone H3 at serine 10. *J Biol Chem*, Vol. 275, No. 28, (Jul 2000), pp. 20980-20984, ISSN 0021-9258

Part 2

Therapeutics

4

A Bromophosphonate Analogue of Lysophosphatidic Acid Surpasses Dacarbazine in Reducing Cell Proliferation and Viability of MeWo Melanoma Cells

Duy Nguyen[1], Oanh Nguyen[1], Honglu Zhang[2], Glenn D. Prestwich[2] and Mandi M. Murph[1]
[1]Department of Pharmaceutical and Biomedical Sciences, The University of Georgia, College of Pharmacy, Georgia,
[2]Department of Medicinal Chemistry, The University of Utah, Salt Lake City, United States of America

1. Introduction

The incidence of melanoma continues to rise, in particular among adult males residing in the U.S. (Jemal, Siegel et al. 2010). Although this disease is treatable in its early stages, diagnosis of or progression to an advanced, metastatic disease stage drastically reduces the prognosis, with few patients surviving 5 years. It is especially disturbing that there is a lack of FDA-approved therapeutics that can adequately treat the disease and very low percentages (5-15%) of patients who will respond to these traditional chemotherapeutics (Thompson, Morton et al. 2004). Even among responders, the response to therapy is usually unsustainable over the long-term, with approximately 10.8% of patients achieving long-term survival (Kim, Lee et al. 2010). Dacarbazine or DTIC is considered the most appropriate cytotoxic chemotherapy, but response rates are poor. Many other single-agents have been tried with response rates ≤18%, these include temozolomide, lomustine, carmustine, cisplatin, carboplatin, vincristine, vinblastine, vindesine, paclitaxel, docetaxel, gemcitabine and topotecan. (Thompson, Morton et al. 2004)

Without patient selection to decipher who belongs to the small portion of responders, the more common approach to therapy is to enroll patients into a clinical trial. Recent trials examining more targeted and selective agents like PLX4032 (Flaherty, Puzanov et al. 2010) and ipilimumab (Hodi, O'Day et al. 2010) have further reinforced this clinical ideology due to the successes observed among some patients. Although the development of chemoresistance is an impediment to achieving cure using these novel agents, they represent the current ideal and a hopeful future for promising targeted therapeutics. Thus, more specific drugs are desirable to increase the options for therapy and improve overall outcomes.

A recently discovered and highly "druggable" method to target melanoma cells is through inhibition of a G protein-coupled receptor (GPCR) that is responsible for viability among melanomas that predominantly express it (Altman, Gopal et al. 2010). This GPCR is called the Lysophosphatidic Acid (LPA) receptor 3 or the LPA3 receptor (Bandoh, Aoki et al. 1999) and is found along the cell surface of specific types of melanomas. In addition, the high-affinity ligand that binds to this GPCR is lysophosphatidic acid (Aoki, Bandoh et al. 2000). Interestingly, the lysophospholipase D that is responsible for the vast majority of the production of LPA from lysophosphatidylcholine is also expressed extracellularly and is a major target in melanoma (Altman et al. 2010; Liu, Murph et al. 2009). This enzyme, autotaxin (ATX), was first isolated from the conditioned medium of melanoma cells and was thought to be responsible for melanoma cell motility (Stracke, Krutzsch et al. 1992). Recent studies have shown that targeting either the LPA3 receptor or ATX effectively reduces melanoma cell viability (Altman et al. 2010). Furthermore, research devoted to producing inhibitors and antagonists targeting the ATX-LPA receptor axis has yielded a large variety of compounds (Albers, Dong et al. 2010; Altman et al. 2010; Baker, Fujiwara et al. 2006; Block, Duff et al. 2010; Hoeglund, Bostic et al. 2010; Hoeglund, Howard et al. 2010; North, Howard et al. 2010; Xu, Yang et al. 2009), suggesting the critical role of this pathway in cancer.

Herein we tested the in vitro capability of another antagonist of the LPA3 receptor and the lysophospholipase D activity of autotaxin, BrP-LPA, among the MeWo melanoma cell line. This compound inhibits the growth of in vivo lung carcinoma and angiogenesis (Xu and Prestwich 2010), but was untested in melanoma, a disease in dire need of additional therapeutics. We compared the BrP-LPA anti diastereoisomer to the BrP-LPA diastereomeric mixture and observed a slight enhancement of activity against MeWo cells using the mixture. Surprisingly, this effect was reduced or absent in the presence of a 24-hour pretreatment with dacarbazine, a traditional alkylating chemotherapeutic agent, suggesting that single-agent therapy is superior. We have observed an in vivo effect on reducing the number of metastatic melanoma lesions in the lungs of mice treated with BrP-LPA, in comparison to control (data not shown). It is unclear whether our in vitro results would extend to in vivo treatment, but if so, then the implications of this study would require naïve patients for clinical trials, an extremely difficult group to have available.

2. Materials and methods

MeWo fibroblast malignant melanoma cells were acquired from ATCC (Manassas, VA) and maintained in Cellgro RPMI (Mediatech, Inc., Manassas, VA) supplemented with 5% fetal bovine serum (Sigma-Aldrich, St Louis, MO). BrP-LPA compounds, the anti diastereoisomer and diastereomeric mixture, were synthesized as previously described (Zhang, Xu et al. 2009) and reconstituted in water prior to use. The alkylating agents temozolomide (TMZ) and dacarbazine (DTIC) were purchased from Sigma-Aldrich.

2.1 Cell viability

MeWo cells were examined for viability by seeding cells (10×10^3) in quadruplicates in 96-well plates. Cells were allowed to attach to the 96-well plate overnight in 5% FBS containing medium prior to the indicated drug treatment and concentration for 36 hours. CellTiter™ Blue reagent (Promega, Madison, WI) was added to plates and cells were incubated at 37°C to assess viability as previously described (Altman et al. 2010; Hasegawa, Murph et al. 2008).

2.2 High-throughput proliferation imaging

To examine the effects of cell proliferation in the presence of monotherapy, 10×10^3 MeWo cells were plated in quadruplicates in 96-well plates. After overnight incubation at 37 °C, the indicated drug and concentration was administered to the cells and the plates were incubated for another 30-40 h. After this incubation the cells were fixed in 2% formaldehyde and stained using the Multiparameter Cytotoxicity II kit (ThermoScientific, Pittsburgh, PA), according to the directions provided by the manufacturer. To obtain the results, the plates were then quantified and visualized using the ArrayScan®VTI HCS Reader (Thermo Scientific). For combination drug treatments, approximately 2,500 MeWo cells were plated in 96-wells and allowed to attach overnight. DTIC was added at the indicated concentration for 24 h followed by the addition of BrP-LPA for 24 h. The cells were fixed and stained using the Multiparameter Cytotoxicity III kit and then following the directions given in the manufacturer's protocol (Thermo Scientific).

2.3 Statistical analysis

Statistical differences in experimental data was determined using analysis of variance (ANOVA) followed by either Tukey's test or Bonferroni's multiple comparison test between groups. Alternatively, single comparisons were calculated using the student's t-test. GraphPad Prism (La Jolla, CA) was used to facilitate the statistical tests performed. $*p < 0.05$ $**p < 0.01$ and $***p < 0.001$ indicate the levels of significance.

3. Results

Figure 1 shows the chemical structures of the two BrP-LPA compounds used. Figure 1A shows the relative anti-configuration of the bromo substituent relative to the natural configuration of the sn-2 hydroxyl of LPA, while Figure 1B shows the diastereomeric mixture of syn- and anti-bromo substituents.

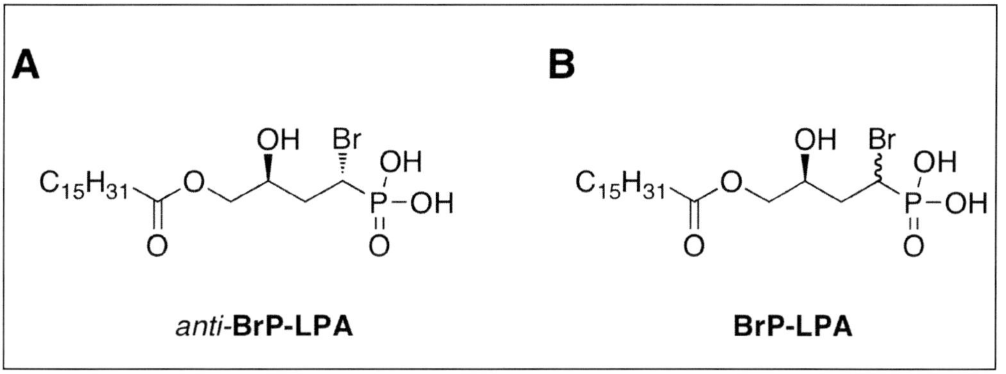

The structures of the anti diastereoisomer of 16:0 BrP-LPA (A) and its diastereomeric mixture (B) are depicted.

Fig. 1. Chemical structures.

We compared these two preparations in a viability curve, which accounts for both proliferation and metabolism, using MeWo melanoma cells. In the viability assay, we measured IC50 values of 17.68 µM and 16.76 µM for the anti diastereoisomer and the diastereomeric mixture, respectively (Figure 2A and 2B). Upon further analysis, the mixture (Figure 1B) consistently demonstrated increased ability to reduce cell viability over anti-BrP-LPA (Figure 1A), especially at the highest concentration (100 µM) tested (Figure 2C).

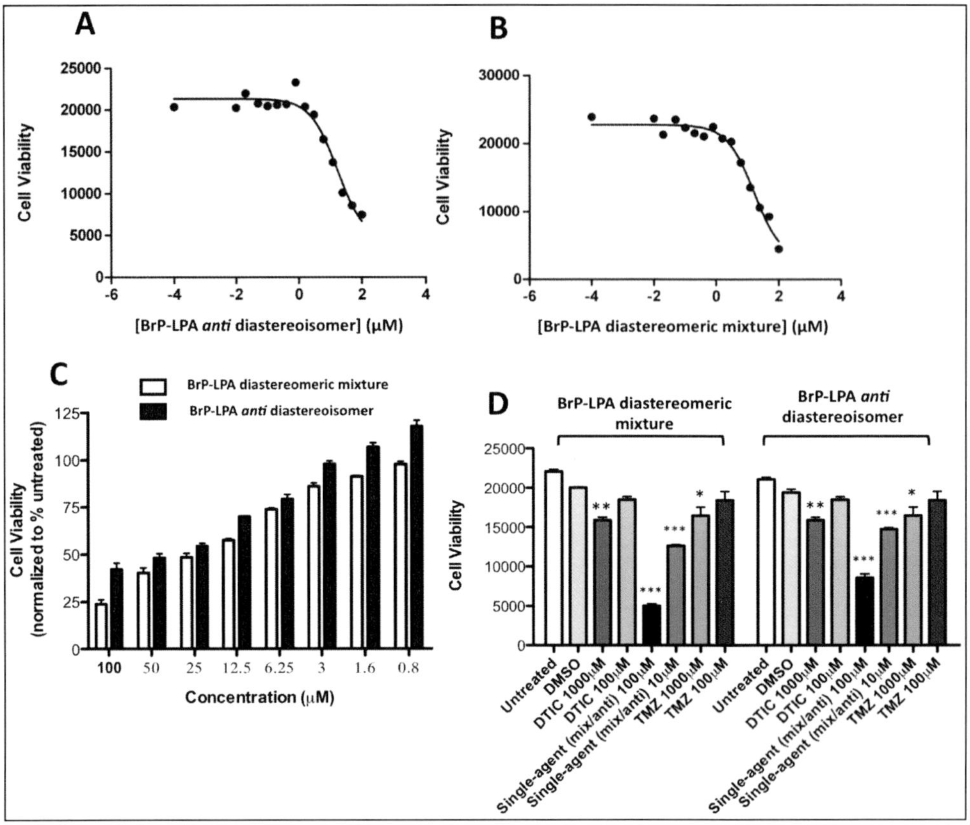

Cell viability assays using MeWo cells treated with increasing doses of the BrP-LPA *anti* diastereoisomer (A) or diastereomeric mixture (B) are log transformed and depicted here. (C) A bar graph showing the range of concentrations used in MeWo cells compares the reduction in viability achieved between the two BrP-LPA reagents. (D) Comparison between the two BrP-LPA reagents and other single-agent treatment with dacarbazine (DTIC) or temozolomide (TMZ) demonstrates potency of the BrP-LPA diastereomeric mixture (100 μM and 10μM) surpasses that achieved by either DTIC or TMZ at higher doses (1000 μM and 100 μM). Similar results are also seen with the BrP-LPA *anti* diastereoisomer. Brackets at the top indicate which single-agent was used. *$p<0.05$, **$p<0.01$ or ***$p<0.001$, compared to DMSO control-treated MeWo cells.

Fig. 2. Single-agent treatment with BrP-LPA compounds reduces cell viability at lower doses than dacarbazine or temozolomide.

We next sought to evaluate how these agents measured up against chemotherapy. In comparison to single-agent BrP-LPA treatment versus traditional alkylating chemotherapy, the BrP-LPA compounds showed more activity in reducing cell viability, even at lower concentrations than the chemotherapy (Figure 2D). For example, 100 μM or 10 μM of BrP-LPA (Figure 1B) was more effective at reducing viability than 1000 μM of dacarbazine (DTIC) or temozolomide (TMZ). At 100 μM of DTIC or TMZ, the modest reduction in viability was not statistically different than diluent control (DMSO). Similar observations occurred with the anti-BrP-LPA (Figure 1A) as well.

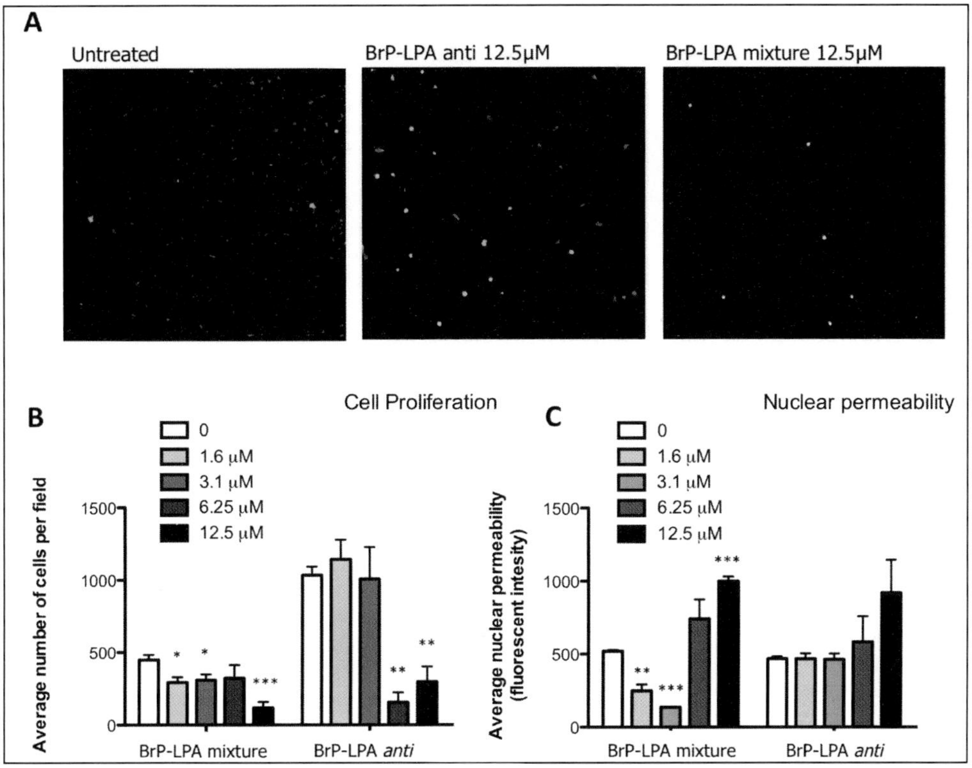

(A) MeWo cells were either untreated, or treated with 12.5 μM BrP-LPA reagents for 36 hours, fixed, processed and stained for immunofluorescence visualization. (B) The average number of cells per field was calculated by automated measurements of quadruplicate well samples using the ArrayScan®VTI HCS Reader, as a measurement of the cell proliferation achieved in the presence of either 0, 1.6, 3.1, 6.25 or 12.5 μM of the BrP-LPA diastereomeric mixture or the *anti* diastereoisomer. (C) Using a nuclear permeability dye, the increase in fluorescence intensity was automatically measured by the ArrayScan®VTI HCS Reader using quadruplicate samples. *$p<0.05$, **$p<0.01$ or ***$p<0.001$, compared to 0 μM or untreated MeWo cells.

Fig. 3. MeWo cell proliferation is reduced after treatment with BrP-LPA reagents.

Since the assay measuring cell viability accounts for both the proliferation and metabolism of cells, we sought to discriminate these two features by looking solely at the rate of in vitro growth or proliferation in the presence of BrP-LPA. After treating MeWo cells for 36 hours in the presence of increasing concentration of drug (Figure 3A), we assessed the number of surviving cells using high-throughput imaging for quantification. Strikingly, even the lowest concentration of the mixture BrP-LPA (Figure 1B) (1.6 μM) showed a significant decrease in the number of cells captured per field compared with untreated cells (Figure 3B). At the highest dose (12.5 μM), an obvious shift in cell number was visually observed (Figure 3A) and was also quantified as statistically significant versus untreated cells (Figure 3B). Although a reduction in cell number was detected among cells treated with the anti-BrP-LPA (1A), the reductions were significant only at 6.25 μM and 12.5 μM. Dying cells display many morphological changes, including nuclear condensation and permeabilization that

can be visualized by an intense increase in the fluorescence intensity of cell nuclei. We quantified nuclear permeability and detected an initial reduction (1.6 µM and 3.1µM), followed by a significant increase at higher concentrations (6.25 µM and 12.5 µM) in MeWo cells treated with the BrP-LPA mixture (Figure 1B) (Figure 3C). Although the results from the anti-BrP-LPA (Figure 1A) were not significant, there did appear to be an increasing trend at higher concentrations (6.25 µM and 12.5 µM).
Due to the favorable results we observed thus far in our analysis, we hypothesized that the combinatorial treatment of BrP-LPA compounds with the alkylating agent DTIC would have superior activity to reduce MeWo cell viability than single-agent BrP-LPA treatment. In contrast, we observed an increase in the number of remaining MeWo cells after 24 hours treatment with DTIC, followed by 24 hours of the BrP-LPA compounds (Figure 4A). We quantified the changes in the loss of cells and determined monotherapy of BrP-LPA to be superior in comparison with combinatorial treatment (Figure 3B and 3C).
Only when DTIC was reduced to 50 µM did the significance return, suggesting that a low enough concentration eliminated the combined inhibition. Similarly, we detected plasma membrane permeability only among DTIC 1000 µM and single-agent anti or mix (10 µM). There was a slight increase in the permeability at 50 µM DTIC and 10 µM of anti or mix, further supporting the observation that the low dose of DTIC eliminates the combined inhibition. Since the drugs were administered 24 hours apart, we hypothesize this is due to the molecular and cellular response to the compound, within the context of proliferation or an effect related to chemoresistance. This could suggest that the BrP-LPA compounds would require chemonaïve patients to achieve therapeutic efficacy, and this group would be incredibly difficult to find.

4. Discussion

Our data suggests, at least in an in vitro comparison, that single-agent or monotherapy using the anti-BrP-LPA (Figure 1A) or the mixed diastereomers BrP-LPA (Figure 1B) is superior at reducing the viability and proliferation of MeWo primary cutaneous melanoma cells than dacarbazine or temozolomide. Although we hypothesized that the mechanism of action for these two different agents would create a synergistic response as others have seen using combinations of dacarbazine with unrelated agents (Jin, Gong et al. 2011), in fact that is not what was observed. While unexpected, our results are similar to what others have also observed using BrP-LPA. Using an in vivo breast cancer model, Zhang et al. reported that the mixed diastereomers BrP-LPA (Figure 1B) alone (10 mg/kg) was superior at reducing tumor burden, compared with taxol alone (10 mg/kg) or taxol followed by BrP-LPA (Zhang et al. 2009). This corroborates our observations and further predicts that similar effects are likely to occur in an in vivo model of melanoma. Indeed, we have tested single-agent BrP-LPA against metastatic melanoma in vivo and measured a significant reduction in the number of lesions in the lungs of animals (data not shown).
The concern over reduced response with combination treatment of a novel agent together with dacarbazine is a major concern since most chemotherapy is now given in combination, even in clinical trials (Chu and DeVita 2008). In our study, we staged the drugs 24 hours apart, yet we still observed a reduction in overall efficacy. Our results are also in agreement with other publications suggesting that dacarbazine selects for a more aggressive phenotype

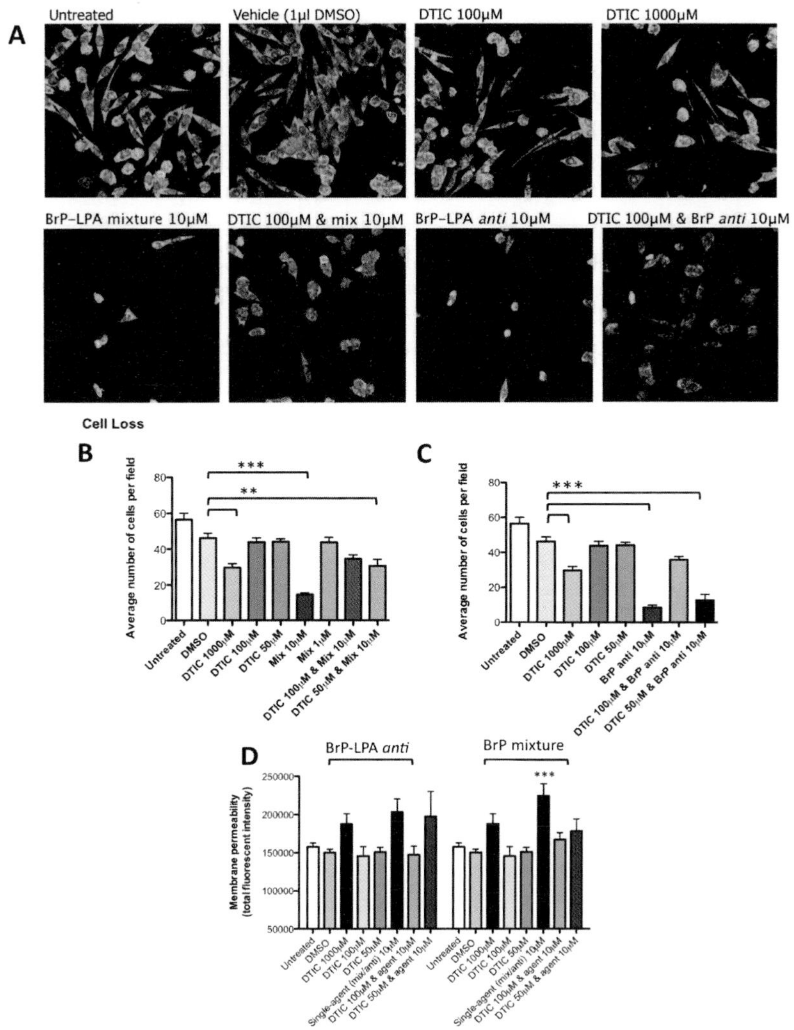

(A) Fluorescent images of MeWo cells treated with the indicated reagents for 24 or 48 h. The combination treatments were staged so that the dacarbazine (DTIC) was added for 24 h prior to the addition of BrP-LPA for an additional 24 h, for a total of 48 h of dacarbazine. The single-agent treatments were for 24 h. (B and C) Cell loss was calculated by measuring the average number of cells lost per field from quadruplicate samples and at least 4 images taken per sample for N=16. The BrP-LPA diastereomeric mixture was used in 'B' and the *anti* diastereoisomer was used in 'C'. (D) Plasma membrane permeability was calculated after staining the MeWo cells with a fluorescent dye capable of penetrating the membrane when small pores or holes provide access for the dye to enter the cell. An increase in the membrane permeability was achieved in the single-agent conditions or when DTIC was very low (50 μM), although statistical significance (***$p<0.001$) was calculated for only the BrP-LPA diastereomeric mixture (10 μM) in comparison with DMSO (1 μM) control using the student's t-test.

Fig. 4. Combination treatment of BrP-LPA reagents with dacarbazine inhibits the reduction in cell loss and proliferation achieved using single-agents.

of melanoma, which may occur through the upregulation of ERK signaling pathways, cytokine release or increased vascular endothelial growth factor (Lev, Onn et al. 2004). In this study we also observed what others have reported in that melanomas are notoriously resistant to therapeutic intervention. Indeed, we also found this to be true after only 24 hours of exposure to dacarbazine, which was unexpected given the short timecourse.

Herein we showed a reduction in cell viability using BrP-LPA compounds over the traditional chemotherapy alkylating agents, even when using BrP-LPA at lower concentrations. This highlights two important points concerning current therapeutics of melanoma. First, the traditional alkylating agents lack sufficient potency against this type of tumor, even when drug delivery is removed from the equation through the use of an in vitro tissue culture model. Second, single-agent BrP-LPA could be far better in generating a reduction in tumor burden and clinical usage than the alkylating agents.

In comparison with other agents that we have tested, the BrP-LPA compounds can generate a more robust effect against certain types of melanoma than thio-ccPA 18:1, which requires a higher dosage in vitro (Altman et al. 2010). Furthermore, in a direct comparison between anti-BrP-LPA (Figure 1A) and the mixed diastereomers BrP-LPA (Figure 1B), we repeatedly observed an enhanced effect of the mixture. Thus far, in vivo studies have not detected any known cytotoxicity of this compound (data not shown), which further indicates its utility. Taken together, this is suggestive of the clinical potential of BrP-LPA in advanced melanoma.

5. Acknowledgments

This work was supported by a grant from the Georgia Cancer Coalition (to M.M.M).
Glenn Prestwich is a scientific advisor for Echelon Biosciences, Inc. and RxBio.

6. References

Albers HM, Dong A, van Meeteren LA, Egan DA, Sunkara M, van Tilburg EW, Schuurman K, van Tellingen O, Morris AJ, Smyth SS, Moolenaar WH, Ovaa H (2010) Boronic acid-based inhibitor of autotaxin reveals rapid turnover of LPA in the circulation. Proc Natl Acad Sci U S A 107: 7257-7262

Altman MK, Gopal V, Jia W, Yu S, Hall H, Mills GB, McGinnis AC, Bartlett MG, Jiang G, Madan D, Prestwich GD, Xu Y, Davies MA, Murph MM (2010) Targeting melanoma growth and viability reveals dualistic functionality of the phosphonothionate analogue of carba cyclic phosphatidic acid. Mol Cancer 9: 140

Aoki J, Bandoh K, Inoue K (2000) A novel human G-protein-coupled receptor, EDG7, for lysophosphatidic acid with unsaturated fatty-acid moiety. Ann N Y Acad Sci 905: 263-266

Baker DL, Fujiwara Y, Pigg KR, Tsukahara R, Kobayashi S, Murofushi H, Uchiyama A, Murakami-Murofushi K, Koh E, Bandle RW, Byun HS, Bittman R, Fan D, Murph M, Mills GB, Tigyi G (2006) Carba analogs of cyclic phosphatidic acid are selective inhibitors of autotaxin and cancer cell invasion and metastasis. J Biol Chem 281: 22786-22793

Bandoh K, Aoki J, Hosono H, Kobayashi S, Kobayashi T, Murakami-Murofushi K, Tsujimoto M, Arai H, Inoue K (1999) Molecular cloning and characterization of a novel human

G-protein-coupled receptor, EDG7, for lysophosphatidic acid. J Biol Chem 274: 27776-27785

Block RC, Duff R, Lawrence P, Kakinami L, Brenna JT, Shearer GC, Meednu N, Mousa S, Friedman A, Harris WS, Larson M, Georas S (2010) The effects of EPA, DHA, and aspirin ingestion on plasma lysophospholipids and autotaxin. Prostaglandins Leukot Essent Fatty Acids 82: 87-95

Chu E, DeVita VT (2008) Physicians' Cancer Chemotherapy Drug Manual. Jones and Bartlett Publishers, Sudbury, MA

Flaherty KT, Puzanov I, Kim KB, Ribas A, McArthur GA, Sosman JA, O'Dwyer PJ, Lee RJ, Grippo JF, Nolop K, Chapman PB (2010) Inhibition of mutated, activated BRAF in metastatic melanoma. N Engl J Med 363: 809-819

Hasegawa Y, Murph M, Yu S, Tigyi G, Mills GB (2008) Lysophosphatidic acid (LPA)-induced vasodilator-stimulated phosphoprotein mediates lamellipodia formation to initiate motility in PC-3 prostate cancer cells. Mol Oncol 2: 54-69

Hodi FS, O'Day SJ, McDermott DF, Weber RW, Sosman JA, Haanen JB, Gonzalez R, Robert C, Schadendorf D, Hassel JC, Akerley W, van den Eertwegh AJ, Lutzky J, Lorigan P, Vaubel JM, Linette GP, Hogg D, Ottensmeier CH, Lebbe C, Peschel C, Quirt I, Clark JI, Wolchok JD, Weber JS, Tian J, Yellin MJ, Nichol GM, Hoos A, Urba WJ (2010) Improved survival with ipilimumab in patients with metastatic melanoma. N Engl J Med 363: 711-723

Hoeglund AB, Bostic HE, Howard AL, Wanjala IW, Best MD, Baker DL, Parrill AL (2010) Optimization of a pipemidic acid autotaxin inhibitor. J Med Chem 53: 1056-1066

Hoeglund AB, Howard AL, Wanjala IW, Pham TC, Parrill AL, Baker DL (2010) Characterization of non-lipid autotaxin inhibitors. Bioorg Med Chem 18: 769-776

Jemal A, Siegel R, Xu J, Ward E (2010) Cancer statistics, 2010. CA Cancer J Clin 60: 277-300

Jin JL, Gong J, Yin TJ, Lu YJ, Xia JJ, Xie YY, Di Y, He L, Guo JL, Sun J, Noteborn MH, Qu S (2011) PTD4-apoptin protein and dacarbazine show a synergistic antitumor effect on B16-F1 melanoma in vitro and in vivo. Eur J Pharmacol 654: 17-25

Kim C, Lee CW, Kovacic L, Shah A, Klasa R, Savage KJ (2010) Long-term survival in patients with metastatic melanoma treated with DTIC or temozolomide. Oncologist 15: 765-771

Lev DC, Onn A, Melinkova VO, Miller C, Stone V, Ruiz M, McGary EC, Ananthaswamy HN, Price JE, Bar-Eli M (2004) Exposure of melanoma cells to dacarbazine results in enhanced tumor growth and metastasis in vivo. J Clin Oncol 22: 2092-2100

Liu S, Murph M, Panupinthu N, Mills GB (2009) ATX-LPA receptor axis in inflammation and cancer. Cell Cycle 8: 3695-3701

North EJ, Howard AL, Wanjala IW, Pham TC, Baker DL, Parrill AL (2010) Pharmacophore development and application toward the identification of novel, small-molecule autotaxin inhibitors. J Med Chem 53: 3095-3105

Stracke ML, Krutzsch HC, Unsworth EJ, Arestad A, Cioce V, Schiffmann E, Liotta LA (1992) Identification, purification, and partial sequence analysis of autotaxin, a novel motility-stimulating protein. J Biol Chem 267: 2524-2529

Thompson, JF, Morton, DL, Kroon, BRB (2004) *Textbook of Melanoma.* Martin Dunitz, Taylor & Francis Group, ISBN:1901865657, London, United Kingdom

Xu X, Prestwich GD (2010) Inhibition of tumor growth and angiogenesis by a lysophosphatidic acid antagonist in an engineered three-dimensional lung cancer xenograft model. Cancer 116: 1739-1750

Xu X, Yang G, Zhang H, Prestwich GD (2009) Evaluating dual activity LPA receptor pan-antagonist/autotaxin inhibitors as anti-cancer agents in vivo using engineered human tumors. Prostaglandins Other Lipid Mediat 89: 140-146

Zhang H, Xu X, Gajewiak J, Tsukahara R, Fujiwara Y, Liu J, Fells JI, Perygin D, Parrill AL, Tigyi G, Prestwich GD (2009) Dual activity lysophosphatidic acid receptor pan-antagonist/autotaxin inhibitor reduces breast cancer cell migration in vitro and causes tumor regression in vivo. Cancer Res 69: 5441-5449

5

Low-Anticoagulant Heparins in the Treatment of Metastasis

Narayanam V. Rao[1,2], Glenn D. Prestwich[2],
John R. Hoidal[1] and Thomas P. Kennedy[3]
[1]*Department of Internal Medicine,*
[2]*Department of Medicinal Chemistry and Center for Therapeutic Biomaterials,*
University of Utah Medical Center, Salt Lake City, Utah,
[3]*Department of Medicine, Georgia Health Sciences University, Augusta, Georgia*
USA

1. Introduction

Metastasis is a spread of cancer cells to a distant location from the primary tumor. This process involves a complex series of events similar to those that occur during inflammation. The events of metastasis can be divided into four major steps. First, cancer cells proliferate and transform to acquire motility and ability to invade basement membrane to reach blood vessels. Second, cancer cells penetrate blood vessels due to increased vascular permeability facilitated by inflammatory mediators and enter the circulation. Third, in the circulation cancer cells are shielded by host cells (platelets and neutrophils) to escape surveillance by immune cells and survive shear forces of the bloodstream. Next, integrin-mediated arrest of circulating cancer cells occurs on the endothelial surface before extravasation. Once cancer cells extravasate, heparanase from cancer cells degrades heparan sulfates of the extra cellular matrix. The cleavage of heparan sulfates release growth factors that stimulate cancer cell growth as well as angiogenesis.

The Receptor for Advanced Glycation Endproducts (RAGE) belongs to the immunoglobulin superfamily of cell surface molecules. The receptor's name, RAGE, was coined for its ability to bind its first described ligand, advanced glycation end products (AGEs), which accumulate in physiological (aging) and pathological disorders such as diabetes (Schmidt et al., 1992). RAGE is a pattern recognition receptor for its ligation to structurally unrelated ligands that include Mac-1, HMGB1 and S100 /calgranulins. Similar to immunoglobulin, RAGE contains an extracellular structure with a V-type binding region and two C-type regions. Immediately following the C-type region is a transmembrane region and a short cytoplasmic domain (Fig. 1). The important roles played by RAGE in inflammation, diabetes, Alzhiemer's disease and cancer have been discussed in detail (Ellerman et al., 2007; Logsdon et al., 2007; Schmidt et al., 2001; Sims et al., 2010; Tang et al., 2010). RAGE is ubiquitously expressed in tissues and inflammatory cells at low levels in homeostasis and its expression is increased in stress conditions. RAGE expression is observed in many tumors, including brain, breast, colon, lung, prostate, pancreatic, ovarian cancers, lymphoma and melanoma (Hsieh et al., 2003; Logsdon et al., 2007) and elevated levels of RAGE have been reported in colon (Sasahira et al., 2005), prostate (Ishiguro et al., 2005) and gastric cancers

(Kuniyasu et al., 2002). In contrast, RAGE levels are down-regulated in lung cancer relative to levels in the normal lung tissue. These observations have led to studies to delineate the pathophysiologic involvement of RAGE in cancer. Notably, AGEs are involved in development and progression of cancers (Abe et al., 2007; Sebekova et al., 2007).

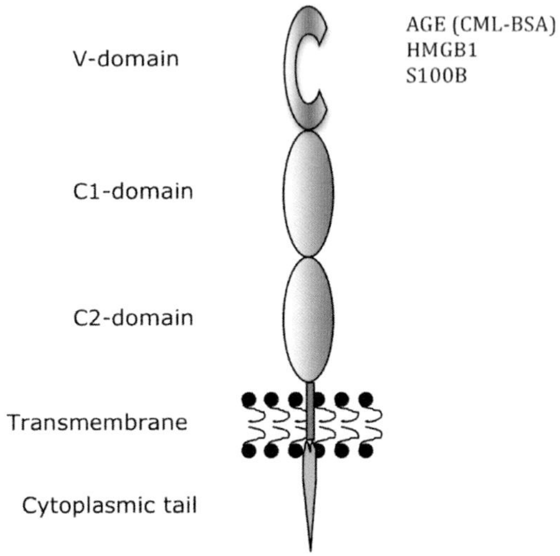

Fig. 1. RAGE domains and ligands involved in cancer. RAGE has ligand-binding V-domain followed by two C-domains of similar to immunoglobulins, a transmembrane region and cytoplasmic tail.

Heparin was discovered in 1916 (McLean, 1916)}, and has been used almost exclusively as an anticoagulant in medicine. However, shortly after its initial discovery, it was reported that heparin had an inhibitory effect on tumor growth in animals (Goerner, 1930). This initial observation led to intensive investigation with regard to heparin's anticancer and anti-metastatic properties (Casu et al., 2010; Casu et al., 2008; Hettiarachchi et al., 1999; Kragh et al., 2005; Kragh & Loechel, 2005; Lapierre et al., 1996; Lever & Page, 2002; Ono et al., 2002; Ornstein & Zacharski, 1999; Smorenburg et al., 1996; Stevenson et al., 2005; Stevenson et al., 2007; Vlodavsky et al., 2006; Yip et al., 2006; Yoshitomi et al., 2004). The usefulness of heparin as an anticancer drug has been hindered by its anticoagulant effect at therapeutic doses required to inhibit cancer growth and spread. The potential of heparin as an anticancer and anti-inflammatory agent led to discovery of a number of low or nonanticoagulant heparins produced by chemical modifications of the heparin polymer itself (Irimura et al., 1986; Lundin et al., 2000; Vlodavsky et al., 1994), sulfation of other natural polymers (Borgenstrom et al., 2007; Kaeffer et al., 1999; Miao et al., 1999) and sulfated heparin-like polymers produced synthetically (Wellstein et al., 1991; Zugmaier et al., 1992). Studies with heparanoids have been limited to animal models. In human studies, heparin has proven beneficial in cancer treatment but its anticoagulant activity has limited its use.

Herein we describe a nonanticoagulant 2-O, 3-O desulfated heparin (ODSH) that retains the anti-inflammatory activities of heparin, including inhibition of P- and L-selectins, heparanase, cationic neutrophil proteases, activation of nuclear factor-κB (NF-κB) and ligation of RAGE by HMGB-1, AGEs and S100 calgranulins (Barry et al., 2010; Lapierre et al., 1996; Rao et al., 2010; Thourani et al., 2000). Also, we describe the first clinical experience with this modified heparin, which has proven safe and low in anticoagulant activity in 137 humans tested to date. Moreover, we present studies demonstrating that ODSH does not cause heparin-induced thrombocytopenia (HIT), a thrombotic syndrome occurring in 3% of individuals receiving heparins (Arepally & Ortel, 2010).

2. Methods

2.1 Production of ODSH

ODSH is a heparin derivative produced for human use under cGMP conditions by the leading U.S. commercial manufacturer of bulk pharmaceutical grade USP heparin, Scientific Protein Laboratories (Wanaukee, WI). It is synthesized by cold alkaline hydrolysis of USP porcine intestinal heparin, as reported (Fryer et al., 1997), which removes the 2-O sulfate groups from iduronic acid residues and the 3-O sulfate groups from the glucosamine residues of the heparin backbone, The N-sulfates, 6-O sulfates, and carboxylates remain intact (Fig.2).

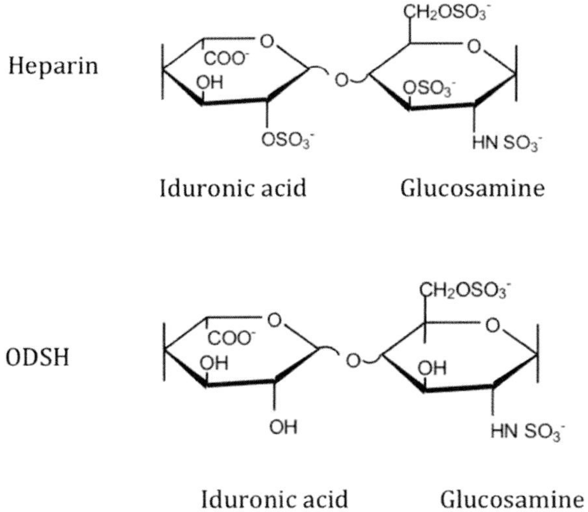

Fig. 2. Sulfate position in disaccharide units of ODSH in comparison to heparin.

2.2 Phase I clinical trials

Two INDs have been opened for intravenous ODSH: #71,356 (under which Phase I safety trials were conducted and pediatric protein losing enteropathy is being studied) and #72,247 (inactive, for a phase II trial in exacerbations of COPD). In the 137 humans who have received intravenous ODSH by bolus and constant infusion for up to 5 days, there have been no serious adverse events, and no decrease in platelet count in any subject to suggest occurrence of HIT, which might have been expected in 2-4 (2-3%) subjects. In Phase I human safety studies (Rao et al., 2010) bolus ODSH was administered safely in doses as high as 20 mg/kg, resulting in lower activated partial thromboplastin times (aPTT) than the usual anticoagulation bolus of unfractionated heparin (80 U/kg, i.e., 0.5 mg/kg at the usual 160 U/mg anti-Xa activity of USP heparin). As part of the Phase I evaluation, ODSH was infused as a bolus of 8 mg/kg followed by continuous intravenous infusion of 0.5 mg/kg/h, adjusted to maintain an aPTT between 40 and 45 seconds (0.64 to 1.39 mg/kg/h final infusion rate).

2.3 Cell culture

U937 monocytes were grown in suspension culture at 37° C in humidified 5% CO_2-95% air in RPMI-1640 supplemented with 10% heat inactivated FBS, 2 mM *L*-glutamine, 1 mM sodium pyruvate, 0.1 mM MEM non-essential amino acids, 100 units/mL penicillin and 100 µg/mL streptomycin. Experiments were performed on cells from passages 1-5. B16F10.1 melanoma cells were grown in Dulbecco's modified Eagle's medium, 10% fetal bovine serum, 100 U/mL penicillin, 100 U/mL streptomycin, 2 mM glutamine and 1 mM sodium pyruvate.

2.4 Adhesion assays

2.4.1 Cell surface binding assays

The effect of heparinoids on binding of U937 monocytes to P-selectin or RAGE was studied in high-bind micro plates coated with 8 µg/mL protein A (50 µL/well) in 0.2 M carbonate-bicarbonate buffer (pH 9.4). Plates were washed with phosphate buffered saline (PBS) containing 1% BSA (PBS-BSA), and P-selectin-Fc or RAGE-Fc chimera (50 µL containing 1 µg) was added to each well and incubated for 2 h at room temperature or overnight at 4° C, respectively. Following incubation, wells were washed twice with PBS-BSA. Fifty µL of heparinoids (0 to 1,000 µg/mL) serially diluted in 20 mM HEPES buffer (containing 125 mM NaCl, 2 mM calcium and 2 mM magnesium) were added to each well and incubated at room temperature for 15 min. As a negative control, 50 µL of 10 mM EDTA was added to select wells to prevent cell binding through sequestration of calcium. At the end of the incubation period, 50 µL of U937 cells (10^5 cells/well, calcein-labeled according to manufacturer's instructions) were added to each well and plates were incubated an additional 30 min at room temperature. The wells were then washed thrice with PBS, and bound cells were lysed by addition of 100 µL of Tris-Triton X-100 buffer. Fluorescence was measured on a microplate reader using excitation of 494 nm and emission of 517 nm.

2.4.2 Solid phase binding assays

Two types of ELISAs were performed, one to observe the binding between RAGE and its ligands, including CML-BSA, HMGB-1 and S100b, and a competitive ELISA to study the ability of ODSH to inhibit/compete for RAGE binding to its ligands.

To confirm RAGE binding to its ligands, polyvinyl 96-well plates were coated with 5 µg/well of specific ligand (CML-BSA, HMGB-1 or S100b calgranulin). Plates were incubated overnight at 4° C and washed thrice with PBS-0.05% Tween-20 (PBST). Next, 50 µL of RAGE from the dilution series ranging from 0.001 to ~ 6 nM was transferred to each respective ligand-coated well and incubated at 37° C for 1 h. Wells were then washed four times with PBST. To detect bound RAGE, 50 µL of anti-RAGE antibody (0.5 µg/mL) was added to each well, the mixture was incubated for 1 h at room temperature, and wells were washed again four times with PBST. HRP-conjugated secondary antibody (50 µL per well) was added, wells were incubated for 1 h at room temperature, and then washed once with PBST. A colorimetric reaction was initiated by addition of 50 µL of TMB and terminated after 15 min by addition of 50 µL of 1 N HCl. Absorbance at 450 nm was read using an automated microplate reader. Binding affinity (K_D) was determined from the plot of absorbance values versus concentrations of RAGE.

RAGE binding to glycated ECM proteins, collagen-I, collagen -IV, fibronectin and laminin coated plates were used. Plates were incubated with 100 µL of 0.15 M glyoxylic acid + 0.45 M sodium cyanoborohydride mixture at 37 °C for 24 hours. At the end of incubation period, the plates were washed with PBST and used for RAGE binding as described above.

For studies of the effect of ODSH or heparin on RAGE binding to its ligands, polyvinyl 96-well plates were coated with specific ligand as described above. Separately, a constant amount of RAGE-Fc chimera (100 µL containing 0.5 µg/mL in PBST containing 0.1% BSA) was incubated with an equal volume of serially diluted ODSH or heparin (0.001 to 1,000 µg/mL in PBST-BSA) overnight at 4° C. The following day, 50 µL of RAGE-heparinoid mix was transferred to each respective ligand-coated well and incubated at 37° C for 2 h. Wells were then washed four times with PBST. Bound RAGE was detected as described above. Absorbance at 450 nm was plotted against concentration of ODSH or heparin. The IC_{50} values were obtained using non-linear regression analysis.

2.5 Elastase and cathepsin G activity assay

The inhibitory activity of heparin and ODSH against HLE and cathepsin G was monitored using the specific chromogenic substrates Suc-Ala-Ala-Val-*p*NA and Suc-Ala-Ala-Pro-Phe-*p*NA, respectively, according to methods previously described (Fryer et al., 1997).

2.6 Mouse model of melanoma lung metastasis

Lung metastasis from melanoma was studied using protocols previously reported by the Varki group (Stevenson et al., 2005). Animal use and husbandry followed protocols approved by the IACUC at the University of Utah. Confluent B16F10 melanoma cells (70-80%) were harvested by brief exposure to trypsin, and washed twice with serum-free medium prior to injection. Living cells were counted with Trypan blue staining prior to injection to insure > 95% viability. Female C57BL/6J mice (n = 6 per group) were injected subcutaneously with 100 µL PBS, heparin (30 mg/kg) or ODSH (30 mg/kg). Thirty min later, 5 x 10^5 B16F10 cells in 200 µL medium were injected intravenously into the lateral tail vein. Mice from each group were injected in alternating order, and cells were resuspended by gently flicking the tube before aspirating the sample for each injection. Twenty-seven days after injection, surviving mice were euthanized. The lungs were removed, perfused intra-tracheally with 10% buffered formalin and photographed. Visible tumor foci were counted independently by two different laboratory personnel blinded with regard to treatment groups, and metastasis quantified in terms of the number of black spots.

3. Results and discussion

3.1 ODSH is a non-anticoagulant heparin that is manufactured at industrial scale and safe from heparin induced thrombocytopenia

The ODSH was manufactured as described in Methods section. Seven serial 1-2 kg batches of material have shown an average molecular mass of 11.7 ± 0.3 kg kDa. ODSH has low affinity for anti-thrombin III (K_D = 339 µM or 4 mg/mL vs. 1.56 µM or 22 µg/mL for heparin) consistent with its low anticoagulant activity. Serial batches of ODSH demonstrated consistently reduced USP (7 ± 0.3 U of anticoagulant activity/mg), anti-Xa (1.9 ± 0.1 U/mg), and anti- IIa (1.2 ± 0.1 U/mg) activities, compared with those of heparin (165-190 U/mg activity for all 3 assays). The current clinical formulation that was used in 137 humans (54 normal and 83 ill patients) is a sterile-filled 20 mL glass vial containing an isotonic 50 mg/mL solution of ODSH in buffered saline. This formulation is cGMP manufactured by Pyramid Laboratories (Costa Mesa, CA). Chemistry and Manufacturing processes are already on file with the FDA in two INDs. A complication of heparin is HIT, which occurs in subjects who produce an activating antibody to the heparin-platelet factor 4 (PF4) complex on the platelet surface, causing thrombocytopenia and thromboembolism (Arepally & Ortel, 2010). In standard serotonin release assays (SRA) performed with human antibodies to the heparin-PF4 complex, heparin triggered release of ^{14}C-serotonin from normal platelets (Fig 3), but ODSH did not trigger HIT at any concentration (Rao et al., 2010).

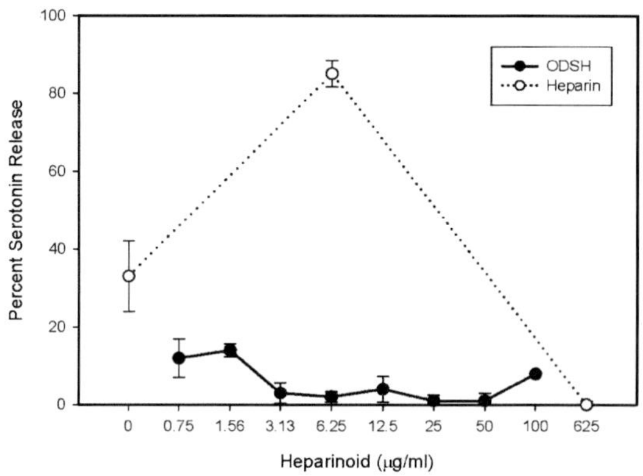

Fig. 3. ODSH does not trigger platelet activation in the serotonin release assay. Normal platelets were loaded with ^{14}C-serotonin and incubated with serum from 3 patients with heparin-PF4 antibodies. Platelets were activated by heparin as a positive control (≥ 20% serotonin release). Rao et al., Am J Physiol Cell Physiol (2010) Am Physiol Soc, used with permission.

3.2 ODSH is safe to use in humans

Two INDs have been opened for intravenous ODSH: #71,356 (under which Phase I safety trials were conducted and pediatric protein losing enteropathy is being studied) and #72,247 (inactive, for a phase II trial in exacerbations of COPD). In the 137 humans who have received intravenous ODSH by bolus and constant infusion for up to 5 days, there have been no serious adverse events, and no decrease in platelet count in any subject to suggest occurrence of HIT, which might have been expected in 2-4 (2-3%) subjects (Arepally & Ortel, 2010). In Phase I human safety studies (Rao et al., 2010) bolus ODSH was administered safely in doses as high as 20 mg/kg, resulting in lower activated partial thromboplastin times (aPTT) than the usual anticoagulation bolus of unfractionated heparin (80 U/kg, i.e., 0.5 mg/kg at the usual 160 U/mg anti-Xa activity of USP heparin). As part of the Phase I evaluation, ODSH was infused as a bolus of 8 mg/kg followed by continuous intravenous infusion of 0.5 mg/kg/h, adjusted to maintain an aPTT between 40 and 45 seconds (0.64 to 1.39 mg/kg/h final infusion rate). This protocol achieved anti-inflammatory plasma ODSH concentrations (≥ 10-20 µg/mL) at doses that did not cause anticoagulation (Fig 4).

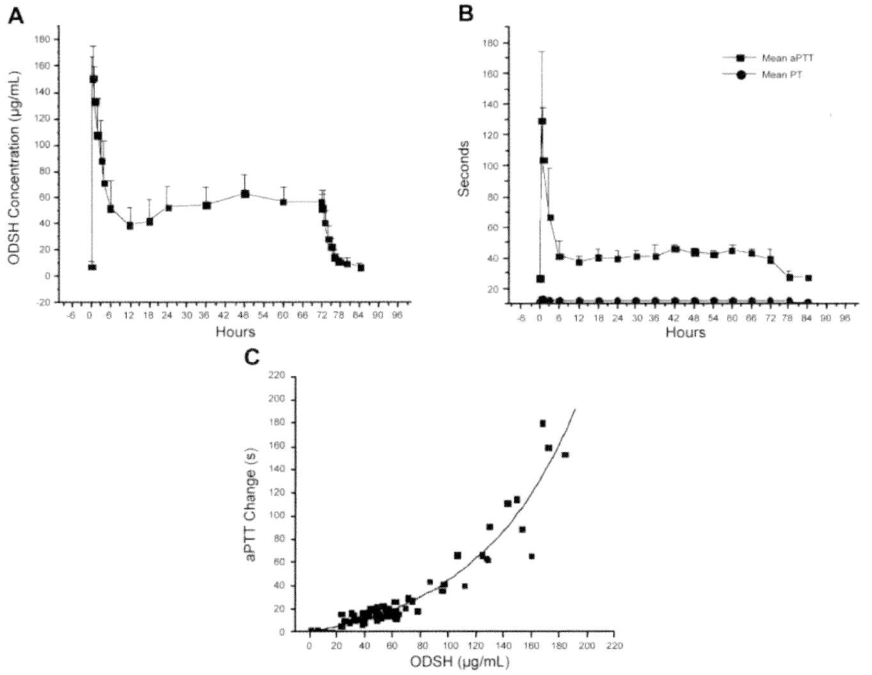

Fig. 4. ODSH infusion in human volunteers achieves anti-inflammatory concentrations before producing anticoagulation. A. Mean (± SD) plasma ODSH levels during study drug infusion, measured by an automated GLP validated assay (Rao et al., 2010). B. Mean (± SD) aPTT and change in prothrombin time (PT) during study drug infusion. C. Relationship between plasma ODSH and change in aPTT from baseline during the 3 day infusion of 8 mg/kg followed by 0.5 mg/kg/h adjusted to maintain aPTT between 40 and 45 seconds. Rao et al., Am J Physiol Cell Physiol (2010) Am Physiol Soc, used with permission.

3.3 ODSH has anti-metastatic and anti-inflammatory activities in vitro

Despite low anticoagulant activity, ODSH retains the strong, broad anti-inflammatory activities and antimetastatic activities of heparin. In metastasis, cancer cells disseminate into the blood circulation and interact with other circulating cells like leukocytes and platelets and also endothelium of vascular wall by selectin-mediated adhesion. The family of selectins includes, P-, L- and E-Selectin, which are expressed on activated platelets, leukocytes and endothelium. Tumor cells express mucins, which are the ligands for selectins, on the cell surface and facilitate cell-cell adhesion. The involvement of selectins in metastasis has been shown in selectin-deficient mouse models (Borsig et al., 2002; Kim et al., 1998; O et al., 2002). Several studies have shown that heparin and heparinoids inhibit selectin-mediated cell adhesion, an important phase of metastasis (Borsig, 2010; Borsig et al., 2001; Borsig et al., 2002; Gao et al., 2006; Ma & Geng, 2000; Maraveyas et al., 2010; Stevenson et al., 2005; Stevenson et al., 2007; Varki, 2007; Wahrenbrock et al., 2003; Wei et al., 2004). To investigate the antimetastatic potency of ODSH, we used U937 cells, a human monocytic leukemia cells. U937 cells express P-selectin ligand, P-selectin glycoprotein ligand-1 (PSGL-1), that functions similar to mucins. We tested the ODSH ability to competitively displace fluorescent-labeled U937 cells adherence to P-selectin via PSGL-1. ODSH inhibited P-selectin with an IC_{50} of 1.1 µg/mL consistent with that of values reported byWang (Wang et al., 2002), who demonstrated that ODSH also inhibits L-selectin-mediated adhesion with an IC_{50} of 3 µg/mL, versus 0.4 µg/mL for heparin (Wang et al., 2002) (Fig. 5).

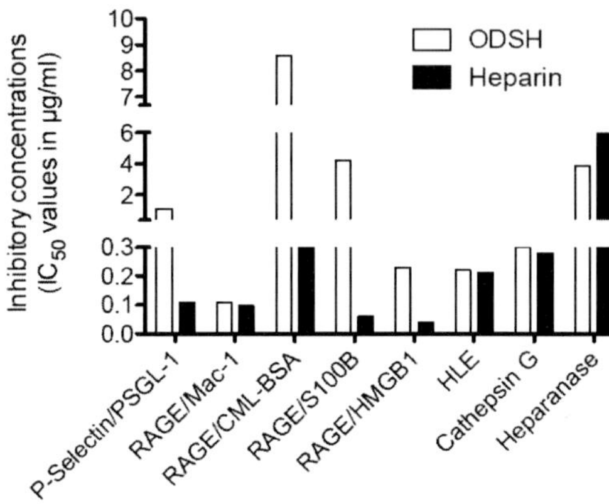

Fig. 5. Anti-inflammatory and anti-metastatic profile of ODSH. The 50% inhibitory concentrations (IC_{50} values) of ODSH to interrupt the receptor ligand pairs, P-selectin/PSGL-1, RAGE/Mac-1, RAGE/CML-BSA, RAGE/S100B and RAGE/HMGB1, interaction are higher than that of heparin. Nonetheless, the IC_{50} concentrations of ODSH required to inhibit HLE, cathepsin G and heparanase activities, the key enzymes involved in the inflammation and metastasis, are similar to the values for heparin. The IC_{50} values of ODSH are higher than that of heparin suggesting that ODSH has lower inhibitory potential than heparin, but the values are much lower than achievable plasma concentration (~200 µg/mL) in humans (see Fig 4). Heparanase data is from (Lapierre et al., 1996).

Though RAGE binds to disparate ligands, we will discuss only the ligands AGE, HMGB1 and S100B that have been evaluated for their role in cancer. RAGE and its ligands are co-expressed in many tumors and the expressed ligands are secreted causing triggering of cellular signaling pathways. This results in expression of cytokines, growth factors, transcription factors, adhesion molecules and NF-kB (Sparvero et al., 2009). Therefore we will focus on the interruption of RAGE-ligand interaction with ODSH.
Several in vitro studies have shown that AGE stimulates growth, proliferation and invasion of cancer cells including melanoma cells (Abe et al., 2004; Yamamoto et al., 1996; Zill et al., 2003; Zill et al., 2001). AGEs are found in extracellular matrix (ECM) proteins (Ling et al., 1998; Mizutari et al., 1997) that can interact with RAGE on tumor cells and enhance RAGE expression causing damage to surrounding tissues. We therefore tested the binding of native and glycated ECM proteins (collagen I, collagen IV, fibronectin and laminin) to RAGE. Results indicate that RAGE binds to native ECM protein with a strong affinity but the affinity is negligibly decreased with glycated ECM proteins. Overall, the K_D values of

RAGE for different ECM proteins are less than 100 ng/mL or <1nM suggesting RAGE on tumor cells might play a role in tumor cell spreading (Fig 6).

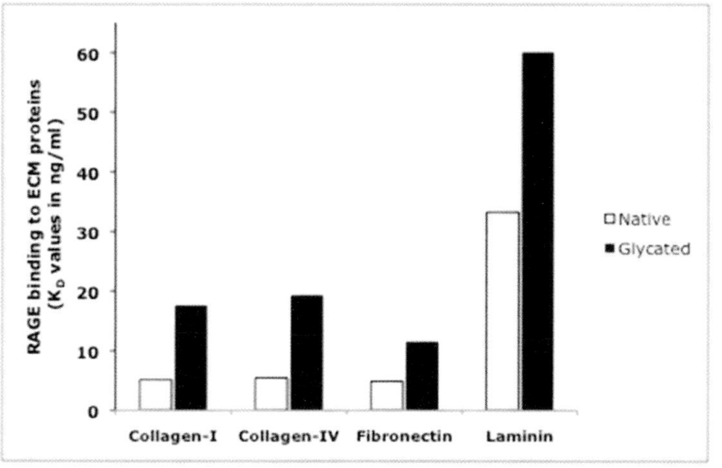

Fig. 6. RAGE binds to AGE-ECM proteins. RAGE binding to ECM proteins was analyzed as described in Methods Section. RAGE bound to native Collagen I, Collagen IV and fibronectin with same affinity but with a lesser affinity to Laminin. The affinity of RAGE for glycated ECM decreased for all the ECM proteins studied but the affinity constants suggest that RAGE binds strongly to ECM proteins even in modified conditions.

In addition, AGE-CML is a common AGE found in vivo (Reddy et al., 1995) and has been detected in tumor tissues (van Heijst et al., 2005). Therefore, we tested potential of ODSH to disrupt the binding between CML-BSA and RAGE as described in methods section. We observed that RAGE bound to CML-BSA with strong affinity (K_D 0.43 nM) and ODSH inhibited the ligation of CML-BSA with IC_{50} of 8.6 µg/mL (Fig 5).

HMGB1 is another ligand for RAGE and both HMGB1 and RAGE have been shown elevated in tumors, including melanoma, colon, prostate, breast and pancreatic cancers (Brezniceanu et al., 2003; Ellerman et al., 2007; Sparvero et al., 2009). Earlier studies by Huttunen et al. suggested that RAGE/HMGB1 signaling might be associated with metastasis (Huttunen et al., 1999; Huttunen et al., 2000). Taguchi et al. found that blockade of HMGB-RAGE signaling suppressed tumor growth as a result of decreased cell migration and invasiveness rather than proliferation or apoptosis (Taguchi et al., 2000). HMGB1 alone or by interaction with NF-kBp65 has been shown to bind specific region of melanocyte inhibitory activity (MIA) promoter in melanocytes and increase the expression of MIA protein, which enhances migration and invasion of tumor cells (Poser et al., 2003; Sasahira et al., 2008). HMGB1 was isolated using heparin-sepharose chromatography (Rauvala & Pihlaskari, 1987) and later was identified to contain a heparin-binding sequence in its amino terminus, suggesting its affinity for heparin (Cardin & Weintraub, 1989). Consistent with these observations, HMGB1 also interacted with carbohydrate chain of syndecan and facilitated cell migration (Rauvala & Rouhiainen, 2010). Syndecan is expressed in normal tissues and tumor tissues but the role of HMGB1 interaction with syndecan in physiological and pathological conditions is not known (Rauvala & Rouhiainen, 2010). Since ODSH is derived from heparin, we tested whether ODSH can interrupt the RAGE-HMB1 ligation. Though HMGB1 binds to RAGE with high affinity (K_D 0.64nM), ODSH inhibited RAGE-HMGB1 interaction with an IC_{50} of 0.23 µg/mL (Figs. 5 and 7).

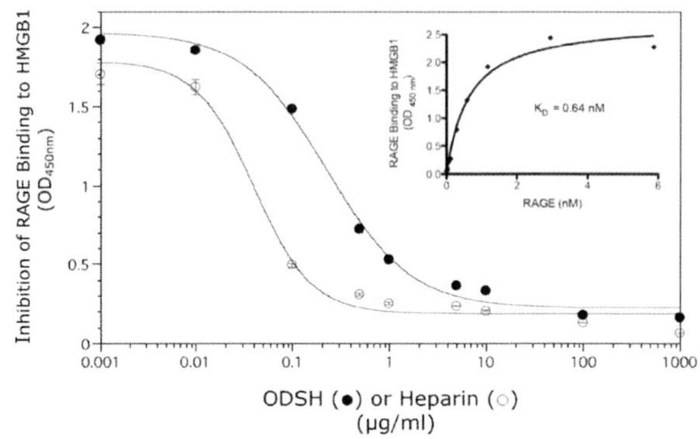

Fig. 7. ODSH and heparin inhibit binding of HMGB-1 to RAGE. HMGB-1 binding to RAGE-Fc chimera was studied using ELISA techniques as described in Methods. RAGE bound to immobilized HMGB-1 in a saturable fashion (*inset*) with a K_D of 0.64 nM. ODSH (•) and heparin (○) inhibit binding of recombinant HMGB-1 to RAGE with IC_{50} values of 0.23 and 0.04 µg/mL, respectively. Rao et al., Am J Physiol Cell Physiol (2010) Am Physiol Soc, used with permission.

S100 proteins are calcium dependent proteins of the EF-hand (helix-loop-helix) type that are differentially located and differentially expressed in a wide variety of cells (Donato, 1999; Donato, 2001; Donato et al., 2009). Among the 25 S100 protein identified, S100b is unique in its location on chromosome 21q22.3 and first one of the group found to ligate to RAGE (Hofmann et al., 1999). S100b is highly expressed in melanoma and considered as possible biomarker for the prognosis of the disease (Harpio & Einarsson, 2004; Salama et al., 2008). We studied the binding affinity of S100b to RAGE. RAGE ligated to S100b with a K_D of 0.45 nM, a value much lower than the affinity range reported (reviewed in (Leclerc et al., 2009)). ODSH inhibited the binding of RAGE to S100b with IC_{50} value of 4.23µg/mL. (Fig 5).
HMGB-1 is released into extracellular milieu as a result of necrosis, apoptosis and secretion. Only HMGB1 released by necrotic cells demonstrates cytokine activity, recruits leukocytes and activates endothelial cell adhesion molecules such as selectins (Dumitriu et al., 2005; Lotze & Tracey, 2005). In cancer, tumor cells undergoing stress are susceptible to death because of factors that include hypoxia, nutrient deprivation and or anticancer treatments (Kepp et al., 2009). These dying cancer cells become a source of HMGB1 (Dong Xda et al., 2007; Scaffidi et al., 2002). Orlova et al (Orlova et al., 2007)) have shown that HMGB1-induced Mac-1 dependent neutrophil recruitment requires the presence of RAGE on neutrophils but not on endothelial cells. Interestingly, three proteins, HMGB1, Mac-1 and RAGE bind to heparin (Diamond et al., 1995; Hanford et al., 2004; Rauvala & Pihlaskari, 1987). We therefore tested Mac-1 dependent binding of U937 cells to immobilized RAGE. ODSH inhibited the adherence of U937 cells to RAGE with IC_{50} values of 0.11 µg/mL (Fig 5).

3.4 ODSH Prevents metastasis in vivo

The vitro studies described above suggested that ODSH, similar to heparin, might interrupt key receptor-ligand interactions involved in metastasis. We therefore investigated the effects of ODSH in experimental melanoma lung metastasis. Heparin significantly decreased lung metastasis at 28 days after melanoma injection, but the same dose of ODSH provided substantially greater reduction of lung metastasis (Fig 8A). ODSH also significantly improved 28-day survival. In contrast to 70% mortality in mice treated with PBS, ~ 70% of ODSH-treated mice survived the experiment (Fig 8B).

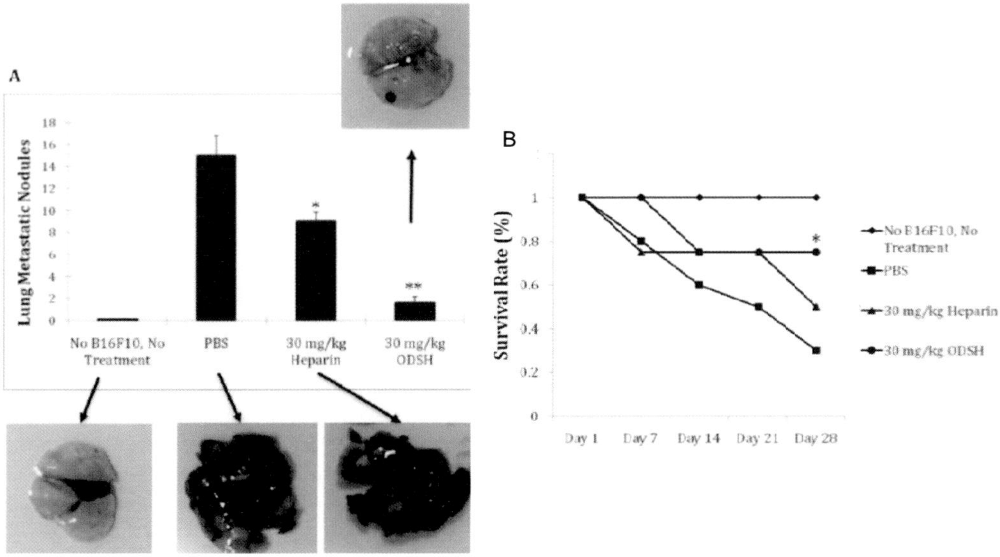

Fig. 8. ODSH inhibits melanoma lung metastasis. Female C57BL/6J mice (n = 6/group) were injected SQ with 100 µL PBS, 30 mg/kg heparin, or 30 mg/kg ODSH. Thirty min later, 5 x 10^5 B16F10 melanoma cells were injected IV into the tail vein. 27 days later surviving mice were euthanized and lungs were removed, fixed, stained and assessed for metastasis by 2 independent observers. A. Heparin (*$P < 0.05$ vs PBS) or ODSH (**$P < 0.01$ vs PBS) significantly reduced metastasis. B. SQ heparin showed little effect on lung metastatic outgrowth but ODSH suppressed metastatic colonization microscopically. C. ODSH improved survival (*$P < 0.05$ vs PBS). Rao et al., Am J Physiol Cell Physiol (2010) Am Physiol Soc, used with permission.

This model is widely used to test the inhibitory capacity of heparin and heparins with no or minimal anticoagulant activity in metastasis (reviewed in (Borsig, 2010). The attenuation of metastasis was attributed to P-selectin and L-selectin as the experimental mice were deficient in selectin but also suggested that there is a selectin-independent mechanism involved. It is not clear whether B16 melanoma cells express mucins on the cells surface to interact with P-selectin, but the expression of RAGE is observed in melanoma cells (Huttunen et al., 2002; Saha et al., 2010). Further, Huttunen et al showed the attenuation of metastasis when B16 cells injected with HMGB1 peptide suggesting the RAGE-mediated tumor cell invasion can be inhibited by competition with RAGE binding ligand such as

ODSH and heparin. In summary, because ODSH interacts with the many receptors, ligands and inhibits enzymes involved in the metastasis, the attenuation of metastasis in the experimental model is due to action of ODSH on multiple sites.

4. Conclusion

A number of fully anticoagulant heparins are commercially available, but their use as a chronic treatment for cancer is dose-limited by their anticoagulant activity. Therapeutic anticoagulant doses of heparin or low molecular weight heparin (Hirsh et al., 2001; Koenig et al., 1998) do not provide sufficiently high plasma drug concentrations to reliably inhibit the selectin-, heparanase- or RAGE-mediated processes (Koenig et al., 1998; Lapierre et al., 1996; Rao et al., 2010; Wang et al., 2002) that are now understood to be important for explaining the benefits of heparins in cancer.

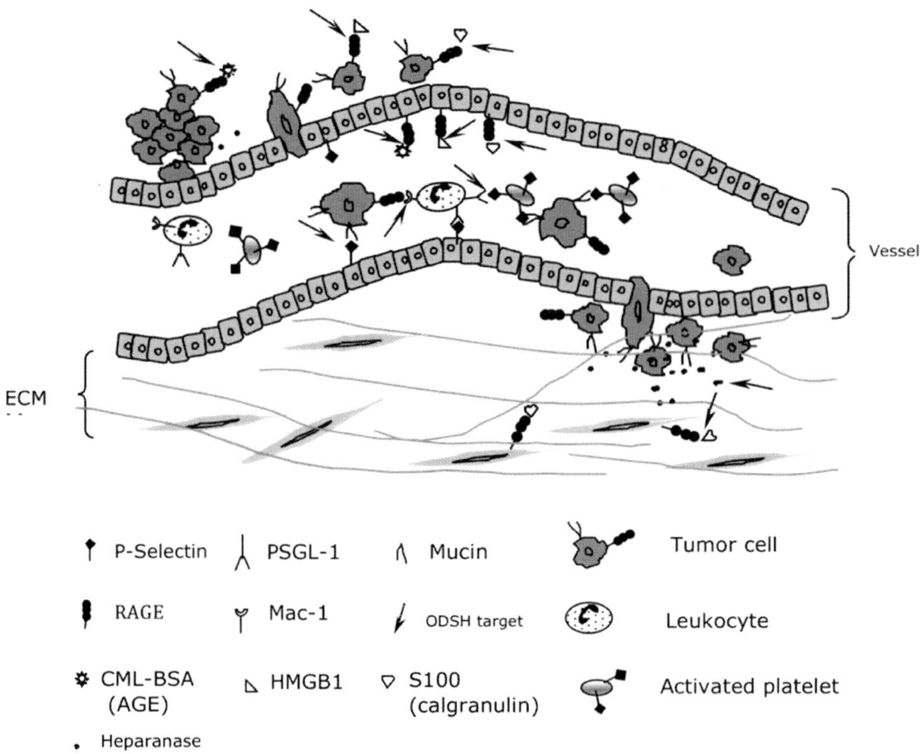

Fig. 9. Potential interference of low anticoagulant ODSH in metastasis. ODSH 1) inhibits heparanse, the enzyme secreted by tumor cells during intravsation and extravsation thus prevent spread of the tumor cells, 2) inhibits the tumor cell mucin (P-selectin ligand) binding to P-selectin on endothelial cells and platelets, 3) inhibits tumor cell RAGE interaction with leukocyte Mac-1, 4) inhibits tumor cell RAGE interaction with its ligands, AGE, HMGB1 and S100b, that are either released by tumor cells within cancer micro environment or by the leukocytes thus prevent sustained signaling for tumor progression, 5) inhibits circulating RAGE ligand interaction with endothelial RAGE.

Of the available low anticoagulant heparin derivatives (Casu et al., 2008; Fryer et al., 1997; Kragh et al., 2005; Kragh & Loechel, 2005; Lapierre et al., 1996; Ono et al., 2002; Rao et al., 2010; Stevenson et al., 2007; Wang et al., 2002; Yoshitomi et al., 2004), only ODSH has been proven safe from major adverse events in humans (Rao et al., 2010) data on file with FDA) and only ODSH is free from the potential to induce HIT (Rao et al., 2010). The concept that P-selectin is the key molecule in metastasis is based on the attenuation of metastasis in animal models. Because of the complex biology of cancer metastasis, it is not easy to identify the specific mediator(s) involved in development of metastatic disease in patients with cancer. In such situation, a compound that can simultaneously target multiple mediators involved in the diseases might have substantial therapeutic value. We have described that non-anticoagulant ODSH, not only targets P-selectin, but additionally is capable of inhibiting the RAGE interaction with its multiple structurally unrelated ligands that play many biological roles in metastasis (Fig. 9). Thus, the results described herein support the notion that low anticoagulant heparin derivatives such as ODSH might prove useful in prevention of metastasis in human cancer.

5. Acknowledgement

We thank Jeanine Walenga and Margaret Prechel for the help with serotonine release assays, Brian Argyle for his expert technical assistance and Xiaoyu Xu for help with lung metastasis animal model. We gratefully acknowledge the expert help of Robert MacArthur and Bradford Walters with phase I studies. The work has been supported by a sponsored research project awarded to the University of Utah by ParinGenix (to N. V. Rao).

6. References

Abe, R., Fujita, Y., & Yamagishi, S. (2007) Angiogenesis and metastasis inhibitors for the treatment of malignant melanoma. *Mini Rev Med Chem,* Vol.7, No.6, pp. 649-661, 1389-5575 (Print) 1389-5575 (Linking)

Abe, R., Shimizu, T., Sugawara, H., Watanabe, H., Nakamura, H., Choei, H., Sasaki, N., Yamagishi, S., Takeuchi, M., & Shimizu, H. (2004) Regulation of human melanoma growth and metastasis by AGE-AGE receptor interactions. *J Invest Dermatol,* Vol.122, No.2, pp. 461-467, 0022-202X (Print) 0022-202X (Linking)

Arepally, G. M., & Ortel, T. L. (2010) Heparin-induced thrombocytopenia. *Annu Rev Med,* Vol.61,pp. 77-90, 1545-326X (Electronic) 0066-4219 (Linking)

Barry, W. H., Zhang, X. Q., Halkos, M. E., Vinten-Johansen, J., Saegusa, N., Spitzer, K. W., Matsuoka, N., Sheets, M., Rao, N. V., & Kennedy, T. P. (2010) Nonanticoagulant heparin reduces myocyte Na+ and Ca2+ loading during simulated ischemia and decreases reperfusion injury. *Am J Physiol Heart Circ Physiol,* Vol.298, No.1, pp. H102-111, 1522-1539 (Electronic) 0363-6135 (Linking)

Borgenstrom, M., Warri, A., Hiilesvuo, K., Kakonen, R., Kakonen, S., Nissinen, L., Pihlavisto, M., Marjamaki, A., Vlodavsky, I., Naggi, A., Torri, G., Casu, B., Veromaa, T., Salmivirta, M., & Elenius, K. (2007) O-sulfated bacterial polysaccharides with low anticoagulant activity inhibit metastasis. *Semin Thromb Hemost,* Vol.33, No.5, pp. 547-556, 0094-6176 (Print) 0094-6176 (Linking)

Borsig, L. (2010) Antimetastatic activities of heparins and modified heparins. Experimental evidence. *Thromb Res,* Vol.125 Suppl 2,pp. S66-71, 1879-2472 (Electronic) 0049-3848 (Linking)

Borsig, L., Wong, R., Feramisco, J., Nadeau, D. R., Varki, N. M., & Varki, A. (2001) Heparin and cancer revisited: mechanistic connections involving platelets, P-selectin, carcinoma mucins, and tumor metastasis. *Proc Natl Acad Sci U S A,* Vol.98, No.6, pp. 3352-3357, 0027-8424 (Print) 0027-8424 (Linking)

Borsig, L., Wong, R., Hynes, R. O., Varki, N. M., & Varki, A. (2002) Synergistic effects of L- and P-selectin in facilitating tumor metastasis can involve non-mucin ligands and implicate leukocytes as enhancers of metastasis. *Proc Natl Acad Sci U S A,* Vol.99, No.4, pp. 2193-2198, 0027-8424 (Print) 0027-8424 (Linking)

Brezniceanu, M. L., Volp, K., Bosser, S., Solbach, C., Lichter, P., Joos, S., & Zornig, M. (2003) HMGB1 inhibits cell death in yeast and mammalian cells and is abundantly expressed in human breast carcinoma. *FASEB J,* Vol.17, No.10, pp. 1295-1297, 1530-6860 (Electronic) 0892-6638 (Linking)

Cardin, A. D., & Weintraub, H. J. (1989) Molecular modeling of protein-glycosaminoglycan interactions. *Arteriosclerosis,* Vol.9, No.1, pp. 21-32, 0276-5047 (Print) 0276-5047 (Linking)

Casu, B., Naggi, A., & Torri, G. (2010) Heparin-derived heparan sulfate mimics to modulate heparan sulfate-protein interaction in inflammation and cancer. *Matrix Biol,* Vol.29, No.6, pp. 442-452, 1569-1802 (Electronic) 0945-053X (Linking)

Casu, B., Vlodavsky, I., & Sanderson, R. D. (2008) Non-anticoagulant heparins and inhibition of cancer. *Pathophysiol Haemost Thromb,* Vol.36, No.3-4, pp. 195-203, 1424-8840 (Electronic) 1424-8832 (Linking)

Diamond, M. S., Alon, R., Parkos, C. A., Quinn, M. T., & Springer, T. A. (1995) Heparin is an adhesive ligand for the leukocyte integrin Mac-1 (CD11b/CD1). *J Cell Biol,* Vol.130, No.6, pp. 1473-1482, 0021-9525 (Print) 0021-9525 (Linking)

Donato, R. (1999) Functional roles of S100 proteins, calcium-binding proteins of the EF-hand type. *Biochim Biophys Acta,* Vol.1450, No.3, pp. 191-231, 0006-3002 (Print) 0006-3002 (Linking)

Donato, R. (2001) S100: a multigenic family of calcium-modulated proteins of the EF-hand type with intracellular and extracellular functional roles. *Int J Biochem Cell Biol,* Vol.33, No.7, pp. 637-668, 1357-2725 (Print) 1357-2725 (Linking)

Donato, R., Sorci, G., Riuzzi, F., Arcuri, C., Bianchi, R., Brozzi, F., Tubaro, C., & Giambanco, I. (2009) S100B's double life: intracellular regulator and extracellular signal. *Biochim Biophys Acta,* Vol.1793, No.6, pp. 1008-1022, 0006-3002 (Print) 0006-3002 (Linking)

Dong Xda, E., Ito, N., Lotze, M. T., Demarco, R. A., Popovic, P., Shand, S. H., Watkins, S., Winikoff, S., Brown, C. K., Bartlett, D. L., & Zeh, H. J., 3rd (2007) High mobility group box I (HMGB1) release from tumor cells after treatment: implications for development of targeted chemoimmunotherapy. *J Immunother,* Vol.30, No.6, pp. 596-606, 1524-9557 (Print) 1524-9557 (Linking)

Dumitriu, I. E., Baruah, P., Manfredi, A. A., Bianchi, M. E., & Rovere-Querini, P. (2005) HMGB1: guiding immunity from within. *Trends Immunol,* Vol.26, No.7, pp. 381-387, 1471-4906 (Print) 1471-4906 (Linking)

Ellerman, J. E., Brown, C. K., de Vera, M., Zeh, H. J., Billiar, T., Rubartelli, A., & Lotze, M. T. (2007) Masquerader: high mobility group box-1 and cancer. *Clin Cancer Res,* Vol.13, No.10, pp. 2836-2848, 1078-0432 (Print) 1078-0432 (Linking)

Fryer, A., Huang, Y. C., Rao, G., Jacoby, D., Mancilla, E., Whorton, R., Piantadosi, C. A., Kennedy, T., & Hoidal, J. (1997) Selective O-desulfation produces nonanticoagulant heparin that retains pharmacological activity in the lung. *J Pharmacol Exp Ther,* Vol.282, No.1, pp. 208-219, 0022-3565 (Print) 0022-3565 (Linking)

Gao, Y., Wei, M., Zheng, S., Ba, X., Hao, S., & Zeng, X. (2006) Chemically modified heparin inhibits the in vitro adhesion of nonsmall cell lung cancer cells to P-selectin. *J Cancer Res Clin Oncol,* Vol.132, No.4, pp. 257-264, 0171-5216 (Print) 0171-5216 (Linking)

Goerner, A. (1930) The influence of anti-clotting agents on transplantation and growth of tumor tissue. *J Lab Clin Med,* Vol.16,pp. 369-372,

Hanford, L. E., Enghild, J. J., Valnickova, Z., Petersen, S. V., Schaefer, L. M., Schaefer, T. M., Reinhart, T. A., & Oury, T. D. (2004) Purification and characterization of mouse soluble receptor for advanced glycation end products (sRAGE). *J Biol Chem,* Vol.279, No.48, pp. 50019-50024, 0021-9258 (Print) 0021-9258 (Linking)

Harpio, R., & Einarsson, R. (2004) S100 proteins as cancer biomarkers with focus on S100B in malignant melanoma. *Clin Biochem,* Vol.37, No.7, pp. 512-518, 0009-9120 (Print) 0009-9120 (Linking)

Hettiarachchi, R. J., Smorenburg, S. M., Ginsberg, J., Levine, M., Prins, M. H., & Buller, H. R. (1999) Do heparins do more than just treat thrombosis? The influence of heparins on cancer spread. *Thromb Haemost,* Vol.82, No.2, pp. 947-952, 0340-6245 (Print) 0340-6245 (Linking)

Hirsh, J., Warkentin, T. E., Shaughnessy, S. G., Anand, S. S., Halperin, J. L., Raschke, R., Granger, C., Ohman, E. M., & Dalen, J. E. (2001) Heparin and low-molecular-weight heparin: mechanisms of action, pharmacokinetics, dosing, monitoring, efficacy, and safety. *Chest,* Vol.119, No.1 Suppl, pp. 64S-94S, 0012-3692 (Print) 0012-3692 (Linking)

Hofmann, M. A., Drury, S., Fu, C., Qu, W., Taguchi, A., Lu, Y., Avila, C., Kambham, N., Bierhaus, A., Nawroth, P., Neurath, M. F., Slattery, T., Beach, D., McClary, J., Nagashima, M., Morser, J., Stern, D., & Schmidt, A. M. (1999) RAGE mediates a novel proinflammatory axis: a central cell surface receptor for S100/calgranulin polypeptides. *Cell,* Vol.97, No.7, pp. 889-901, 0092-8674 (Print) 0092-8674 (Linking)

Hsieh, H. L., Schafer, B. W., Sasaki, N., & Heizmann, C. W. (2003) Expression analysis of S100 proteins and RAGE in human tumors using tissue microarrays. *Biochem Biophys Res Commun,* Vol.307, No.2, pp. 375-381, 0006-291X (Print) 0006-291X (Linking)

Huttunen, H. J., Fages, C., Kuja-Panula, J., Ridley, A. J., & Rauvala, H. (2002) Receptor for advanced glycation end products-binding COOH-terminal motif of amphoterin inhibits invasive migration and metastasis. *Cancer Res,* Vol.62, No.16, pp. 4805-4811, 0008-5472 (Print) 0008-5472 (Linking)

Huttunen, H. J., Fages, C., & Rauvala, H. (1999) Receptor for advanced glycation end products (RAGE)-mediated neurite outgrowth and activation of NF-kappaB require the cytoplasmic domain of the receptor but different downstream signaling pathways. *J Biol Chem,* Vol.274, No.28, pp. 19919-19924, 0021-9258 (Print) 0021-9258 (Linking)

Huttunen, H. J., Kuja-Panula, J., Sorci, G., Agneletti, A. L., Donato, R., & Rauvala, H. (2000) Coregulation of neurite outgrowth and cell survival by amphoterin and S100 proteins through receptor for advanced glycation end products (RAGE) activation. *J Biol Chem,* Vol.275, No.51, pp. 40096-40105, 0021-9258 (Print) 0021-9258 (Linking)

Irimura, T., Nakajima, M., & Nicolson, G. L. (1986) Chemically modified heparins as inhibitors of heparan sulfate specific endo-beta-glucuronidase (heparanase) of metastatic melanoma cells. *Biochemistry,* Vol.25, No.18, pp. 5322-5328, 0006-2960 (Print) 0006-2960 (Linking)

Ishiguro, H., Nakaigawa, N., Miyoshi, Y., Fujinami, K., Kubota, Y., & Uemura, H. (2005) Receptor for advanced glycation end products (RAGE) and its ligand, amphoterin are overexpressed and associated with prostate cancer development. *Prostate,* Vol.64, No.1, pp. 92-100, 0270-4137 (Print) 0270-4137 (Linking)

Kaeffer, B., Benard, C., Lahaye, M., Blottiere, H. M., & Cherbut, C. (1999) Biological properties of ulvan, a new source of green seaweed sulfated polysaccharides, on cultured normal and cancerous colonic epithelial cells. *Planta Med,* Vol.65, No.6, pp. 527-531, 0032-0943 (Print) 0032-0943 (Linking)

Kepp, O., Tesniere, A., Schlemmer, F., Michaud, M., Senovilla, L., Zitvogel, L., & Kroemer, G. (2009) Immunogenic cell death modalities and their impact on cancer treatment. *Apoptosis,* Vol.14, No.4, pp. 364-375, 1573-675X (Electronic) 1360-8185 (Linking)

Kim, Y. J., Borsig, L., Varki, N. M., & Varki, A. (1998) P-selectin deficiency attenuates tumor growth and metastasis. *Proc Natl Acad Sci U S A,* Vol.95, No.16, pp. 9325-9330, 0027-8424 (Print) 0027-8424 (Linking)

Koenig, A., Norgard-Sumnicht, K., Linhardt, R., & Varki, A. (1998) Differential interactions of heparin and heparan sulfate glycosaminoglycans with the selectins. Implications for the use of unfractionated and low molecular weight heparins as therapeutic agents. *J Clin Invest,* Vol.101, No.4, pp. 877-889, 0021-9738 (Print) 0021-9738 (Linking)

Kragh, M., Binderup, L., Vig Hjarnaa, P. J., Bramm, E., Johansen, K. B., & Frimundt Petersen, C. (2005) Non-anti-coagulant heparin inhibits metastasis but not primary tumor growth. *Oncol Rep,* Vol.14, No.1, pp. 99-104, 1021-335X (Print) 1021-335X (Linking)

Kragh, M., & Loechel, F. (2005) Non-anti-coagulant heparins: a promising approach for prevention of tumor metastasis (review). *Int J Oncol,* Vol.27, No.4, pp. 1159-1167, 1019-6439 (Print) 1019-6439 (Linking)

Kuniyasu, H., Oue, N., Wakikawa, A., Shigeishi, H., Matsutani, N., Kuraoka, K., Ito, R., Yokozaki, H., & Yasui, W. (2002) Expression of receptors for advanced glycation end-products (RAGE) is closely associated with the invasive and metastatic activity of gastric cancer. *J Pathol,* Vol.196, No.2, pp. 163-170, 0022-3417 (Print) 0022-3417 (Linking)

Lapierre, F., Holme, K., Lam, L., Tressler, R. J., Storm, N., Wee, J., Stack, R. J., Castellot, J., & Tyrrell, D. J. (1996) Chemical modifications of heparin that diminish its anticoagulant but preserve its heparanase-inhibitory, angiostatic, anti-tumor and anti-metastatic properties. *Glycobiology,* Vol.6, No.3, pp. 355-366, 0959-6658 (Print) 0959-6658 (Linking)

Leclerc, E., Fritz, G., Vetter, S. W., & Heizmann, C. W. (2009) Binding of S100 proteins to RAGE: an update. *Biochim Biophys Acta,* Vol.1793, No.6, pp. 993-1007, 0006-3002 (Print) 0006-3002 (Linking)

Lever, R., & Page, C. P. (2002) Novel drug development opportunities for heparin. *Nat Rev Drug Discov,* Vol.1, No.2, pp. 140-148, 1474-1776 (Print) 1474-1776 (Linking)

Ling, X., Sakashita, N., Takeya, M., Nagai, R., Horiuchi, S., & Takahashi, K. (1998) Immunohistochemical distribution and subcellular localization of three distinct specific molecular structures of advanced glycation end products in human tissues. *Lab Invest,* Vol.78, No.12, pp. 1591-1606, 0023-6837 (Print) 0023-6837 (Linking)

Logsdon, C. D., Fuentes, M. K., Huang, E. H., & Arumugam, T. (2007) RAGE and RAGE ligands in cancer. *Curr Mol Med,* Vol.7, No.8, pp. 777-789, 1566-5240 (Print) 1566-5240 (Linking)

Lotze, M. T., & Tracey, K. J. (2005) High-mobility group box 1 protein (HMGB1): nuclear weapon in the immune arsenal. *Nat Rev Immunol,* Vol.5, No.4, pp. 331-342, 1474-1733 (Print) 1474-1733 (Linking)

Lundin, L., Larsson, H., Kreuger, J., Kanda, S., Lindahl, U., Salmivirta, M., & Claesson-Welsh, L. (2000) Selectively desulfated heparin inhibits fibroblast growth factor-induced mitogenicity and angiogenesis. *J Biol Chem,* Vol.275, No.32, pp. 24653-24660, 0021-9258 (Print) 0021-9258 (Linking)

Ma, Y. Q., & Geng, J. G. (2000) Heparan sulfate-like proteoglycans mediate adhesion of human malignant melanoma A375 cells to P-selectin under flow. *J Immunol,* Vol.165, No.1, pp. 558-565, 0022-1767 (Print) 0022-1767 (Linking)

Maraveyas, A., Johnson, M. J., Xiao, Y. P., & Noble, S. (2010) Malignant melanoma as a target malignancy for the study of the anti-metastatic properties of the heparins. *Cancer Metastasis Rev,* Vol.29, No.4, pp. 777-784, 1573-7233 (Electronic) 0167-7659 (Linking)

McLean, J. (1916) The thromboplastic action of cephalin. *American Journal of Physiology,* Vol.41,pp. 250-257,

Miao, H. Q., Elkin, M., Aingorn, E., Ishai-Michaeli, R., Stein, C. A., & Vlodavsky, I. (1999) Inhibition of heparanase activity and tumor metastasis by laminarin sulfate and synthetic phosphorothioate oligodeoxynucleotides. *Int J Cancer,* Vol.83, No.3, pp. 424-431, 0020-7136 (Print) 0020-7136 (Linking)

Mizutari, K., Ono, T., Ikeda, K., Kayashima, K., & Horiuchi, S. (1997) Photo-enhanced modification of human skin elastin in actinic elastosis by N(epsilon)-(carboxymethyl)lysine, one of the glycoxidation products of the Maillard reaction. *J Invest Dermatol,* Vol.108, No.5, pp. 797-802, 0022-202X (Print) 0022-202X (Linking)

O, I., Otvos, L., Kieber-Emmons, T., & Blaszczyk-Thurin, M. (2002) Role of SA-Le(a) and E-selectin in metastasis assessed with peptide antagonist. *Peptides,* Vol.23, No.5, pp. 999-1010, 0196-9781 (Print) 0196-9781 (Linking)

Ono, K., Ishihara, M., Ishikawa, K., Ozeki, Y., Deguchi, H., Sato, M., Hashimoto, H., Saito, Y., Yura, H., Kurita, A., & Maehara, T. (2002) Periodate-treated, non-anticoagulant heparin-carrying polystyrene (NAC-HCPS) affects angiogenesis and inhibits subcutaneous induced tumour growth and metastasis to the lung. *Br J Cancer,* Vol.86, No.11, pp. 1803-1812, 0007-0920 (Print) 0007-0920 (Linking)

Orlova, V. V., Choi, E. Y., Xie, C., Chavakis, E., Bierhaus, A., Ihanus, E., Ballantyne, C. M., Gahmberg, C. G., Bianchi, M. E., Nawroth, P. P., & Chavakis, T. (2007) A novel pathway of HMGB1-mediated inflammatory cell recruitment that requires Mac-1-integrin. *EMBO J,* Vol.26, No.4, pp. 1129-1139, 0261-4189 (Print) 0261-4189 (Linking)

Ornstein, D. L., & Zacharski, L. R. (1999) The use of heparin for treating human malignancies. *Haemostasis,* Vol.29 Suppl S1,pp. 48-60, 0301-0147 (Print) 0301-0147 (Linking)

Poser, I., Golob, M., Buettner, R., & Bosserhoff, A. K. (2003) Upregulation of HMG1 leads to melanoma inhibitory activity expression in malignant melanoma cells and contributes to their malignancy phenotype. *Mol Cell Biol,* Vol.23, No.8, pp. 2991-2998, 0270-7306 (Print) 0270-7306 (Linking)

Rao, N. V., Argyle, B., Xu, X., Reynolds, P. R., Walenga, J. M., Prechel, M., Prestwich, G. D., MacArthur, R. B., Walters, B. B., Hoidal, J. R., & Kennedy, T. P. (2010) Low anticoagulant heparin targets multiple sites of inflammation, suppresses heparin-induced thrombocytopenia, and inhibits interaction of RAGE with its ligands. *Am J Physiol Cell Physiol,* Vol.299, No.1, pp. C97-110, 1522-1563 (Electronic) 0363-6143 (Linking)

Rauvala, H., & Pihlaskari, R. (1987) Isolation and some characteristics of an adhesive factor of brain that enhances neurite outgrowth in central neurons. *J Biol Chem,* Vol.262, No.34, pp. 16625-16635, 0021-9258 (Print) 0021-9258 (Linking)

Rauvala, H., & Rouhiainen, A. (2010) Physiological and pathophysiological outcomes of the interactions of HMGB1 with cell surface receptors. *Biochim Biophys Acta,* Vol.1799, No.1-2, pp. 164-170, 0006-3002 (Print) 0006-3002 (Linking)

Reddy, S., Bichler, J., Wells-Knecht, K. J., Thorpe, S. R., & Baynes, J. W. (1995) N epsilon-(carboxymethyl)lysine is a dominant advanced glycation end product (AGE) antigen in tissue proteins. *Biochemistry,* Vol.34, No.34, pp. 10872-10878, 0006-2960 (Print) 0006-2960 (Linking)

Saha, A., Lee, Y. C., Zhang, Z., Chandra, G., Su, S. B., & Mukherjee, A. B. (2010) Lack of an endogenous anti-inflammatory protein in mice enhances colonization of B16F10 melanoma cells in the lungs. *J Biol Chem,* Vol.285, No.14, pp. 10822-10831, 1083-351X (Electronic) 0021-9258 (Linking)

Salama, I., Malone, P. S., Mihaimeed, F., & Jones, J. L. (2008) A review of the S100 proteins in cancer. *Eur J Surg Oncol,* Vol.34, No.4, pp. 357-364, 1532-2157 (Electronic) 0748-7983 (Linking)

Sasahira, T., Akama, Y., Fujii, K., & Kuniyasu, H. (2005) Expression of receptor for advanced glycation end products and HMGB1/amphoterin in colorectal adenomas. *Virchows Arch,* Vol.446, No.4, pp. 411-415, 0945-6317 (Print) 0945-6317 (Linking)

Sasahira, T., Kirita, T., Oue, N., Bhawal, U. K., Yamamoto, K., Fujii, K., Ohmori, H., Luo, Y., Yasui, W., Bosserhoff, A. K., & Kuniyasu, H. (2008) High mobility group box-1-inducible melanoma inhibitory activity is associated with nodal metastasis and lymphangiogenesis in oral squamous cell carcinoma. *Cancer Sci,* Vol.99, No.9, pp. 1806-1812, 1349-7006 (Electronic) 1347-9032 (Linking)

Scaffidi, P., Misteli, T., & Bianchi, M. E. (2002) Release of chromatin protein HMGB1 by necrotic cells triggers inflammation. *Nature,* Vol.418, No.6894, pp. 191-195, 0028-0836 (Print) 0028-0836 (Linking)

Schmidt, A. M., Vianna, M., Gerlach, M., Brett, J., Ryan, J., Kao, J., Esposito, C., Hegarty, H., Hurley, W., Clauss, M., & et al. (1992) Isolation and characterization of two binding proteins for advanced glycosylation end products from bovine lung which are present on the endothelial cell surface. *J Biol Chem,* Vol.267, No.21, pp. 14987-14997, 0021-9258 (Print) 0021-9258 (Linking)

Schmidt, A. M., Yan, S. D., Yan, S. F., & Stern, D. M. (2001) The multiligand receptor RAGE as a progression factor amplifying immune and inflammatory responses. *J Clin Invest,* Vol.108, No.7, pp. 949-955, 0021-9738 (Print) 0021-9738 (Linking)

Sebekova, K., Wagner, Z., Schupp, N., & Boor, P. (2007) Genomic damage and malignancy in end-stage renal failure: do advanced glycation end products contribute? *Kidney Blood Press Res,* Vol.30, No.1, pp. 56-66, 1420-4096 (Print) 1420-4096 (Linking)

Sims, G. P., Rowe, D. C., Rietdijk, S. T., Herbst, R., & Coyle, A. J. (2010) HMGB1 and RAGE in inflammation and cancer. *Annu Rev Immunol,* Vol.28,pp. 367-388, 1545-3278 (Electronic) 0732-0582 (Linking)

Smorenburg, S. M., Griffini, P., Tiggelman, A. B., Moorman, A. F., Boers, W., & Van Noorden, J. F. (1996) alpha2-Macroglobulin is mainly produced by cancer cells and not by hepatocytes in rats with colon carcinoma metastases in liver. *Hepatology,* Vol.23, No.3, pp. 560-570, 0270-9139 (Print) 0270-9139 (Linking)

Sparvero, L. J., Asafu-Adjei, D., Kang, R., Tang, D., Amin, N., Im, J., Rutledge, R., Lin, B., Amoscato, A. A., Zeh, H. J., & Lotze, M. T. (2009) RAGE (Receptor for Advanced Glycation Endproducts), RAGE ligands, and their role in cancer and inflammation. *J Transl Med,* Vol.7, 17, 1479-5876 (Electronic) 1479-5876 (Linking)

Stevenson, J. L., Choi, S. H., & Varki, A. (2005) Differential metastasis inhibition by clinically relevant levels of heparins--correlation with selectin inhibition, not antithrombotic activity. *Clin Cancer Res,* Vol.11, No.19 Pt 1, pp. 7003-7011, 1078-0432 (Print) 1078-0432 (Linking)

Stevenson, J. L., Varki, A., & Borsig, L. (2007) Heparin attenuates metastasis mainly due to inhibition of P- and L-selectin, but non-anticoagulant heparins can have additional effects. *Thromb Res,* Vol.120 Suppl 2,pp. S107-111, 0049-3848 (Print) 0049-3848 (Linking)

Taguchi, A., Blood, D. C., del Toro, G., Canet, A., Lee, D. C., Qu, W., Tanji, N., Lu, Y., Lalla, E., Fu, C., Hofmann, M. A., Kislinger, T., Ingram, M., Lu, A., Tanaka, H., Hori, O., Ogawa, S., Stern, D. M., & Schmidt, A. M. (2000) Blockade of RAGE-amphoterin signalling suppresses tumour growth and metastases. *Nature,* Vol.405, No.6784, pp. 354-360, 0028-0836 (Print) 0028-0836 (Linking)

Tang, D., Kang, R., Zeh, H. J., 3rd, & Lotze, M. T. (2010) High-mobility group box 1 and cancer. *Biochim Biophys Acta,* Vol.1799, No.1-2, pp. 131-140, 0006-3002 (Print) 0006-3002 (Linking)

Thourani, V. H., Brar, S. S., Kennedy, T. P., Thornton, L. R., Watts, J. A., Ronson, R. S., Zhao, Z. Q., Sturrock, A. L., Hoidal, J. R., & Vinten-Johansen, J. (2000) Nonanticoagulant heparin inhibits NF-kappaB activation and attenuates myocardial reperfusion injury. *Am J Physiol Heart Circ Physiol,* Vol.278, No.6, pp. H2084-2093, 0363-6135 (Print) 0363-6135 (Linking)

van Heijst, J. W., Niessen, H. W., Hoekman, K., & Schalkwijk, C. G. (2005) Advanced glycation end products in human cancer tissues: detection of Nepsilon-(carboxymethyl)lysine and argpyrimidine. *Ann N Y Acad Sci,* Vol.1043,pp. 725-733, 0077-8923 (Print) 0077-8923 (Linking)

Varki, A. (2007) Trousseau's syndrome: multiple definitions and multiple mechanisms. *Blood,* Vol.110, No.6, pp. 1723-1729, 0006-4971 (Print) 0006-4971 (Linking)

Vlodavsky, I., Abboud-Jarrous, G., Elkin, M., Naggi, A., Casu, B., Sasisekharan, R., & Ilan, N. (2006) The impact of heparanese and heparin on cancer metastasis and angiogenesis. *Pathophysiol Haemost Thromb,* Vol.35, No.1-2, pp. 116-127, 1424-8832 (Print) 1424-8832 (Linking)

Vlodavsky, I., Mohsen, M., Lider, O., Svahn, C. M., Ekre, H. P., Vigoda, M., Ishai-Michaeli, R., & Peretz, T. (1994) Inhibition of tumor metastasis by heparanase inhibiting species of heparin. *Invasion Metastasis,* Vol.14, No.1-6, pp. 290-302, 0251-1789 (Print) 0251-1789 (Linking)

Wahrenbrock, M., Borsig, L., Le, D., Varki, N., & Varki, A. (2003) Selectin-mucin interactions as a probable molecular explanation for the association of Trousseau syndrome with mucinous adenocarcinomas. *J Clin Invest,* Vol.112, No.6, pp. 853-862, 0021-9738 (Print) 0021-9738 (Linking)

Wang, L., Brown, J. R., Varki, A., & Esko, J. D. (2002) Heparin's anti-inflammatory effects require glucosamine 6-O-sulfation and are mediated by blockade of L- and P-selectins. *J Clin Invest,* Vol.110, No.1, pp. 127-136, 0021-9738 (Print) 0021-9738 (Linking)

Wei, M., Tai, G., Gao, Y., Li, N., Huang, B., Zhou, Y., Hao, S., & Zeng, X. (2004) Modified heparin inhibits P-selectin-mediated cell adhesion of human colon carcinoma cells to immobilized platelets under dynamic flow conditions. *J Biol Chem,* Vol.279, No.28, pp. 29202-29210, 0021-9258 (Print) 0021-9258 (Linking)

Wellstein, A., Zugmaier, G., Califano, J. A., 3rd, Kern, F., Paik, S., & Lippman, M. E. (1991) Tumor growth dependent on Kaposi's sarcoma-derived fibroblast growth factor inhibited by pentosan polysulfate. *J Natl Cancer Inst,* Vol.83, No.10, pp. 716-720, 0027-8874 (Print) 0027-8874 (Linking)

Yamamoto, Y., Yamagishi, S., Hsu, C. C., & Yamamoto, H. (1996) Advanced glycation endproducts-receptor interactions stimulate the growth of human pancreatic cancer cells through the induction of platelet-derived growth factor-B. *Biochem Biophys Res Commun,* Vol.222, No.3, pp. 700-705, 0006-291X (Print) 0006-291X (Linking)

Yip, G. W., Smollich, M., & Gotte, M. (2006) Therapeutic value of glycosaminoglycans in cancer. *Mol Cancer Ther,* Vol.5, No.9, pp. 2139-2148, 1535-7163 (Print) 1535-7163 (Linking)

Yoshitomi, Y., Nakanishi, H., Kusano, Y., Munesue, S., Oguri, K., Tatematsu, M., Yamashina, I., & Okayama, M. (2004) Inhibition of experimental lung metastases of Lewis lung carcinoma cells by chemically modified heparin with reduced anticoagulant activity. *Cancer Lett,* Vol.207, No.2, pp. 165-174, 0304-3835 (Print) 0304-3835 (Linking)

Zill, H., Bek, S., Hofmann, T., Huber, J., Frank, O., Lindenmeier, M., Weigle, B., Erbersdobler, H. F., Scheidler, S., Busch, A. E., & Faist, V. (2003) RAGE-mediated MAPK activation by food-derived AGE and non-AGE products. *Biochem Biophys Res Commun,* Vol.300, No.2, pp. 311-315, 0006-291X (Print) 0006-291X (Linking)

Zill, H., Gunther, R., Erbersdobler, H. F., Folsch, U. R., & Faist, V. (2001) RAGE expression and AGE-induced MAP kinase activation in Caco-2 cells. *Biochem Biophys Res Commun,* Vol.288, No.5, pp. 1108-1111, 0006-291X (Print) 0006-291X (Linking)

Zugmaier, G., Lippman, M. E., & Wellstein, A. (1992) Inhibition by pentosan polysulfate (PPS) of heparin-binding growth factors released from tumor cells and blockage by PPS of tumor growth in animals. *J Natl Cancer Inst,* Vol.84, No.22, pp. 1716-1724, 0027-8874 (Print) 0027-8874 (Linking)

6

Novel Antifolates as Produgs for the Treatment of Melanoma

Jose Neptuno Rodriguez-Lopez[1], Luis Sanchez-del-Campo[1], Magali Saez-Ayala[1], Maria F. Montenegro[1] and Juan Cabezas-Herrera[2]

[1]*Department of Biochemistry & Molecular Biology A, University of Murcia,*
[2]*Research Unit of Clinical Analusis Service, University Hospital Virgen de la Arrixaca*
Spain

1. Introduction

Malignant melanoma is a deadly disease in which standard treatment options have remained remarkably static over the past 30 years (Sullivan & Atkins, 2009). At present, the incidence of melanoma continues to increase despite public health initiatives that have promoted protection against the sun. Thus, during the past ten years, the incidence and annual mortality of melanoma has increased more rapidly than any other cancer and according to an American Cancer Society estimate, there will have been approximately 68,720 new cases of invasive melanoma diagnosed in 2009 in the United States, which resulted in approximately 8,650 deaths (American Cancer Society, 2009). Unfortunately, the increase in incidence has not been paralleled by the development of new therapeutic agents with a significant impact on survival. Although many patients with melanoma localized to the skin are cured by surgical excision, increased time to diagnosis is associated with higher stage of disease, and those with regional lymphatic or metastatic disease respond poorly to conventional radiation and chemotherapy with 5-year survival rates ranging from 10 to 50% (Tawbi & Buch, 2010). Currently, limited therapeutic options exist for patients with metastatic melanomas, and all standard combinations currently used in metastasis therapy have low efficacy and poor response rates. One example of the complications involved in melanoma chemotherapy is the limited effectiveness of antifolates. Although methotrexate (MTX), the most frequently used antifolate, is an efficient drug for several types of cancer, it is not active against melanoma (Kufe et al., 1980). Undoubtedly, unravelling the mechanism of the resistance of melanomas to this drug could help to improve current therapeutic approaches. Moreover, it could help to develop a novel generation of antifolate drugs that overcome resistance problems and present low toxicity for the prophylaxis and treatment of melanoma.

2. Mechanisms of resistance of melanoma to classical antifolates

Dihydrofolate reductase (DHFR; 5,6,7,8-tetrahydrofolate: $NADP^+$ oxidoreductase, EC 1.5.1.3) catalyzes the reduction of 7,8-dihydrofolate (DHF) to 5,6,7,8-tetrahydrofolate (THF) in the presence of coenzyme NADPH as follows: DHF + NADPH + H+ → THF + NADP+. This enzyme is necessary for maintaining intracellular pools of THF and its derivatives which are essential cofactors in one-carbon metabolism. Coupled with thymidylate synthase (Lockshin et al., 1979), it is directly involved in thymidylate (dTMP) production through a *de novo* pathway. DHFR is therefore pivotal in providing purines and pyrimidine precursors for the biosynthesis of DNA, RNA and amino acids. In addition, it is the target enzyme (Blakley, 1969) for antifolate drugs such as the antineoplastic drug MTX and the antibacterial drug trimethoprim (TMP). The mechanisms of resistance to MTX have been extensively studied, mainly in experimental tumors propagated *in vitro* and *in vivo* (Kufe et al., 1980; Zhao & Goldman, 2003; Assaraf, 2007); however, the specific basis for the resistance of melanoma cells to MTX is unclear. During decades the mechanism of resistance of melanoma to MTX was associated with general mechanisms of resistance detected in other epithelial cancer cell including reduced cellular uptake of this drug, high intracellular levels of DHFR and/or insufficient rate of MTX polyglutamylation, which diminishes long-chain MTX polyglutamates from being preferentially retained intracellularly (Assaraf, 2007). However, recently, a melanoma-specific mechanism of resistance to cytotoxic drugs, including MTX, has been described (Chen et al., 2006; Sánchez-del-Campo et al., 2009a; Xie et al., 2009). Experiments from our laboratory and others provide evidences that melanosomes contribute to the refractory properties of melanoma cells by sequestering cytotoxic drugs and increasing melanosome-mediated drug export. Concretely, we have described that folate receptor α (FRα)-endocytotic transport of MTX facilitates drug melanosomal sequestration and cellular exportation in melanoma cells, which ensures reduced accumulation of MTX in intracellular compartments (Sánchez-del-Campo et al., 2009a).

An important observation in this study was that MTX was a cytostatic agent on melanoma cells. These cells were resistant to MTX-induced apoptosis but responded to the drug by arresting their growth. A similar response was observed when the murine B16/F10 melanoma cell line was grown in low folate. After 3 days in folate-deficient medium the cells had restricted proliferative activity and also increased their metastatic potential (Branda et al., 1988). Taking this into consideration, the results indicate that MTX might also induce depletion of intracellular reduced folate coenzymes by reducing their transport though the FRα and/or competing with them for the reduced folate carrier (RFC). Melanoma cells may be highly sensitive to intracellular depletion of folate coenzymes, and in this situation may enter into a "latent" state. This form of melanoma should indeed be highly resistant to MTX, since antifolate drugs are more effective on fast-dividing cells, which require continuous DNA synthesis. Most likely, the high increases of DHFR expression in cells treated with MTX (Kufe et al., 1980) would represent an adaptation mechanism that allows cells to survive with low intracellular concentrations of folate coenzymes. Increasing the recycling of folate molecules the cells would maintain other cellular functions that are dependent on folate coenzymes, such as the synthesis of purines, pyrimidines, amino acids and methylation reactions. The presence of this "latent" form of melanoma should be critical for the resistance to MTX during *in vivo* therapies. Although MTX chemotherapy could initially halt the development of the tumor, after clearance of the drug from the body the melanoma cells may reinitiate their progression, possibly with an increased metastatic potential (Branda et al., 1988).

A defect in intracellular folate retention is another recognized mechanism of drug resistance (Assaraf, 2007; Gaukroger et al., 1983; Kufe et al., 1980; Zhao and Goldman, 2003). In addition to a decrease in antifolate polyglutamylation, melanoma cells may also export cytotoxic drugs by melanosome sequestration (Chen et al., 2006). The results presented in this study indicated that drug exportation was an operative mechanism of resistance to MTX in melanoma cells. Although the mechanism by which cytotoxic drugs are sequestered into melanosomes remains unclear, we demonstrated that MTX-melanosome trapping may be a consequence of its FRα-endosomal transport (Sánchez-del-Campo et al., 2009a). To test the importance of this process on the resistance of melanoma to antifolates, we silenced the expression of the melanosomal structural protein gp100/Pmel17, which is known to play a critical role in melanosome biogenesis (Theos et al., 2005). Recently, Xie and collaborators (2009) provided the first direct evidence that disruption of the process of normal melanosome biogenesis, by mutation of gp100/Pmel17, increased sensitivity to cisplatin. We also observed that effective silencing of gp100/Pmel17 significantly increased the sensitivity of melanoma cells to MTX, favouring MTX-induced apoptosis. This observation strongly supports the hypothesis which indicates that melanosome biogenesis is a specialization of the endocytic pathway (Raposo and Marks, 2002; 2007); however, the exact mechanism by which MTX induces abnormal trafficking of early endosomes in melanoma cells, favoring the exportation of melanosomes, is still unclear. Whether MTX blocks the formation of carrier vesicles operating between early and late endosomes, inhibits the delivery of endocytosed material from endosomes to lysosomes, promoting, thus, the generation of exosomes (Raposo and Marks, 2007) and/or induces a failure of lysosomal acidification, which is essential for normal endocytosis (Liang et al., 2003), remains to be determined.

To explore the relationship between MTX exportation and melanosome trafficking, we studied the possible interaction of MTX with melanin (Sánchez-del-Campo et al., 2009a). Such interaction was confirmed by incubating this drug with synthetic 3,4-dihydroxyphenylalanine (DOPA)-melanin. Importantly, folic acid and 5-methyl-THF, the natural source of cellular folates, did not appear to interact with synthetic DOPA-melanin. A comparison of the interaction of several folates (folic acid and 5-methyl-THF) and antifolates (MTX and aminopterin) with synthetic DOPA-melanin indicated that the double amino group of the pterin ring is an important molecular requirement for the drug-melanin interaction. Therefore, the physiological importance of the high affinity of melanin for antifolates, such as MTX and aminopterin, for drug melanosomal sequestration is also another important issue that remains to be addressed. Endocytic transport of molecules involves several processes, including the fusion of early and late endosomes and the dissociation of receptor-ligand complexes through the acidic pH of preformed vesicles (Sabharanjak and Mayor, 2004). After melanosome biogenesis from MTX-loaded endosomes, dissociated MTX could be trapped in the melanosomes by its interaction with melanins. In contrast, folate substrates would not be sequestered in melanosomes due to their low affinities for melanin; facilitated by the acidic pH of this organelle, uncharged reduced folates would leave the melanosome by passive diffusion and reach the cytosol, where they would become available for cellular functions. Therefore, elucidation of the molecular basis for the (anti)folate interaction with melanins could have important therapeutic implications, and this study might be used as a guide for the synthesis of new antifolates or for using existing antifolates in ways that escape melanin trapping.

In addition to these cellular mechanisms of resistance to MTX in melanoma, other mechanism that includes liver transformation of the drug has also been reported. A paradoxical response of malignant melanoma to MTX *in vivo* and *in vitro* has been described (Gaukroger et al., 1983). The authors observed that MTX showed consistent cytotoxicity for melanoma cells *in vitro* but was ineffective at equivalent concentrations *in vivo*. MTX undergoes oxidation to its primary metabolite 7-hydroxy-MTX (7-OH-MTX) in the liver by the enzyme aldehyde oxidase (Assaraf, 2007) and therefore, this transformation has been proposed as a novel mechanism of resistance to explain this paradox (Gaukroger et al., 1983; Assaraf, 2007). In contrast to the large body of literature available on the multiple modalities of MTX resistance, very little is known regarding the ability of 7-OH-MTX to provoke antifolate-resistance phenomena that may disrupt MTX activity. Recent studies seem to indicate that 7-OH-MTX which exceeds by far MTX in the plasma of MTX-treated patients can provoke distinct modalities of antifolate-resistance that severely compromise the efficacy of the parent drug MTX (Joerger et al., 2006).

3. The antifolate activity of tea catechins

Recent studies have presented data that show a variety of biological activities of tea catechins, compounds which constitute about 15% (dry weight) of green tea (Mukhtar & Ahmad, 2000; Fujiki et al., 2002). Green tea catechins include: (-)-epigallocatechin gallate (EGCG), (-)-epigallocatechin (EGC), (-)-epicatechin gallate (ECG) and (-)-epicatechin (EC). EGCG is the most abundant (one 240 mL cup of brewed tea contains up to 200 mg EGCG), and many health benefits, including antioxidant, antibiotic and antiviral activities, have been attributed to this compound (Yam et al., 1998; Mabe et al., 1999; Hamilton-Miller, 2001). Some authors consider EGCG alone to be the active anticancer component, while others suggest that other tea constituents also have antiproliferative or anticarcinogenic properties (Jung & Ellis, 2001). Green tea extracts have been shown *in vitro* to stimulate apoptosis of various cancer cell lines, including prostate, lymphoma, colon, and lung (Yang et al., 2000; Mukhtar & Ahmad, 2000; Jung & Ellis, 2001; Gupta et al., 2003). Moreover, EGCG was reported to inhibit tumour invasion and angiogenesis, processes that are essential for tumour growth and metastasis (Jung & Ellis, 2001). Despite great efforts during the last two decades to understand the anticarcinogenic activity of tea, the exact mechanism(s) of action are not well defined. Therefore, deciphering the molecular mechanism by which green tea or its polyphenols impart their antiproliferative effects could be important and may result in improved opportunities for the treatment of cancer.

Based on the observation that classical (MTX) and non-classical (TMP) antifolate compounds possess similar chemical structures to some tea polyphenols (Navarro-Perán et al., 2005a), we started to work on the hypothesis that tea catechins could inhibit DHFR activity. Suppression of DNA synthesis by tea catechins could explain many of the observed effects on cancer inhibition by these compounds. Recently, we have shown that ester bonded gallate catechins isolated from green tea, such as EGCG and ECG are potent inhibitors of DHFR activity *in vitro* at concentrations found in the serum and tissues of green tea drinkers (0.1–1.0 μM) (Navarro-Perán et al., 2005b). EGCG exhibited the kinetic characteristics of a slow-binding inhibitor of DHF reduction with bovine liver DHFR but of a classical, reversible, competitive inhibitor with chicken liver DHFR. Structural modelling showed that EGCG can bind to human DHFR in a similar orientation to that observed for a number of structurally characterized DHFR inhibitor complexes (Fig. 1) (Navarro-Perán et al., 2005a). These results suggested that EGCG could act as an antifolate compound in the same way as MTX and TMP. Since these first reports describing the inhibition of DHFR by tea polyphenols, several studies by us and other laboratories have reported that EGCG inhibits DHFR from a variety of biological sources (Navarro-Martínez et al., 2005; 2006; Navarro-Perán et al., 2007; Hannewald et al., 2008; Kao et al., 2008; Spina et al., 2008; Sánchez-del-

Campo et al., 2010a). Recently, a screening of DHFR-binding drugs by MALDI-TOFMS demonstrated that EGCG is an active inhibitor of DHFR and has a relative affinity between that of pyrimethamine and MTX (Hannewald et al., 2008).

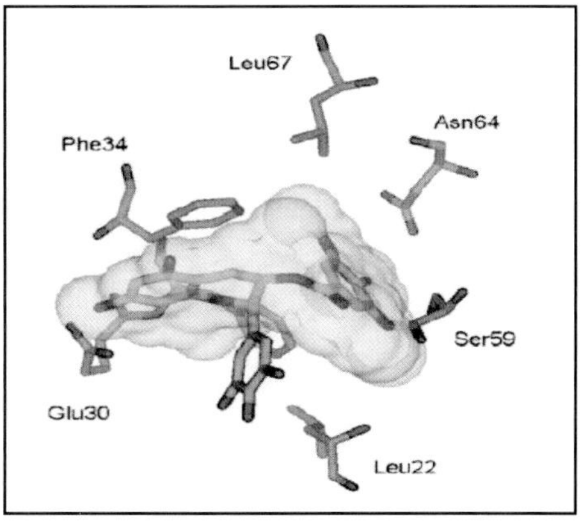

Fig. 1. View of EGCG modeled into the folate-binding site of human DHFR (Navarro-Perán et al., 2005a). Carbon atoms of the ECG ligand and surrounding protein are colored green and grey respectively. Residue Phe-31, located behind the EGCG, is unlabelled. Four different ligands from human and chicken DHFR crystal structures were used to define a binding envelope, shown in cyan; these were placed in a common orientation by superimposing backbone atoms from a common set of protein residues located around the ligands. Ligands from the following PDB structure files were used; 1DR1 (biopterin), 1S3V (TQD), 1S3W, and 1DLR. The figure was prepared using ViewerLite software.

Other studies have been focused in understand weather the antifolate activity of tea catechins could explain their anti-inflammatory and antitumoral properties (Navarro-Perán et al., 2007; Navarro-Perán et al., 2008). The most common use of MTX is as an anticancer drug, although the drug is also considered to have anti-inflammatory and immuno-suppressive properties with accompanying activity against autoimmune disorders (Cutolo et al., 2001). Inflammation is central to our fight against pathogens, but if it is not ordered and timely the resulting chronic inflammation may contribute to diseases such as arthritis, heart attacks and Alzheimer's disease. A functional link between chronic inflammation and cancer has long been suspected (Aggarwal, 2004; Balkwill & Coussens, 2004). This link is of great interest in the context of this chapter because green tea has shown remarkable anti-inflammatory activity (Sueoka et al., 2001). Understanding the mechanisms by which EGCG imparts this effect could be of importance for explaining the epidemiological data on the prophylactic effects of diets high in gallate polyphenols for certain forms of cancer. Most solid tumors contain many non-malignant cells, including immune cells and blood-vessel cells, which are important in inflammation, although the crucial molecular pathways that permit communication between abnormally growing cancer cells and these inflammatory cells remain unknown. A mouse model of inflammation-associated cancer now points to the involvement of the gene transcription factor NF-κB and the inflammatory mediator known as TNF-α in cancer progression (Pikarsky et al., 2004). Several of the anti-inflammatory effects of MTX and other antifolates can be explained by the suppression of NF-κB activation, a multisubunit factor known to play a role in inflammation, immune modulation and cell proliferation.

Although the mechanism by which antifolates modulate NF-κB activation has remained unclear for some time, recent investigations have demonstrated that MTX could inhibit the TNF-α-induced NF-κB activation though the release of adenosine (Cutolo et al., 2001; Majumdar & Aggarwal, 2001). By lowering THF cofactors, MTX inhibits two steps of the purine synthesis pathway: the conversion of GAR to FGAR and the conversion of AICAR to FAICAR. Excess AICAR inhibits the conversion of AMP to IMP by AMP deaminase, while AMP is rapidly converted to adenosine by surface expressed ecto-5′ nucleotidase. Adenosine is a potent endogenous regulator of a variety of physiological processes through specific receptors on the cell surface and binds to four different types of G protein-coupled cell surface molecules, termed the A_1, A_2A, A_2B, and A_3 adenosine receptors (Linden, 2001). After binding to the cell surface receptors, adenosine alters the immune cell production of soluble mediators such as cytokines, free radicals, and arachidonic acid metabolites (Majumdar & Aggarwal, 2001). Although MTX is widely used for the treatment of inflammatory and autoimmune diseases, its use as a chemopreventive agent is precluded, even at low doses, due to its adverse side effects. However, there is no evidence for such side effects as a result of the regular consumption of tea. The finding that EGCG shares mechanisms of action with MTX could be of interest, and suggests that the regulation of chronic inflammation by EGCG could represents a strong possibility to explain the epidemiological data concerning the green tea's prophylactic effects on certain forms of cancer (Yang et al., 2000). To check our hypothesis that the anti-inflammatory properties of EGCG could be related to its antifolate action and whether adenosine and its receptors are involved in EGCG action, we investigated the EGCG-induced suppression of NF-κB in Caco-2 cell monolayer, which acted as a model of the human intestinal epithelium (Navarro-Perán et al., 2008). We observed that EGCG, by inhibiting DHFR, can disturb the metabolism of this vitamin in Caco-2 cells, producing the release of adenosine and the suppression of NF-κB. The data suggest that by modulating NF-κB activation, EGCG might not only combat inflammation, but also cancer. Since by reducing chronic inflammation there is a strong possibility of modulating tumorogenesis, these results could be of importance for explaining tea's cancer preventive effects.

4. Synthetic catechins as antifolate prodrugs against melanoma

Despite the excellent properties of tea catechins, they have at least one limitation, their low bioavailability (Nakagawa & Miyazawa, 1997). Factors influencing this low bioavailability could be related to their low stability in neutral or slightly alkaline solutions and their inability to cross cellular membranes (Hong et al., 2002). In an attempt to solve such bioavailability problems, we first synthesized a 3,4,5-trimethoxybenzoyl analogue of ECG [3-O-(3,4,5-trimethoxybenzoyl)-(-)-epicatechin, TMECG] (Sánchez-del-Campo et al., 2008). This compound was successfully synthesized following the five-step reaction sequence shown in Fig. 2, starting from the commercially available catechin. In comparing the antiproliferative activity of TMECG on several human and mouse cancer cell lines, we noticed that this compound was much more active on melanoma cells than on normal human melanocytes and other epithelial cancer cell lines from breast, lung and colon cancers (Sánchez-del-Campo et al., 2008; Sánchez-del-Campo et al., 2009b). Next, we designed experiments to throw light on the elevated activity of TMECG on melanoma cell lines. As one of the most striking differences between melanoma and other epithelial cells is the presence of tyrosinase in melanoma, we wondered whether TMECG cytotoxicity against melanoma might be mediated by cellular tyrosinase activation. The results indicated that tyrosinase oxidized TMECG to its corresponding o-quinone, which quickly evolved through a series of chemical reactions to a quinone methide (QM), which showed high stability over a wide pH range (Fig. 3).

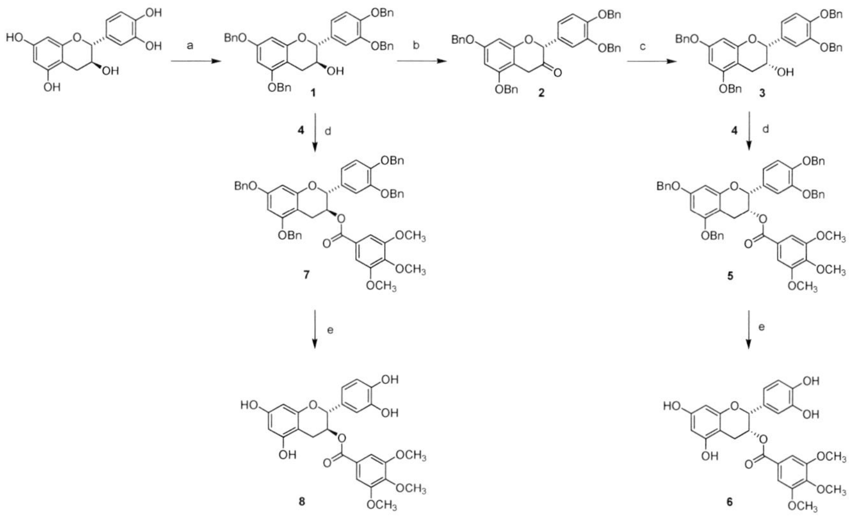

Fig. 2. Synthesis of TMECG (6) and TMCG (8). Reagents and conditions: (a) benzyl bromide, K_2CO_3, N,N-dimethylformamide, -10ºC to rt; (b) Dess-Martin periodinane, moist CH_2Cl_2, rt; (c) L-Selectride, n-Bu_4NCl, THF, -78ºC; (d) 3,4,5-trimethoxybenzoyl chloride, 4, CH_2Cl_2, DMAP, rt; (e) H_2, 20% Pd/C, THF/MeOH, rt.

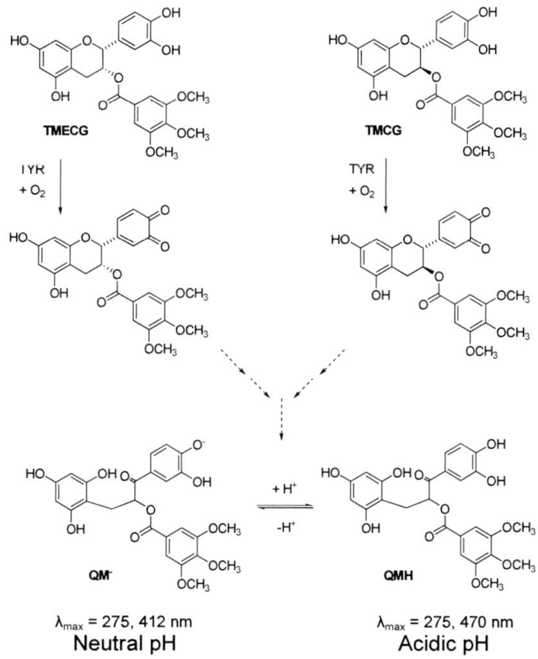

Fig. 3. Reaction sequences indicating the oxidation of TMECG and TMCG by tyrosinase and the formation of quinone methide (QM) species.

The TMECG-QM was found to be a potent irreversible inhibitor of human DHFR, and this highly stable product may be responsible for TMECG's high activity against melanoma cells (Sánchez-del-Campo et al., 2009b). To explain the irreversibility on the binding of TMECG-QM to human DHFR, we performed *in silico* molecular modelling experiments. TMECG bound to human DHFR in a similar way to that described for EGCG binding (Navarro-Perán et al., 2005a), with specific hydrogen bonding interactions, most notably involving Glu-30 (Fig. 4). However, the open structure of QM increases its molecular flexibility, and it adopts a different conformation in the active site of human DHFR (Fig. 4). QM maintained the hydrogen bond with the Glu-30 side chain (O · · · ·O distance 1.99 Å), but three new interactions were detected. The other phenolic group of ring A forms a hydrogen bond with Ile-7, whereas the other two hydrogen bonds formed between two oxygens of the methoxy groups of ring D and Ser-59 and Ile-60. This strong interaction between QM and different residues of the protein could explain the irreversibility of the inhibitor-protein complex.

Prodrugs are compounds that must be transformed before exhibiting their pharmacological action. They are often divided into two groups: those designed to increase bioavailability to improve the pharmacokinetics of antitumor agents, and those designed to deliver antitumor agents locally (Rooseboom et al., 2004). TMECG could, therefore, be considered an anticancer prodrug on melanoma since it showed both of these characteristics. Therapies with TMECG would increase bioavailability and would achieve high melanoma drug concentrations. The soft antifolate character (Graffner-Nordberg et al., 2004) of the prodrug (TMECG), its specific activation on melanoma cells and the fact that antifolates are more active on fast-dividing cancer cells make this compound ideal for the prevention and treatment of this skin pathology.

However, the synthesis of TMECG is difficult and results in low yields. Therefore, we synthesized a related-epimer compound with catechin configuration [3-O-(3,4,5-trimethoxybenzoyl)-(-)-catechin (TMCG)] (Fig. 2) (Sáez-Ayala et al., 2011). As observed in this figure TMECG and TMCG share the first synthesis step, but the yields of the other synthetic steps were significantly different. The overall yield of TMCG in the two steps of alkylation and deprotection was 88%; however, the overall yield of TMECG in the four steps of epimerisation of C-3 (oxidation and reduction), alkylation and deprotection was 16%. The difference between these yields was due to the limiting stereoselective reduction of compound 2 (Fig. 2), which gives moderate yield and purity and requires further purifications lowering the yield. Because of the absence of the limiting reduction step, the synthesis of TMCG was simpler (only three steps) and more economical (only common reagents). Since the active product of TMECG in melanoma is its QM derivative, we hypothesized that both TMECG and TMCG should have similar activity against these cancer cells (Sáez-Ayala et al., 2011). Oxidation of TMCG and TMECG by tyrosinase is predicted to generate the same final product because proton-catalysed hydrolysis of ring C would generate a freely rotating carbon (C-3), which should prevent epimeric differences in the QM product (Fig. 3). To confirm that TMECG and TMCG generate the same quinonic product after tyrosinase oxidation, both substrates were oxidised *in vitro* using mushroom tyrosinase as a catalyst. The final products of the corresponding oxidations were analysed and compared using several spectroscopic techniques. Tyrosinase oxidised TMECG and TMCG to stable final products, which varied in colour from yellow to orange depending on pH. The products had similar spectroscopic properties, with λmax at 275/412 nm at acidic pH and 275/470 nm at higher pH values (pKa = 6.9). Thus, the UV-Vis spectroscopy data indicated that, as represented in Fig. 3, both TMEGC and TMCG generated the same QM product after tyrosinase oxidation. Mass spectroscopy confirmed these results, and the spectra of both final oxidation products exhibited the same molecular ion peak. High-performance liquid chromatography-mass spectrometry (HPLC-MS) revealed that the molecular weights of the compounds were 498.7 (for TMECG) and 498.8 (for TMCG), which correspond to the calculated mass of the QM product depicted in Fig. 3. Both molecules were analysed by MS/MS and produced the same daughter ion peaks at m/z 363 and m/z 287, corresponding to the loss of the dihydroxybenzoyl moiety and the trimethoxybenzoyl moiety, respectively.

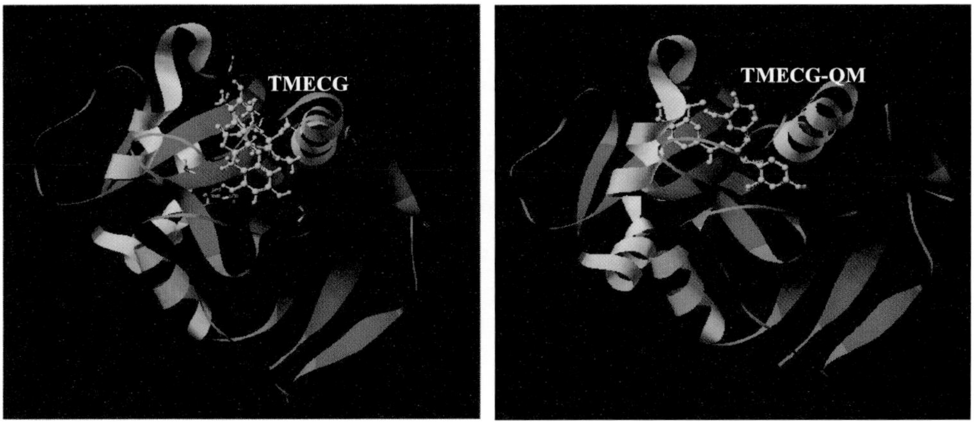

Fig. 4. Molecular modelling for the binding of TMECG and TMECG-QM to human DHFR.

5. Antitumoral activity of TMECG in melanoma

5.1 TMECG inhibits folate metabolism and transport in melanoma

The folate cycle plays a central role in cell metabolism. Among its important functions are the delivery of one-carbon units to the methionine cycle for use in methylation reactions, and the synthesis of pyrimidines and purines. Several enzymes, including DHFR, TS and methyltetrahydrofolate reductase (MTHFR), participate in the activation and regeneration of folic acid coenzymes. Several studies have shown that the protein and mRNA levels of TS and DHFR are higher in tumor tissues and cancer cells than in their normal counterpart (Kufe et al., 1980; Rahman et al., 2004). Tumors with high levels of these enzymes are thought to undergo more active cellular proliferation, which, in turn, is associated with tumor invasiveness and metastasis. Having demonstrated the strong *in vitro* inhibition of human DHFR by QM, further experiments were designed to test its antifolate activity in culture systems. To investigate whether TMECG could interfere with folate metabolism in cancer cells, the levels of expression of these folate cycle genes were analyzed in melanoma SK-MEL-28 cells using real time PCR (Sánchez-del-Campo et al., 2008). As observed in other tumor tissues and cells, the genes involved in the metabolism of folic acid were highly overexpressed in melanoma cells compared with normal melanocytes. The levels of DHFR, TS and MTHFR mRNAs were calculated to be about 400-, 22- and 4-fold higher, respectively, in melanoma cells than in normal melanocytes. Treatment of SK-MEL-28 with TMECG produced a substantial and rapid downregulation of these genes, involving significant changes in the mRNA levels of the genes at 24 h of treatment. DHFR, TS and

MTHFR mRNA levels were similar to that detected in normal melanocyte cells after 5 days of TMECG treatment. The data indicated that TMECG disturbs the folate metabolism in melanoma cells and suggest that this might be the mechanism by which TMECG induces cell growth inhibition and death.

It is widely accepted that antifolates block the *de novo* biosynthesis of thymine, purines and pyrimidines by inhibiting the synthesis of THF, an essential cofactor in these biosynthetic pathways, and that the administration of exogenous reduced folates, such as leucovorin (5-formyl-THF), or growing the cells in an HT-medium, effectively prevent antifolate cytotoxicity in mammalian cells. We observed that TMECG was more active on cells growing in a normal culture medium than in an HT medium (Sánchez-del-Campo et al., 2009b); however, leucovorin did not "rescue" SK-MEL-28 cells from TMECG-induced death. Recently, it has been reported that natural tea catechins inhibit folate transport in Caco-2 cells, which might be partly responsible for their antifolate activity (Alemdaroglu et al., 2007). Therefore, to understand the different response of SK-MEL-28 to leucovorin- and HT-treatments, and to prove or discard the *in vivo* antifolate activity of TMECG, the status of the RFC, the major protein involved in the transport of reduced folates, was analyzed in this cell line. RFC mRNA expression was significantly higher in SK-MEL-28 than in normal human melanocytes (8.9 times), but treating SK-MEL-28 with TMECG strongly downregulated RFC gene expression. The time-dependent effect of TMECG on SK-MEL-28 was studied using RT PCR, and the data indicated that cells responded quickly to TMECG treatment with a more than 80% reduction in RFC expression 24 h after treatment. Protein levels of this transporter correlated with gene expression (Sánchez-del-Campo et al., 2009b). This finding could explain why leucovorin did not affect TMECG treatments. As demonstrated, TMECG highly down-regulated the RFC and, therefore, SK-MEL-28 cells became practically impermeable to leucovorin during TMECG treatment and can not, therefore, restore the reduced folate levels in the cells.

5.2 TMECG downregulates DHFR expression in melanoma

As described for other cancer cell lines, DHFR is overexpressed in melanoma (Kufe et al., 1980). The level of DHFR polyA+ mRNA in these melanoma cells was estimated to be 400 to 500 times higher than in normal human melanocytes, resulting in increased DHFR protein content (Sánchez-del-Campo et al., 2009b). An increase in DHFR expression/activity after antifolate treatment has been recognized as a mechanism of resistance of cancer cells to antineoplastic drugs. As expected, treatment of SK-MEL-28 with MTX resulted in a significant increase of DHFR mRNA and protein. However, treatment of SK-MEL-28 with TMECG rapidly reduced DHFR mRNA and protein to normal levels. The efficient down-regulation of DHFR by TMECG is evidence of its proposed antifolate activity. The lack of reduced folate coenzyme recycling by DHFR could be one of the reasons for its *in vivo* activity.

The mechanism by which TMECG-QM downregulates DHFR expression in melanoma has been studied in more detail (Sánchez-del-Campo et al., 2010b). TMECG-QM has a dual action on these cells. First, it acts as a potent antifolate compound, disrupting folate metabolism and increasing intracellular oxidized folate coenzymes, such as DHF, which is a non-competitive inhibitor of dihydropterine reductase, an enzyme essential for tetrahydrobiopterin (H_4B) recycling. Such inhibition results in H_4B deficiency, endothelial nitric oxide synthase (eNOS) uncoupling and superoxide production. Second, TMECG-QM acts as an efficient superoxide scavenger and promotes intra-cellular H_2O_2 accumulation. We presented evidence that TMECG markedly reduces melanoma H_4B and NO bioavailability and that TMECG action is abolished by the eNOS inhibitor Nω-nitro-L-arginine methyl ester or the H_2O_2 scavenger catalase, which strongly suggested H_2O_2-dependent DHFR downregulation (Sánchez-del-Campo et al., 2010b). It is this duality that may be of importance for TMECG action. Classical antifolate compounds are very effective in inhibiting DHFR but the lack of an antioxidant property may be the cause of the lack of DHFR downregulation. In cells treated with antifolates, the common effect is the overexpression of DHFR, which may be responsible for cell resistance to antifolates and is probably the reason that these compounds fail to treat melanoma (Zhao & Goldman, 2003). In addition, antioxidant therapies have little effect on melanoma. It is interesting to speculate that unsatisfactory outcomes of some of these antioxidant therapies are partially due to their ineffectiveness in uncoupling the eNOS reaction (Chalupsky & Cai, 2005).

5.3 TMECG induces apoptosis in melanoma cells

To investigate whether the metabolic changes induced by TMECG resulted in the apoptosis of melanoma cells, melanoma cell lines were treated for seven days with different concentrations of this compound and the degree of apoptosis induction was evaluated using a DNA fragmentation assay (Sánchez-del-Campo & Rodríguez-López, 2008). The results indicated that the reduced viability of melanoma cells in the presence of TMECG was indeed due to apoptosis induction. The data also indicated that normal melanocytes were highly resistant to TMECG-induced apoptosis, which is a highly desirable feature for potential antitumoral agents. TMECG-induced apoptosis was studied in greater detail using the SK-MEL-28 cell line. SK-MEL-28 cells exposed to 50 μM TMECG for seven days showed evident signs of cellular damage. Morphological changes included cell shrinkage, loss of cell-cell contact and the fragmentation of plasmatic and nuclear membranes (Fig. 5). Another feature of apoptotic cell death, the activation of caspase-3, was evaluated by a colorimetric activity assay and Western blot analysis. The cells treated with TMECG showed significantly higher caspase-3 activity. Immunoblot analysis confirmed caspase-3 activation (Fig. 5). The Bcl-2 family proteins play a critical regulatory role through their interacting pro- and anti-apoptotic members, which integrate a wide array of upstream survival and distress signals to decide the fate of cells. Bax and Bcl-2 proteins are the key elements of this protein family. As reported for EGCG (Nihal et al., 2005), TMECG treatment resulted in a decrease in anti-apoptotic Bcl-2 and an increase in proapoptotic Bax at the levels of mRNA and protein, thereby resulting in a significant increase in the Bax/Bcl-2 ratio that favors apoptosis. Immunohistochemistry results also indicated that TMECG treatment caused mitochondrial translocation of Bax, which is a common response of cancer cells subject to certain apoptotic stimuli (Choi & Singh, 2005).

In general, melanoma cells are quite resistant to apoptosis and it has recently been shown that these cells can avoid suicide by inactivating the apoptosis protease-activating factor-1 (Apaf-1) gene, which is one step further on from p53 in the apoptosis pathway (Soengas et al., 2001). It was proposed that Apaf-1 inactivation involves the addition of methyl groups to cytosine nucleotides in DNA and the removal of acetyl groups from the hystone proteins that bundle DNA into the compressed form seen in the nucleus. *In vivo*, loss of expression of Apaf-1 has been associated with tumor progression, suggesting that Apaf-1 inactivation may provide a selective survival advantage to neoplastic cells (Soengas et al., 2001). To

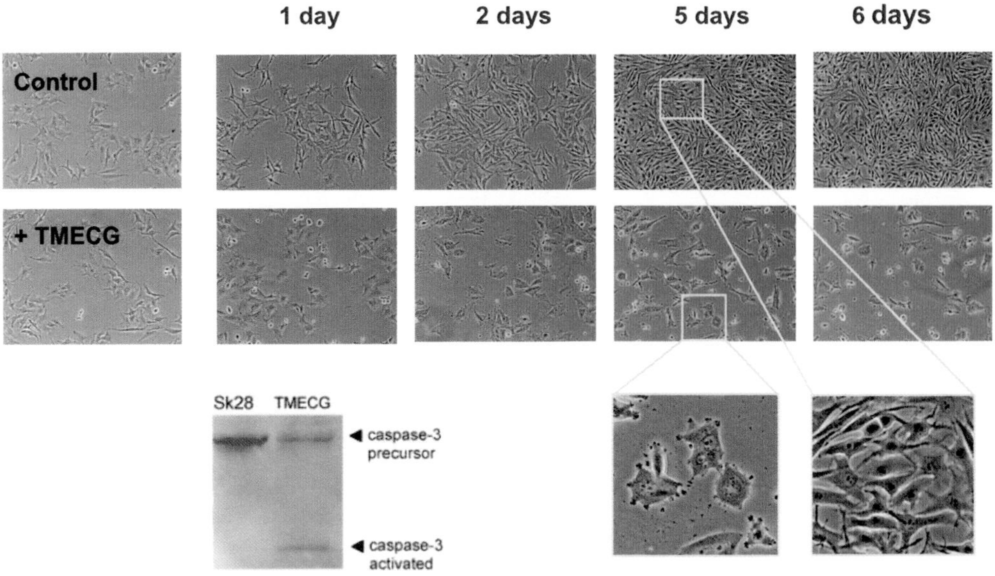

Fig. 5. Apoptosis of SK-MEL-28 induced by TMECG visualized by the morphological aspect of untreated SK-MEL-28 cells compared with those subject to treatment with 50 μM TMECG. The effect of TMECG on the protein content of caspase-3 in SK-MEL-28 was visualized by Western blot analysis in control cells (Sk28) and those treated with TMECG. Cells were treated for 7 days with 50 μM TMECG

evaluate the participation of Apaf-1 in SK-MEL-28 apoptosis during TMECG treatment, its mRNA and protein levels were determined by PCR and Western blot, respectively (Sánchez-del-Campo & Rodríguez-López, 2008). Apaf-1 mRNA and protein were detected in SK-MEL-28 and their levels were essentially the same than those detected in normal human melanocytes. This data indicated that, although methylation of Apaf-1 has been proposed as a mechanism for controlling its expression, TMECG, which decreased cellular methylation in SK-MEL-28 cells, was not able to produce Apaf-1 activation. These results are in accordance with others which found that drugs acting on different mechanisms did not induce or upregulate the expression of Apaf-1 at the levels of mRNA and protein (Zanon et al., 2004).

5.4 TMEGC inhibits growth and metastasis of induced melanoma tumors in mice

To check whether TMECG was pharmacologically active in *in vivo* situations and to study the possible inactivation of TMECG in the body, we performed experiments to test the effectiveness of this compound in induced melanoma tumors in mice. The group receiving TMECG therapy showed significantly longer survival times than the control group (Fig. 6). Moreover, we observed that tumor growth was significantly reduced by the treatment with TMECG but not with MTX (Fig. 6). The observation that TMECG-treated animals survived with larger tumors indicated that treatment could also reduce the metastasis of primary tumors. To confirm this, a third group was inoculated with B16 melanoma cells and treated with TMECG for 21 days (median survival time of the control group). After this time the animals were sacrificed and a post-mortem examination of the lungs was performed to search for metastatic lesions. Secondary metastasis in the lungs was more frequent in control mice (Fig. 6), while treatment with TMECG drastically reduced lung metastasis. The lungs of the control animals showed prominent tumor nodules around the terminal bronchioles. These tumour nodules were composed of polygonal tumor cells with a prominent nucleolus. Intracellular melanin deposition and clear areas of necrosis were also detected. The lungs of the TMECG-treated tumor-bearing animals showed no significant tumor mass. The alveoli and pleura were tumor free, and the alveolar passage was lined with healthy ciliated columnar epithelial cells.

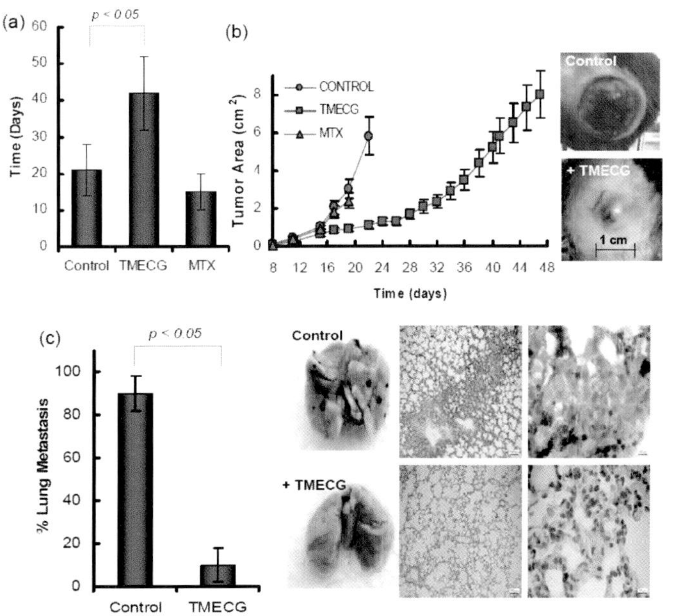

Fig. 6. Inhibition of melanoma growth and metastasis by TMECG: (a) Median survival time following tumor implantation; (b) Mean tumor size in C57/B16 mice bearing B16 melanomas. (c) Rate of metastasis in postmortem and histological examination of lungs showing general aspect and histopathological analysis of lungs from C57/B16 mice bearing the B16 melanoma in control and TMECG-treated animals (Sánchez-del-Campo et al., 2009b).

5.5 Proposed mechanism for the activation and antitumoral activity of TMEGC on melanoma

Taken in consideration all these observations a mechanism for the activation, cellular distribution and action of TMECG and its products may now be proposed (Fig. 7). Although TMECG efficiently binds to DHFR, we hypothesized that this hydrophobic compound would cross the cell membrane without needing to bind to folate transporters. Therefore, the most plausible transport mechanism for this lipophilic drug is passive diffusion across the plasma membrane in a manner driven solely by the concentration gradient (Fig. 7a). Its independence from folate transporters means that TMECG may avoid transport-mediated resistance mechanisms (Ma et al., 2000). In fact, TMECG downregulated RFC but, far from

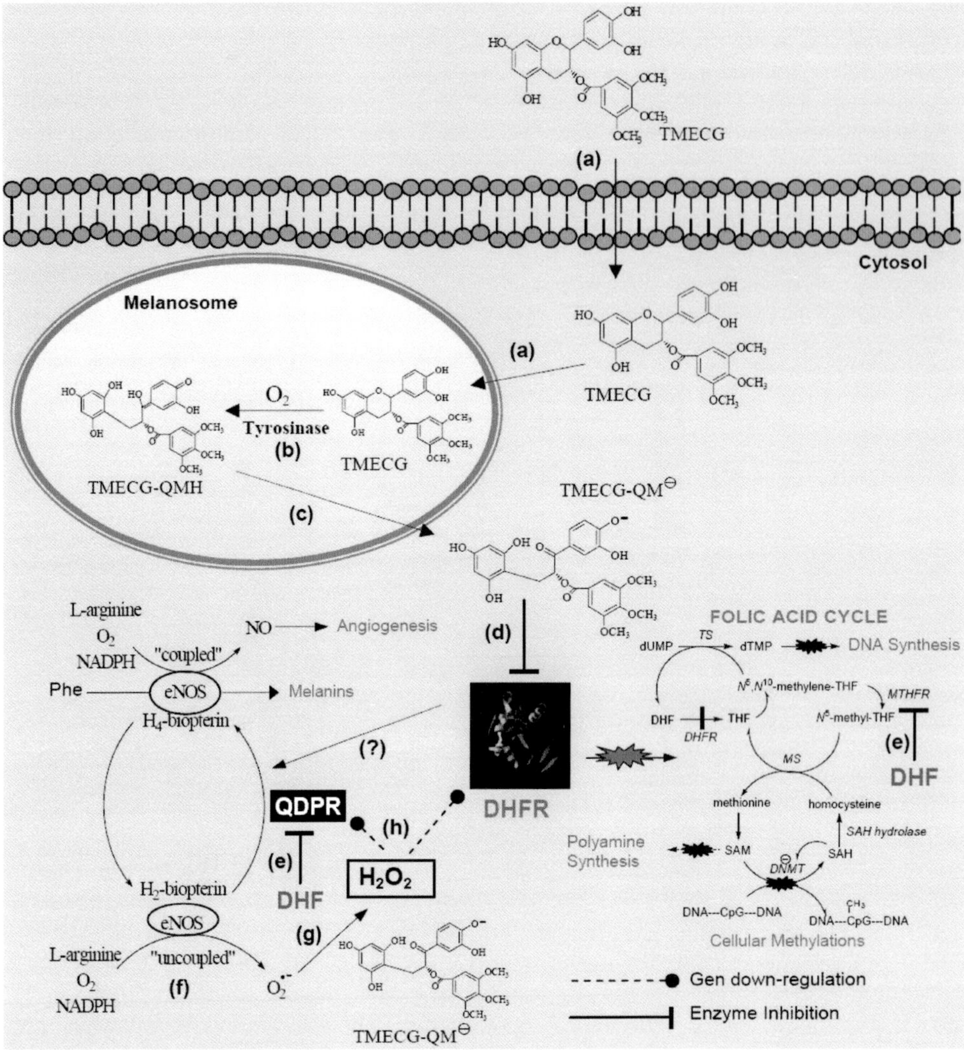

Fig. 7. Schematic mechanism underlying activation, cellular distribution and action of TMECG in melanoma cells (Sánchez-del-Campo et al., 2010b).

being a disadvantage, this could represent an important advantage for its antiproliferative action. Downregulation of RFC would reduce intracellular folate pools, reducing competition reactions with the active form of TMECG and the molecular target, DHFR. Subsequent transport to the melanosome by a concentration gradient would facilitate its tyrosinase-catalyzed oxidation and transformation to the corresponding QM (Fig. 7b). Observations from our laboratory indicated that TMECG or TMECG-QM did not interact with DOPA-melanins, which may avoid melanosomal trapping. Because of the low pH of this organelle, the predominant form is QMH, which, due to its high stability and the absence of formal charge, would exit the melanosome and enter the cytosol (Fig. 7c). Under the slightly basic pH of the cytosol, the anionic form of QM would be the predominant form, and it would be trapped in this compartment due to its formal negative charge. This retention mechanism would represent another advantage with respect to antifolates that require polyglutamylation for cellular retention. This would be even more essential in cancer cell environments, in which folate requirements lead to an increase in the cellular THF-cofactor pools. As the THF-cofactor pool is increased, there is a feedback inhibition of folate polyglutamylation, which results in the accumulation of easily exported compounds (Tse & Moran, 1998). Once in the cytosol, TMECG-QM may inhibit DHFR activity and, in addition, lead to the downregulation of DHFR (Fig. 7d-h). The finding that tyrosinase is highly overexpressed in melanoma cells with respect to normal melanocytes might also influence the degree, the specificity and the duration of the antifolate inhibitory effect of TMECG-QM. Finally, the data on the effectiveness of TMECG in mouse melanoma models indicates that TMECG is bioavailable for cancer cells and avoids not only cellular mechanisms of resistance to antifolates but also mechanisms related with body drug inactivation.

6. Combined therapies to improve the activity of synthetic catechins in melanoma

The combination of several drugs to improve the clinical efficiency of the treatments is a common strategy for the fighting of pathological bacteria. For instance, TMP is used in combination with sulphonamides as a therapy against multiple bacterial infections. These are treatment based in the metabolic attack of the bacteria, where TMP inhibits the recycling of folic acid coenzymes and the sulphonamide inhibits the synthesis of folic acid. Conventional chemotherapy treatments against cancer have shown important clinical limitations and, therefore, it would be of interest to develop new and more efficient strategies for the treatment of this fatal pathology. The metabolic attack of cancer cells could be an interesting perspective. The identification of metabolic and signalling pathways essential for tumour growth and dissemination, but less important for healthy cells, could guide the development of new cancer therapies. The combination of several drugs to target several metabolic and/or signalling pathways could increase the efficiency of the treatments. Recently, it has been observed that the major catechin presented in green tea, EGCG, showed synergic activity with other drugs commonly used for the treatment of several cancers and in some cases EGCG sensitizes cancer cells to other treatments (Liu et al., 2001; Farabegoli et al., 2007). The identification of synthetic catechins as antifolate compounds can help the design of more directed combined therapies against melanoma since the folic acid has multiple connections with metabolic and signalling pathways. Thus, we started this application targeting the methionine cycle in melanoma using TMECG in combination with other drugs (Fig. 8).

Malignant tumors are characterized by a high rate of growth. Tumor cells drain the energy of the host, particularly glucose but also amino acids. Methionine is an essential amino acid with at least four major functions (Fig. 8) (Cellarier et al., 2003). First, methionine participates in protein synthesis. Second, methionine is a precursor of glutathione, a tripeptide that reduces reactive oxygen species, thereby protecting cells from oxidative stress (Anderson, 1998). Third, it is required for the formation of polyamines, which have far-ranging effects on nuclear and cell division (Thomas & Thomas, 2001). Fourth, methionine is the major source of the methyl groups necessary for the methylation of DNA and other molecules (Cellarier et al., 2003). It is important to bear in mind the well-established connection of the methionine cycle with two crucial cell metabolites, folic acid

and adenosine (Fig. 8). Folic acid acts as the fuel for the methionine cycle, which, after transformation by folate cycle enzymes such as DHFR, TS and MTHFR, forms 5-methyl-THF, the cofactor of methionine synthase (MS), the enzyme responsible for methionine synthesis (Fig. 8). Adenosine, in contrast, is a product of the methionine cycle, and is produced at high concentrations in tumor cells. The efficient intracellular elimination of this product by adenosine-transforming enzymes, such as adenosine deaminase (ADA), or its transport out of the cells by specific adenosine transporters, including the equilibrate nucleoside transporters (ENTs), is of vital importance for cancer cell survival.
The efficacy of antifolates in treating cancer is widely attributed to the subsequent decrease in nucleotide production, but in addition to these effects, antifolate treatment has also been linked to a decrease in cellular methylation. We observed that TMECG modulated the expression of genes involved in methionine metabolism, cellular methylation and glutathione synthesis in melanoma cells (Sánchez-del-Campo & Rodríguez-López, 2008). Having elucidated the effects of TMECG on the melanoma folate and methionine cycles, we designed therapeutical strategies to increase its effectiveness. Combinations of TMECG with S-adenosylmethionine (SAM) or compounds that modulate the intracellular concentration of adenosine strongly increase the antiproliferative effects of TMECG. The ability of TMECG to target multiple aspects related with melanoma survival, with a high degree of potency, points to its clinical value in melanoma therapy.

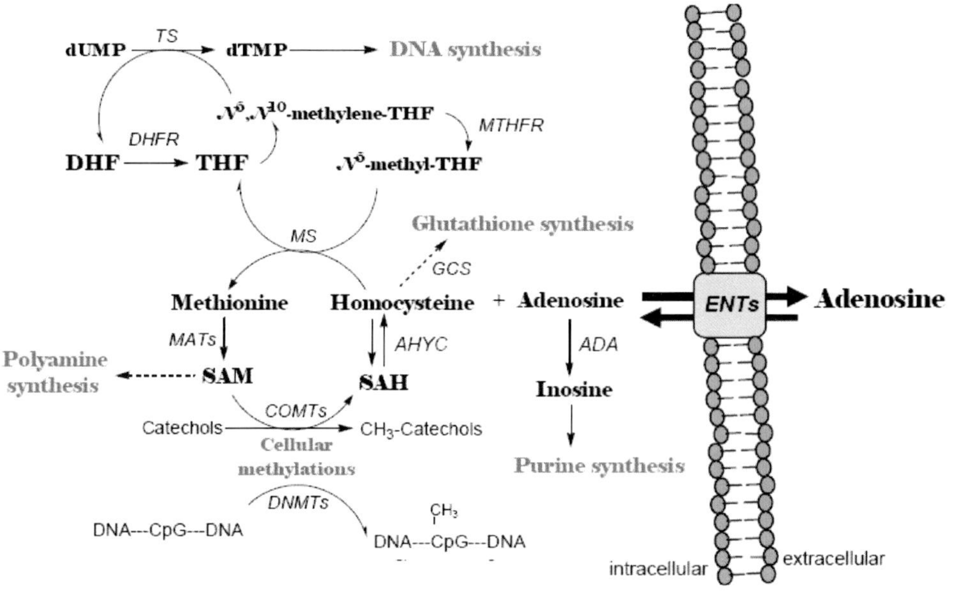

Fig. 8. The methionine cycle and its connections with several metabolic and survival cell pathways. Abbreviations: ADA, adenosine deaminase; AHYC, S-adenosylhomocysteine hydrolase; COMT, catechol-*O*-methyltransferase; DHF, dihydrofolate; DHFR, dihydrofolate reductase; DNMT, DNA methyltransferase; ENT, equilibrative nucleoside transporter; GCS, γ-glutamylcysteine synthetase; MAT, methionine adenosyltransferase; MS, methionine synthase; MTHFR, 5,10-methylenetetrahydrofolate reductase; SAH, S-adenosylhomocysteine; SAM, S-adenosylmethionine; THF, tetrahydrofolate; TS, thymine synthase.

6.1 SAM enhances the antiproliferative effects of TMECG

Having analyzed the ability of TMECG to disrupt the methionine cycle, we designed several strategies to completely block this pathway. The first strategy was to inhibit methionine adenosyltransferase-2A (MAT2A) enzyme (Fig. 8). MAT2A shows a very low K_m for methionine (4-10 μM) and, in tissues that predominantly express MAT2A, the rate of SAM synthesis is near maximal and relatively unaffected by fluctuations in methionine concentration and, thus, MAT2A can work even a very low concentration of methionine. Another kinetic characteristic of MAT2A is that this enzyme is strongly inhibited by SAM, its reaction product (IC_{50} = 60 μM) (Sullivan & Hoffman, 1983). We hypothesized that, by increasing intracellular SAM concentration in the presence of TMECG, two consecutive steps in the methionine cycle, the synthesis of methionine and the synthesis of SAM, could be blocked (Fig. 8). Only high concentrations of SAM (up to 100 μM) affected SK-MEL-28 growth in accordance with its calculated IC_{50} towards MAT2A. However, in the presence of TMECG, lower concentrations of SAM showed a synergistic behavior with this antifolate compound. Thus, the combination 20 μM SAM with 50 μM TMECG efficiently inhibited the growth of SK-MEL-28. The results indicated that when MAT2A is working at limiting concentrations of methionine in the presence of TMECG, it is highly susceptible to inhibition by low SAM concentrations.

6.2 Strategies to increase the intracellular concentration of adenosine in the presence of TMECG

As observed in Fig. 8, adenosine is a direct product of the methionine cycle, and is produced in high concentration when the cycle is highly active. Any resulting excess of adenosine may not be a problem for cancer cells. Adenosine is efficiently metabolized by specific enzymes such as ADA and adenosine kinase (ADK) before being used for purine nucleotide synthesis, which is even more necessary for DNA synthesis in these highly proliferating cells. Finally, excess adenosine can be transported out of the cells by ENTs, bidirectional transporters that allow adenosine release and uptake by facilitating diffusion along its concentration gradient. However, in the presence of an antifolate compound, adenosine accumulation might represent a severe problem for the cell. Depletion of 5-methyl-THF would result in the production of high concentrations of S-adenosylhomocysteine (SAH), which strongly inhibits cellular methyltransferases. This inhibition would produce an accumulation of SAM, which would inhibit the MAT2A reaction. We hypothesized that accumulation of adenosine in the presence of TMECG may block the methionine cycle at three levels: the synthesis of methionine, the methylase reaction and the synthesis of SAM (Fig. 8). Adenosine flux across the cellular membrane depends on the concentration gradients between extra- and intracellular nucleoside levels (Tabrizchi & Bedi, 2001). Therefore, we first tried to increase the extracellular concentration of adenosine. Adenosine alone had no detectable effect on SK-MEL-28 growth at the studied concentrations (up to 500 μM) but, in the presence of TMECG, adenosine had a significant synergistic effect, enhancing the antiproliferative action of this antifolate compound. A combination of 50 μM adenosine with 50 μM TMECG was seen to completely inhibit the growth of SK-MEL-28.

Although adenosine is currently used for the treatment of several cardiovascular diseases, its use as a therapeutic agent is restricted, since it is rapidly metabolized to inosine and AMP, which limits its ability to exert a systemic effect. Therefore, we planned other strategy to accumulate adenosine in melanoma cells using dipyridamole. This drug suppresses adenosine transport by inhibiting ENTs. Moreover, it also inhibits the enzyme ADA, which normally breaks down adenosine into inosine. We hypothesized that inhibition of ENTs and ADA in melanoma cells would result in an intracellular accumulation of adenosine, which, in the presence of TMECG-accumulated homocysteine, would produce an effective blockage of the methionine cycle. Dipyridamole alone inhibited SK-MEL-28 growth with a calculated IC_{50} (at 5 days) of 20 μM. However, in the presence of 50 μM TMECG, the IC_{50}-value fell to less than 1 μM. A combination of 5 μM dipyridamole with 50 μM TMECG had a deadly effect on melanoma cells. The results pointed to the possibility of using this combination treatment against malignant melanoma.

6.3 Methionine depletion for melanoma treatment: Conclusions

Conventional chemotherapy treatments have shown their limits, especially for patients with advancer cancer. New therapeutic strategies must be identified, and the metabolic abnormalities of cancer cell open up such opportunities (Cellarier et al., 2003). Many human cancer cells lines and primary tumors have an absolute need for methionine, an essential amino acid. In contrast, normal cells are relatively resistant to exogenous methionine restriction. We show that melanoma cells are highly dependent on methionine. The resistance of melanomas to general chemotherapies and their avoidance of cellular suicide or resistance to apoptosis is primarily related with the high activity of the methionine cycle in these cells, which permits the methylation of specific genes and activation of different survival pathways. Blockage of the methionine cycle by the new antifolate, TMECG, is an effective therapy for melanoma. The specific activity of TMECG on melanoma methionine cycle was confirmed by the high synergy found with compounds that uncoupled adenosine metabolism in these cells. In conclusion, our results show that TMECG is a potent antitumor agent that modulates multiple aspects of melanoma metabolism and survival, including the folic acid and the methionine cycles and the methylation status of the cells. This broad spectrum of antitumor activities in conjunction with low toxicity underlies the translational potential of TMECG and suggests it may be used as part of a therapeutic strategy against melanoma. A combination with other compounds that modulate melanoma methionine cycle, such as SAM, adenosine or dipyridamole, represents another promising strategy to combat this malignant skin pathology.

7. Conclusions

Several investigations indicate that natural and synthetic polyphenols may well be beneficial, not only in the prevention but also in the treatment of cancer. Antifolates are usually used as chemotherapeutic agents for certain types of cancer. Although antifolates such as MTX attack proliferating tissues selectively, they are also toxic to normal cells. Deleterious side effects are seen against tissues that proliferate as part of their normal function; such tissues include intestinal mucosa, hair cells, and components of the immune system. The "soft" character of polyphenols could be developed for use in the treatment of cancer with significantly reduced side effects compared to those of the DHFR inhibitors currently in use in chemotherapy such as MTX. Moreover, we have demonstrated that synthetic derivatives of ECG, TMECG and TMCG, might be considered a treatment for melanoma. Disruption of the cell folate cycle by these compounds and their active products may explain many of the molecular and cellular effects described for these synthetic polyphenols on melanoma cells because antifolates exert their action by disturbing the nucleic acid metabolism of cancer cells, including its synthesis, methylation and stability (Navarro-Perán et al., 2007; Sánchez-del-Campo & Rodríguez-López, 2008). We define them as *new generation antifolates* because they maintain the ability to inhibit DHFR and disrupt folate metabolism but show significant and important differences from other classical and non-classical antifolates. TMECG was seen to be active not only in melanoma cells in culture but was also effective in an animal model, where it inhibited growth and metastasis of preformed tumors. An additional advantage of these compounds is their *prodrug character*, which would favour its specific activity against melanoma cells and prevent unspecific side effects in rapidly dividing healthy cells. In addition, the multiple connections of the folic acid cycle with many metabolic and signalling pathways in melanoma cells could open the way for the development of new combined and directed therapies against this elusive skin pathology.

8. Acknowledgements

Research described was supported in part by a grant from Ministerio de Ciencia e Innovación (MICINN) (Project SAF2009-12043-C02-01). J.C-H is contracted by the Translational Cancer Research Group (Fundación para la Formación e Investigación Sanitarias). M.S-A has a fellowship from MICINN. M.F.M is contracted by an agreement with the Fundación de la Asociación Española contra el Cáncer (FAECC). L.S-d-C has a postdoctoral fellowship from Fundación Séneca (Región de Murcia) for application in the Ludwig Institute for Cancer Research, Nuffield Department of Clinical Medicine, University of Oxford, Headington, Oxford, UK.

9. References

Aggarwal, B.B. (2004). Nuclear factor-κB: the enemy within. *Cancer Cell*, Vol.6, No.3, pp.203-208.

Alemdaroglu, N.C.; Wolffram, S.; Boissel, J.P.; Closs, E.; Spahn-Langguth, H. & Langguth, P. (2007). Inhibition of folic acid uptake by catechins and tea extracts in Caco-2 cells. *Planta Medica*, Vol.73, No.1, pp.27-32.

American Cancer Society (2009). Cancer Facts & Figures. Atlanta: American Cancer Society.

Anderson, M.E. (1998). Glutathione: an overview of biosynthesis and modulation. *Chemico-Biological Interactions*, Vol.111-112, pp.1-14.

Assaraf, Y.G. (2007). Molecular basis of antifolate resistance. *Cancer & Metastasis Reviews*, Vol.26, No.1, pp.153-181.

Balkwill, F. & Coussens, L.M. (2004). An inflammatory link. *Nature*, Vol.431, No.7007, pp.405-406.

Blakley, R.L. (1969). The Biochemistry of Folic Acid and Related Pteridines, Elsevier, New York.

Branda, R.F.; McCormack, J.J.; Perlmutter, C.A.; Mathews, L.A. & Robison, S.H. (1988). Effects of folate deficiency on the metastatic potential of murine melanoma cells. *Cancer Research*, Vol.48, No.16, pp.4529-4534.

Cellarier, E.; Durando, X.; Vasson, M.P.; Farges, M.C.; Demiden, A.; Maurizis, J.C.; Madelmont, J.C. & Chollet, P. (2003). Methionine dependency and cancer treatment. *Cancer Treatment Reviews*, Vol.29, No.6, pp.489-499.

Chalupsky, K. & Cai, H. (2005). Endothelial dihydrofolate reductase: critical for nitric oxide bioavailability and role in angiotensin II uncoupling of endothelial nitric oxide synthase. *Proceedings of the National Academy of Sciences USA*, Vol.102, No.25, pp.9056-9061.

Chen, K.G.; Valencia, J.C.: Lai, B.; Zhang, G.; Paterson, J.K.; Rouzaud, F.; Berens, W.; Wincovitch, S.M.; Garfield, S.H.; Leapman, R.D.; Hearing, V.J. & Gottesman, M.M. (2006). Melanosomal sequestration of cytotoxic drugs contributes to the intractability of malignant melanomas. *Proceedings of the National Academy of Sciences USA*, Vol.103, No.26, pp.9903-9907.

Choi, S. & Singh, S.V. (2005). Bax and Bak are required for apoptosis induction by sulforaphane, a cruciferous vegetable-derived cancer chemopreventive agent. *Cancer Research*, Vol.65, No.5, pp.2035-2043.

Cutolo, M.; Sulli, A.; Pizzorni, C.; Seriolo, B. & Straub, R.H. (2001). Anti-inflammatory mechanisms of methotrexate in rheumatoid arthritis. *Annals of the Rheumatic Diseases*, Vol.60, No.8, pp.729-735.

Farabegoli, F.; Barbi, C.; Lambertini, E. & Piva, R. (2007). (-)-Epigallocatechin-3-gallate downregulates estrogen receptor alpha function in MCF-7 breast carcinoma cells. *Cancer Detection and Prevention*, Vol.31, No.6, pp.499-504.

Fujiki, H.; Sugunuma, M.; Imai, K. & Nakachi, K. (2002). Green tea: cancer preventive beverage and/or drug. *Cancer Letters*, Vol.188, No.1-2, pp.9-13.

Gaukroger, J.; Wilson, L.; Stewart, M.; Farid, Y.; Habeshaw, T.; Harding, N. & Mackie, R. (1983). Paradoxical response of malignant melanoma to methotrexate *in vivo* and *in vitro*. *British Journal of Cancer*, Vol.47, No.5, pp.671-679.

Graffner-Nordberg, M.; Kolmodin, K.; Aqvist, J.; Queener, S.F. & Hallberg, A. (2004). Design, synthesis, and computational affinity prediction of ester soft drugs as inhibitors of dihydrofolate reductase from *Pneumocystis carinii*. *The European Journal of Pharmaceutical Sciences*, Vol.22, No.1, pp.43-54.

Gupta, S.; Hussain, T. & Makhtar, H. (2003). Molecular pathway for (-)epigallocatechin-3-gallate-induced cell arrest and apoptosis of human prostate carcinoma cells. (2003). *Archives of Biochemitry & Biophysics*, Vol.410, No.1, pp.177-185.

Hamilton-Miller, J.M.T. (2001). Anti-cariogenic properties of tea (*Camellia sinensis*). *Journal of Medical Microbiology*, Vol.50, No.4, pp.299-302.

Hannewald, P.; Maunit, B. & Muller, J.F. (2008). Screening of DHFR-binding drugs by MALDI-TOFMS. *Analytical and Bioanalytical Chemistry*, Vol.392, No.7-8, pp.1335-1344.

Hong, J.; Lu, H.; Meng, X.; Ryu, J.H.; Hara, Y. & Yang, C.S. (2002). Stability, cellular uptake, biotransformation, and efflux of tea polyphenol (-)-epigallocatechin-3-gallate in HT-29 human colon adenocarcinoma cells. *Cancer Research*, Vol.62, No.24, pp.7241-7246.

Joerger, M.; Huitema, A.D.; van den Bongard, H.J.; Baas, P.; Schornagel, J.H.; Schellens, J.H. & Beijnen, J.H. (2006). Determinants of the elimination of methotrexate and 7-hydroxy-methotrexate following high-dose infusional therapy to cancer patients. *British Journal of Clinical Pharmacology*, Vol.62, No.1, pp.71-80.

Jung, Y.D. & Ellis, L.M. (2001). Inhibition of tumour invasion and angiogenesis by epigallocatechin gallate (EGCG), a major component of green tea. *International Journal of Experimental Pathology*, Vol.82, No.6, pp.309-316.

Kao, T.T.; Wang, K.C.; Chang, W.N.; Lin, C.Y.; Chen, B.H.; Wu, H.L.; Shi, G.Y.; Tsai, J.N. & Fu, T.F. (2008). Characterization and comparative studies of zebrafish and human recombinant dihydrofolate reductases--inhibition by folic acid and polyphenols. *Drug Metabolism and Disposition*, Vol.36, No.3, pp.508-516.

Kufe, D.W.; Wick, M.M. & Abelson, H.T. (1980). Natural resistance to methotrexate in human melanomas. *Journal of Investigative Dermatology*, Vol.75, No.4, pp.357-359.

Liang, X.J.; Shen, D.W.; Garfield, S. & Gottesman, M.M. (2003). Mislocalization of membrane proteins associated with multidrug resistance in cisplatin-resistant cancer cell lines. *Cancer Research*, Vol.63, No.18, pp.5909-5916.

Linden, J. (2001). Molecular approach to adenosine receptors: Receptor-mediated mechanisms of tissue protection. *The Annual Review of Pharmacology & Toxicology*, Vol.41, pp.775-787.

Liu, J.D.; Chen, S.H.; Lin, C.L.; Tsai, S.H. & Liang, Y.C. (2001). Inhibition of melanoma growth and metastasis by combination with (-)-epigallocatechin-3-gallate and dacarbazine in mice. *Journal of Cellular Biochemistry*, Vol.83, No.4, pp.631-642.

Lockshin, A.; Moran, R.G. & Danenberg, P.V. (1979). Thymidylate synthetase purified to homogeneity from human leukemic cells. *Proceedings of the National Academy of Sciences USA*, Vol.76, No.2, pp.750-754.

Ma, D.; Huang, H. & Moscow, J.A. (2000). Down-regulation of reduced folate carrier gene (RFC1) expression after exposure to methotrexate in ZR-75-1 breast cancer cells. *Biochemical & Biophysical Research Communications*, Vol.279, No.3, pp.891-897.

Mabe, K.; Yamada, M.; Oguni, I. & Takahashi, T. (1999). *In vitro* and *in vivo* activities of tea catechins against *Helicobacter pylori*. *Antimicrobial Agents Chemotherapy*, Vol.43, No.7, pp.1788-1791.

Majumdar, S. & Aggarwal, B.B. (2001). Methotrexate suppresses NF-κB activation through inhibition of IκBα phosphorylation and degradation. *The Journal of Immunology*, Vol.167, No.5, pp.2911-2920.

Mukhtar, H. & Ahmad, N. (2000). Tea polyphenols: prevention of cancer and optimizing health. *The American Journal of Clinical Nutrition*, Vol.71, No6., pp.1698S-1702S.

Nakagawa, K. & Miyazawa, T. (1997). Chemiluminescence-high-performance liquid chromato-graphic determination of tea catechin, (-)-epigallocatechin 3-gallate, at picomole levels in rat and human plasma. *Analytical Biochemistry*, Vol.248, No.1, pp.41-49.

Navarro-Martínez, M.D.; García-Cánovas, F. & Rodríguez-López, J.N. (2006). Tea polyphenol epigallocatechin-3-gallate inhibits ergosterol synthesis by disturbing folic acid metabolism in *Candida albicans*. *Journal of Antimicrobial Chemotherapy*, Vol.57, No.6, pp.1083-1092.

Navarro-Martínez, M.D.; Navarro-Perán, E.; Cabezas-Herrera, J.; Ruiz-Gómez, J.; García-Cánovas, F. & Rodríguez-López, J.N. (2005). Antifolate activity of epigallocatechin gallate against *Stenotrophomonas maltophilia*. *Antimicrobial Agents Chemotherapy*, Vol.49, No.7, pp.2914-2920.

Navarro-Perán, E.; Cabezas-Herrera, J.; García-Cánovas, F.; Durrant, M.C.; Thorneley, R.N.F. & Rodríguez-López, J.N. (2005a). The antifolate activity of tea catechins. *Cancer Research*, Vol. 65, No. 6, pp.2059-2064.

Navarro-Perán, E.; Cabezas-Herrera, J.; Hiner, A. N. P.; Sadunishvili, T.; García-Cánovas, F. & Rodríguez-López, J. N. (2005b). Kinetics of the inhibition of bovine liver dihydrofolate reductase by tea catechins: origin of slow-binding inhibition and pH studies. *Biochemistry*, Vol.44, No20, pp.7512-7525.

Navarro-Perán, E.; Cabezas-Herrera, J.; Sánchez del Campo, L. & Rodríguez-López, J. N. (2007). Effects of folate cycle disruption by the green tea polyphenol epigallocatechin-3-gallate. *International Journal of Biochemistry & Cell Biology*, Vol.39, No.12, pp.2215-2225.

Navarro-Perán, E.; Cabezas-Herrera, J.; Sánchez del Campo, L.; Garcia-Canovas F. & Rodríguez-López, J.N. (2008). The anti-inflammatory and anti-cancer properties of epigallocatechin-3-gallate are mediated by folate cycle disruption, adenosine release and NF-κB suppression. *Inflammation Research*, Vol.57, No.10, pp.472-478.

Nihal, M.; Ahmad, N.; Mukhtar, H. & Wood, G.S. (2005). Anti-proliferative and proapoptotic effects of (-)-epigallocatechin-3-gallate on human melanoma: possible implications for the chemoprevention of melanoma. *International Journal of Cancer*, Vol.114, No.4, pp.513-521.

Pikarsky, E.; Porat, R.M.; Stein, I.; Abramovitch, R.; Amit, S.; Kasem, S.; Gutkovich-Pyest, E.; Urieli-Shoval, S.; Galun, E. & Ben-Neriah, Y. (2004). NF-κB functions as a tumour promoter in inflammation-associated cancer. *Nature*, Vol.431, No. 7007, pp.461-466.

Rahman, L.; Voeller, D.; Rahman, M.; Lipkowitz, S.; Allegra, C.; Barrett, J. C.; Kaye, F. J. & Zajac-Kaye, M. (2004). Thymidylate synthase as an oncogene: a novel role for an essential DNA synthesis enzyme. *Cancer Cell*, Vol.5, No.4, pp.341-351.

Raposo, G. & Marks, M.S. (2002). The dark side of lysosome-related organelles: specialization of the endocytic pathway for melanosome biogenesis. *Traffic*, Vol.3, No.4, pp.237-248.

Raposo, G. & Marks, M.S. (2007). Melanosomes-dark organelles enlighten endosomal membrane transport. *Nature Reviews Molecular Cell Biology*, Vol.8, No.10, pp.786-797.

Rooseboom, M.; Commandeur, J.N.M. & Vermeulen, N.P.E. (2004). Enzyme-catalyzed activation of anticancer prodrugs. *Pharmacological Reviews*, Vol.56, No.1, pp.53-102.

Sabharanjak, S. & Mayor, S. (2004). Folate receptor endocytosis and trafficking. *Advanced Drug Delivery Reviews*, Vol.56, No.8, pp.1099-1109.

Sáez-Ayala, M.; Sánchez-del-Campo, L.; Montenegro, M.F.; Chazarra, S.; Tárraga, A.; Cabezas-Herrera, J. & Rodríguez-López, J.N. (2011). Comparison of a Pair of Synthetic Tea-Catechin-Derived Epimers: Synthesis, Antifolate Activity, and Tyrosinase-Mediated Activation in Melanoma. *ChemMedChem*, Vol.6, No.3, pp.440-449.

Sánchez-del-Campo, L. & Rodríguez-López, J.N. (2008). Targeting the methionine cycle for melanoma therapy with 3-*O*-(3,4,5-trimethoxybenzoyl)-(-)-epicatechin. *International Journal of Cancer*, Vol.123, No.10, pp.2446-2455.

Sánchez-del-Campo, L.; Chazarra, S.; Montenegro, M.F.; Cabezas-Herrera, J. & Rodríguez-López, J.N. (2010b). Mechanism of dihydrofolate reductase downregulation in melanoma by 3-*O*-(3,4,5-trimethoxybenzoyl)-(-)-epicatechin. *Journal of Cellular Biochemistry*, Vol.110, No.6, pp.1399-1409.

Sánchez-del-Campo, L.; Montenegro, M.F.; Cabezas-Herrera, J. & Rodríguez-López, J.N. (2009a). The critical role of alpha-folate receptor in the resistance of melanoma to methotrexate. *Pigment Cell & Melanoma Research*, Vol.22, No.5, pp.588-600.

Sánchez-del-Campo, L.; Otón, F.; Tárraga, A.; Cabezas-Herrera, J.; Chazarra, S. & Rodríguez-López, J.N. (2008). Synthesis and biological activity of a 3,4,5-trimethoxybenzoyl ester analogue of epicatechin-3-gallate. *Journal of Medicinal Chemistry*, Vol.51, No.7, pp.2018-2016.

Sánchez-del-Campo, L.; Sáez-Ayala, M.; Chazarra, S.; Cabezas-Herrera, J. & Rodríguez-López, J.N. (2010a). Binding of natural and synthetic polyphenols to human dihydrofolate reductase. *International Journal of Molecular Sciences*, Vol.10, No.12, pp.5398-5410.

Sánchez-del-Campo, L.; Tárraga, A.; Montenegro, M.F.; Cabezas-Herrera, J. & Rodríguez-López, J.N. (2009b). Melanoma activation of 3-*O*-(3,4,5-trimethoxybenzoyl)-(-)-epicatechin to a potent irreversible inhibitor of dihydrofolate reductase. *Molecular Pharmaceutics*, Vol.6, No.3, pp.883-894.

Soengas, M.S.; Capodieci, P.; Polsky, D.; Mora, J.; Esteller, M.; Opitz-Araya, X.; McCombie, R.; Herman, J.G.; Gerald, W.L.; Lazebnik, Y.A.; Cordón-Cardó, C. & Lowe, S.W. (2001). Inactivation of the apoptosis effector Apaf-1 in malignant melanoma. *Nature*, Vol.409, No.6817, 207-211.

Spina, M.; Cuccioloni, M.; Mozzicafreddo, M.; Montecchia, F.; Pucciarelli, S.; Eleuteri, A.M.; Fioretti, E. & Angeletti, M. (2008). Mechanism of inhibition of wt-dihydrofolate reductase from *E. coli* by tea epigallocatechin-gallate. *Proteins*, Vo.72, No.1, pp.240-251.

Sueoka, N.; Suganuma, M.; Sueoka, E.; Okabe, S.; Matsuyama, S.; Imai, K.; Nakachi, K. & Fujiki H. (2001). A new function of green tea: prevention of lifestyle-related diseases. *Annals of the New York Academy of Sciences*, Vol.928, pp.274-280.

Sullivan, D.M. & Hoffman, J.L. (1983). Fractionation and kinetic properties of rat liver and kidney methionine adenosyltransferase isozymes. *Biochemistry*, Vol.22, No.7, pp.1636-1641.

Sullivan, R.J. & Atkins, M.B. (2009). Molecular-targeted therapy in malignant melanoma. *Expert Review of Anticancer Therapy*, Vol.9, No.5, pp.567-581.

Tabrizchi, R. & Bedi, S. (2001). Pharmacology of adenosine receptors in the vasculature. *Pharmacology & Therapeutics*, Vol.91, No.2, pp.133-147.

Tawbi, H.A. & Buch, S.C. (2010). Chemotherapy resistance abrogation in metastatic melanoma. *Clinical Advances in Hematology & Oncology*, Vol.8, No.4, pp.259-266.

Theos, A.C.; Truschel, S.T.; Raposo, G. & Marks, M.S. (2005). The Silver locus product Pmel17/gp100/Silv/ME20: controversial in name and in function. *Pigment Cell Research*, Vol.18, No.5, pp.322-336.

Thomas, T. & Thomas, T.J. (2001). Polyamines in cell growth and cell death: molecular mechanisms and therapeutic applications. *Cellular & Molecular Life Sciences*, Vol.58, No.2, pp.244-258.

Tse, A. & Moran, R.G. (1998). Cellular folates prevent polyglutamation of 5, 10-dideaza-tetrahydrofolate. A novel mechanism of resistance to folate antimetabolites. *The Journal of Biological Chemistry*, Vol.273, No.40, pp.25944-25952.

Xie, T.; Nguyen, T.; Hupe, M. & Wei, M.L. (2009). Multidrug resistance decreases with mutations of melanosomal regulatory genes. *Cancer Research*, Vol. 69, No.3, pp.992-999.

Yam, T.S.; Hamilton-Miller, J.M.T. & Shah, S. (1998). The effect of a component of tea (*Camellia sinensis*) on methicillin resistance, PBP2' synthesis, and beta-lactamase production in *Staphylococcus aureus*. *Journal of Antimicrobial Chemotherapy*, Vol.42, No.2, pp.211-216.

Yang, F.; Chung, J.Y.; Yang, G.Y.; Li, C.; Meng, X. & Lee, M.J. (2000). Mechanisms of inhibition of carcinogenesis by tea. *Biofactors*, Vol.13, No.1-4, pp.73-79.

Zanon, M.; Piris, A.; Bersani, I.; Vegetti, C.; Molla, A.; Scarito, A. & Anichini, A. (2004). Apoptosis protease activator protein-1 expression is dispensable for response of human melanoma cells to distinct proapoptotic agents. *Cancer Research*, Vol.64, No.20, pp.7386-7394.

Zhao, R. & Goldman, I.D. (2003). Resistance to antifolates. *Oncogene*, Vol.22, No.47, pp.7431-7457.

7

The Potential of Triterpenoids in the Treatment of Melanoma

J. Sarek[1,2], M. Kvasnica[3], M. Vlk[2,4], M. Urban[5],
P. Dzubak[6] and M. Hajduch[6]

[1]*Dept. of Org. Chem., IMTM, Faculty of Sciences, Palacky University, Olomouc,*
[2]*Betulinines – Chemical group, Stribrna Skalice,*
[3]*IOCB, Academy of Sciences, Prague,*
[4]*Dept. of Nuclear Chemistry, Faculty of Nuclear Sciences and Physical Engineering, CTU, Prague,*
[5]*Dept. of Chem. and Bioch., Univ. of Colorado at Boulder, Colorado,*
[6]*Lab. of Exp. Medicine, IMTM, Faculty of Medicine and Dentistry, Palacky University and University Hospital in Olomouc, Olomouc*
[1,2,3,4,6]*Czech Republic;*
[5]*USA*

1. Introduction

Malignant melanoma can be currently allocated within the list of the most serious diseases with high mortality, every year, over 50,000 patients with this diagnosis die worldwide (Pirard & Vries, 2007). In addition, its incidence (200,000 per year worldwide) (Mathers *et al.*, 2001) is still increasing due to deteriorating environmental factors (increased exposure to UV light, unhealthy lifestyle, pollution etc.). Chemotherapy is one of the most important therapeutic modalities of this diagnosis however, despite significant advances in the field of contemporary medicine and a broad portfolio of medicaments in use, the treatment success rate is still insufficient. For these reasons, scientific and pharmaceutical communities have intensively investigated new compounds that could be applied as new drugs for this devastating disease.

Triterpenes - substances abundant in natural sources belong to a group of isoprenoids, compounds made of 6 isoprene building units. They have a wide spectrum of pharmacological activities (Dzubak *et al.*, 2006), of which the most noteworthy are: antiviral, anti-inflammatory, antiulcerogenic, antimicrobial, anticariogenic and most importantly anticancer activity. Betulinic acid (1) and many other triterpenes have been known over a century, however, until recently their selective cytotoxic activity against human melanoma cells was undiscovered (Cichewicz & Kouzi, 2004; Eiznhamer & Xu, 2004; Salvador, 2010). The extract of *Vauquelinia corymbosa* (Fig. 1) showed significant cytotoxic activity against a cell line of lymphocytic leukemia P-388 in the work of Trumbull by 1976 and betulinic acid (1) along with uvaol and ursolic acid were supposed to be responsible for it (Trumbull *et al.*, 1976). Despite that, the fundamental study of selective cytotoxic activity of acid 1 against human melanoma cells MEL-1 with IC_{50} values in the range between 0.5 - 1.5 µg/mL was reported by Pisha and his team (Pisha *et al.*, 1995) incredible 19 years after Trumbull's paper. A large number of natural triterpenes have been isolated and many more semi-synthetic compounds have been prepared from them since then. Plenty of these derivatives also showed cytotoxic activity against melanoma cells (Salvador, 2010).

In this chapter (**Isolated pentacyclic triterpenes** and **Semi-synthetic triterpenoids**), there will be a summary of representatives from both natural and semi-synthetic lupane triterpenoids with cytotoxic activity against melanoma cells that were studied during the past fifteen years. Current knowledge of the mechanisms of action of the leading representatives, results and aspects of *in vivo* tests and clinical trials will be discussed here. Betulinic acid (1) will be given the most attention as it is historically the first known triterpene with activity against melanoma. Betulinic acid (1) is currently in the second phase of clinical trials for treatment of dysplastic nevus and therefore, it has a high potential to be used in future clinical practice.

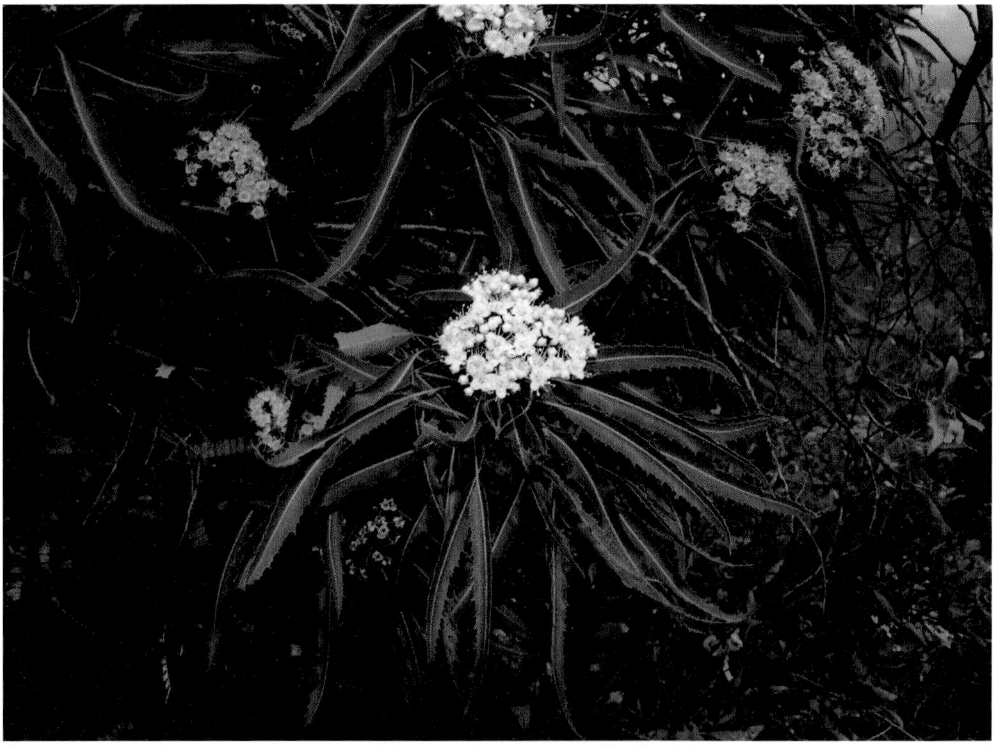

Fig. 1. *Vauquelinia corymbosa* (Photo: Dr. Carlos Gerardo Velazco Macías)

2. Anticancer effects of triterpenoids used for treatment of melanoma

To date, several hundred triterpenoid compounds with significant *in vitro* cytotoxic activity against a variety of cancer cell lines have been found (Salvador, 2010) however; few of them were screened against human melanoma lines such as MEL-1, -2, -3, -4. Most of the triterpenes that actually were tested and showed interesting activity against melanoma cell lines were derivatives of lupane. That is why this chapter will be focused on lupane triterpenoids with anti-melanoma activity and they will be divided into two groups 1) isolated pentacyclic triterpenoids, meaning they were isolated from a natural source and 2) semi-synthetic triterpenoids that were obtained by modification of natural compounds using chemical reactions or biotransformations.

2.1 Isolated pentacyclic triterpenes

Natural appearance and properties of betulinic acid (1)

Betulinic acid (1) is a natural triterpene with extraordinarily high activity against human melanoma and is found throughout the plant kingdom (e.g. genus *Betulla, Ziziphus, Syzigium, Diospiros, Paeonia*) (Cichewicz & Kouzi, 2004). When isolated as a pure compound, this natural pentacyclic triterpene appears to be snow-white crystalline odorless and tasteless powder that is almost insoluble in water (Cichewicz & Kouzi, 2004; Glassby, 1982; Simonsen & Ross, 1957).

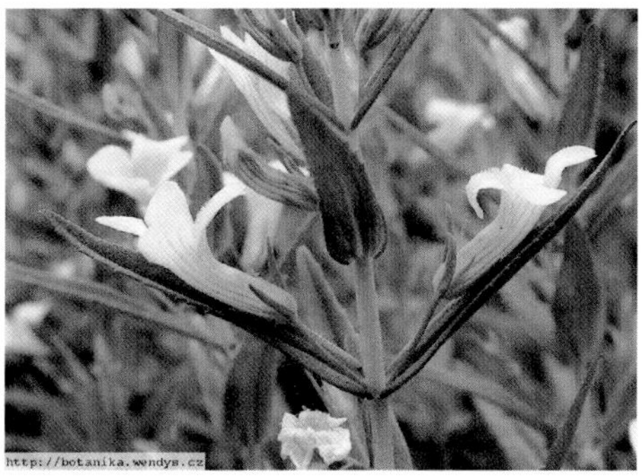

Fig. 2. *Gratiola officinalis* (photo: http://botanika.wendys.cz);

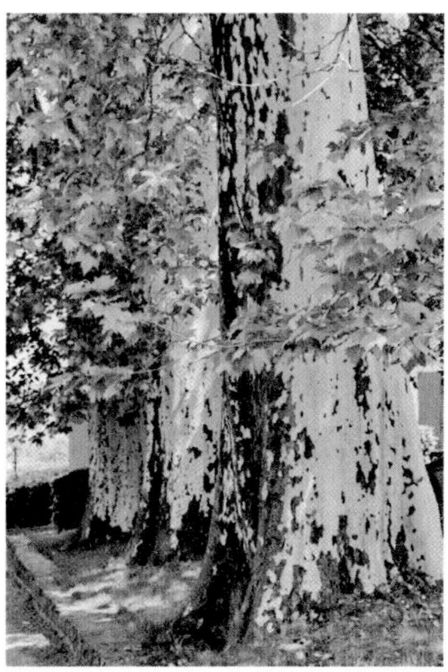

Fig. 3. *Platanus acerifolia* (photo: www.shutterstock.com);

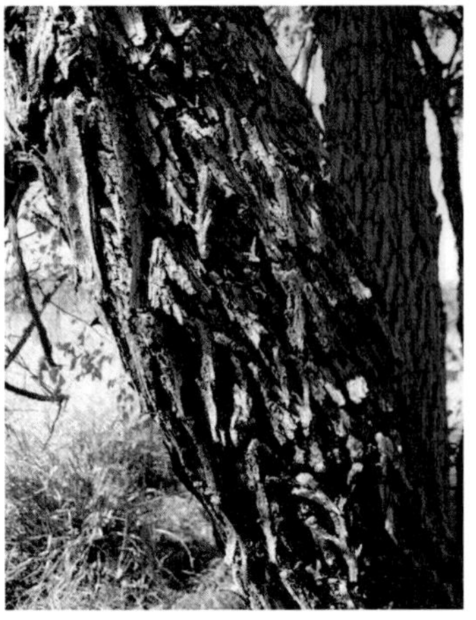

Fig. 4. *Ziziphus Mauritiana* - bark (photo: http://en.wikipedia.org)

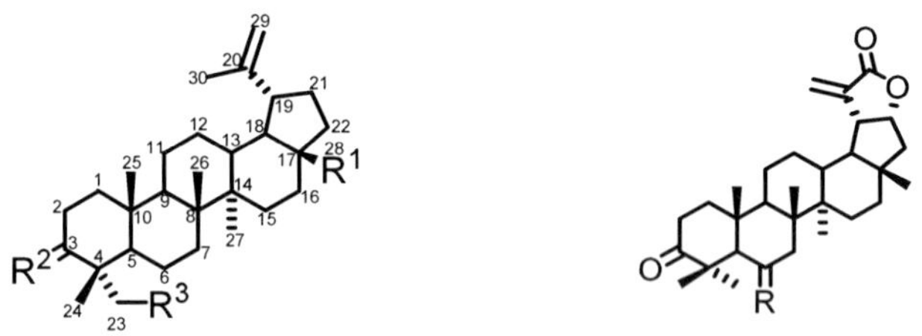

1: $R^1 = CO_2H$, $R^2 = \beta\text{-OH}, \alpha\text{-H}$, $R^3 = H$
2: $R^1 = CO_2H$, $R^2 = \beta\text{-OH}, \alpha\text{-H}$, $R^3 = OH$
3: $R^1 = CH_2OH$, $R^2 = \beta\text{-OH}, \alpha\text{-H}$, $R^3 = H$
4: $R^1 = COH$, $R^2 = \beta\text{-OH}, \alpha\text{-H}$, $R^3 = H$
5: $R^1 = CO_2H$, $R^2 = O$, $R^3 = H$

6: R = H, H
7: R = O

Fig. 5.

The first isolation of the compound currently known as betulinic acid (1) was described by Retzlaff in 1902 (Retzlaff, 1902; Simonsen & Ross, 1957), who extracted the yet unknown substance from *Gratiola officinalis* (Fig. 2) which he called "graciolon". In 1925, betulinic acid (1) was independently obtained from the bark of plane trees *Platanus acerifolia* (Fig. 3) by Zellner and Ziffer (Simonsen & Ross, 1957; Zellner & Ziffer, 1925) using either extraction or sublimation. The authors named it after its source "platanolic acid" and did not recognize its true identity. Similarly, the same compound was isolated from *Florida Cornus* (Fig. 6) during the dissertation research of Soliman who, in 1939 first called it "cornolic acid". However, soon he and his co-workers identified it correctly as betulinic acid (1) (Robertson *et al.*, 1939). In 1944, Barton and Jones used physical constants to correctly identify "graciolon" as betulinic acid (1) (Barton & Jones, 1944) and in 1948, Bruckner and co-workers identified (Bruckner *et al.*, 1948) "platanolic acid" as betulinic acid (1) as well. Demonstrating, that betulinic acid (1) is widely spread throughout nature and that its identification was often accompanied with many problems during the 20th century.

Acid 1 is accessible from plane tree and birch bark on an industrial scale since both types of bark contain several percent of it. In addition to the extraction procedures (Cichewicz & Kouzi, 2004; Simonsen & Ross, 1957; Urban *et al.*, 2004), several industrial processes were developed to manufacture (Csuk *et al.*, 2006; Krasutsky *et al.*, 2003, 2006; Pezzuto *et al.*, 2007) betulinic acid (1) from betulin (3), a triterpene far more abundant (up to 30 %) in birch bark (e.g. *Betula pendula*; Fig. 7) than the acid, which makes it far more profitable process. This is especially useful in northern European countries, Russia, Canada, where paper mills mostly use birches to produce cellulose pulp and where over 40 tons of birch bark (Krasutsky, 2005, 2006; Sarek, 2008) is produced daily, with 6 tons a day being burned as a cheap fuel (5-7 USD per ton; 7-11 MJ/kg). Using birch bark as a cheap source of betulin can provide the industry with a less expensive source of betulinic acid (Csuk *et al.*, 2006; Krasutsky, 2003, 2006; Pezzuto, 2007). With these procedures, there should not be a significant problem with manufacturing betulinic acid (1) on a multi ton scale. The best known industrial process to convert betulin (3) into betulinic acid (1) is based on conversion of it into aldehyde 4 (Csuk *et al.*, 2006; Krasutsky *et al.*, 2006a, 2006b, 2006c) followed by oxidation (Csuk *et al.*, 2006; Krasutsky *et al.*, 2006) of aldehyde 4 to betulinic acid (1). Older patented procedures (Pezzuto *et al.*, 2007) that use oxidation of betulin (3) with Jones reagent into betulonic acid (5) followed by selective reduction are not preferable because they use toxic Cr(VI) compounds in large quantities and also a 3α-epimeric product originates as a by-product (Pezzuto, 2007) which makes the isolation and purification far too expensive.

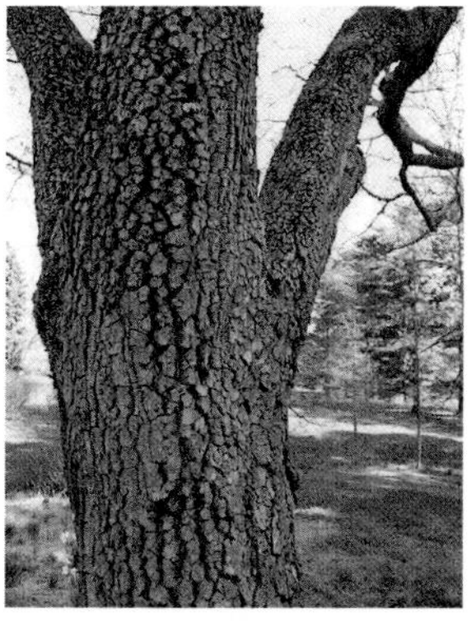

Fig. 6. *Florida cornus* - bark (photo: http://en.wikipedia.org);

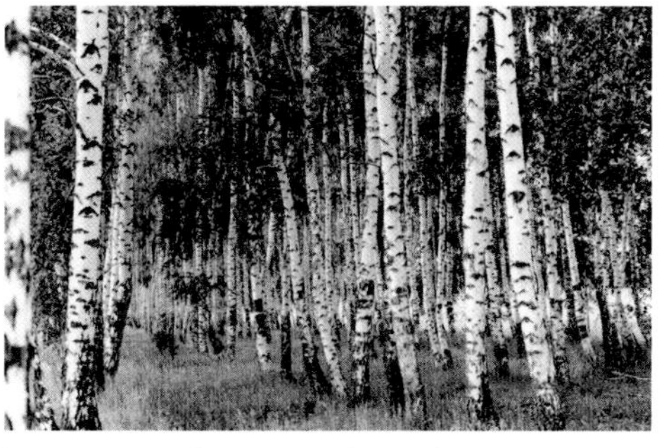

Fig. 7. Betula pendula (photo: www.shutterstock.com)

Antitumor activities of acid 1 against human melanoma cells

Despite acid 1 having been isolated in 1902, its cytotoxic effects were not found until the examination of cytotoxicity of various *Vaquelinia corymbosa* (Fig. 1) extracts against lymphocytic leukemia cells P-388 by Trumbull in 1976 (Trumbull *et al.*, 1976). Approximately 19 years later, Pisha and his co-workers (Pisha *et al.*, 1995) published their findings of selective cytotoxic effects of betulinic acid (1) extracted from stem bark of *Ziziphus Mauritiana* (Lamnaceae, Fig. 4) against human melanoma cells Mel-1, -2, -3, -4. Furthermore, this work investigated the mechanism of action by flow-cytometry (Pisha *et al.*, 1995), and it was found that acid 1 induced selective apoptosis of tumor cells Mel-2, which remained in G0/G1 phase. Moreover, induction of apoptosis was evident from the emergence of sub-G1 apoptotic peak (Ap) in DNA histograms and its increase between 56-72 h after application. Direct perturbation of the mitochondria by betulinic acid (1) was observed by (Fulda *et al.*, 1998) and this type of activity was also found when the cancer cells were treated by various triterpene scaffolds without limitation to the melanoma cells. Despite extensive research, the molecular target of betulinic acid (1) has not yet been identified. Only from some published pathway alterations like Bcl-2 and NF-kB modulation and antiangiogenic activity were some speculations about the target able to be made (Selzer *et al.*, 2000, 2002). There is a plethora of information about the activity of potent derivatives of betulinic acid (1) (e.g. NVX-207, PA-457) in *in vitro* and *in vivo* models but it seems to be a reality, that small changes in the chemical structure could lead to significant differences in specificity and mechanisms of action (Keller *et al.*, 2001; Suh *et al.*, 1999; Willmann *et al.*, 2009).
Another advantage of using acid 1 in cancer therapy is its very low toxicity in a Hippocratic screens at doses of 200 and 400 mg per kg body weight in animal models (Pisha *et al.*, 1995). In a study published by Pisha, intraperitoneal application of acid 1 to mice in six doses of 500 mg/kg every fourth day and six doses of 250 mg/kg every third day were accepted without any signs of toxicity (Cichewicz & Kouzi, 2004). In vitro studies showed that the only symptom of high doses of acid 1 was an increase of intracellular-free calcium, and this increase was only associated with a small decrease in cell viability (Cichewicz & Kouzi, 2004). Very low toxicity and significant antitumor activity give acid 1 a very favorable therapeutic index (Cichewicz & Kouzi, 2004). These findings thrust common triterpenes - betulinic acid (1) - to the center of interest within scientific groups studying antitumor activities and mechanisms of action, and pharmaceutical companies interested in chemotherapeutics (e.g. BMS).

Other anticancer activities and studies

Acid 1 has presented promising antitumor activity against a variety of tumor cell lines such as malignant brain-tumor (Fulda *et al*, 1999), neuroectodermal (Zuco *et al.*, 2002), human chronic myelogenous leukemia (CML) 562 (Gopal *et al.*, 2005) and many other cell lines derived from the most prevalent human cancer types (lung, colorectal, breast, prostate and cervical cancer (Kessler *et al.*, 2007; Zuco, 2002). Furthermore selective cytotoxicity against tumor cell lines in comparison with normal cells has been confirmed (Hata *et al.*, 2002).
Pulsatilic acid (2), a compound isolated from *Pulsatilla chinensis* is another example of a triterpene highly cytotoxic against mouse melanoma cell line B16 (Bi *et al.*, 2007; Liu *et al*, 2004; Zhou *et al.*, 2007). Pulsatilic acid (2) is a little less active than acid 1 (53 μmol/L for acid 1 and 83 μmol/L for acid 2) (Bi *at al.*, 2007).
The last type of natural pentacyclic triterpenes active against melanoma are ochraceolides, compounds with modified E-ring. Ochraceolides A (6) and C (7) were isolated together with

other lupane derivatives from *Kokoona ochracea* and their activity against line UISO-MEL-2 was approximately 15 µmol/L (Ngassapa *et al.*, 1991).

Synergisms of acid 1 with cytostatics and other effects.

Animal and cell based studies (Sawada *et al.*, 2004; Selzer *et al.*, 2000; Wachsberger *et al.*, 2002) have focused on investigating the synergic anticancer activities of various doses of acid 1 and vincristine (Fig. 8), radio therapy, lowering pH, or hyperthermia. A significant increase in the efficiency of radio therapy against human melanoma cells was demonstrated when combined with dossing of betulinic acid (1). Response of melanoma cells to betulinic acid (1) alone or in combination with irradiation was studied by Selzer and co-workers (Selzer *et al.*, 2000). Analysis of tumor cell survival following the treatment by acid 1 combined with an application of ionizing γ irradiation (dose of 2 Gy, within the range used in clinical therapy) indicates that betulinic acid (1) and irradiation have an additive effect on the inhibition of colony-forming ability. It is possible that acid 1 can target tumor cells that are resistant to ionizing radiation.

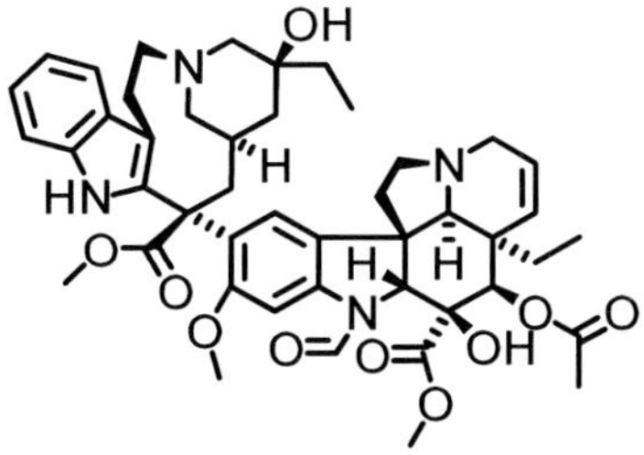

Fig. 8. Vincristine

In another study, Japanese authors looked at the influence of combination of betulinic acid (1) and vincristine on mice melanoma B16F *in vitro* and *in vivo* (Sawada *et al.*, 2004). Based on fast apoptosis of those melanoma cells, the authors suggested an existence of a synergic effect between acid 1 and vincristine, they found, that each substance causes inhibition of cell cycle in different phases: betulinic acid (1) in G1 phase and vincristine in G2/M phase (Sawada *et al.*, 2004). An application of both compounds *in vivo* increased suppression of lung metastasis of melanoma cells in a model C57BL/6 in mice, in comparison to vincristine only. Authors proclaimed that acid 1 is a suitable complement to the chemotherapy of malignant melanoma (Sawada *et al.*, 2004).
Wachsberger *et al* reported an influence of antitumor activity of compound 1 together with application of hyperthermia and lower pH in human melanoma cells DB-1 (Wachsberger *et al.*, 2002). They found that percentage of survived tumor cells during the combined application of acid 1 and hyperthermia of 42°C for two hours decreased with respect of used pH 7.3, 6.7 and 6.3 from 5 %, 9 %, to 2 %.

In vivo studies and the clinical trials of betulinic acid (1)

Based on promising *in vitro* and *in vivo* activity of betulinic acid (1) in melanocarcinoma cells and tumors in animal models, human clinical trials were induced. Some considerations were taken in regard to actinic keratosis (AKs), which represents the initial intraepidermal manifestation of keratinocyte abnormal transformation that may potentially progress to small cell carcinoma. In a randomised trial, Huyke (Huyke *et al.*, 2009) treated 45 patients (with <10 AKs each) either with a topical betulin-based oleogel twice daily, or cryotherapy, or a combination of the two. Treatment with betulin-based oleogel was well-tolerated and showed efficacy in treating AKs. Continued controlled studies on larger sample sizes investigating the use of betulinic acid for the treatment of nonmelanoma skin cancer are warranted. Phase I and II clinical trials evaluating the topical application of betulinic acid (1) in the treatment of dysplastic nevi with moderate to severe dysplasia are currently ongoing (www.clinicalstrials.gov). Clinical trials with acid (1) have not been completed to date.

Overview of other biological activities of acid 1

It should be stated that betulinic acid (1) also has other interesting biological activities, especially, anti-HIV (Fujioka *et al.*, 1994; Mayaux *et al.*, 1994) and anti-inflammatory (Huang *et al.*, 1995; Mukherjee *et al.*, 1997; Recio *et al.*, 1995a, 1995b; Yasukawa *et al.*, 1991). The anti-HIV activity of betulinic acid (1) and its derivatives was first described by two independent research groups (Fujioka *et al.*, 1994; Mayaux *et al.*, 1994). Since then, several researchers prepared, published and often patented a large number of novel derivatives (Jacob *et al.*, 2010; Salzwedel *et al.*, 2010) with significant activity against HIV (EC_{50} < 1 nM). Among these derivatives, three main groups are worth mentioning. First 3β-*O*-acyl derivatives of betulinic acid that inhibit the maturation of HIV virus (Kashiwada *et al.*, 1996). 3β-*O*-3′,3′-dimethylsuccinylbetulinic acid (8), also known as PA-457 or bevirimat is the most important representative of this group.

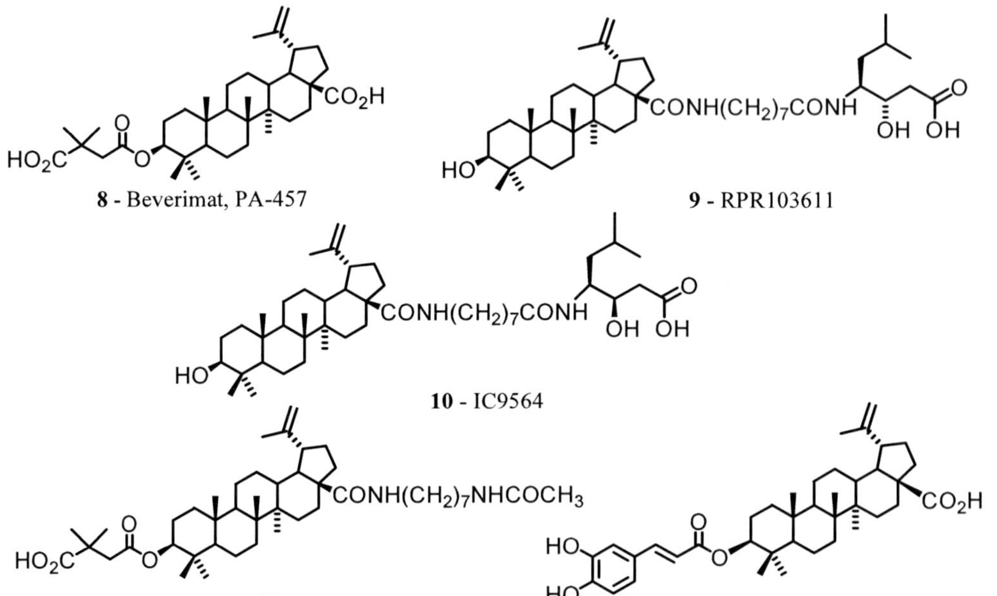

8 - Beverimat, PA-457

9 - RPR103611

10 - IC9564

11

12

Fig. 9.

The companies Panacos (Salzwedel *et al.*, 2010) and Myriad (Jacob *et al.*, 2010) found bevirimat to be active against HIV in vivo which sent the compound to phase IIa of clinical trials under registry number NCT01026727 (US National Institute of Health). Not only does

Bevirimat (Jacob *et al.*, 2010; Kashiwada *et al.*, 1996; Salzwedel *et al.*, 2010) show very high anti-HIV activity (EC_{50} ~ 0.35 nM) but it also has a very low toxicity (typical for betulinic acid derivatives) which together puts the value of its therapeutic index over 20,000. Another advantage of bevirimat is that to date no resistance to it has been recorded. The second group of anti-HIV active compounds are 28-amides (Evers *et al.*, 1996; Soler *et al.*, 1996; Sun *et al.*, 2002) of betulinic acid that block the entry of the virion into cells. The most important amide derivatives (Holz-Smith *et al.*, 2001; Sun *et al.*, 2002) are compounds 9 and 10 also known as RPR103611 and IC9564. The third group is represented by compounds that combine both of the previously mentioned mechanizms of activity (Huang *et al.*, 2006) because they contain a combination of both pharmacophors - acyl group in the position 3β and 28-amide group. Those compounds were discovered most recently and the most active is ([(N-[3β-*O*-(3´,3´-dimethylsuccinyl)lup-20(29)-en-28-oyl]-7-aminoheptyl)-carbamoyl]methane) (11) which showed activity about 20 times higher than Bevirimat in *in vitro* tests (Huang *et al.*, 2006).

Yasukawa was the first to describe anti-inflammatory activity of betulinic acid (1) (Yasukawa *et al.*, 1991) and relevant inhibition effect against TPA –induced inflammation was found at concentration of 5 μM (Huang *et al.*, 1995; Mukherjee *et al.*, 1997; Recio *et al.*, 1995a, 1995b). Promising anti-inflammatory activity has also been found in 3β−*O*-caffeoyl betulinic acid (12) by Fuchino group (Fuchino *et al.*, 1995, 1996, 1998). This compound is one of the components of birch bark. Last but not least, betulinic acid (1) is commonly used in the cosmetic industry. It is usually used in concentrations of 50-500 mg per gram to prevent and help treat UV-induced skin cancer, to reduce signs of cellulitide and to stimulate collagen synthesis in skin-care products. It's also used to prevent sunlight-caused signs of aging, wrinkles, and blotches and to improve skin homogeneity and pigmentations. (Bradbury *et al.*, 1997a, 1997b, 1997c)

2.2 Semi-synthetic triterpenoids with activity against melanoma

The very poor solubility of acid 1 in water based media (< 1 μmol/L) (Cichewicz & Kouzi, 2004; Symon *et al.*, 2005), high hydrophobicity (*log P*) (Srivastava *et al.*, 2002) and unsuitable pK parameters (absorption, distribution, metabolism and elimination), along with strong antitumor potential (Pisha *et al.*, 1995) and low acute toxicity (Cichewicz & Kouzi, 2004) motivated a number of scientific institutions to synthesize derivatives, pro-drugs and formulations of betulinic acid (1) that could retain the activity and low toxicity, but improve the afore mentioned properties. The following semi-synthetic derivatives might be divided into three groups: simple derivatives of natural triterpenes (2.2.1), derivatives obtained by biotransformation procedures of betulinic acid (1) (2.2.2) and triterpenoids with modification of lupane skeleton (2.2.3).

2.2.1 Derivatives of natural triterpenes (acids 1, 2 and betulin (3))

Several functional groups can be used for the derivatization of acid 1, such as the secondary hydroxyl group in the position 3β, a neopentyl 28-carboxyl moiety in the location 17 and finally, a double bond located between carbons 20 and 29. As both hydroxyl and carboxyllic groups are sterically hindered, common derivatization processes usually don't work very well or fail completely. A typical example is the esterification of 28-carboxylic group. The reaction does not work with alcohols at all; acid catalysis or use of DCC does not help either.

Using alkyl bromides or iodides and alkali carbonates or DBU as the basis in DMF are the most effective conditions to introduce an ester to 28-carboxyl group. Analogously, simple alkali hydrolysis of alkyl betulinates does not work and to release a free acid from its ester, it is necessary to apply drastic conditions such as reflux with potassium hydroxide in ethylene glycol or nucleophilic deprotection using lithium iodide in collidines under reflux. For the purposes of this chapter, the compounds that are modified at more than one site of the skeleton are classified according to significance of the modification. Also, many cytotoxic compounds with no data about their activity on melanoma lines are not included in this chapter.

Derivatization of betulinic (1) and pulsatillic acid (2) in position 28

Cytotoxicity of various types of esters of betulinic acid (1) is very well researched. In the past, researchers found that the cytotoxicity of betulinic acid decreases by forming alkyl or aryl esters from 28-carboxylic group. (Kim *et al.*, 1998, 2001; Kvasnica *et al.*, 2005; Urban *et al.*, 2004, 2005). One of the explanations of this fact is that free carboxyl group is responsible for the activity and the hydrolysis of its esters is extremely difficult and requires extreme conditions which are caused by sterical hinderance of the neopentyl-type group. Curiously, difficulties with the hydrolysis were not observed at similar β,γ-unsaturated esters (*e.g.* compound 13, Fig. 10) (Sarek *et al.*, 2005) which suggests that a different reaction mechanism might exist to cleave them, so those difficulties are probably specific for alkyl and aryl esters and for acids with unmodified E-ring. Very detailed studies of the dependency of cytotoxicity on the type of the ester in position 28 of betulinic acid (1) have been published in literature (Kvasnica *et al.*, 2005; Urban *et al.*, 2005) The authors demonstrated that methyl, ethyl, and benzyl esters are an order of magnitude less active than the free acid 1.

A different situation was observed at substituted alkyl esters of acid 1 and 2 (Bi *et al.*, 2007; Urban *et al.*, 2005). Urban *et al.* compared the cytotoxicity of methyl-, pivaloyloxymethyl-, and acetoxymethyl- esters of betulinic and betulonic acid 15 - 22 on broad scale of cancer cell lines. They found that while methyl- and pivaloyloxymethyl- group significantly decrease the activity, the Acm-esters were either as active as the starting acids or better. The Acm group is therefore a suitable derivatization group that could possibly be useful to synthesize prodrugs. Another good property of Acm is that it increases hydrophilicity.

A completely new type of esters was published by Effenberger *et al.* who synthesized esters from a variety of monoterpenes, sesquiterpenes, and betulinic acid with carboxylic and hydroxyethylene derivatives of thymoquinone (Effenberger *et al.*, 2010). However, 28-esteric derivative 23 was about 7 times less active against the cell line 518A2 than the free acid 1 (Effenberger *et al.*, 2010). A SARS study done by Bi *et al.* who investigated the activity of alkenyl, alkynyl and hydroxyalkyl esters of pulsatillic acid 24 - 29 against several tumor cell lines. The authors included *in vivo* experiments using the most active allyl ester 24 and the starting acid 2 on mice in H22 and B16 models. The *in vitro* experiments showed that all prepared esters were more active than the starting acid 2 against line B16 and also that 6-hydroxyethylester was only slightly better than the acid 2 on the same line. *In vivo* experiments brought even more exciting results when they showed that allyl pulsatillate 24 (applied as intraperitoneal DMSO solution) caused a larger reduction of the mass of a tumor than the free acid 2. Its activity was actually comparable to cyclophosphamide which is a commercially used cytostatic.

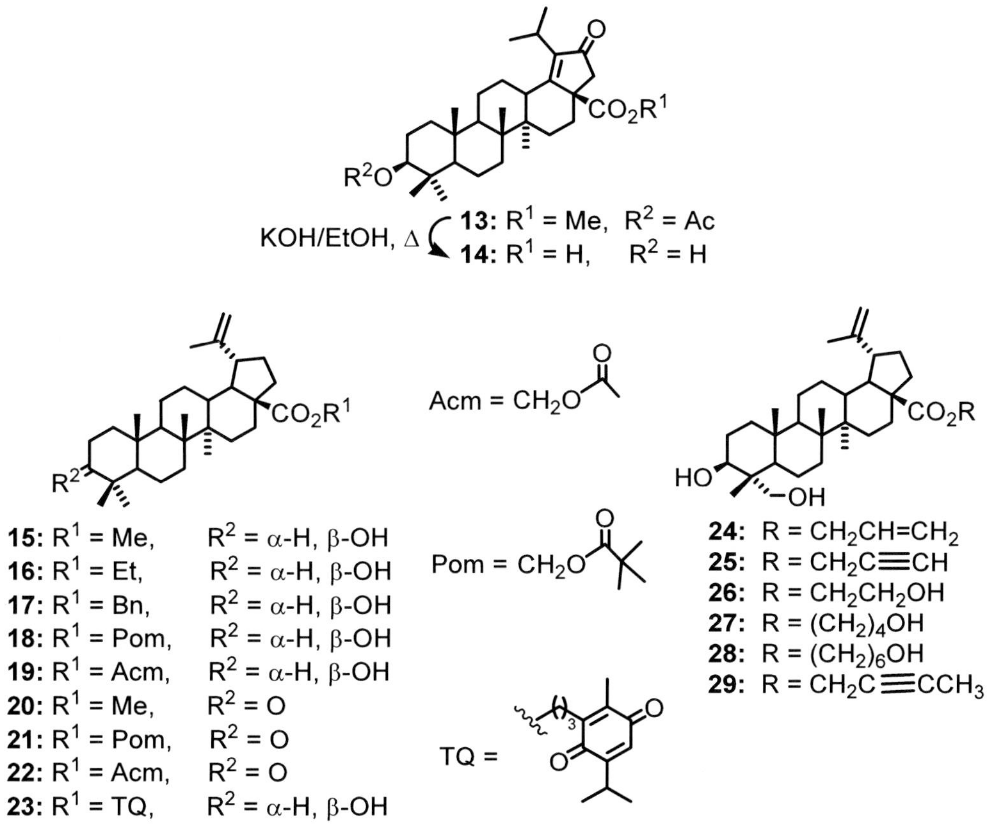

Fig. 10.

Willmann *et al.* brought even more promising results using the compound 30 - NVX-207 that is an ester of acetylbetulinic acid with tris(hydroxymethyl)aminomethane (TRIS). The compound was highly active *in vitro* against 15 cancer cell lines including human melanoma 518A2 and the activity was between 2.6 µmol/L on 518A2 and 5.6 µmol/L on fibrosarcoma HAT 1080. Those initial experiments were followed by a phase I/II animal clinical study on canine patients with spontaneous currently untreatable tumors using intralesional and surrounding tissue application of NVX-207. Five dogs bearing tumors of different histogenetic origine (squamous cell carcinoma, soft tissue sarcoma, mammary carcinoma and adenocarcinoma of the scent gland of the paw) were treated. The complete response to the therapy was observed in two dogs, almost complete remission (90% reduction), stable disease (50% response) and 30% percent reduction was observed in the remaining cases. No systemic side effects and minor local side effects (mild local discomfort) after infiltration of the tumors were observed (Willmann *et al.*, 2009).

Another large group of activated esters are esters with sugars, sometimes improperly called glycosides. The cytotoxicity of these compounds has not been studied thoroughly and the few examples in literature (Gauthier *et al.*, 2009a, 2009b; Pakulski *et al.*, 2009) do not show activity against melanoma cell lines. The only conclusion that can be made is that esters where a terpene is connected to a single saccharide unit are far less active than the free acid. An example of this is - β-D-glucopyranosyl betulinate (31) (Gauthier *et al.*, 2009a, 2009b) which has activity lower than the activity of betulinic acid (1) by an order of magnitude. Despite this, a study which researched the cytotoxicity of bidesmosidic saponines showed that the saccharide component bound as an ester is an important part of the pharmacophore because its removal caused significant drop of activity. The study contained pulsatillic glycosides 32 isolated from *Schefflera rotundifolia* (Cioffi *et al.*, 2003).

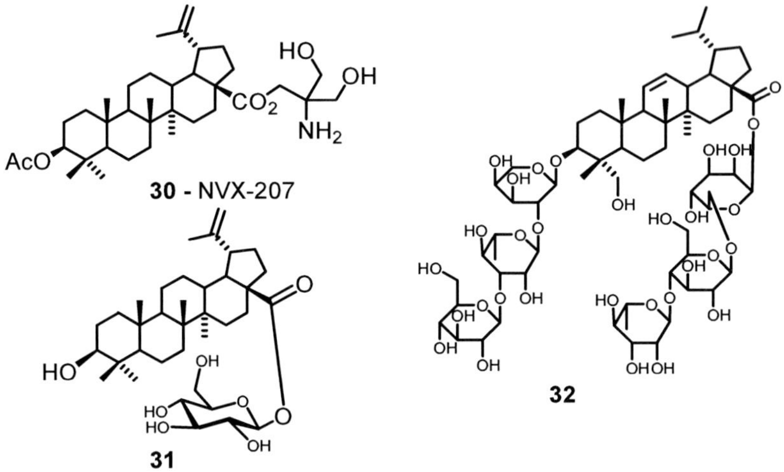

Fig. 11.

Amides represent another type of carboxylic acid derivative. Their antitumor activity is usually high and their hydrophilicity makes their use in *in vivo* tests very easy (Jeong *et al.*, 1999; Willmann *et al.*, 2009). Jeong published a very complex SARS study about the cytotoxic activity of conjugates of betulinic acid (1) with natural amino acids along with a toxicity study on fibroblasts and basic studies of solubility. The best results against MEL-2 cell line were found using conjugates of betulinic acid with alanine - 33 and 35; although the compounds were somewhat toxic against fibroblasts. While the conjugates of betulinic acid with valine 34, 37 and glycine 36 were less active than those with alanine 33 and 35; they were completely non toxic. The glycine conjugate 36 was also the most hydrophilic of the studied compounds. The authors tested the solubility of the conjugates with a very simple method. They prepared solutions of each studied compound in DMSO and kept diluting those solutions with water until they started to precipitate. While the most active alanine derivative 33 could be diluted up to 50 times, the glycine conjugate 36 could be diluted 100 times. Despite the fact, that the cytotoxicity of the glycine conjugate 36 was the same as the activity of free betulinic acid (1) (4.2 μmol/L), the conjugate 36 is far more soluble in water and that makes it a very suitable candidate for *in vivo* testing.

Another type of derivative that showed cytotoxicity against melanoma lines was quaternary ammonium salts (Biedermann *et al.*, 2010; Sarek *et al.*, 2008). The strong antitumor activity of quaternary ammonium salts of four terpenic acids (betulinic (1), dihydrobetulinic (38), platanic (39) and 21-oxoacid 14) on a panel of 11 cancer cell lines has been demonstrated in the literature (Sarek *et al.*, 2008). The salts were obtained by a two step reaction of a terpenic acid with 1,2-dibromoethane followed by a quaternization with a corresponding amine (trimethylamine, triethylamine, pyridine). The best cytotoxicity was obtained with quaternary salts of triethylamine - compound 40 and 41. The dihydrobetulinic salt 41 is currently being tested on melanoma lines and has shown activity between 1.6 μmol/L against the line UAAC 62 and 14.6 μmol/L against the line M14 (see Tab. 4). Salts 40 and 41 are also very hydrophilic which makes it easy to dissolve them (55 mg/mL of vehiculum) in media based on water and moreover, their oral accessibility makes them ideal candidates for *in vivo* testing on animals.

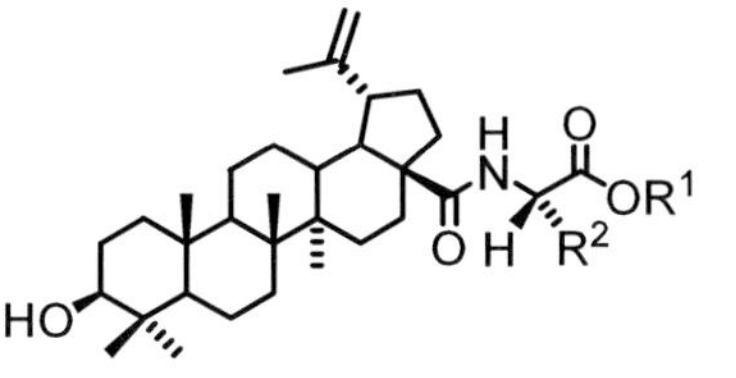

33: R^1 = H, R^2 = Me
34: R^1 = Me, R^2 = $CH(CH_3)_2$
35: R^1 = Me, R^2 = Me
36: R^1 = H, R^2 = H
37: R^1 = H, R^2 = $CH(CH_3)_2$

Fig. 12.

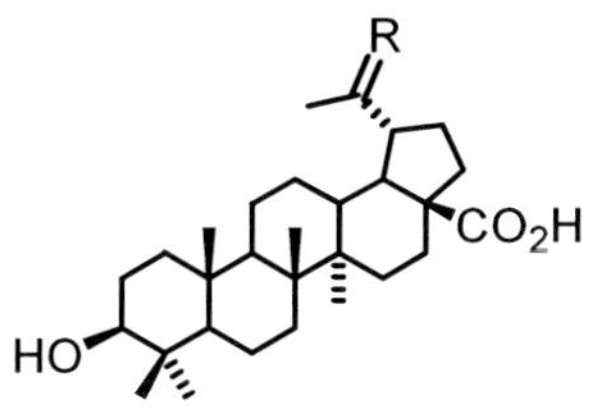

38: R = CH_3,H
39: R = O,

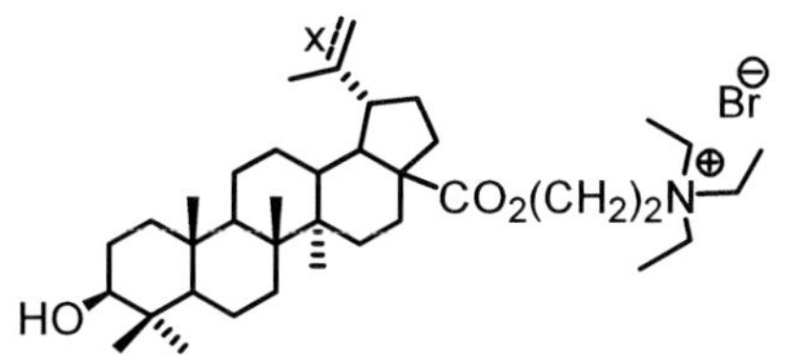

40: x = double bond
41: x = single bond

Fig. 13.

The final group of carboxylic derivatives consists of compounds with aldehydic or hydroxymethyl group in position 17 because they can be prepared by simple reduction step from carboxylic acids. Those compounds are actually more easily synthesized from betulin (3) than from betulinic acid (1). It was shown that the carbonyl group (aldehyde or carboxylic acid) is essential for cytotoxicity because while aldehydes are active, 28-hydroxyderivatives are generally not. This fact was well documented in the work (Hata *et al.*, 2003) in which betulinal (4) had activity 10.6 μmol/L, and acid 1 6.5 μmol/L against melanoma cell line SK-MEL-2. However, if another part of the molecule of 28-hydroxyderivatives is modified, the activity may increase. The best examples are glycosides of betulin (3) that are very active on melanoma B-16F, especially when position 3β was glycosylated. Curiously, 28-*O*-glycosides were inactive (Gauthier *et al.*, 2006). Among β-D-glucoside, α-D-arabinoside, and α-L-rhamnoside 42 – 44 (Fig. 13), the last listed was the most active against B16-F1 cell line (18 μmol/L, which is just slightly worse than acid 1 with an activity of 16 μmol/L) (Gauthier *et al.*, 2006). There are no results for bisdesmosidic saponines on melanoma cell lines, however, work of Gauthier describes similar trend on another lines (most active is betulin-3β,28-*O*-bis(α-L-rhamnoside) 45 (Gauthier *et al.*, 2009a).

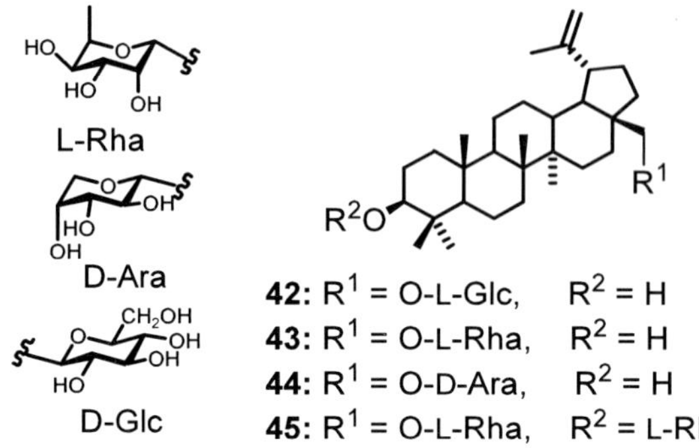

42: R^1 = O-L-Glc, R^2 = H
43: R^1 = O-L-Rha, R^2 = H
44: R^1 = O-D-Ara, R^2 = H
45: R^1 = O-L-Rha, R^2 = L-Rha

Fig. 14.

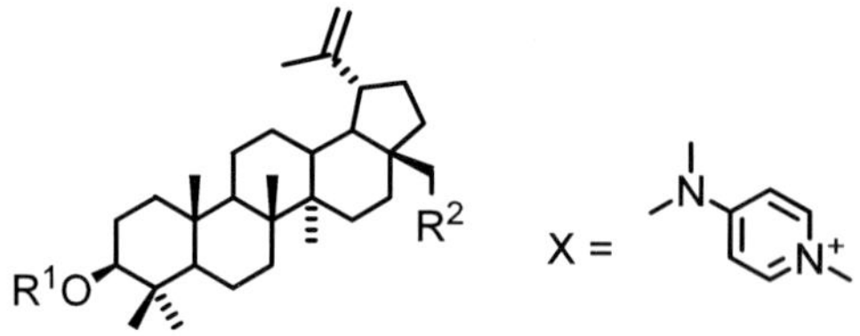

46: $R^1 = OCOCH_2X^+Br^-$; $R^2 = OH$
47: $R^1 = OCO(CH_2)_3X^+Br^-$; $R^2 = OCOCH_2)_3X^+Br^-$
48: $R^1 = OCOCH_2X^+Cl^-$; $R^2 = OH$
49: $R^1 = OCO(CH_2)_2X^+Cl^-$; $R^2 = OCO(CH_2)_2X^+Cl^-$
50: $R^1 = OCOCH(C_2H_5)X^+Br^-$; $R^2 = OCOCH(C_2H_5)X^+Br^-$
51: $R^1 = OCOCH(CH_3)X^+Cl^-$; $R^2 = OCOCH(CH_3)X^+Cl^-$
52: $R^1 = OCOCH_2X^+Cl^-$; $R^2 = OCOCH_2X^+Cl^-$
53: $R^1 = OCOCH_2X^+Br^-$; $R^2 = OCOCH_2X^+Br^-$
54: $R^1 = CONHCH_2CH_3$; $R^2 = OCONHCH_2CH_3$
55: R^1 = Ac; R^2 = OH
56: R^1 = H; R^2 = OAc
57: R^1 = Ac; R^2 = OAc

Fig. 15.

Dimethylaminopyridine quaternary ammonium derivatives of betulin 46 – 53 showed strong activities of 0.3 - 2.6 μmol/L on cell lines WM3211 a WM793 and again, the 3β,28-bisfunctional derivatives were more active than the monofunctional (Holy *et al.*, 2010). Also bis(carbamoyl) derivatives had strong activity against 518A2 when bis(ethylcarbamate) 54 was almost as active as betulinic acid (1) (about 8 μmol/L). Common acyl derivatives such as 55 - 57 acetates cause a complete extinction of any cytotoxic activity (Gauthier *et al.*, 2006).

Derivatization of betulinic acid (1) and betulin (3) in position 3β

This heterogeneous group of derivatives contains C-3 glycosides, 3β-*O*-acyl derivatives, 3-oxo compounds and their derivatives (ketones, oximes), and products of reduction of nitrogen derivatives (3β-amines). As already mentioned in the previous chapter, antitumor activity of triterpenoid saponins is relatively well explored (Gauthier *et al.*, 2006, 2009a, 2009b; Pakulski *et al.*, 2009; Thibeault *et al.*, 2007) however there is not much data for the melanoma line (Gauthier *et al.*, 2006; Pakulski *et al.*, 2009).

The situation with betulinic acid 3β-glycosides reminds the situation with esters of betulinic acid (1) with sugars. 3β-*O*-α-L-rhamnopyranoside 59 is the most active glycoside with activity of 3.9 μmol/L against metastatic murine melanoma line B-16F1. Glycoside 59 is approximately 4 times more active than acid 1 itself (Gauthier *et al.*, 2006). Approximately the same activity as betulinic acid (1) was found in case of its 3β-*O*-α-D-arabinopyranoside 60, while 3β-*O*-β-D-glucopyranoside 58 was 2 times less active than the 3β-*O*-α-L-rhamnopyranoside 59 (Gauthier *et al.*, 2006). In the same work, an inverse relation for glycosides of methyl betulinate (15) is also documented; 3β-*O*-β-glucopyranoside 58 was the most active from them. (Gauthier *et al.*, 2006)

(Pakulski *et al.*, 2009) investigated the antitumor efficacy of mannopyranosides and 3,6-branched trimannopyranosides, which were stereoselectively prepared from the natural triterepenes - betulin (3), and betulinic acid (1). Although it is a synthetically attractive method, the mannosylation did not bring any significant effect against melanoma. 3β-*O*-α-D-mannopyranoside 61 and 28-*O*-α-D-mannopyranoside 62 showed very poor results against malign melanoma line G 361 and trimannopyranosides were not active as well.

2-Deoxygalactosides and 2-deoxyglucosides (Sarek *et al.*, 2009), prepared from a large group of highly oxidized lupane hydroxyderivatives by stereospecific additions of corresponding glycals, have significant antitumor activity. The above mentioned 2-deoxyglucosides were effective against a wide range of cancer cell lines, including MDR (Sarek *et al.*, 2009). Recently, we tested the anticancer effectiveness of derivative 64 against melanoma lines where activity reached approximately 20 μmol/L (Tab. 4). This group of saponins is promising because peracetylated analogues have an order of magnitude better activity than free 2-deoxyglycosides (Sarek *et al.*, 2009). 2-deoxyglycosides are very hydrophilic in character which makes them readily soluble in aqueous media and easily applicable in *in vivo* conditions, e.g. compound 64 up to 68 mg/mL (Sarek *et al.*, 2007). It was shown on mice that 2-deoxyglycosides are orally bioavailable which is possibly result of their hydrophilicity (Sarek *et al.*, 2007), and that makes them promising candidates for anticancer drugs. An example of a natural highly active glycoside of betulinic acid is 3β-*O*-α-L-arabinopyranoside 63 isolated from *Schefflera rotundifolia*, which has an activity of 0.55 μmol/L against mouse fibrosarcoma line and also shows a combination of glycoside and saccharide ester in molecule.

Acyl derivatives of betulinic acid (1) and betulin (3) are a large group of semisynthetic derivatives known especially for their antiviral effects while their cytotoxicity is much lower than that of hydroxyderivatives. This fact dramatically improves their therapeutic index for testing anti-HIV activity (Krasutsky *et al.*, 2006; Fujioka *et al.*, 1994, Mayaux *et al.*, 1994). A comparison of activity of betulinic (1) and dihydrobetulinic acid (38) with their acetates is described in (Kim *et al.*, 2001; Mukherjee *et al.*, 2004). Tests with SK-MEL-2 and M14-MEL lines showed that the acetylation of hydroxyderivatives causes either a small decrease or no change in cytotoxicity (Kim *et al.*, 2001). This fact is in good agreement with the work, where the influence of the 3β-*O*-acetyl group on cytotoxicity of broader group of triterpenoides 65 - 67 was studied (Mukherjee *et al.*, 2004; Sarek *et al.*, 2005). In the work of Chien *et al.*, the cytotoxicity of natural 3β-*O*-acyl derivatives of betulinic acid 68 - 71 isolated from *Strychnos vanprukii Craib* was investigated against MEL2 line. Cytotoxicity of feruoyl 68, 69 and coumaroyl 70, 71 derivatives was approximately 3 times worse than the free acid 1 (Chien *et al.*, 2004).

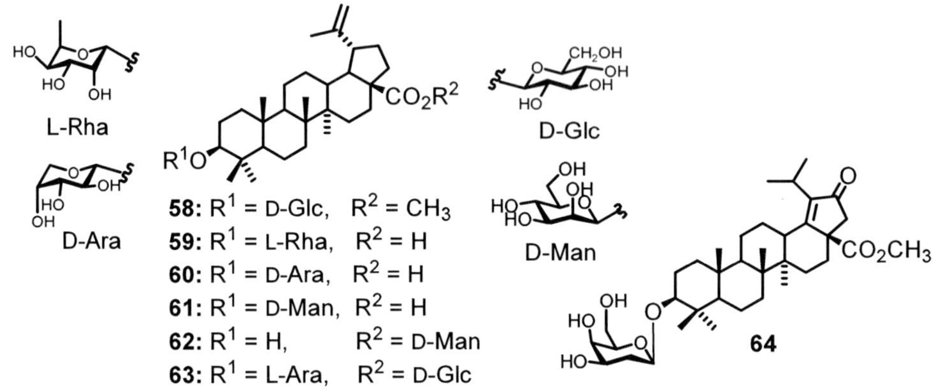

Fig. 16.

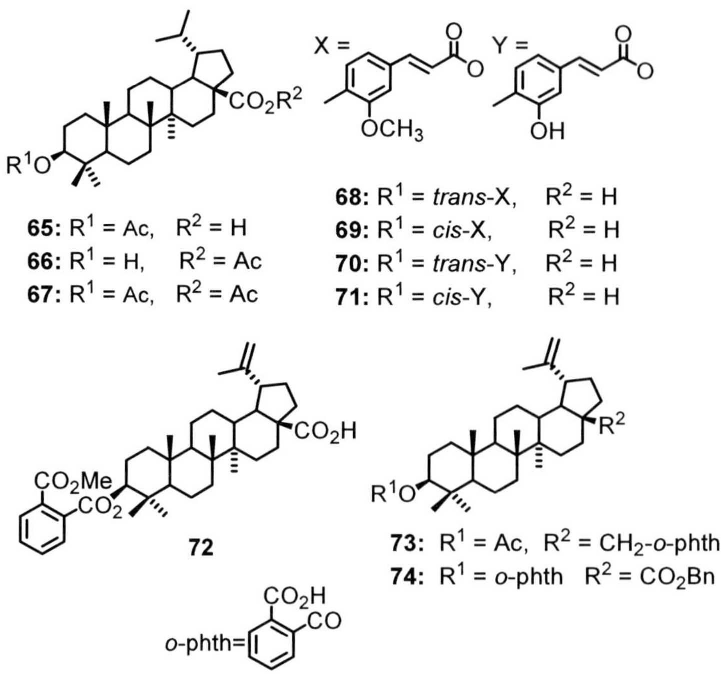

Fig. 17.

The last type of 3β-*O*-acyl derivatives of betulinic acid (1) with described cytotoxicity against the human melanoma line SK MEL2 is represented by phthalates 72 - 74 prepared by (Kvasnica *et al.*, 2005). A SARS study (Kvasnica *et al.*, 2005) of cytotoxicity of hemiphthalates and phthalates of betulinic acid (1) and betulin (3) and their esters against SK MEL2 line shows that the more lipophilic the phthalate ester is, the more active the hemiphthalate is and thus the difference in the activities of the ester is higher. The best activity was reached by derivatives 72 and 74 which was 10 times more active than benzyl betulinate (17) (Fig. 9) itself and a little more active than the free acid 1. Another convenient feature of hemiphthalates is their high hydrophilicity allowing their easy dissolution in aqueous media and their use in *in vivo* tests (Krasutsky *et al.*, 2006; Sarek *et al.*, 2007).

The final group consists of derivatives of 3-oxo acids 5, 75, 76 and their mostly nitrogenous analogues 77 - 81. It is known that oxidation of the 3β-hydroxy group to the oxo group increases the cytotoxicity against the human melanoma line MEL-2. (Kim *et al.*, 1998) While in the pair of betulinic acid (1) - betulonic acid (5) the change is relatively insignificant (1.2 vs. 0.9 μmol/L), the difference is almost an order of magnitude (5.8 vs. 0.7 μmol/L) large in the case of dihydrobetulinic acid (38) - dihydrobetulonic acid (75), which makes dihydrobetulonic acid (75) about twice more effective against MEL-2 than betulinic acid (1) itself (Kim *et al.*, 1998). Analogous results were obtained in cytotoxicity tests of oxidation products of pulsatillic acid (2) (Liu *et al.*, 2004; Zhou *et al.*, 2007). Pulsatillonic acid (76) showed higher activity against B16 line than the original pulsatillic acid (2) (Liu *et al.*, 2004; Zhou *et al.*, 2007). Oxime derivatives of both acids 77 and 80 showed the cytotoxicity against MEL-2 an order of magnitude lower than oxo acids 5 and 75, methyloxime analogues 78 and 81 were two orders of magnitude less active (Kim *et al.*, 1998). In contrast, the 3β-amino analogue 79 obtained by reductive ammination of betulonic acid (5) showed anti-MEL-2 activity comparable with betulinic acid (1) (Kim *et al.*, 1998). The nitrogenous derivatives of betulinic acid (1) in position 3β can also include carbamoyl derivatives 82 – 84 synthesized according to the literature (Kommera *et al.*, 2010). While the 3β-phenylcarbamoyl derivative of betulinic acid - 83 - was active against 518A2, 3β-ethyl carbamates 82, 84 showed activity comparable to or better than betulinic acid (1). Strong antitumor activity against a radial-phase WM3211 and a vertical-phase melanoma WM793 was also found in the case of the quaternary salt 85 with DMAP, with activity 2.6 respectively 5.7 μmol/L.

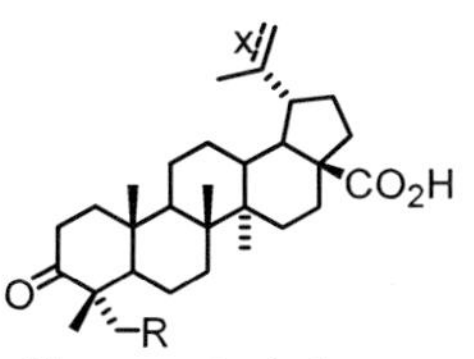

75: R = H, x = single b.
76: R = OH, x = double b

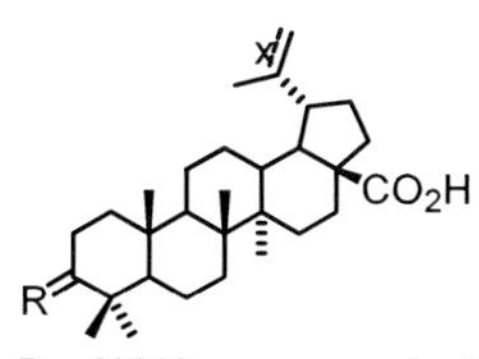

77: R = NOH, x = double b.
78: R = $NOCH_3$, x = double b.
79: R = β-NH_2, α-H; x = double b.
80: R = NOH, x = single b.
81: R = $NOCH_3$, x = single b.

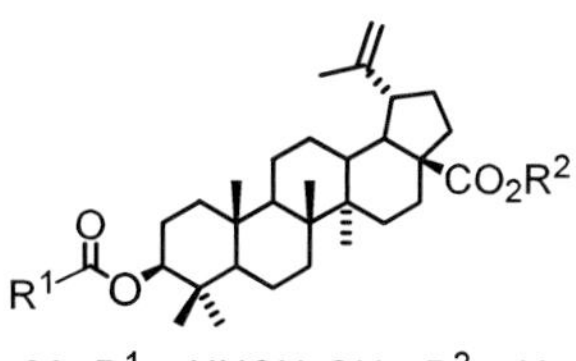

82: R^1 = $NHCH_3CH_2$, R^2 = H
83: R^1 = NHPh, R^2 = H
84: R^1 = $NHCH_3CH_2$, R^2 = CH_3
85: R^1 = $CH_2X^+Br^-$, R^2 = H
where X see Fig. 15

Fig. 18.

Modification of skeleton of betulinic acid (1) on the isopropenyl side chain

An addition of hydrogen, respectively hydrogenation of 20(29)-double bond, represents the simplest modification on the isopropenyl side chain as well as a simple way to isotopically label the terpenic skeleton with either deuterium or tritium. Although the hydrogenation of a terminal double bond seems easy to be done, experiments show the contrary, because 20(29)-double bond is disubstituted. Under the standard conditions - using hydrogen on Pd/C, it is possible to achieve a selective debenzylation of benzyl betulinate (17), without 20(29)-double bond to be hydrogenated (Kvasnica *et al.*, 2005). As mentioned above, dihydrobetulinic acid (38) is approximately four times less active than betulinic acid (1) against the line MEL-2, whereas the cytotoxicity of oxidized forms, such as dihydrobetulonic (75) and betulonic acid (5) is almost identical. These data show that 20(29) dihydroderivatives are comparably active to their unsaturated analogs (Biedermann *et al.*, 2010; Sarek *et al.*, 2007).

Among the other explored addition reaction to 20(29)-double bond, there is the addition of halogene (Mukherjee *et al.*, 1997) or dihalocarbene (Symon *et al.*, 2005). In the study of Mukherjee's *et al.*, cytotoxic activity (except melanoma lines) of the products of addition of bromine to betulonic (5), betulinic (1), and acetylbetulinic (65) acids (e.g. 86 - 87, Fig. 19) was explored and the best results were achieved using 20,29–dibromo-3β-*O*-acetylbetulinic acid (87) which activity was about the same as betulinic acid (1). A Russian team tested the activity of formerly prepared addition adducts 88 and 89 of dichloro- and dibromocarbene to betulinic acid (1) against human melanoma cells Colo 38 and Bro.92. The best results were achieved with a dichloroderivative 88 with the activity on Bro line slightly better than the activity of acid 1, nevertheless the authors claimed that the high lipophilicity of synthesized derivatives complicated *in vitro* tests, therefore further tests of the derivatization of these non-polar compounds were suggested (Symon *et al.*, 2005).

Another option to modify the isopropenyl side chain is substitution, respectively allylic oxidation. Introducing alcohol moieties into the location 30 might be carried out either by allylic bromination using NBS followed by nucleofilic substitution (Kim *et al.*, 2001) or allylic oxidation followed with reduction (Biedermann *et al.*, 2005). The most unique compound among these oxygenated derivatives is the unsaturated aldehyde 90, synthesized by allylic oxidation of acid 1 by selenium dioxide. Aldehyde 90 disposes of strong multispectral antitumor activity, including melanoma lines B16, B16F, SK-MEL2 a MEL-3 (9.3, 12.4, 17.7 and 3.7 μmol/L; also see Tab. 4), and except for B16F, it is several times stronger than acid 1 (Sarek *et al.*, 2003). Corresponding allylic alcohol 91 and its methyl ether 92 had a similar acitivity of 20 μmol/L on SK-MEL2 lines (Kim *et al.*, 2001). 3,30-Diamino derivatives synthesized by (Mar *et al.*, 2010) showed strong proapoptotic effect against panel of seven tumors lines, include SK-MEL-2. Derivative 93 was reported to have two times better cytotoxic effect against SK-MEL2 than acid 1 itself and furthermore this compound is highly hydrophilic and therefore it is easily applicable for *in vivo* tests (Mar *et al.*, 2010).

Finally, compounds formed by oxidative cleavage of the double bond 20(29) should be mentioned (Kim *et al.*, 2001). Evaluated anti SK-MEL2 activity of platanic acid (39) (and its derivatives), obtained by the oxidative cleavage of the double bond using ruthenium tetraoxide (which provide mostly products expected from ozonolysis under standard conditions) was published in Kim's study. Platanic acid (39), alcohol 94 and oxime 95 did not show significant cytotoxicity on SK-MEL2 (Kim *et al.*, 2001).

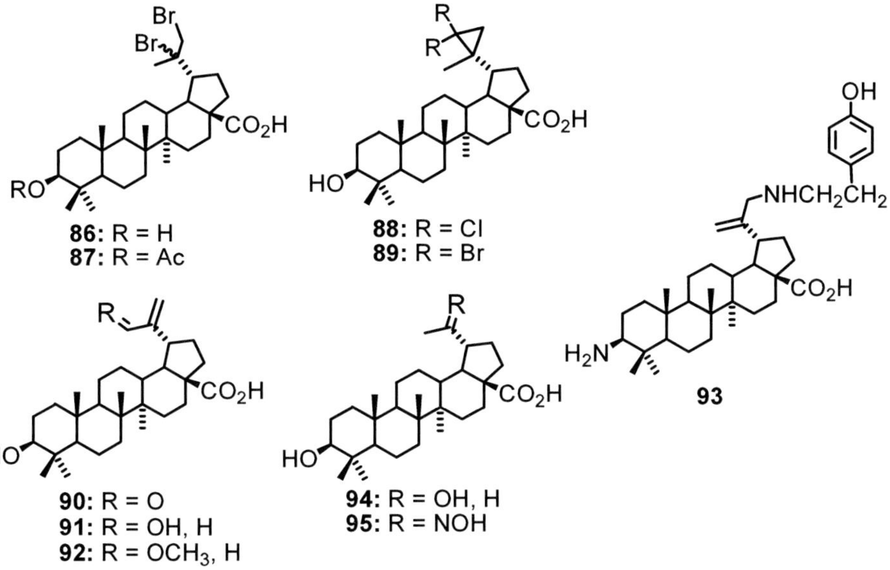

86: R = H
87: R = Ac
88: R = Cl
89: R = Br
90: R = O
91: R = OH, H
92: R = OCH_3, H
93
94: R = OH, H
95: R = NOH

Fig. 19.

2.2.2 Derivatives obtained by biotransformation procedures of betulinic acid (1)

Several papers have described the biotransformation (Chatterjee *et al.*, 1999, 2000; Kouzi *et al.*, 2000) of betulinic acid (1) and the biological activity of those biotransformation products 96 - 102. In Fig. 20, the biotransformation products of different bacterial strains are clearly shown.

The bacterial biotransformation usually produces compounds that would be very difficult to obtain using classical chemical approaches. An example of such compounds is a group of hydroxyderivatives with hydroxyl groups in positions 1, 6, 7, 11 and 15, sometimes the hydroxylation is accompanied by an oxidation in position 3 or an esterification in position 28 by the glucopyranosyl residue. Monohydroxyderivatives 99, 100, as well as betulonic acid (5) showed an order of magnitude better activity during cytotoxicity screening against the Mel-2 cancer line (pleural fluid) than betulinic acid (1) itself, whereas their activity against the Mel-1 cancer line (lymph node) was an order of magnitude worse. 1,7-Dihydroxyderivative 102, 6,7-dihydroxyderivative 98, and 7,15-dihydroxyderivative 96 as well as 7-hydroxyderivative 97 (Kouzi *et al.*, 2000) or glucopyranosyl ester 101 did not show any significant activity against either Mel-1 or Mel-2 cancer lines.

These SARS studies of biotransformation products of acid 1 show that the hydroxylation of the lupane skeleton has a positive impact on antimelanoma activity only if it does not occur in position 7 or 15. Inactivity of β-D-glucopyranosyl ester 101 is possibly caused by the difficulties with hydrolysis of this ester function.

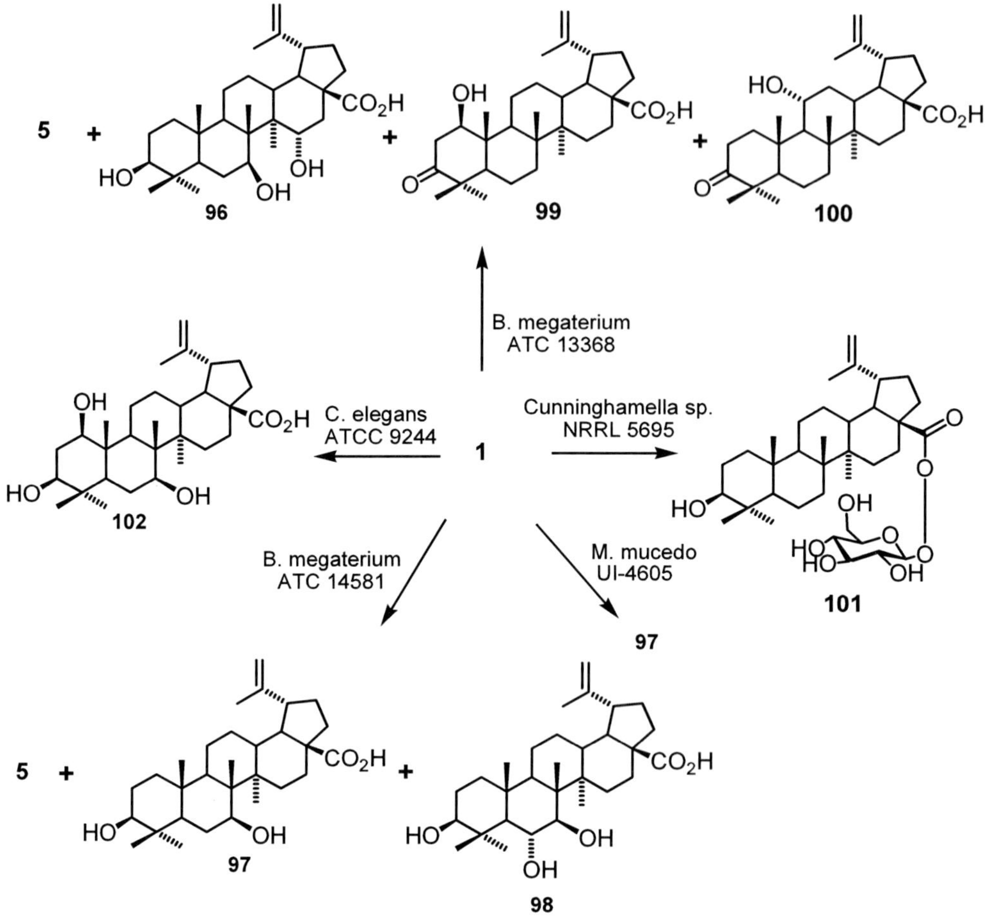

Fig. 20. Biotransformation of betulinic acid (1)

2.2.3 Triterpeoids with modification of lupane skeleton (at ring A or E)

Oxidative modification and cleavage on A-ring of betulinic acid (1)

A detailed study of the cytotoxicity of the products of oxidation of betulinic acid (1) on A-ring was published in paper (Urban *et al.*, 2004). The authors firstly oxidized betulinic acid (1) using chromium(VI) oxide to obtain betulonic acid (5) that was further oxidized with air or oxygen in the presence of potassium tert-butoxide in tert-butylalcohol. That way, either diosphenol 103 or lactol 105 was obtained. Diosphenol 103 was then oxidized with hydrogen peroxide in basic conditions to give A-seco triacid 106, reduction of this triacid afforded A-seco triol 107 and dehydratation of the same triacid gave a 7-membered anhydride 108 (Urban *et al.*, 2004). Curiously, diosphenol 103 only occurs in its enolfom which had not been known before as some literature displays it as a diketone structure that actually does not exist. Derivatives of diosphenol 103, A-seco triol 107 and 7-membered anhydride 108 were the most cytotoxic active compounds from this group. Their cytotoxicity was firstly measured on five cancer cell lines (none of them melanoma) and the active derivatives of diosphenol 103 was then tested on three more lines including human melanoma SK-Mel2. More recent tests of the diosphenol derivatives 104 against three melanoma lines in groups of Sarek and Hajduch resulted in activity about 7-10 times worse than betulinic acid (1). Tab 4.

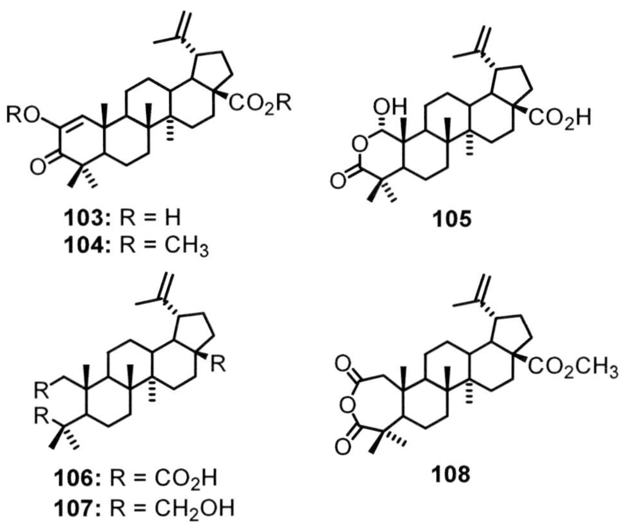

Fig. 21.

Condensation reactions at A-ring

This special chapter will discuss aldehydes and β-ketoesters, the products of Claisen condensation of triterpenoid 3-oxoderivatives with formates and carbonates. Both aldehydes and β-ketoesters are in their enolforms probably due to the boat conformation of the A-ring. Those β-dicarbonyl compounds are a good starting material for synthesis of various heterocycles and for many other substitution reactions. A very complex evaluation of activity of A-homo derivatives was published in work (You *et al.*, 2003). Probably the most interesting was 109 a cytotoxic lupane analogue of a promising anticancer drug CDDO, mainly because it's structural motif seems to be the universal pharmacophor of the cytotoxicity in pentacyclic triterpenes (Suh *et al.*, 1999; You *et al.*, 2003). This derivative is the most active compound from a group of three very promising structures - chloroderivative 110, aldehyde 111, and nitrile 109, which activities against melanoma cell lines SK-MEL-2 a B16-F10 were an order of magnitude better than the activity of betulinic acid (1) (You *et al.*, 2003). These compounds are actually also an exemption from the rule that the 28-alkyl esters are inactive because prepared methyl esters are almost as active as free acids (You *et al.*, 2003).
Heterocyclic derivatives are another type of compounds with homologous carbon atoms bound to the A-ring of the terpenic skeleton (Kumar *et al.*, 2008; Urban *et al.*, 2007; You *et al.*, 2003). You *et al.* published results of the testing of cytotoxic activity of four isoxazole derivatives 112 - 115, prepared by a condensation of aldehydes with hydroxylamine against cell lines SK-MEL-2 a B16-F10. The isoxazoles were strongly cytotoxic only when 28-carboxylic acid was free (compounds 112 and 114). In an article (Urban *et al.*, 2007), a

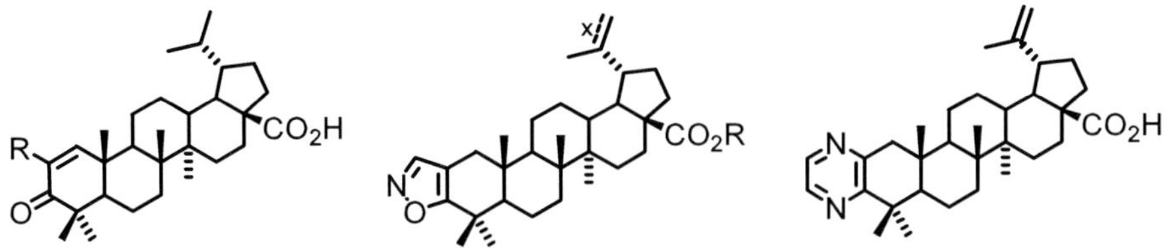

109: R = CN
110: R = Cl
111: R = CHO

112: R = H, x = double b.
113: R = CH_3, x = double b.
114: R = H, x = single b.
115: R = CH_3, x = single b.

116

Fig. 22.

synthesis of triterpenoid pyrazines from betulonic (5) and dihydrobetulonic acid (75) and their cytotoxic activity on 9 cancer cell lines including SK-MEL2 was published. The compounds were obtained by a reaction of 3-oxoacids with ethylenediamine, followed by aromatization of the intermediate dihydropyrazine (Urban *et al.*, 2007). Despite the fact that these pyrazines (e.g. 116) were more cytotoxic against many cancer cell lines than betulinic acid (1), they were four fold less active against the melanoma cell line SK-MEL2. A conclusion is ambiguous, a 2,3 annealing of a pyrazine cycle to the lupane skeleton increases the cytotoxic activity against some cancer cell lines while vanishes the activity against others, such as melanoma (Urban *et al.*, 2007). Analogous quinoxalines (benzopyrazines) were inactive at all. Urban *et al.* also confirmed that there is a strong dependence of the cytotoxicity on the type of ester at 28 carboxylic group. As mentioned before, the Acm esters were generally as active as free acids. Another kind of heterocycles were described in work (Kumar *et al.*, 2008), who prepared and performed a large SARS study with 2,3-annealed indole derivatives of betulinic (1) and betulonic acid (5), prepared by Fisher reaction. The article contains over 30 indole derivatives that were tested on a panel of 8 cancer cell lines, however, not including melanoma. Despite that, a general conclusion can be made that an introduction of the indol heterocycle to a terpene improves the cytotoxicity when both N-1 and C-28 positions remain free. An exception from this assumption is the most active derivative 117 (Kumar *et al.*, 2008) which is conjugated with glycine through C-28 but that is not surprising with respect to high activity of compound 36.

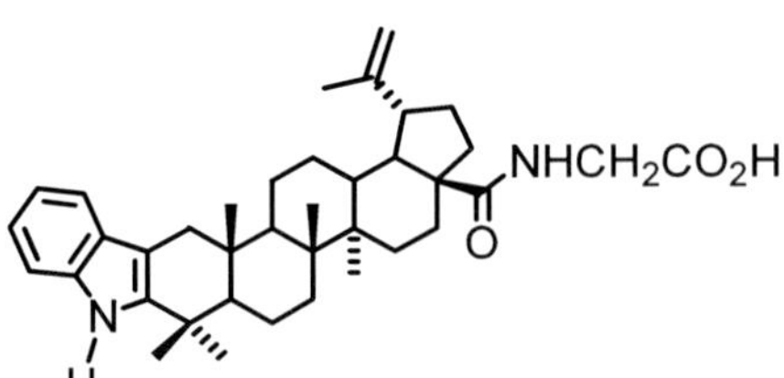

117

Fig. 23.

Modification of the ring E

First semi-synthetic anticancer lupane and 18,19-seco lupane derivatives with modified ring E (referred to as Betulinines) to be published were compounds derived from 18-lupene that contained either intact E-ring and oxygen functional groups in the positions 21 and 22, or cleaved E-ring and 18,19-diketone system (Sarek *et al.*, 2003). The group of Betulinines contains several compounds with significant antitumor activity against wide range of cancer cell lines, including MDR and melanoma lines (SK-MEL-2 MEL-3, B-16, B-16F), diketones 118, and 119 and triketone 126 were among the best. Diketone 118, which is on the other tumor lines much more active than the acid 1, has shown activity in melanoma lines about three times worse than acid 1; Tab. 2, 4 (Sarek *et al.*, 2003). Compounds with pyrazine and quinoxaline heterocycle condensed to the E-ring were not as active as compounds 118, 119, and 126 (Urban *et al.*, 2007). Last but not least, we should mention quaternary ammonium salt 120 was the most active.

Taraxastane derivatives - heterobetulinic acid (121) and heterobetulonic acid (122) should be formally included in this chapter. The acid 121 was firstly isolated from *Calyptranthes pallens*, (Lobo-Echeverri *et al.*, 2005) but it is also available synthetically from betulin (3) in five steps (Bradbury & Mingjun, 2007), which include a rearrangement of lupane skeleton to taraxastane. Heterobetulinic acid (121) showed antitumor activity against melanoma lines M14 UACC62 and SK MEL 5 comparable to or slightly better than that of betulinic acid (1), Tab. 4.

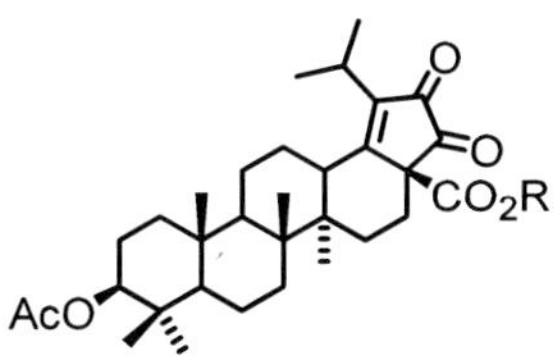

118: R = CH_3
119: R = Acm

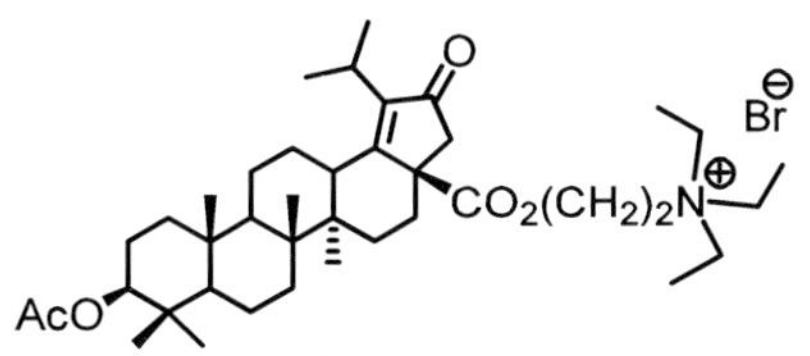

120

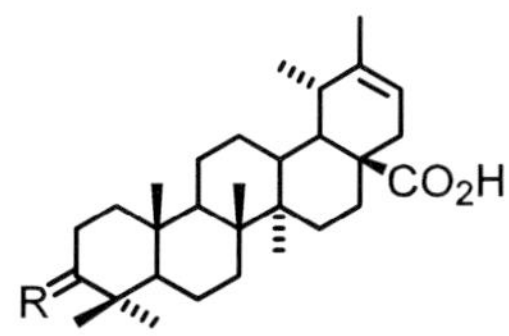

121: R = β-OH, α-H
122: R = O

Fig. 24.

Des-E lupane derivatives

Des-E lupane derivatives represent the ultimate synthetic step in the oxidative cleavage/degradation of the ring E of the 21,22-dioxolupane compounds using ruthenium(VIII) oxide. (Sarek *et al.*, 2003) described several des-E-lupane compounds, most important are the γ-keto and β-keto acids 123, 124 and methyleneketone 125. They are also named Betulinines. β-Keto acid 124 (also called JS8) is the most promising anticancer drug within this group, based on the values of cytotoxic activity against more than 30 lines including MDR (the cytotoxicity was 1.28 μmol/L for MEL-3, 4.3 μmol/L for M14, and 1.16 μmol/L for SK-MEL-2; Tab. 4) (Sarek *et al.*, 2003). It is essential to mention that, according to data from flow cytometry, JS8 causes selective apoptosis of tumor cells with rate comparable to the commercial cytostatic diterpenic drug paclitaxel. It was found that JS8 has a unique and new mechanism of action with primary target located in mitochondria. Compound JS8 is also very interesting from the chemical point of view, because it is a β-keto acid that are known to be extremely unstable because they tend to decarboxylate spontaneously. Despite that, JS8 is relatively stable compound when stored at reduced temperature and it is probably due to a significant steric hindrance of the labile carboxyl group. As a tetracyclic pentanorlupane derivative, JS8 is very hydrophilic in comparison to the full-sized triterpenes, and so it is readily soluble in aqueous media (maximum solubility is 68 mg/mL) (Sarek *et al.*, 2007). In conclusion, JS8 is highly antitumor compound, it has favorable solubility for the *in vivo* tests;

its structure, activity and manufacturing procedure has been patented (Fisher *et al.*, 2003) and therefore it has a great chance to become an anticancer drug. Methyleneketone 125, one of the two degradation products of JS8, has similarly strong antitumor properties (activity against M14 was 4.3 μmol/L and against SK-MEL 5 was 3.4 μmol/L; Tab. 4) (Sarek *et al.*, 2007).

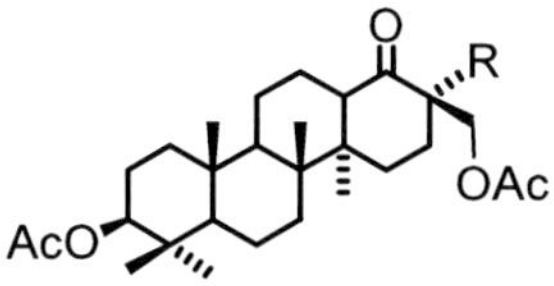

123: R = CH_2CO_2H
124: R = CO_2H

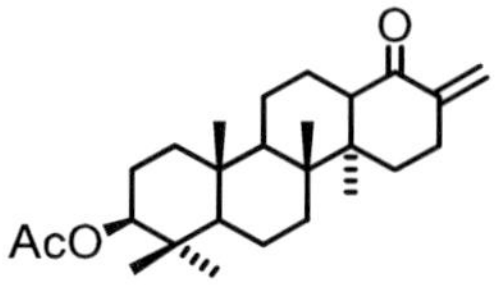

125

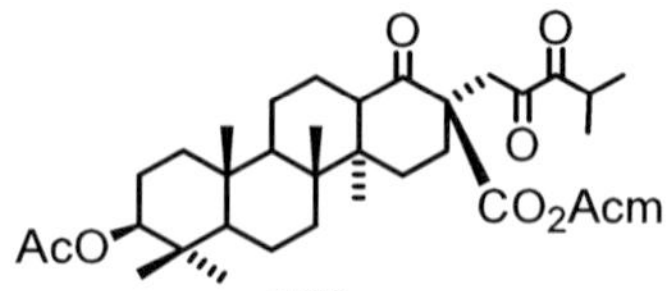

126

Fig. 25.

3. Conclusions and future directions

Despite the fact that betulinic acid (**1**) was first isolated in 1902, it took another forty years to solve its structure and to identify that several compounds obtained from natural sources by other research groups were identical to it. Trumbull *et al.* was the first to discover the interesting cytotoxic activity of betulinic acid (**1**) in 1976 when he studied a chloroform extract of *Vauquelinia corymbosa* against lymphocytic leukemia cells anti-P-388. He suggested that uvaol, ursolic acid, and betulinic acid (**1**) are the components responsible for the cytotoxicity. After that, it took another 19 years until Pisha *et al.* confirmed that the activity is caused by betulinic acid (**1**) and these authors were first to report that the cytotoxicity is selective against human melanoma cells. This fact sparked intensive research and gave the oncologists hope for the birth of a new drug to combat the insidious disease with steadily increasing incidence.

During early 90th of the last century, the scientists stood at the starting line - they had a natural substance with a quite complicated structure and available only in limited quantities from precious natural sources, however, the compound had strong and selective activity against melanoma and very low toxicity. The main disadvantage seemed to be its unfavorable pharmacokinetic parameters. After solving the difficulties with the availability of acid **1** by developing its synthetic procedure from betulin (**3**), the use of betulinic acid (**1**) was given a real dimension. As a result, several hundred semi-synthetic lupane analogues were published up today, derivatives of betulinic acid (**1**), pulsatillic acid (2), and betulin (**3**), many of those showed significant anticancer effects. They are more hydrophilic and their pharmacokinetic profile is improved. Some of them were tested *in vitro* on activity against human or murine melanoma cells and three of them were tested *in vivo*.

There are several tens of derivatives with promising activity against melanoma cells *in vitro*; the most significant are artificially modified compounds as pulsatillates **24** - **29**; NVX-207 (**30**); conjugates of acid **1** with amino acids **33**, **36**, **37**; quaternary ammonium salts **40**, **41** and **46** - **53**, **85**; some glycosides (the best showed to be: **32**, **58**, **59** and **64**); hemiphtalates **72**, **74**; carbamate **54**; compounds with modified isopropenyl chain (acid **90**, **93**, methoxyderivative **92** and alcohol **91**); compounds with modified A-ring (most active were compounds that have an EWG group in the location 2 of the 3-oxo lupane skeleton or the EWG with a multiple bond in conjugation with 3-oxo group - the best are **109** - **112**, **114** and **117**); compounds with modified E-ring where active was diketone **118** and heterobetulinic acid (**121**); and finally, the des-E-derivatives JS8 (**124**) and methyleneketone **125**.

Betulinic acid (1) itself is now in phase II of clinical trials against dysplastic nevus, compound NVX-207 (**30**) was tested on dogs with particularly good results and pulsatillate **24** was successfully tested on the mice models. These *in vivo* data together with current industrial availability of betulinic acid (**1**) and a variety of its active derivatives with improved hydrophilicity and a reasonable solubility in water-based media gives this group of natural compounds high potential to become a new generation of cytostatic drugs to combat a malignant melanoma.

4. Tables of activities

Compound	B16	B16-F1	MEL-1	MEL-2
1	53.5	16.1	6.3	1.3
2	83.0	—	—	—
3	—	13.8	—	—
5	—	—	31.8	0.1
13	—	210.1	—	244.1
14	—	—	—	160.0
15	—	26.0	—	—
16	—	—	—	217.9
17	—	—	—	NA
24	80.5	—	—	—
25	72.9	—	—	—
26	80.9	—	—	—
27	66.0	—	—	—
28	41.1	—	—	—
29	63.2	—	—	—
30	—	—	—	—
31	—	—	NA	NA
33	—	—	—	2.9
34	—	—	—	4.1
35	—	—	—	6.8
36	—	—	—	8.0
37	—	—	—	18.1
38	-	-	-	12.7
42	—	>248	—	—
43	—	>228	—	—
44	—	>175	—	—
55	—	—	—	247.0
56	—	—	—	223.7
58	—	7.1	—	—
59	—	3.9	—	—
60	—	11.0	—	—
68	—	—	—	3.4
69	—	—	—	3.4
70	—	—	—	4.2
71	—	—	—	3.7
72	—	—	—	13.4
73	—	—	—	24.9
74	—	—	—	90.0
75	-	-	-	1.5
77	—	—	—	2.4
78	—	—	—	8.3
79	—	—	—	1.3
80	—	—	—	2.2
81	—	—	—	NA

Table 1.

Compound	B16-F1	MEL-1	MEL-2	M14-MEL
91	-	-	18.0	-
92	-	-	20.0	-
93	-	-	3.0	-
96	-	NA	NA	-
97	-	14.1	14.1	-
98	-	21.5	33.3	-
99	-	NA	0.5	-
100	-	NA	0.4	-
102	-	NA	NA	-
103	-	-	23.0	-
109	2.7	-	1.5	-
110	3.0	-	0.21	-
111	0.55	-	0.50	-
112	6.1	-	31.2	-
114	3.1	-	2.2	-
116	-	-	98.0	-
118	67.9	-	65.3	-
119	NA	-	NA	-
123	11.5	-	19.9	-
124	0.4	-	1.2	4.3
125	0.7	-	2.1	-
126	34.3	-	223.7	-

Table 2.

Compound	518A2	Colo38	Bro	WM3211	WM793
15	28.8	—	—	—	—
30	2.6	—	—	—	—
46	—	—	—	0.6	2.5
47	—	—	—	0.7	1.3
48	—	—	—	0.3	1.9
49	—	—	—	0.6	0.8
50	—	—	—	0.3	0.5
51	—	—	—	0.5	0.5
52	—	—	—	0.4	0.4
53	—	—	—	0.5	0.5
54	8.18	—	—	—	—
82	17.8	—	—	—	—
83	51.5	—	—	—	—
84	16.7	—	—	—	—
85	—	—	—	2.6	5.7
87	—	10	10	—	—
88	—	> 10	> 10	—	—

Table 3.

Compound	M14	UACC 62	SK MEL 5
1	5.4	5.0	4.5
38	16.7	22.3	4.7
41	14.6	1.6	2.2
64	21.1	19.0	18.4
75	12.7	12.6	9.3
90	9.2	5.8	6.9
104	54.0	29.8	27.6
116	41.2	14.7	6.3
118	15.8	14.7	11.3
121	6.2	4.6	3.5
122	45.8	13.9	6.4
124	4.9	3.5	3.8
125	4.3	3.5	3.4

Table 4.

Table 1-4: Table 1-3 - cytotoxicity (IC_{50} in μM) of published compounds against melanoma cell lines; Table 4 - cytotoxicity (IC_{50} in μM) selected semisynthetic lupane derivatives against melanoma cell lines which are part of the NCI60 cell lines panel and are therefore well characterized and further studied, e.g. cell line M14 is bearing the mutated p53 protein. NA is not active.

5. Acknowledgment

This study was supported partially by the Czech Science Foundation (305/09/1216 and 301/09/P433), by grant from EHP/Norway (CZ0099) and by the Ministry of Education of the Czech Republic (MSM 6840770040). Special thanks to Dr. Carlos Gerardo Velazco Macías from Áreas Naturales Protegidas, Parques y Vida Silvestre de Nuevo León for providing photos of plants and Andrew Olson for text corrections. The infrastructural part of this project (IMTM) was supported from the Operational Program Research and Development for Innovations (project CZ.1.05/2.1.00/01.0030).

6. References

Akihisa, T.; Takamine Y.; Yoshizumi, K.; Tokuda, H.; Kimura, Y.; Ukiya, M.; Nakahara, T.; Yokochi, T.; Ichiishi E. & Nishino, H. (2002). Microbial transformations of two lupane-type triterpenes and anti-tumor-promoting effects of the transformation products. *Journal of Natural Products*, Vol. 65, No. 3, pp. 278–282, ISSN 0163-3864.

Barton, D. H. R. & Jones, E. R. H. (1944). Optical rotatory power and structure in triterpenoid, compounds. Application of the method of molecular rotation differences. *Journal of the Chemical Society*, pp. 659 - 665.

Bi, Y.; Xu, J.; Wu, X.; Ye, W.; Yuan, S. & Zhang, L. (2007). Synthesis and cytotoxic activity of 17-carboxylic acid modified 23-hydroxy betulinic acid ester derivatives. *Bioorganic & Medicinal Chemistry Letters*, Vol. 17, No. 5, pp. 1475-1478, ISSN 0960 - 894X.

Biedermann, D.; Eignerova, B.; Hajduch, M. & Sarek, J. (2010) Synthesis and Evaluation of Biological Activity of the Quaternary Ammonium Salts of Lupane-, Oleanane-, and Ursane-Type Acids. *Synthesis-Stuttgart*, Vol. 42, No. 22, 3839-3848, ISSN 0039-7881.

Biedermann, D.; Sarek, J.; Klinot, J.; Hajduch, M. & Dzubak, P. (2005). Fluorination of Betulinines and Other Triterpenoids with DAST. *Synthesis-Stuttgart*, Vol 37, No. 7, pp. 1157-1163, ISSN 0039-7881.

Bradbury, B. J. & Mingjun, H. (2007). Substituted Taraxastanes Useful for Treating Viral Infections, WO 2007098247, Filling date 20.2. 2007.

Bradbury, B. J.; Soper, S. J.; Kaczvinsky J. R.; Bailey, D. L.; Gale, C. D. (1997) Method for Regulating Hair Growth, DE 19,532,006, pub. date 1997-09-17.

Bradbury, B. J.; Soper, S. J.; Kaczvinsky J. R.; Bailey, D. L.; Gale, C. D (1997). Compositions which contain terpenes for regulating hair growth, JP 09087156, pub. Date 1997-07-15.

Bradbury, B. J.; Soper, S. J.; Kaczvinsky J. R.; Bailey, D. L.; Gale, C. D (1997). Compositions which contain terpenes for regulating hair growth,JP 10025236, 1998-07-17.

Bruckner, V.; Kovács, J. & Koczka, I. (1948). Occurrence of Betulinic Acid in the Bark of the Plane Tree. *Journal of the Chemical Society*, pp. 948 – 951.

Chatterjee, P.; Pezzuto, J. M. & Kouzi, S. A. (1999). Glucosidation of betulinic acid by Cunninghamella species. *Journal of Natural Products*, Vol. 62, No. 5, pp. 761–763, ISSN 0163-3864.

Chatterjee, P.; Kouzi, S. A.; Pezzuto, J. M. & Hamann, M. T. (2000). Biotransformation of the antimelanoma agent betulinic acid by Bacillus megaterium ATCC 13368. *Applied and environmental microbiology*, Vol. 66, No. 9, pp. 3850–3855, ISSN 0099-2240.

Chien, N. Q. ; Hung, N. V. ; Santarsiero, B. D.; Mesecar, A. D.; Cuong, N. M.; Soejarto, D. D.; Pezzuto, J. M.; Fong, H. H. S.; Tan, G. T. (2004). New 3-O-Acyl Betulinic Acids from Strychnos vanprukii Craib. *Journal of Natural Products,* Vol. 67, No 6, pp. 994–998, ISSN 0163-3864.

Clark, A. M. & Hufford, C. D. (1991). Use of microorganisms for the study of drug metabolism: An update. *Medicinal Research Reviews*, Vol. 11, No. 5, pp. 437–501, ISSN 0198-6325.

Cichewicz, R. H. & Kouzi, S. A. (2004). Chemistry, biological activity, and chemotherapeutic potential of betulinic acid for the prevention and treatment of cancer and HIV infection. *Medicinal Research Reviews*, Vol. 24, No. 1, pp. 90-114, ISSN 0198-6325.

Cioffi, G.; Braca, A.; Autore, G.; Morelli, I. ; Pinto, A.; Venturella, F. & De Tommasi, N. (2003). Cytotoxic saponins from Schefflera fagueti. *Planta Medica*, Vol. 69, No. 8, pp. 750 – 756, ISSN 0032-0943.

Csuk, R.; Schmuck, K. & Schäfer, R. (2006). A practical synthesis of betulinic acid. *Tetrahedron Letters*, Vol. 47, No. 49, pp. 8769-8770, ISSN 0040-4039.

Dzubak, P.; Hajduch, M.; Vydra, V.; Hustova, A.; Kvasnica, M.; Biedermann, D.; Markova, L.; Urban, M. & Sarek, J. (2006). Pharmacological activities of natural triterpenoids and their therapeutic implications. *Natural Product Reports*, Vol. 23, No. 3, pp. 394-411, ISSN 0265-0568.

Effenberger, K.; Breyer, S. & Schobert, R. (2010). Terpene Conjugates of the Nigella sativa Seed-Oil Constituent Thymoquinone with Enhanced Efficacy in Cancer Cells. *Chemistry and Biodiversity*, Vol. 7, No. 1, pp 129-139, ISSN 1612-1872.

Eiznhamer, D. & Xu, Z. (2004). Betulinic acid: A promissing anticancer candidate. *Idrugs*, Vol. 7, No. 4, pp. 359-373, ISSN 1369-7056.

Evers, M.; Poujade, C.; Soler, F.; Ribeill, Y.; James, C.; Lelievre, Y.; Gueguen, J.-C.; Reisdorf, D. & Morize, I. (1996). Betulinic acid derivatives: A new class of human immunodeficiency virus type 1 specific inhibitors with a new mode of action. *Journal of Medicinal Chemistry*, Vol. 39, No. 5, pp. 1056–1068, ISSN 0022-2623.

Fischer, P. M.; Sarek, J.; Blaney, P. M.; Collier, P. & Fergusson J. R. (2003) Medicament. PCT Int. Patent Appl. WO03045971 A2, 2003-06-05.

Fuchino, H.; Satoh, T. & Tanaka, N. (1995). Chemical Evaluation of Betula Species in Japan .1. Constituents of Betula-Ermanii. *Chemical & Pharmaceutical Bulletin*, Vol. 43, No. 11, pp. 1937–1942, ISSN 0009-2363.

Fuchino, H.; Satoh, T. & Tanaka, N. (1996). Chemical evaluation of Betula species in Japan .3. Constituents of Betula maximowicziana. *Chemical & Pharmaceutical Bulletin*, Vol. 44, No. 9, pp. 1748–1753, ISSN 0009-2363.

Fuchino, H.; Satoh, T.; Shimizu, M. & Tanaka, N. (1998). Chemical evaluation of Betula species in Japan. IV. Constituents of Betula davurica *Chemical & Pharmaceutical Bulletin*, Vol. 46, No. 1, pp. 166–168, ISSN 0009-2363.

Fujioka, T.; Kashiwada, Y.; Kilkuskie, R. E.; Cosentino, L. M.; Ballas, L. M.; Jiang, J. B.; Janzen, W. P.; Chen, I. S. & Lee, K. H. (1994). Anti-Aids Agents .11. Betulinic Acid and Platanic Acid as Anti-Hiv Principles from Syzigium-Claviflorum, and the Anti-Hiv Activity of Structurally Related Triterpenoids. *Journal of Natural Products*, Vol. 57, No. 2, pp. 243–247, ISSN 0163-3864.

Fulda, S.; Jeremias, I.; Steiner, H. H.; Pietsch, T. & Debatin, K. M. (1999). Betulinic acid: A new cytotoxic agent against malignant brain-tumor cells. *International Journal of Cancer*, Vol. 82, No. 3, pp. 435 - 441, ISSN 0020 - 7136.

Fulda, S.; Scaffidi, C.; Susin, S. A.; Krammer, P. H.; Kroemer, G.; Peter, M. E. & Debatin, K. M. (1998). Activation of mitochondria and release of mitochondrial apoptogenic factors by betulinic acid. *Journal of Biological Chemistry*, Vol 273, No. 51, pp. 33942-33948, ISSN 0021-9258.

Gauthier, C.; Legault, J.; Girard-Lalancette, K.; Mshvildadze V. & Pichette, A. (2009). Haemolytic acitivity, cytotoxicity and membrane cell permeabilization of semi-synthetic and natural lupane- and oleanane-type saponins. *Bioorganic & Medicinal Chemistry*, Vol. 17, No. 5, pp. 2002-2008, ISSN0968-0896.

Gauthier, C.; Legault, J.; Lavoie, S.; Rondeau, S.; Tremblay, S. & Pichette, A. (2009). Synthesis and Cytotoxicity of Bidesmosidic Betulin and Betulinic Acid Saponins. *Journal of Natural Products*, Vol. 72, No. 1, pp. 72-81, ISSN 0163-3864.

Gauthier, C.; Legault, J.; Lebrun M.; Dufour P.; S. & Pichette, A. (2006). Glycosidation of lupane-type triterpenoids as potent in vitro cytotoxic agents. *Bioorganic & Medicinal Chemistry*, Vol. 14, No. 19, pp. 6713-6725, ISSN 0968-0896.

Glasby, J. S. (1982). *Encyclopedia of the Terpenoids*, John Wiley, ISBN 0471279862 (0-471-27986-2), New York.

Gopal, D. V. R.; Narkar, A. A.; Badrinath, Y.; Mishra, K. P. & Joshi, D. S. (2005). Betulinic acid induces apoptosis in human chronic myelogenous leukemia (CML) cell line K-562 without altering the levels of Bcr-Abl. *Toxicology Letters*, Vol. 155, No. 3, pp. 343 - 351, ISSN 0378 - 4274.

Hata, K.; Hori, K. & Takahashi, S. (2002). Differentiation- and apoptosis-inducing activities by pentacyclic triterpenes on a mouse melanoma cell line. *Journal of Natural Products*, Vol. 65, No. 5, pp. 645 - 648, ISSN 0163 - 3864.

Hata, K.; Hori, K.; Ogasawara, H. & Takahashi, S. (2003). Anti-leukemia activities of Lup-28-al-20(29)-en-3-one, a lupane triterpene. *Toxicology Letters*, Vol. 143, No. 1, pp. 1–7, ISSN 0378-4274.

Holy, J.; Kolomitsyna, O.; Krasutsky, D.; Oliviera, J. P. & Perkins, E. (2010). Dimethylaminopyridine derivatives of lupane triterpenoids are potent disruptors of mitochondrial structure and function. *Bioorganic & Medicinal Chemistry*, Vol. 18, No. 18, pp. 6080-6088, ISSN 0968-0896.

Holz-Smith, S. L.; Sun, I. C.; Jin, L.; Matthews, T. J.; Lee, K.- H. & Chen, C. H. (2001). Role of human immunodeficiency virus (HIV) type 1 envelope in the anti-HIV activity of the betulinic acid derivative IC9564. Antimicrobial Agents and Chemotherapy, Vol. 45, No. 1, pp. 60–66, ISSN 0066-4804.

Huang, C.; Tunon, H. & Bohlin, L. (1995). Anti-inflammatory compounds isolated from Menyanthes trifoliata L. *Yao Xue Xue Bao*, Vol. 30, No. 8, pp. 621–626, ISSN 0513-4870.

Huang, L.; Ho, P.; Lee, K.-H. & Chen, C. – H. (2006). Synthesis and anti-HIV activity of bi-functional betulinic acid derivatives. *Bioorganic & Medicinal Chemistry*, Vol. 14, No. 7, pp. 2279–2289, ISSN 0968-0896.

Jacob, J. S.; Richards, J.; Augustine, J. G. & Milea, J. S. (2010). Liquid Bevirimat Dosage Forms for Oral Administration, US 2010216751, pub. date 2010-08-26.

Jeong, H.-J.; Chai, H.-B.; Park, S.-Y. & Kim, D. S. H. L. (1999). Preparation of amino acid conjugates of betulinic acid with activity against human melanoma. Bioorg. *Bioorganic & Medicinal Chemistry Letters*, Vol. 9, No. 8, pp. 1201-1204, ISSN 0960 - 894X.

Kashiwada, Y.; Hashimoto, F.; Cosentino, L. M.; Chen, C.-H.; Garrett, P. E. & Lee, K. H. (1996). Betulinic acid and dihydrobetulinic acid derivatives as potent anti-HIV agents. *Journal of Medicinal Chemistry*, Vol. 39, No. 5, pp. 1016–1017, ISSN 0022-2623.

Kasperczyk, H.; La Ferla-Bruhl, K.; Westhoff, M. A.; Behrend, L.; Zwacka, R. M.; Debatin, K. M. & Fulda, S. (2005). Betulinic acid as new activator of NF-kappaB: molecular mechanisms and implications for cancer therapy. *Oncogene*, Vol. 24, No. 46, pp. 6945-6956, ISSN 0950-9232.

Keller, P. W.; Adamson, C. S.; Heymann, J. B.; Freed, E. O. & Steven, A. C. (2011). HIV-1 maturation inhibitor bevirimat stabilizes the immature Gag lattice. *Journal of Virology*, Vol. 85, No. 4, pp. 1420-1428, ISSN 0022-538X.

Kessler, J. H.; Mullauer, F. B.; de Roo, G. M. & Medema, J. P. (2007). Broad in vitro efficacy of plant-derived betulinic acid against cell lines derived from the most prevalent human cancer types. *Cancer Letters*, Vol. 251, No. 1, pp. 132 - 145, ISSN 0304 - 3835.

Kim, D. S. H.; Pezzuto, J. M. & Pisha, E. (1998). Synthesis of betulinic acid derivatives with activity against human melanoma. *Bioorganic & Medicinal Chemistry Letters*, Vol. 8, No. 13, pp. 1707 - 1712, ISSN 0960 - 894X.

Kim, J.-Y.; Koo, H.-M. & Kim, D. S. H. L. (2001). Development of C-20 modified betulinic acid derivatives as antitumor agents. *Bioorganic & Medicinal Chemistry Letters*, Vol. 11, No. 17, pp. 2405 - 2408, ISSN 0960 - 894X.

Kommera, H.; Kaluderovič, G.; Dittrich, . Kalbitz, J.; Drager, B.; Mueller, T. & Paschke, R. (2010). Carbamate derivatives of betulinic acid and betulin with selective cytotoxic activity. *Bioorganic & Medicinal Chemistry Letters*, Vol. 20, No. 11, pp. 3409-3412, ISSN 0960 - 894X.

Kouzi, S. A.; Chatterjee, P.; Pezzuto, J. M. & Hamann, M. T. (2000). Microbial transformations of the antimelanoma agent betulinic acid. *Journal of Natural Products*, Vol. 63, No. 12, pp. 1653-1657, ISSN 0163-3864.

Krasutsky, P. A. & Munshi, K. (2006). Synthesis of Betulonic and Betulinic Aldehydes. WO2006133314 (A2), pub. date 2006-12-14

Krasutsky, P. A.; Khotkevych, A. B.; Puschenikov, A. & Rudnitskaya, A. (2006). Electrochemical Method for the Production of Betuline Aldehyde. WO2006105357, pub. date 2006-10-05.

Krasutsky, P. A. (2006). Birch bark research and development. *Natural Product* Reports, Vol. 23, No. 3, pp. 919-942, ISSN 0265 - 0568.

Krasutsky, P. A.; Carlson, R. M.; Nestrenko, V. V.; Kolomitsyn, I. V. & Edwardson, C. F. (2005). Birch bark processing and the isolation of natural products from birch bark, US2005158414, pub. date. 2005-07-21.

Krasutsky, P. A.; Carlson, R. M. & Nestrenko, V. V. (2003). Methods for manufacturing betulinic acid, US2003073858, pub. date. 2003-04-17.

Krasutsky, P. A.; Puschenikov, A. & Sergeeva, T. (2006). Selective Oxidation of Triterpenes Employing TEMPO. WO2006105354, pub. date 2006-10-05.

Kumar, V.; Rani, N.; Aggarwal, P.; Sanna, K. V.; Singh, A. T.; Jaggi, M.; Joshi, N.; Sharma, P. K.; Irchhaiya, R. & Burman, A. C. (2008). Synthesis and cytotoxic activity of heterocyclic ring-substituted betulinic acid derivatives. *Bioorganic & Medicinal Chemistry Letters*, Vol. 18, No. 18, pp. 5058-5062, ISSN 0960 - 894X.

Kvasnica, M.; Sarek, J.; Klinotova, E.; Dzubak, P. & Hajduch, M. (2005). Synthesis of Phthalates of Betulinic Acid and Betulin with Cytotoxic Activity. *Bioorganic & Medicinal Chemistry*, Vol. 13, No. 10, pp. 3447-3454, ISSN 0968-0896.

Liu, W.-K.; Ho, J. C. K.; Cheung, F. W. K.; Liu, B. P. L.; Ye, W.-C. & Che, Ch.-T. (2004). Apoptotic activity of betulinic acid derivatives on murine melanoma B16 cell line. *European Journal of Pharmacology*, Vol. 498, No. 1-3, pp. 71-78, ISSN 0014-2999.

Lobo-Echeverri, T.; Rivero-Cruz, J. F.; Su, B.-N.; Chai, H.-B.; Cordell, G. A.; Pezzuto, J. M.; Swanson, S. M.; Soejarto, D. D. & Kinghorn, D. A. (2005). Constituents of the Leaves and Twigs of Calyptranthes pallens Collected from an Experimental Plot in Southern Florida. Journal of Natural Products, Vol. 68, No. 4, pp. 577-580, ISSN 0163-.3864.

Mar, A. A.; Szotek, E. L.; Koohang, A.; Flavin, W. P.; Eiznhamer, D. A.; Flavin, M. T. & Xu, Z.-Q. (2010). Synthesis, proapoptotic screening, and structure-activity relationships of novel aza-lupane triterpenoids. *Bioorganic & Medicinal Chemistry Letters*, Vol. 20, No. 18, pp. 5389-5393, ISSN 0960-894X.

Mathers, C. D.; Boshi-Pinto, C.; Lopez, A. D. & Murray, C. JL. (2001). Cancer incidence, mortality, and survival by site for 14 regions of the world, in: *Global Programme on evidence for Health Policy Discussion Paper No. 13 (World Health Organization)*, 16. 04. 2011, Available from: http://www.who.int/healthinfo/global_burden_disease/data_sources_methods/en/

Mayaux, J.-F.; Bousseau, A.; Pauwels, R.; Huet, T.; Henin, Y.; Dereu, N., Evers, M.; Soler, F.; Paujado, C.; De Clereq, E. & Le Pecq, J. (1994). Triterpene Derivatives That Block Entry of Human-Immunodeficiency-Virus Type-1 into Cells. *Proceedings of the National Academy of Sciences of the United States of America*, Vol. 91, No. 9, pp. 3564 - 3568, ISSN 0027-8424.

Mayer, R. (1996). Three Lupane Derivatives from *Leptospermum scoparium*. *Archiv der Pharmazie*, Vol. 329, No. 10, 447 - 450.

Mukherjee, P. K.; Saha, K.; Das, J.; Pal, M. & Saha, B. P. (1997). Studies on the anti-inflammatory activity of rhizomes of Nelumbo nucifera. *Planta Medica*, Vol. 63, No. 4, pp. 367–369, ISSN 0032-0943.

Mukherjee, R.; Jaggi, M.; Rajendran, P.; Siddiqui, M. J. A.; Srivastava, S. K.; Vardhan, A. & Burman, A. (2004). Betulinic acid and its derivatives as anti-angiogenic agents. *Bioorganic & Medicinal Chemistry Letters*, Vol. 14, No. 9, pp. 2181 - 2184, ISSN 0960 - 894X.

Ngassapa, O. D.; Soejarto, D. D. & Che, Ch.-T. (1991). New Cytotoxic Lupane Lactones from Kokoona-Ochracea. *Journal of Natural Products*, Vol 54, No. 5, pp. 1353-1359, ISSN 0163-3864.

Pakulski, Z. A.; Cmoch, P.; Oklestkova, J. & Strnad, M. (2009). Saccharide lupane derivatives, their use and pharmaceuticals compositions containing these derivatives. PCT/CZ2009/000007, filling date 2009-01-28.

Pezzuto, J. N.; Kosmeder, J. W.; Xu, Ze-Qi; Zhou, N. E. & Goldsmith, M. E. (2007). Method of preparing and use of prodrugs of betulinic acid derivatives, US 2007072835, pub. date 2007-03-29.

Pirard, P. & de Vries, E. (May 2007). Incidence of melanoma in people aged under 55 years, in: *European Environment and Health Information System*, 16. 04. 2011, Available from: http://www.euro.who.int/en/what-we-do/data-and-evidence/environment-and-health-information-system-enhis/publications/pre-2009/enhis-fact-sheets-2007/incidence-of-melanoma-in-people-aged-under-55-years-enhis-2007-fact-sheet-4.2

Pisha, E.; Chai, H.; Lee, I-S.; Chagwedera, T. E.; Farnsworth, N. R.; Cordell, G. A.; Beecher, C. W. W.; Fong, H. H. S.; Kinghorn, A. D.; Brown, D. M.; Wain, M. C.; Wall, M. E.; Hieken, T. J.; Das Gupta, T. K. & Pezzuto, J. M. (1995). Discovery of Betulinic Acid as a Selective Inhibitor of Human-Melanoma That Functions by Induction of Apoptosis. *Nature Medicine*, Vol. 1, No. 10, pp. 1046 – 1051, ISSN 1078-8956.

Recio, M.; Giner, R.; Manez, S. & Rios, J. (1995). Structural Requirements for the Antiinflammatory Activity of Natural Triterpenoids. *Planta Medica*, Vol. 61, No. 2, pp. 182 – 185, ISSN 0032-0943.

Recio, M. d. C.; Giner, R. M.; Manez, S.; Gueho, J.; Julien, H. R.; Hostettmann, K.; & Rios, J. L. (1995). Investigations on the Steroidal Antiinflammatory Activity of Triterpenoids from Diospyros-Leucomelas. *Planta Medica*, Vol. 61, No. 1, pp. 9–12, ISSN 0032-0943.

Retzlaff, F. (1902). Ueber Herba Gratiolae. *Archiv der Pharmazie*, Vol. 240, No. 8, pp. 561-568.

Robertson, A.; Soliman, G. & Owen, E. (1939). Polyterpenoid compounds - Part I Betulic acid from Cornus floridal, L. *Journal of the Chemical Society*, pp. 1267 – 1273.

Salzwedel, K.; Li, F.; Wild, C. T.; Allaway, G. P. & Freed, E. O. (2010). Inhibition of HIV-1 Replication by Disruption of the Processing of the Viral Capsid-Spacer Peptide 1 Protein, US2010221264, pub. date 2010-09-02.

Salvador, J. A. R. (2010). *Pentacyclic Triterpenes as Promising Agents in Cancer,* Nova Science Publishers, Inc., ISBN 978-1-61122-835-9, Hauppauge NY.

Sarek, J.; Biedermann, D. & Hajdúch, M. (2008). Triterpenoids derivatives for cancer treatment and preparation thereof. CZ 301158, filing date 2008-09-01.

Sarek, J.; Hajduch, M.; Novakova, K.; Svoboda, M.; Spacilova, P.; Kubelka, T. & Biedermann D. (2007). Method of preparation of a soluble formulation of water-insoluble pentacyclic and tetracyclic terpenoids, a soluble formulation of a pentacyclic or tetracyclic terpenoid and a pharmaceutical composition containing this soluble formulation. PCT/CZ2007/000088, 2007-09-25.

Sarek, J.; Hajduch, M. & Svoboda, M. (2008). Method of preparation and isolation of betulin diacetate from birch bark from paper mills and its optional processing to betulin patent CZ 301038, pub. date 2008-10-29.

Šarek, J.; Klinot, J.; Bražinová, S.; Džubák, P.; Klinotová, E.; Nosková, V.; Křeček, V.; Kořínková, G.; Thomson, J. O.; Janošťáková, A.; Wang, S.; Parsons, S.; Fischer, P. M.; Zhelev, N. Z. & Hajdúch, M. (2003). New Lupane Derived Compounds with

Pro-Apoptotic activity: Synthesis and Structure-Activity Relationships. *Journal of Medicinal Chemistry*, Vol. 46, No. 25, pp. 5402 - 5415, ISSN 0022-2623.

Sarek, J.; Kvasnica, M.; Urban, M.; Klinot, J.; & Hajduch, M. (2005). Correlation of Cytotoxic Activity of Betulinines and their Hydroxy Analogues. *Bioorganic & Medicinal Chemistry Letters*, Vol. 15, No. 19, pp. 4196 - 4200, ISSN 0960 - 894X.

Sarek, J.; Spacilova, P. & Hajduch, M. (2009). Triterpenoid 2-deoxy glycosides, method of preparation thereof and use thereof as medicaments. PCT/CZ2009/000132, 2009-11-06.

Sawada, N.; Kataoka, K.; Kondo, K.; Arimochi, H.; Fujino, H.; Takahashi, Y.; Miyoshi, T.; Kuwahara, T.; Monden, Y. & Ohnishi, Y. (2004). Betulinic acid augments the inhibitory effects of vincristine on growth and lung metastasis of B16F10 melanoma cells in mice. *British Journal of Cancer*, Vol. 90, No. 8, pp. 1672 - 1678, ISSN 0007 - 0920.

Selzer, E.; Pimentel, E.; Wacheck, W.; Schlegel, W.; Pehamberger, H.; Jansen, B. & Kodym, R. (2000). Effects of betulinic acid alone and in combination with irradiation in human melanoma cells. *The Journal of Investigative Dermatology*, Vol. 114, No. 5, pp. 935 - 940, ISSN 0022 - 202X.

Selzer, E.; Thallinger, C.; Hoeller, C.; Oberkleiner, P.; Wacheck, V.; Pehamberger, H. & Jansen, B. (2002). Betulinic acid-induced Mcl-1 expression in human melanoma--mode of action and functional significance. *Molecular Medicine*, Vol. 8, No. 12, pp. 877-884, ISSN 1076-1551.

Simonsen, J. & Ross, W. C. J. (1957). *The terpenes, vol. V* (1st edition), Cambridge University Press, ISBN 0521064740, New York.

Soler, F.; Poujade, C.; Evers, M.; Carry, J. - C.; Henin, Y.; Bousseau, A.; Huet, T.; Pauwels, R. & De Clercq, E. (1996). Betulinic acid derivatives: A new class of specific inhibitors of human immunodeficiency virus type 1 entry. *Journal of Medicinal Chemistry*, Vol. 39, No. 5, pp. 1069–1083, ISSN 0022-2623.

Srivastava, A. K.; Shakeel, M. & Khan, A. A. (2002). QSAR studies on anti HIV-1N-substituted betulinic acid amides. *Indian Journal of Chemistry Section B-Organic Chemistry Including Medicinal Chemistry*, Vol. 41, No. 2, pp. 436–439, ISSN 0376-4699.

Suh, N; Wang, Y; Honda, T; Gribble, G. W.; Dmitrovsky, E; Hickey, W. F.; Maue, R. A.; Place, A. E.; Porter, D. M.; Spinella, M. J.; Williams, C. R.; Wu, G.; Dannenberg, A. J.; Flanders, K. C.; Letterio, J. J.; Mangelsdorf, D. J.; Nathan, C. F.; Nguyen, L.; Porter, W. W.; Ren, R. F.; Roberts, A. B.; Roche, N. S.; Subbaramaiah, K. & Sporn, M. B. (1999). A novel synthetic oleanane triterpenoid, 2-cyano-3,12-dioxoolean-1,9-dien-28-oic acid, with potent differentiating, antiproliferative, and anti-inflammatory activity. *Cancer Research*, Vol. 59, No 2, pp. 336-41, ISSN 0008-5472.

Sun, I.-C.; Chen, C. H.; Kashiwada, Y.; Wu, J. – H.; Wang, H. – K. & Lee, K.-H. (2002). Anti-AIDS agents 49. Synthesis, anti-HIV, and anti-fusion activities of IC9564 analogues based on betulinic acid. *Journal of Medicinal Chemistry*, Vol. 45, No. 19, pp. 4271–4275, ISSN 0022-2623.

Symon, A. V.; Veselova, N. N.; Kaplun, A.P.; Vlasenkova, N. K.; Fedorova, G.A.; Lyutik, A.I.; Gerasimova, G. K. & Shvets, V. I. (2005). Synthesis and antitumor activity of cyclopropane derivatives of betulinic and betulonic acids. *Russian journal of Bioorganic chemistry*, Vol. 31, No. 3, pp. 286-291, ISSN 1068-1620.

Takada, Y. & Aggarwal, B. B. (2003). Betulinic acid suppresses carcinogen-induced NF-kappa B activation through inhibition of I kappa B alpha kinase and p65 phosphorylation: abrogation of cyclooxygenase-2 and matrix metalloprotease-9. *Journal of Immunology*, Vol. 171, No. 6, pp. 3278-3286, ISSN 0022-1767.

Thibeault, D.; Gauthier, C.; Legault, J.; Bouchard J.; Dufour P.; S. & Pichette, A. (2007). Synthesis and structure-activity relationship study of cytotoxic germanicane- and lupane-type 3 beta-O-monodesmosidic saponins starting from betulin *Bioorganic & Medicinal Chemistry*, Vol. 15, No. 18, pp. 6144-6157, ISSN 0968-0896.

Thurnher, D.; Turhani, D.; Pelzmann, M.; Wannemacher, B.; Knerer, B.; Formanek, M.; Wacheck, V. & Selzer, E. (2003). Betulinic acid: a new cytotoxic compound against malignant head and neck cancer cells. *Head and Neck-Journal for the Sciences and Specialties of the Head and Neck*, Vol. 25, No. 9, pp. 732-740, ISSN 1043-3074.

Trumbull, E. R.; Bianchi, E.; Eckert, D. J.; Wiedhopf, R. M. & Cole, J. R. (1976). Tumor Inhibitory Agents from Vauquelinia-Corymbosa (Rosaceae). *Journal of Pharmaceutical Sciences*, Vol. 65, No. 9, pp. 1407 - 1408, ISSN 0022-3549.

Urban, M.; Sarek, J.; Kvasnica, M.; Tislerova, I & Hajduch, M. (2007). Triterpenoid pyrazines and benzopyrazines with cytotoxic activity. Journal *of Natural Products*, Vol. 70, No. 4, pp. 526-532, ISSN 0163-3864.

Urban, M.; Sarek, J.; Klinot, J.; Korinkova, G. & Hajduch, M. (2004). Synthesis of A-seco derivatives of betulinic acid with cytotoxic activity. *Journal of Natural Products*, Vol. 67, No. 7, pp. 1100 -1105, ISSN 0163 - 3864.

Urban, M.; Sarek, J.; Tislerova, I.; Dzubak, P. & Hajduch, M. (2005). Influence of Esterification and Modification of A-ring in a Group of Lupane Acids on their Cytotoxicity. *Bioorganic and Medicinal Chemistry*, Vol. 13, No. 19, pp. 5527 - 5535, ISSN 0968-0896.

Urban, M.; Sarek, J.; Klinot, J.; Korinkova, G. & Hajduch, M. (2004). Synthesis of A-seco derivatives of betulinic acid with cytotoxic activity. *Journal of Natural Products*, Vol. 67, No. 7, pp. 1100 -1105, ISSN 0163 - 3864.

US National Institute of Health. Available in: http://www.clinicaltrials.gov/ct2/results?term=bevirimat

Wachsberger, P. R.; Burd, R.; Wahl, M. L.; Leeper & D. B. (2002). Betulinic acid sensitization of low pH adapted human melanoma cells to hyperthermia. *International Journal of Hyperthermia*, Vol. 18, No. 2, pp. 153 - 164, ISSN 0265 - 6763.

Willmann, M.; Wacheck, V.; Buckley, J.; Nagy, K.; Thalhammer, J.; Paschke, R.; Triche, T.; Jansen, B. & Selzer, E. (2009). Characterization of NVX-207, a novel betulinic acid-derived anti-cancer compound. *European journal of clinical investigation*, Vol. 39, No. 5, pp. 384-394, ISSN 1365-2362.

Yasukawa, K.; Takido, M.; Matsumoto, T.; Takeuchi, M. & Nakagawa, S. (1991). Sterol and Triterpene Derivatives from Plants Inhibit the Effects of a Tumor Promoter, and Sitosterol and Betulinic Acid Inhibit Tumor-Formation in Mouse Skin 2-Stage Carcinogenesis. *Oncology*, Vol. 48, No. 1, pp. 72–76, ISSN 0030-2414.

You, Y.J.; Kim, Y.; Nam, N.-H. & Ahm, B.-Z. (2003). Snythesis and cytotoxick activity of A-ring Modified Betulinic Acid Derivatives. *Bioorganic & Medicinal Chemistry Letters*, Vol. 13, No. 19, pp. 3137-3140, ISSN 0960 - 894X.

Zellner, J. & Ziffer, J. (1925). "Plantanolsäure" aus der Rinde von *Platanus orientalis* L. *Monatshefte Chemie*, Vol. 46, 323-325 (1925).

Zhou, J. P.; Li, D.; Wu, X. M.; Ye, W. C. & Zhang, L. Y. (2007). Synthesis and antitumor activity of derivatives of 23-hydroxybetulinic acid. *Chinese Chemistry Letters*, Vol. 18, No. 10 1195-1198, ISSN 1001-8417.

Zuco, V.; Supino, R.; Righetti, S. C.; Cleris, L.; Marchesi, E.; Gambacorti-Passerini, C. & Formelli, F. (2002). Selective cytotoxicity of betulinic acid on tumor cell lines, but not on normal cells. *Cancer Letters*, Vol. 175, No. 1, pp. 17 - 25, ISSN 0304 - 3835.

Part 3

Molecular Signaling

8

New Molecular Targets for the Systemic Therapy of Melanoma

Kausar Begam Riaz Ahmed and Michael A. Davies
The University of Texas MD Anderson Cancer Center
USA

1. Introduction

Melanoma is one of the most deadly forms of skin cancer. The incidence of melanoma has been steadily increasing over the last several decades. It is estimated that in 2010 68,130 adults were diagnosed with melanoma, and 8,700 patients died of this disease (Jemal et al.). Melanoma is highly curable when it is diagnosed at early stages. However, patients with distant metastases have a median overall survival of only 6-8 months (Balch et al. 2009). Chemotherapy regimens have not improved survival in patients with metastatic melanoma, and immunotherapies have generally benefited only a small percentage of patients (Koon and Atkins 2006). Thus, there is a critical need to develop more effective therapeutic approaches for this disease. Recently, dramatic results have been reported with agents that specifically target proteins or pathways that are aberrant in this disease, such as *BRAF* and *c-KIT* (Flaherty et al. ; Hodi et al. 2008). These results support the rationale for continued investigation into the molecular events that characterize and contribute to melanoma. This review will describe existing knowledge about several of the molecules and pathways that have been implicated in melanoma, and review the results of clinical studies focused on these targets.

2. Melanoma molecular targets

Melanoma has traditionally been classified based on the clinical and pathological features of the tumor. The most commonly observed type of melanoma is cutaneous melanoma (CM), arising from skin with either intermittent or chronic sun exposure. While ultraviolet radiation likely has a significant causative role in these tumors, its role in certain other subtypes is less clear. Cutaneous melanomas can arise in areas with limited sun/UV radiation exposure such as palms, soles and the area under nails (acral lentiginous melanoma). Other melanomas arise from mucosal surfaces of the body, including the upper aerodigestive, gastrointestinal, and genitourinary tracts, and are termed mucosal melanomas. Melanomas also originate from melanocytes in the uveal tract of the eye (uveal/ocular melanoma). In addition to anatomic differences, recent research has demonstrated that the different melanoma subtypes are characterized by distinct regions of DNA copy number gain and loss (Curtin et al. 2005). This finding suggested that each of these tumor types could be characterized by distinct molecular mechanisms, a hypothesis that is also supported by the marked variance of recently described oncogenic mutations across the different melanoma subtypes.

2.1 RAS/RAF/MAPK pathway

The RAS/RAF/MAPK cascade is a critical growth and survival signaling pathway in cells. The pathway is generally triggered by activation of cell surface receptor(s) [i.e., receptor tyrosine kinases (RTK), G-protein coupled receptors (GPCR), etc] following ligand binding or cell-to-cell contact. The receptors induce activation of RAS through guanine exchange factors (GEFs), which promote the exchange of RAS-GDP to RAS-GTP. GTP-bound RAS recruits and activates the RAF (A-, B- and C-RAF) family of serine-threonine kinases, which then phosphorylate and activate Mitogen Activated Kinase Kinase [MAPKK or MAP/ERK kinase (MEK)]. Phosphorylated MEK, which is also a kinase, activates the downstream Extracellular Regulatory Kinase (ERK1/2 or P44/42 MAPK) through phosphorylation. Once activated, ERK translocates to the nucleus where it regulates the expression of several genes involved in differentiation, survival and proliferation by phosphorylating transcription factors such as ETS, MYC etc. The MAPK pathway also regulates the apoptotic machinery in cells through post-translational regulation of BAD, BIM, MCL-1 and BCL-2 proteins (George, Thomas, and Hannan).

In addition to RAF, the RAS proteins activate several other effectors that contribute to the pro-survival and proliferative phenotype, including phospholipase C (PLC), phosphatidyl inositol-3-Kinase (PI3K), Ral, Rac and Rho-GTPases. Mutations in the *RAS* family genes (*HRAS, NRAS* and *KRAS*) have been detected in approximately one-third of all cancers, including pancreatic, colon, leukemia and thyroid cancers (Bos et al. 1987; Bos et al. 1985; Almoguera et al. 1988; Forrester et al. 1987; Padua, Barrass, and Currie 1985). Activating mutations of *RAS* have been reported in 15-20% of melanomas, and almost exclusively involve the *NRAS* isoform (Tsao et al. 2000). *NRAS* mutations are highly conserved in melanoma, as over 90% of the detected mutations occur in codons 12, 13 and 61 (Hocker and Tsao 2007). *NRAS* mutations occur in 26% of cutaneous and 14% of mucosal melanomas, but only in 4% of acral and less than 1% of uveal melanomas (Hocker and Tsao 2007). Mutant RAS proteins have very little GTPase activity, and thus remain constitutively active. This results in aberrant regulation of its downstream signaling pathways and subsequent uncontrolled cell proliferation and survival. RAS also promotes suppression of $p16^{INK4a}$ and p53 in melanoma models, and knockdown of mutated *H-RAS* (*H-Ras*^{V12G}) using siRNAs in an doxycycline inducible melanoma mouse model resulted in tumor regression (Chin et al. 1997; Chin et al. 1999).

Activating mutations in the serine/threonine kinase *BRAF* were first reported by Davies and colleagues in 2002, who demonstrated in a small cohort of tumors and cancer cell lines that 66% of melanomas harbored somatic mutations in *BRAF*, which were also detected in smaller fractions of gliomas, colon and ovarian cancer samples. A recent meta-analysis reported *BRAF* mutations in 43% of melanoma clinical specimens and 65% of human melanoma cell lines (Hocker and Tsao 2007). *BRAF* mutations were detected most frequently in cutaneous melanomas (42.5%), but were markedly less common in acral (18.1%), mucosal (5.6%), and uveal (<1%) melanomas. Some studies have also reported significantly lower rates of *BRAF* mutations in cutaneous melanomas with chronic sun damage (Curtin et al. 2005), but this has not been recapitulated in other studies (Handolias, Salemi et al. 2010). Approximately 40 different *BRAF* mutations have been identified in melanoma. The most frequent mutation (approximately 90% of mutations in clinical samples) arises due to a T→A transversion in position 1799 of the *BRAF* gene (T1799A) resulting in the substitution of glutamic acid for valine at position 600 ($BRAF^{V600E}$) of the BRAF protein acid, which has markedly increased catalytic activity compared to the wild-type BRAF protein (Davies et al. 2002; Wan et al. 2004; Hocker and Tsao 2007). Interestingly, some of the *BRAF* mutations that have been detected in cancer do not increase the catalytic activity of the BRAF protein, but still result in hyperactivation of MEK and ERK through efficient dimerization with other RAF isoforms (Garnett et al. 2005; Heidorn et al. 2010).

In melanoma, activating *BRAF* and *NRAS* mutations are almost always mutually exclusive, but overlap can occur with non-activating *BRAF* mutations (Heidorn et al. 2010; Tsao et al. 2004). While *BRAF* mutations are extremely common in melanoma, there is significant evidence that they must be complemented by additional genetic events in melanomagenesis. Pollock *et al* (2002) reported that the $BRAF^{V600E}$ mutation is detectable in 82% of benign nevi, which have virtually no malignant potential. In addition, expression of the $BRAF^{V600E}$ mutation alone in melanocytes failed to induce transformation in several preclinical models, including zebrafish and mice (Patton et al. 2005). Invasive lesions were only seen when other molecules were inactivated concurrently, such as p16/Ink4a, p53, and *PTEN* or *p53* (Dankort et al. 2009; Chudnovsky et al. 2005).

The dual specificity kinases MEK1/2 that lie downstream of BRAF are activated in majority of the cancers with deregulated RAS/RAF/MAPK signaling. The MEK kinases phosphorylate ERK1/2 downstream and mediate cell survival signaling through MAPK signaling cascade. Emery *et al.* (2009), using random mutagenesis and massive parallel sequencing approaches identified mutations in the drug binding and regulatory domains of MEK1 kinase that led to increased phosphorylation of ERK and a MEK inhibitor-resistance phenotype. Subsequently, *MEK1* point mutations P124L and C121S have been detected in melanoma patients who progressed after initial clinical responses to MEK or BRAF inhibitors (Wagle et al. ; Emery et al. 2009). To date no *MEK1* or *MEK2* mutations have been reported *de novo* in melanoma.

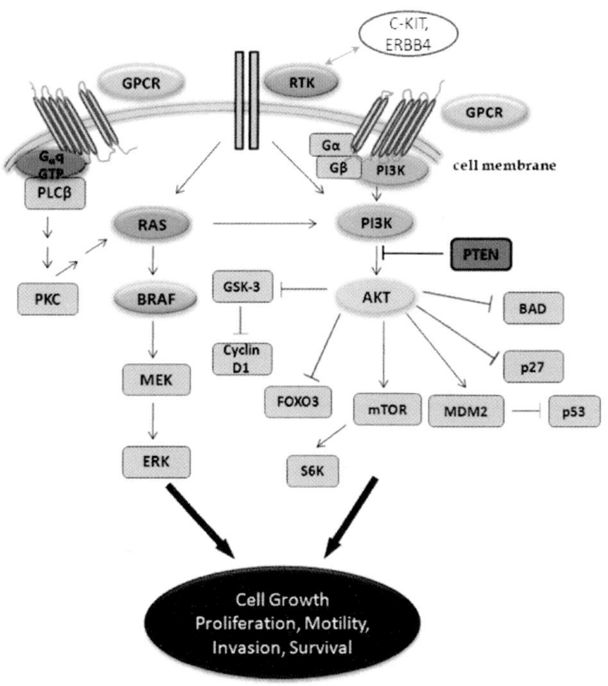

Fig. 1. Molecular targets in melanoma. The diagram illustrates pathways that are affected by prevalent genetic alterations in melanoma.

2.2 PI3K/AKT/mTOR pathway

The PI3K/AKT/mTOR pathway is one of the most important intracellular signaling pathways. The pathway regulates many important cellular processes, including proliferation, differentiation, motility, metabolism, survival, invasion and intracellular transport (Engelman, Luo, and Cantley 2006). The Phosphatidyl Inositol-3 Kinases (PI3K) are a family of lipid kinases that are composed of an adaptor/regulatory subunit (i.e. p85) and a catalytic unit (i.e. p110). Similar to RAS/RAF/ERK, the PI3K/AKT/mTOR pathway is activated by a variety of signals, including receptor tyrosine kinases and RAS proteins. Activation of PI3K results in phosphorylation of phosphatidylinositols in the cell membrane at the 3′-hydroxyl group. This reaction generates the lipid species PI $(3,4)P_2$ and $PI(3,4,5)P_3$. PI $(3,4)P_2$ and $PI(3,4,5)P_3$ act as second messengers, recruiting proteins that contain a pleckstrin homology (PH) domain to the cell membrane, such as the serine/threonine kinases AKT and PDK1. Upon recruitment to the cell membrane, AKT is phosphorylated at two critical residues, serine 473 and threonine 308. Once phosphorylated, the activated AKT translocates to the cytosol where it promotes cell proliferation and survival by phosphorylating numerous substrate proteins including mTOR, GSK3, FOXO, and BAD, among others.

The activity of the PI3K/AKT/mTOR pathway is normally controlled by the lipid phosphatase PTEN (Phosphatase and Tensin Homolog), which dephosphorylates phosphatidyl inositols (PI) at the 3′ position, thereby inhibiting PI3K-mediated signaling (Maehama and Dixon 1998). PTEN, which is a tumor suppressor, is inactivated in a variety of tumor types, through both genetic and epigenetic mechanisms (Li et al. 1997; Myers et al. 1998; Mirmohammadsadegh et al. 2006). Tumors with loss of PTEN are characterized by markedly increased basal activation of AKT (Davies et al. 1999; Davies et al. 1998; Davies et al. 2009).

In melanoma, *PTEN* loss is observed in up to 20% of tumors and 30% of melanoma cell lines (Tsao et al. 1998; Tsao, Mihm, and Sheehan 2003; Tsao et al. 2000). This prevalence is primarily defined for cutaneous melanomas; the prevalence in other subtypes is poorly described. Similar to BRAF, loss of PTEN appears to be mutually exclusive with the presence of an *NRAS* mutation in melanoma tumors and cell lines. While this pattern suggests functional redundancy, quantitative analysis of AKT activation demonstrated that PTEN loss correlated with significantly higher levels of phosphorylated AKT than *NRAS* mutations in both clinical specimens and cell lines (Davies et al. 2009). In contrast to NRAS, PTEN loss frequently occurs in melanomas with a concurrent activating *BRAF* mutation (Tsao et al. 2000; Goel et al. 2006; Tsao et al. 2004). The functional nature of this pattern is supported by mouse studies, which demonstrated that crossing mice with the $BRAF^{V600E}$ mutation in melanocytes with mice that harbour PTEN loss resulted in frankly invasive and metastatic melanomas, which did not occur with either lesion alone (Dankort et al. 2009).

In addition to loss of PTEN, the PI3K/AKT/mTOR pathway may also be activated by gene amplifications and gain of function mutations in other pathway components. Rare activating mutations in *PI3KCA* have been detected in 2-3% of melanomas (Omholt et al. 2006). Studies by Stahl *et al*, identified activation of AKT3 in 43 to 60% of sporadic melanomas, which was associated with an increase in copy number of the *AKT3* gene along with a simultaneous decreased activity of PTEN, either due to loss or haploinsufficiency of the *PTEN* gene. Knockdown of *AKT3* by siRNA induced apoptosis and reduced melanoma tumor development (Stahl et al. 2004). Davies *et al* recently also reported rare gain of function point mutations in the regulatory pleckstrin homology domains of *AKT1* and *AKT3* (*AKT1 E17K,*

AKT3 E17K) in ~2% melanoma cell lines and tumor specimens (Davies et al. 2008). Every melanoma with an *AKT1* or *AKT3* mutation also had a concurrent *BRAF* mutation.

2.3 Receptor tyrosine kinases

Activating mutations or amplifications of receptor tyrosine kinases are implicated in multiple tumor types, including gastrointestinal stromal tumors (GIST) (*c-KIT*), breast (*HER2/neu*), and lung (*EGFR*) cancers. However, until recently there has been little evidence of significant aberrations in melanoma. The relatively low rate of *BRAF* and *NRAS* mutations in non-cutaneous melanomas led to focused searches for other oncogenic drivers in these tumor types. Comparative genome hybridization (CGH) analysis identified selective amplification of the 4q12 chromosomal region in acral and mucosal melanomas (Curtin et al. 2005). Detailed analysis of the genes in this region identified focal amplifications of the *c-KIT* gene (Curtin et al. 2006). C-KIT is a receptor tyrosine kinase which is affected by activating mutations in ~80% of GISTs (Hirota et al. 1998). Subsequent to the discovery of gene amplifications, sequencing demonstrated that the *c-KIT* gene is also frequently mutated in the same melanoma subtypes in which amplifications had been detected(Curtin et al. 2006). Overall, *c-KIT* gene amplification or mutation was identified in 39% of mucosal and 36% of acral melanomas. Among cutaneous melanomas, *c-KIT* gene alterations were also detected in 28% of cutaneous melanomas with chronic sun damage (CSD), but no *c-KIT* gene aberrations were reported in cutaneous melanomas without CSD (Curtin et al. 2006). However, other studies have reported lower rates of *c-KIT* alterations in cutaneous melanomas with CSD (Handolias, Salemi et al. 2010). The mutations in *c-KIT* gene generally affect the same exons that are mutated in GIST, although the distribution in melanoma shows a higher prevalence of mutations in exons associated with resistance to many c-KIT inhibitors. Interestingly, while most *c-KIT* mutations in GIST are short insertions or deletions, the overwhelming majority of changes in melanoma are point mutations, with the most common event being the L576P substitution at exon 11 of the juxtamembrane region (Beadling et al. 2008). The finding of activating *c-KIT* mutations was surprising, as previous reports had demonstrated that although c-KIT is essential for the development of normal melanocytes, c-KIT activation suppressed the growth of melanoma cells, and melanoma progression was associated with loss of c-KIT expression (Huang et al. 1996; Lassam and Bickford 1992). However, the lack of mutations in *c-KIT* in cutaneous melanomas suggests that other lineage-specific genetic or environmental factors in the non-cutaneous melanocytes may critically interact with the *c-KIT* mutations.

More recently, high-throughput sequencing analysis of all protein kinases identified novel somatic mutations in 19 different genes (Prickett et al. 2009). The most frequently mutated gene was *ERBB4* (24 missense mutations in 15 patients; 19% prevalence in the cohort), which encodes a receptor tyrosine kinase that is a member of the epidermal growth factor receptor family (EGFR, HER2, HER3). *ERBB4* mutations have previously been reported in lung, colon, stomach and breast cancers (Soung et al. 2006; Ding et al. 2008). Interestingly, the mutations in the melanomas were distributed throughout the entire *ERBB4* gene. Despite this unusual pattern for an activating event, Pickett et al., found that every tumor-derived mutation *ERBB4* tested had higher levels of receptor tyrosine kinase activity, promoted anchorage independent growth, and induced cellular transformation (Prickett et al. 2009). In contrast to the distinct patterns seen with other mutations, *ERBB4* mutations were not mutually exclusive with *BRAF* or *NRAS* mutations. Further investigation is needed to gain a better understanding of the role of ERBB4 in melanoma, and to understand the therapeutic potential of inhibitors against this target.

2.4 G proteins

Heterotrimeric guanine nucleotide-binding proteins (G proteins) are a diverse family of proteins that regulate and propagate signals from G-Protein Coupled Receptors (GPCRs) that are expressed at the cell membrane. The complex of G-proteins and GPCRs activate several key signaling pathways involved in cell survival, proliferation, and transformation. There is growing evidence that this family of genes may play a significant role in certain subtypes of melanoma.

A role for G proteins in melanoma was first suggested by a preclinical study that was designed to identify genes that promote melanin synthesis and pigmentation in mice. Two different G protein alpha subunits, *GNAQ* and *GNA11*, were identified in this screen (Van Raamsdonk et al. 2004). In order to determine the clinical relevance of these genes in patients, panels of melanomas and nevi were then screened for alterations in these genes. Remarkably, point mutations in *GNAQ* were identified in ~50% of primary uveal melanomas (Onken et al. 2008; Van Raamsdonk, Bezrookove, Green, Bauer, Gaugler, O/'Brien et al. 2009). *GNAQ* mutations were also identified in 50-80% of blue nevi, and in 6% of rare lesions called nevi of Ota, which are associated with an increased risk of uveal melanoma (Van Raamsdonk, Bezrookove, Green, Bauer, Gaugler, O/'Brien et al. 2009). In contrast, no *GNAQ* mutations were identified in cutaneous melanomas without chronic sun damage, acral melanomas, or mucosal melanomas; 1 of 27 cutaneous melanomas with chronic sun damage tested had a mutation. Further sequencing identified point mutations of *GNA11* in 32% of primary uveal melanomas, all of which were mutually exclusive with *GNAQ* mutations (Van Raamsdonk et al. 2010). Interestingly, analysis of a cohort of uveal melanoma metastases identified a higher prevalence of *GNA11* (56%) than *GNAQ* (22%) mutations. Overall, somatic mutations in *GNAQ* and *GNA11* were detected in over 80% of all uveal melanomas analyzed (Van Raamsdonk, Bezrookove, Green, Bauer, Gaugler, O'Brien et al. 2009).

Over 90% of the reported mutations in *GNAQ* and *GNA11* affect the Q209 residue. This occurs in a RAS-like domain of these proteins, and is specifically analogous to the Q61 residue that is the most common site of point mutations in the *RAS* gene. Functional studies of the Q209L mutation in both *GNAQ* and *GNA11* demonstrated that this mutation promotes anchorage independent growth, tumorigenicity, and activation of the RAS/RAF/MAPK pathway (Van Raamsdonk, Bezrookove, Green, Bauer, Gaugler, O/'Brien et al. 2009; Van Raamsdonk et al. 2010). These findings suggest that these mutations may obviate the requirement for *BRAF* or *NRAS* mutations, which are virtually non-existant in uveal melanomas (Cohen et al. 2003; Rimoldi et al. 2003). Studies to determine the various functions of *GNAQ* and *GNA11* mutations in uveal melanoma, and determine the therapeutic potential of inhibiting these genes or their effectors, are currently ongoing.

In addition to these mutations in uveal melanoma, high-throughput sequencing for mutations in G protein family members in cutaneous melanomas identified 18 non-synonymous somatic mutations in G protein subunits spanning seven genes (Cardenas-Navia et al.). Mutations were identified in *GNA12, GNG10, GNAZ, GNG14, GNA15, GNA11, and GNB3* (Cardenas-Navia et al.). Further work needs to be done to understand the pathways and processes affected by these mutations.

2.5 Other affected genes

Alterations in several regulators of cell cycle progression have also been implicated in melanoma. Allelic alterations in *CDK4* and *CCND1* have been reported in melanoma (Curtin et al. 2005; Smalley et al. 2008). Inactivation of the tumor suppressor *p53,* which is associated with DNA damage and metabolic stress, has also been reported. (Yang, Rajadurai, and Tsao 2005; Jonsson et al. 2007). P53 may also be functionally inactivated by loss of function of $p16^{INK4a}/p14^{ARF}$ genes (Pomerantz et al. 1998; Stott et al. 1998; Zhang, Xiong, and Yarbrough 1998). Loss of function of $p16^{INK4a}/p14^{ARF}$ is present in most familial melanomas (Cannon-Albright et al. 1992; Goldstein et al. 2007). Loss of both *p16* and *p14* is seen in both melanoma cell lines and primary tumors and is a selection factor for the survival of melanoma cells *in vitro* (Daniotti et al. 2004; Rakosy et al. 2008). However, currently there are no therapies in place to restore the expression of these tumor suppressors.

A comparative genetic analysis of melanomas with other tumor types identified selective amplifications of the gene encoding the microphthalmia-associated transcription factor (*MITF*) in melanoma (Garraway et al. 2005). *MITF* is a transcription factor that regulates many genes associated with melanin production and melanocyte development (Levy, Khaled, and Fisher 2006). Initial studies demonstrated the MITF could function as an oncogene, and was able to cooperate with the mutant *BRAF* gene to induce transformation of normal melanocytes (Garraway et al. 2005). Amplification of the MITF locus occurs in 10-20% melanomas, and subsequent studies have also detected rare somatic mutations in the gene in melanomas (Cronin et al. 2009).

3. Clinical targeting of activated pathways in melanoma

The treatment of many cancers has changed dramatically due to an improved understanding of the genes and pathways that contribute to the aggressive nature of many of these diseases. The discovery of activating events in kinase signaling pathways in melanoma rapidly led to clinical testing of a number of targeted therapies for this disease. The early results illustrate both the promise and challenge of this strategy.

3.1 The RAS/RAF/MAPK pathway

The high prevalence of mutations in components of the RAS/RAF/MAPK pathway in melanoma, particularly in the most common subtype (cutaneous), strongly supports the rationale to test the clinical efficacy of drugs against it. After the discovery of activating *BRAF* mutations (Davies et al. 2002), the first drug against the pathway to be tested clinically was sorafenib. Sorafenib is a small molecule that inhibits a number of kinases, including BRAF, CRAF, vascular endothelial growth factor receptor (VEGFR), platelet derived growth factor receptor (PDGFR), and c-Kit (Strumberg 2005). Preclinical studies demonstrated that sorafenib slowed the growth of melanoma xenografts with activating *BRAF* mutations, but did not result in tumor eradication (Karasarides et al. 2004). Subsequently, in a single-agent phase II trial, treatment with sorafenib resulted in only 1 clinical response among 34 evaluable patients (Eisen et al. 2006). More promising results were observed in a phase I trial that tested the safety of combined treatment with sorafenib, carboplatin, and paclitaxel. Ten clinical responses were observed, all of which occurred in patients with metastatic melanoma [n=24; 40% overall response rate (ORR)] (Flaherty et al. 2008). Of note, the clinical benefit among the melanoma patients did not correlate with the presence of activating *BRAF* mutations. Despite these promising results, a subsequent randomized phase III trial of treatment with carboplatin and paclitaxel with or without sorafenib definitively showed that sorafenib did not improve the ORR or progression-free survival (PFS) that was achieved with the chemotherapy agents alone (Hauschild et al. 2009). Combined with preclinical studies that showed the high prevalence of *BRAF* mutations in benign nevi, and induction of cellular senescence only following expression of mutant *BRAF* in normal melanocytes, these results raised doubts about the value of *BRAF* as a therapeutic target.

The identification of mutant *BRAF* as a therapeutic target in melanoma has now been confirmed by clinical trials with potent, selective second-generation BRAF inhibitors. PLX4032 (vemurafenib) is a small molecule that has an *in vitro* IC50 for the $BRAF^{V600E}$ protein of ~ 10 nM. This is one log lower than the IC50 for the wild-type BRAF protein, and 2-3 logs lower than the IC50 for other related kinases (Tsai et al. 2008). Experiments in xenografts models demonstrated that PLX4720, a closely related compound used for preclinical studies, eradicated melanomas with a $BRAF^{V600E}$ mutation (Yang et al. 2010). More importantly, the phase I trial of PLX4032 in patients with advanced melanoma reported an unconfirmed ORR of 81% among patients with the $BRAF^{V600E}$ mutation (Flaherty et al. 2010). The selectivity of the agent *in vivo* is supported by the relatively mild toxicity of the drug, which was well-tolerated by patients. In addition, no clinical responses were observed in the 5 patients included in the trial who had a wild-type *BRAF* gene. In fact, 4 of those patients demonstrated clinical progression of disease at their initial restaging. This clinical finding is consistent with work in preclinical models that demonstrated that treatment of human melanoma cell lines with a wild-type *BRAF* gene with PLX4720 and other selective *BRAF* inhibitors resulted in hyperactivation of MEK and MAPK, and increased growth of cancer cells *in vitro* and *in vivo* (Halaban et al. 2010; Hatzivassiliou et al. 2010; Heidorn et al. 2010; Poulikakos et al. 2010). A second selective inhibitor of the $BRAF^{V600E}$ protein, GSK2118436, has demonstrated similar activity, with a 62% ORR in phase I testing in advanced melanoma patients with a *BRAF* mutation (Kefford et al. 2010).

While the high response rate with minimal toxicity with PLX4032 and GSK2118436 is unprecedented, it is now becoming clear that resistance will be a major problem with these agents. In the phase I trial of PLX4032, virtually all patients who responded clinically went on to develop disease progression, with a median duration of response of approximately 7 months (Flaherty et al. 2010). While the experience with resistance to targeted therapies in other diseases made it reasonable to hypothesize that secondary *BRAF* mutations could cause this, to date the analysis of tumors and cell lines with secondary resistance to selective BRAF inhibitors have failed to identify any such mutations (Nazarian et al. 2010; Villanueva et al. 2010). Instead, cells lines and tumors have developed changes that either maintain activation of the RAS/RAF/MAPK pathway in the presence of the BRAF inhibitors, or changes that allow cells to survive even when that pathway is inhibited. Mechanisms that result in continued activation of the RAS/RAF/MAPK pathway include (1) concurrent *NRAS* or *MEK1* mutation (Nazarian et al. 2010; Wagle et al.), (2) induction of the serine-threonine kinase COT1 (Johannessen et al. 2010), or (2) utilization of all 3 RAF isoforms to activate MEK (Villanueva et al. 2010). Mechanisms that result in resistance to cell killing despite continued inhibition of MEK and MAPK generally implicate activation of the PI3K-AKT pathway, either through the increased expression of receptor tyrosine kinases or through the loss of PTEN (Nazarian et al. 2010; Villanueva et al. 2010). Activation of the PI3K-AKT pathway by loss of PTEN also results in *de novo* resistance to cell killing by BRAF inhibitors, but the relationship between PTEN loss and clinical responsiveness in patients has yet to be determined (Paraiso et al. 2011).

In addition to BRAF inhibitors, MEK inhibitors have shown promise in the treatment of metastatic melanoma. The initial presentation of the preliminary results of the phase I trial of GSK1120212, an orally available MEK inhibitor with a very long half life, reported a 40% ORR response among patients with metastatic melanoma (Infante et al. 2010). This response rate is higher than previous reports with other MEK inhibitors, such as AZD6244 (Dummer et al. 2008). Preclinical studies demonstrated that, similar to the results with BRAF inhibitors, loss of PTEN correlates with increased resistance to cell killing by MEK inhibitors (Gopal et al. 2010). Interestingly, several cells with normal PTEN expression but similar resistance developed activation of the PI3K-AKT pathway following treatment with MEK inhibitors. This compensatory mechanism, which was mediated by the insulin-like growth factor-1 receptor, gives further support to the rationale for testing the effects of targeted therapy combinations to improve clinical results with both BRAF and MEK inhibitors.

3.2 c-KIT

Imatinib, a small molecule inhibitor of a number of kinases, is approved by the FDA for the first-line treatment of metastatic GISTs, which are characterized by a high (~80%) prevalence of activating mutations in the *c-KIT* gene. This clinical experience gave cause for optimism for the use of imatinib in melanoma, a mesenchymal tumor like GIST with very poor responsiveness to cytotoxic chemotherapies. Prior to the identification of *c-KIT* mutations in acral and mucosal melanomas, three different phase II trials with imatinib were conducted in advanced melanoma patients (Kim et al. 2008; Ugurel et al. 2005; Wyman et al. 2006). The cumulative ORR was only 1.5% for these trials. However, the patients overwhelmingly consisted of patients with cutaneous primary melanomas, and thus were unlikely to harbor activating *c-Kit* mutations.

There are now several case reports describing impressive clinical responses to c-KIT inhibitors in melanoma patients with mutations in the *c-KIT* gene (Handolias, Hamilton et al. 2010; Hodi et al. 2008). In addition, relatively large clinical trials are ongoing testing the efficacy of c-KIT inhibitors in this patient population. An initial report from one of the imatinib trials reported an ORR of approximately 50% among patients with *c-KIT* mutations, but 0 of 10 patients with only gene amplification of the wild-type gene responded (Fisher et al. 2010). In addition, while c-KIT inhibitors have induced some durable responses, other dramatic responses have lasted for only a few months (Woodman et al. 2009). Thus, the further development of therapies for melanoma patients with *c-KIT* mutations will likely require an improved understanding of mechanisms of resistance to these agents, and combinatorial approaches.

Affected Gene	Subtypes Affected	Classes of Inhibitors
BRAF	Cutaneous >> Acral > Mucosal	Selective BRAF inhibitors Non-Selective BRAF Inhibitors MEK inhibitors
NRAS	Cutaneous > Acral > Mucosal	Farnesyl transferase inhibitors
PI3K/PTEN/AKT	(Undefined)	AKT inhibitors PI3K inhibitors Dual PI3K/mTOR inhibitors mTORC1/2 inhibitors
c-KIT	Mucosal > Acral >> Cutaneous	c-KIT inhibitors
ERBB4	(Undefined)	HER-family inhibitors
GNAQ, GNA11	Uveal	MEK inhibitors

Table 1. Molecular Targets in Melanoma

4. Summary

The testing and treatment of melanoma patients is evolving rapidly due to an improved understanding of the genes and pathways that are genetically altered in this disease. The dramatic responses of melanoma patients with *BRAF* and *c-KIT* mutations to inhibitors against these targets demonstrate the power and benefit of research to uncover the underpinnings of cancer. However, the early experience with these targets has also illuminated the challenges of this approach.

There is a clear need to improve our understanding of the factors that are present at baseline that allow resistance to occur to BRAF and c-KIT inhibitors, as well as changes that evolve over time to manifest the resistance. An improved understanding of pre-treatment factors that facilitate the eventual emergence of resistance may suggest rational combinatorial approaches that can prevent resistance from developing. Such factors may also serve as markers that clinically distinguish patients who need combinatorial treatments, which are likely to incur additional toxicities, from those who may achieve significant benefit from single-agent therapy. Similarly, determining the changes that evolve over time and correlate with functional resistance will also suggest rational combinatorial approaches that can be used after single-agent therapies fail. While it is reasonable to hypothesize that many of the critical mechanisms that underlie resistance will involve changes in signaling pathways in the tumors, the possibility of other factors should not be dismissed. For example, recent research has demonstrated that targeted therapies against the RAS/RAF/MAPK pathway can influence both the ability of immune cells to recognize melanomas, and their proliferation and survival (Boni et al. 2010). As immunotherapies have been associated with relatively low response rates but durable benefit when they occur, it is possible that strategies that combine such approaches with targeted therapies may have synergistic clinical benefit.

While there are now clearly defined challenges for patients with *BRAF* and *c-KIT* mutations, the picture remains much less clear for other patients. To date, effective treatment strategies for tumors with mutations in *RAS* family members have not been validated clinically. Research clearly needs to be undertaken to develop such approaches for patients with *NRAS* mutations, and perhaps the analogous mutations in *GNAQ* and *GNA11* in uveal melanomas. Furthermore, a significant number of patients (i.e. ~30% of cutaneous melanomas) do not have a detectable mutation in *BRAF, NRAS,* or *c-KIT*. As has been described here, the number of other mutations that have been identified in melanoma is now rapidly increasing, but the functions and therapeutic implications of many of these events remain poorly characterized. It is highly likely that many more events will be identified in the future, as the first whole-genome sequencing effort revealed almost 200 non-synonymous coding region substitutions in a single patient-derived melanoma (Pleasance et al. 2010). Unraveling the functional interactions and significance of the multiple mutations that are present in each tumor will require extensive testing and innovation. In addition, additional pathways, such as metabolism, oxidative stress, and angiogenesis likely play key functional roles, and may be important therapeutic targets without being directly involved by genetic alterations.

Overall, recent discoveries have provided new hope and therapeutic options for patients with melanoma. These advances highlight the potential of translational research, and provide the impetus for continued research of this highly aggressive disease.

5. Acknowledgements

M.A.D. reports receiving research funding from AstraZeneca, GlaxoSmithKline, and Merck. M.A.D. is supported by a Career Development Award from the American Society of Clinical Oncology, a Young Investigator Award from the Melanoma Research Alliance, and is the Goodfellow Scholar of the MD Anderson Cancer Center Physician Scientist Program.

6. References

Almoguera, C., D. Shibata, K. Forrester, J. Martin, N. Arnheim, and M. Perucho. 1988. Most human carcinomas of the exocrine pancreas contain mutant c-K-ras genes. *Cell* 53 (4):549-54.

Balch, C. M., J. E. Gershenwald, S. J. Soong, J. F. Thompson, M. B. Atkins, D. R. Byrd, A. C. Buzaid, A. J. Cochran, D. G. Coit, S. Ding, A. M. Eggermont, K. T. Flaherty, P. A. Gimotty, J. M. Kirkwood, K. M. McMasters, M. C. Mihm, Jr., D. L. Morton, M. I. Ross, A. J. Sober, and V. K. Sondak. 2009. Final version of 2009 AJCC melanoma staging and classification. *J Clin Oncol* 27 (36):6199-206.

Beadling, C., E. Jacobson-Dunlop, F. S. Hodi, C. Le, A. Warrick, J. Patterson, A. Town, A. Harlow, F. Cruz, 3rd, S. Azar, B. P. Rubin, S. Muller, R. West, M. C. Heinrich, and C. L. Corless. 2008. KIT gene mutations and copy number in melanoma subtypes. *Clin Cancer Res* 14 (21):6821-8.

Boni, Andrea, Alexandria P. Cogdill, Ping Dang, Durga Udayakumar, Ching-Ni Jenny Njauw, Callum M. Sloss, Cristina R. Ferrone, Keith T. Flaherty, Donald P. Lawrence, David E. Fisher, Hensin Tsao, and Jennifer A. Wargo. 2010. Selective BRAFV600E Inhibition Enhances T-Cell Recognition of Melanoma without Affecting Lymphocyte Function. *Cancer Research*:-.

Bos, J. L., E. R. Fearon, S. R. Hamilton, M. Verlaan-de Vries, J. H. van Boom, A. J. van der Eb, and B. Vogelstein. 1987. Prevalence of ras gene mutations in human colorectal cancers. *Nature* 327 (6120):293-7.

Bos, J. L., D. Toksoz, C. J. Marshall, M. Verlaan-de Vries, G. H. Veeneman, A. J. van der Eb, J. H. van Boom, J. W. Janssen, and A. C. Steenvoorden. 1985. Amino-acid substitutions at codon 13 of the N-ras oncogene in human acute myeloid leukaemia. *Nature* 315 (6022):726-30.

Cannon-Albright, L. A., D. E. Goldgar, L. J. Meyer, C. M. Lewis, D. E. Anderson, J. W. Fountain, M. E. Hegi, R. W. Wiseman, E. M. Petty, A. E. Bale, and et al. 1992. Assignment of a locus for familial melanoma, MLM, to chromosome 9p13-p22. *Science* 258 (5085):1148-52.

Cardenas-Navia, L. I., P. Cruz, J. C. Lin, S. A. Rosenberg, and Y. Samuels. Novel somatic mutations in heterotrimeric G proteins in melanoma. *Cancer Biol Ther* 10 (1):33-7.

Chin, L., J. Pomerantz, D. Polsky, M. Jacobson, C. Cohen, C. Cordon-Cardo, J. W. Horner, 2nd, and R. A. DePinho. 1997. Cooperative effects of INK4a and ras in melanoma susceptibility in vivo. *Genes Dev* 11 (21):2822-34.

Chin, L., A. Tam, J. Pomerantz, M. Wong, J. Holash, N. Bardeesy, Q. Shen, R. O'Hagan, J. Pantginis, H. Zhou, J. W. Horner, 2nd, C. Cordon-Cardo, G. D. Yancopoulos, and R.

A. DePinho. 1999. Essential role for oncogenic Ras in tumour maintenance. *Nature* 400 (6743):468-72.

Chudnovsky, Y., A. E. Adams, P. B. Robbins, Q. Lin, and P. A. Khavari. 2005. Use of human tissue to assess the oncogenic activity of melanoma-associated mutations. *Nat Genet* 37 (7):745-9.

Cohen, Y., N. Goldenberg-Cohen, P. Parrella, I. Chowers, S. L. Merbs, J. Pe'er, and D. Sidransky. 2003. Lack of BRAF mutation in primary uveal melanoma. *Invest Ophthalmol Vis Sci* 44 (7):2876-8.

Cronin, Julia C., John Wunderlich, Stacie K. Loftus, Todd D. Prickett, Xiaomu Wei, Katie Ridd, Swapna Vemula, Allison S. Burrell, Neena S. Agrawal, Jimmy C. Lin, Carolyn E. Banister, Phillip Buckhaults, Steven A. Rosenberg, Boris C. Bastian, William J. Pavan, and Yardena Samuels. 2009. Frequent mutations in the MITF pathway in melanoma. *Pigment Cell Melanoma Res* 22 (4):435-444.

Curtin, J. A., K. Busam, D. Pinkel, and B. C. Bastian. 2006. Somatic activation of KIT in distinct subtypes of melanoma. *J Clin Oncol* 24 (26):4340-6.

Curtin, J. A., J. Fridlyand, T. Kageshita, H. N. Patel, K. J. Busam, H. Kutzner, K. H. Cho, S. Aiba, E. B. Brocker, P. E. LeBoit, D. Pinkel, and B. C. Bastian. 2005. Distinct sets of genetic alterations in melanoma. *N Engl J Med* 353 (20):2135-47.

Daniotti, M., M. Oggionni, T. Ranzani, V. Vallacchi, V. Campi, D. Di Stasi, G. D. Torre, F. Perrone, C. Luoni, S. Suardi, M. Frattini, S. Pilotti, A. Anichini, G. Tragni, G. Parmiani, M. A. Pierotti, and M. Rodolfo. 2004. BRAF alterations are associated with complex mutational profiles in malignant melanoma. *Oncogene* 23 (35):5968-77.

Dankort, D., D. P. Curley, R. A. Cartlidge, B. Nelson, A. N. Karnezis, W. E. Damsky, Jr., M. J. You, R. A. DePinho, M. McMahon, and M. Bosenberg. 2009. Braf(V600E) cooperates with Pten loss to induce metastatic melanoma. *Nat Genet* 41 (5):544-52.

Davies, H., G. R. Bignell, C. Cox, P. Stephens, S. Edkins, S. Clegg, J. Teague, H. Woffendin, M. J. Garnett, W. Bottomley, N. Davis, E. Dicks, R. Ewing, Y. Floyd, K. Gray, S. Hall, R. Hawes, J. Hughes, V. Kosmidou, A. Menzies, C. Mould, A. Parker, C. Stevens, S. Watt, S. Hooper, R. Wilson, H. Jayatilake, B. A. Gusterson, C. Cooper, J. Shipley, D. Hargrave, K. Pritchard-Jones, N. Maitland, G. Chenevix-Trench, G. J. Riggins, D. D. Bigner, G. Palmieri, A. Cossu, A. Flanagan, A. Nicholson, J. W. Ho, S. Y. Leung, S. T. Yuen, B. L. Weber, H. F. Seigler, T. L. Darrow, H. Paterson, R. Marais, C. J. Marshall, R. Wooster, M. R. Stratton, and P. A. Futreal. 2002. Mutations of the BRAF gene in human cancer. *Nature* 417 (6892):949-54.

Davies, M. A., D. Koul, H. Dhesi, R. Berman, T. J. McDonnell, D. McConkey, W. K. Yung, and P. A. Steck. 1999. Regulation of Akt/PKB activity, cellular growth, and apoptosis in prostate carcinoma cells by MMAC/PTEN. *Cancer Res* 59 (11):2551-6.

Davies, M. A., Y. Lu, T. Sano, X. Fang, P. Tang, R. LaPushin, D. Koul, R. Bookstein, D. Stokoe, W. K. Yung, G. B. Mills, and P. A. Steck. 1998. Adenoviral transgene expression of MMAC/PTEN in human glioma cells inhibits Akt activation and induces anoikis. *Cancer Res* 58 (23):5285-90.

Davies, M. A., K. Stemke-Hale, E. Lin, C. Tellez, W. Deng, Y. N. Gopal, S. E. Woodman, T. C. Calderone, Z. Ju, A. J. Lazar, V. G. Prieto, K. Aldape, G. B. Mills, and J. E.

Gershenwald. 2009. Integrated Molecular and Clinical Analysis of AKT Activation in Metastatic Melanoma. *Clin Cancer Res* 15 (24):7538-7546.

Davies, M. A., K. Stemke-Hale, C. Tellez, T. L. Calderone, W. Deng, V. G. Prieto, A. J. Lazar, J. E. Gershenwald, and G. B. Mills. 2008. A novel AKT3 mutation in melanoma tumours and cell lines. *Br J Cancer* 99 (8):1265-8.

Ding, L., G. Getz, D. A. Wheeler, E. R. Mardis, M. D. McLellan, K. Cibulskis, C. Sougnez, H. Greulich, D. M. Muzny, M. B. Morgan, L. Fulton, R. S. Fulton, Q. Zhang, M. C. Wendl, M. S. Lawrence, D. E. Larson, K. Chen, D. J. Dooling, A. Sabo, A. C. Hawes, H. Shen, S. N. Jhangiani, L. R. Lewis, O. Hall, Y. Zhu, T. Mathew, Y. Ren, J. Yao, S. E. Scherer, K. Clerc, G. A. Metcalf, B. Ng, A. Milosavljevic, M. L. Gonzalez-Garay, J. R. Osborne, R. Meyer, X. Shi, Y. Tang, D. C. Koboldt, L. Lin, R. Abbott, T. L. Miner, C. Pohl, G. Fewell, C. Haipek, H. Schmidt, B. H. Dunford-Shore, A. Kraja, S. D. Crosby, C. S. Sawyer, T. Vickery, S. Sander, J. Robinson, W. Winckler, J. Baldwin, L. R. Chirieac, A. Dutt, T. Fennell, M. Hanna, B. E. Johnson, R. C. Onofrio, R. K. Thomas, G. Tonon, B. A. Weir, X. Zhao, L. Ziaugra, M. C. Zody, T. Giordano, M. B. Orringer, J. A. Roth, M. R. Spitz, Wistuba, II, B. Ozenberger, P. J. Good, A. C. Chang, D. G. Beer, M. A. Watson, M. Ladanyi, S. Broderick, A. Yoshizawa, W. D. Travis, W. Pao, M. A. Province, G. M. Weinstock, H. E. Varmus, S. B. Gabriel, E. S. Lander, R. A. Gibbs, M. Meyerson, and R. K. Wilson. 2008. Somatic mutations affect key pathways in lung adenocarcinoma. *Nature* 455 (7216):1069-75.

Dummer, R., C. Robert, P. Chapman, J. Sosman, M. R. Middleton, L. Bastholt, K. Kemsley, M. V. Cantarini, C. Morris, and J. M. Kirkwood. 2008. AZD6244 (ARR-142886) vs temozolomide (TMZ) in patients with advanced melanoma: an open-label, randomized, multicenter, phase II study. *J Clin Oncol* 26 (May 20 supplement):9033.

Eisen, T., T. Ahmad, K. T. Flaherty, M. Gore, S. Kaye, R. Marais, I. Gibbens, S. Hackett, M. James, L. M. Schuchter, K. L. Nathanson, C. Xia, R. Simantov, B. Schwartz, M. Poulin-Costello, P. J. O'Dwyer, and M. J. Ratain. 2006. Sorafenib in advanced melanoma: a Phase II randomised discontinuation trial analysis. *Br J Cancer* 95 (5):581-6.

Emery, C. M., K. G. Vijayendran, M. C. Zipser, A. M. Sawyer, L. Niu, J. J. Kim, C. Hatton, R. Chopra, P. A. Oberholzer, M. B. Karpova, L. E. MacConaill, J. Zhang, N. S. Gray, W. R. Sellers, R. Dummer, and L. A. Garraway. 2009. MEK1 mutations confer resistance to MEK and B-RAF inhibition. *Proc Natl Acad Sci U S A* 106 (48):20411-6.

Engelman, J. A., J. Luo, and L. C. Cantley. 2006. The evolution of phosphatidylinositol 3-kinases as regulators of growth and metabolism. *Nat Rev Genet* 7 (8):606-19.

Fisher, D. E., R. Barnhill, F. S. Hodi, M. Herlyn, G. Merlino, E. Medrano, B. Bastian, T. M. Landi, and J. Sosman. 2010. Melanoma from bench to bedside: meeting report from the 6th international melanoma congress. *Pigment Cell Melanoma Res* 23 (1):14-26.

Flaherty, K. T., I. Puzanov, K. B. Kim, A. Ribas, G. A. McArthur, J. A. Sosman, P. J. O'Dwyer, R. J. Lee, J. F. Grippo, K. Nolop, and P. B. Chapman. Inhibition of mutated, activated BRAF in metastatic melanoma. *N Engl J Med* 363 (9):809-19.

Flaherty, Keith T., Igor Puzanov, Kevin B. Kim, Antoni Ribas, Grant A. McArthur, Jeffrey A. Sosman, Peter J. O'Dwyer, Richard J. Lee, Joseph F. Grippo, Keith Nolop, and Paul

B. Chapman. 2010. Inhibition of Mutated, Activated BRAF in Metastatic Melanoma. *New England Journal of Medicine* 363 (9):809-819.

Flaherty, Keith T., Joan Schiller, Lynn M. Schuchter, Glenn Liu, David A. Tuveson, Maryann Redlinger, Chetan Lathia, Chenghua Xia, Oana Petrenciuc, Sunil R. Hingorani, Michael A. Jacobetz, Patricia A. Van Belle, David Elder, Marcia S. Brose, Barbara L. Weber, Mark R. Albertini, and Peter J. O'Dwyer. 2008. A Phase I Trial of the Oral, Multikinase Inhibitor Sorafenib in Combination with Carboplatin and Paclitaxel. *Clinical Cancer Research* 14 (15):4836-4842.

Forrester, K., C. Almoguera, K. Han, W. E. Grizzle, and M. Perucho. 1987. Detection of high incidence of K-ras oncogenes during human colon tumorigenesis. *Nature* 327 (6120):298-303.

Garnett, M. J., S. Rana, H. Paterson, D. Barford, and R. Marais. 2005. Wild-type and mutant B-RAF activate C-RAF through distinct mechanisms involving heterodimerization. *Mol Cell* 20 (6):963-9.

Garraway, Levi A., Hans R. Widlund, Mark A. Rubin, Gad Getz, Aaron J. Berger, Sridhar Ramaswamy, Rameen Beroukhim, Danny A. Milner, Scott R. Granter, Jinyan Du, Charles Lee, Stephan N. Wagner, Cheng Li, Todd R. Golub, David L. Rimm, Matthew L. Meyerson, David E. Fisher, and William R. Sellers. 2005. Integrative genomic analyses identify MITF as a lineage survival oncogene amplified in malignant melanoma. *Nature* 436 (7047):117-122.

George, A. J., W. G. Thomas, and R. D. Hannan. The renin-angiotensin system and cancer: old dog, new tricks. *Nat Rev Cancer* 10 (11):745-59.

Goel, V. K., A. J. Lazar, C. L. Warneke, M. S. Redston, and F. G. Haluska. 2006. Examination of mutations in BRAF, NRAS, and PTEN in primary cutaneous melanoma. *J Invest Dermatol* 126 (1):154-60.

Goldstein, A. M., M. Chan, M. Harland, N. K. Hayward, F. Demenais, D. T. Bishop, E. Azizi, W. Bergman, G. Bianchi-Scarra, W. Bruno, D. Calista, L. A. Albright, V. Chaudru, A. Chompret, F. Cuellar, D. E. Elder, P. Ghiorzo, E. M. Gillanders, N. A. Gruis, J. Hansson, D. Hogg, E. A. Holland, P. A. Kanetsky, R. F. Kefford, M. T. Landi, J. Lang, S. A. Leachman, R. M. MacKie, V. Magnusson, G. J. Mann, J. N. Bishop, J. M. Palmer, S. Puig, J. A. Puig-Butille, M. Stark, H. Tsao, M. A. Tucker, L. Whitaker, and E. Yakobson. 2007. Features associated with germline CDKN2A mutations: a GenoMEL study of melanoma-prone families from three continents. *J Med Genet* 44 (2):99-106.

Gopal, Y. N., W. Deng, S. E. Woodman, K. Komurov, P. Ram, P. D. Smith, and M. A. Davies. 2010. Basal and treatment-induced activation of AKT mediates resistance to cell death by AZD6244 (ARRY-142886) in Braf-mutant human cutaneous melanoma cells. *Cancer Res* 70 (21):8736-47.

Halaban, R., W. Zhang, A. Bacchiocchi, E. Cheng, F. Parisi, S. Ariyan, M. Krauthammer, J. P. McCusker, Y. Kluger, and M. Sznol. 2010. PLX4032, a selective BRAF(V600E) kinase inhibitor, activates the ERK pathway and enhances cell migration and proliferation of BRAF melanoma cells. *Pigment Cell Melanoma Res* 23 (2):190-200.

Handolias, D., A. L. Hamilton, R. Salemi, A. Tan, K. Moodie, L. Kerr, A. Dobrovic, and G. A. McArthur. 2010. Clinical responses observed with imatinib or sorafenib in melanoma patients expressing mutations in KIT. *Br J Cancer* 102 (8):1219-1223.

Handolias, D., R. Salemi, W. Murray, A. Tan, W. Liu, A. Viros, A. Dobrovic, J. Kelly, and G. A. McArthur. 2010. Mutations in KIT occur at low frequency in melanomas arising from anatomical sites associated with chronic and intermittent sun exposure. *Pigment Cell Melanoma Res* 23:210-215.

Hatzivassiliou, G., K. Song, I. Yen, B. J. Brandhuber, D. J. Anderson, R. Alvarado, M. J. Ludlam, D. Stokoe, S. L. Gloor, G. Vigers, T. Morales, I. Aliagas, B. Liu, S. Sideris, K. P. Hoeflich, B. S. Jaiswal, S. Seshagiri, H. Koeppen, M. Belvin, L. S. Friedman, and S. Malek. 2010. RAF inhibitors prime wild-type RAF to activate the MAPK pathway and enhance growth. *Nature*.

Hauschild, Axel, Sanjiv S. Agarwala, Uwe Trefzer, David Hogg, Caroline Robert, Peter Hersey, Alexander Eggermont, Stephan Grabbe, Rene Gonzalez, Jens Gille, Christian Peschel, Dirk Schadendorf, Claus Garbe, Steven O'Day, Adil Daud, J. Michael White, Chenghua Xia, Kiran Patel, John M. Kirkwood, and Ulrich Keilholz. 2009. Results of a Phase III, Randomized, Placebo-Controlled Study of Sorafenib in Combination With Carboplatin and Paclitaxel As Second-Line Treatment in Patients With Unresectable Stage III or Stage IV Melanoma. *J Clin Oncol* 27 (17):2823-2830.

Heidorn, Sonja J., Carla Milagre, Steven Whittaker, Arnaud Nourry, Ion Niculescu-Duvas, Nathalie Dhomen, Jahan Hussain, Jorge S. Reis-Filho, Caroline J. Springer, Catrin Pritchard, and Richard Marais. 2010. Kinase-Dead BRAF and Oncogenic RAS Cooperate to Drive Tumor Progression through CRAF. *Cell* 140 (2):209-221.

Hirota, S., K. Isozaki, Y. Moriyama, K. Hashimoto, T. Nishida, S. Ishiguro, K. Kawano, M. Hanada, A. Kurata, M. Takeda, G. Muhammad Tunio, Y. Matsuzawa, Y. Kanakura, Y. Shinomura, and Y. Kitamura. 1998. Gain-of-function mutations of c-kit in human gastrointestinal stromal tumors. *Science* 279 (5350):577-80.

Hocker, T., and H. Tsao. 2007. Ultraviolet radiation and melanoma: a systematic review and analysis of reported sequence variants. *Hum Mutat* 28 (6):578-88.

Hodi, F. S., P. Friedlander, C. L. Corless, M. C. Heinrich, S. Mac Rae, A. Kruse, J. Jagannathan, A. D. Van den Abbeele, E. F. Velazquez, G. D. Demetri, and D. E. Fisher. 2008. Major response to imatinib mesylate in KIT-mutated melanoma. *J Clin Oncol* 26 (12):2046-51.

Huang, S., M. Luca, M. Gutman, D. J. McConkey, K. E. Langley, S. D. Lyman, and M. Bar-Eli. 1996. Enforced c-KIT expression renders highly metastatic human melanoma cells susceptible to stem cell factor-induced apoptosis and inhibits their tumorigenic and metastatic potential. *Oncogene* 13 (11):2339-47.

Infante, J. R., L. A. Fecher, S. Nallapareddy, M. S. Gordon, K. T. Flaherty, D. S. Cox, D. J. DeMarini, S. R. Morris, H. A. Burris, and W. Messersmith. 2010. Safety and efficacy results from the first time in humans study of the oral MEK1/2 inhibitor GSK1120212. *J Clin Oncol*.

Jemal, A., R. Siegel, J. Xu, and E. Ward. Cancer statistics, 2010. *CA Cancer J Clin* 60 (5):277-300.

Johannessen, Cory M., Jesse S. Boehm, So Young Kim, Sapana R. Thomas, Leslie Wardwell, Laura A. Johnson, Caroline M. Emery, Nicolas Stransky, Alexandria P. Cogdill, Jordi Barretina, Giordano Caponigro, Haley Hieronymus, Ryan R. Murray, Kourosh Salehi-Ashtiani, David E. Hill, Marc Vidal, Jean J. Zhao, Xiaoping Yang, Ozan Alkan, Sungjoon Kim, Jennifer L. Harris, Christopher J. Wilson, Vic E. Myer, Peter M. Finan, David E. Root, Thomas M. Roberts, Todd Golub, Keith T. Flaherty, Reinhard Dummer, Barbara L. Weber, William R. Sellers, Robert Schlegel, Jennifer A. Wargo, William C. Hahn, and Levi A. Garraway. 2010. COT drives resistance to RAF inhibition through MAP kinase pathway reactivation. *Nature* 468 (7326):968-972.

Jonsson, G., C. Dahl, J. Staaf, T. Sandberg, P. O. Bendahl, M. Ringner, P. Guldberg, and A. Borg. 2007. Genomic profiling of malignant melanoma using tiling-resolution arrayCGH. *Oncogene* 26 (32):4738-48.

Karasarides, M., A. Chiloeches, R. Hayward, D. Niculescu-Duvaz, I. Scanlon, F. Friedlos, L. Ogilvie, D. Hedley, J. Martin, C. J. Marshall, C. J. Springer, and R. Marais. 2004. B-RAF is a therapeutic target in melanoma. *Oncogene* 23 (37):6292-8.

Kefford, Richard F., H. Arkenau, M. P. Brown, M. Milward, J. R. Infante, G. V. Long, D. Ouellet, M. Curtis, P. F. Lebowitz, and G. S. Falchook. 2010. Phase I/II study of GSK2118436, a selective inhibitor of oncogenic mutant BRAF kinase, in patients with metastatic melanoma and other solid tumors. *J Clin Oncol* 28 (15s):8503.

Kim, K. B., O. Eton, D. W. Davis, M. L. Frazier, D. J. McConkey, A. H. Diwan, N. E. Papadopoulos, A. Y. Bedikian, L. H. Camacho, M. I. Ross, J. N. Cormier, J. E. Gershenwald, J. E. Lee, P. F. Mansfield, L. A. Billings, C. S. Ng, C. Charnsangavej, M. Bar-Eli, M. M. Johnson, A. J. Murgo, and V. G. Prieto. 2008. Phase II trial of imatinib mesylate in patients with metastatic melanoma. *Br J Cancer* 99 (5):734-40.

Koon, H., and M. Atkins. 2006. Autoimmunity and immunotherapy for cancer. *N Engl J Med* 354 (7):758-60.

Lassam, N., and S. Bickford. 1992. Loss of c-kit expression in cultured melanoma cells. *Oncogene* 7 (1):51-6.

Levy, C., M. Khaled, and D. E. Fisher. 2006. MITF: master regulator of melanocyte development and melanoma oncogene. *Trends Mol Med* 12 (9):406-14.

Li, J., C. Yen, D. Liaw, K. Podsypanina, S. Bose, S. I. Wang, J. Puc, C. Miliaresis, L. Rodgers, R. McCombie, S. H. Bigner, B. C. Giovanella, M. Ittmann, B. Tycko, H. Hibshoosh, M. H. Wigler, and R. Parsons. 1997. PTEN, a putative protein tyrosine phosphatase gene mutated in human brain, breast, and prostate cancer. *Science* 275 (5308):1943-7.

Maehama, T., and J. E. Dixon. 1998. The tumor suppressor, PTEN/MMAC1, dephosphorylates the lipid second messenger, phosphatidylinositol 3,4,5-trisphosphate. *J Biol Chem* 273 (22):13375-8.

Mirmohammadsadegh, A., A. Marini, S. Nambiar, M. Hassan, A. Tannapfel, T. Ruzicka, and U. R. Hengge. 2006. Epigenetic silencing of the PTEN gene in melanoma. *Cancer Res* 66 (13):6546-52.

Myers, M. P., I. Pass, I. H. Batty, J. Van der Kaay, J. P. Stolarov, B. A. Hemmings, M. H. Wigler, C. P. Downes, and N. K. Tonks. 1998. The lipid phosphatase activity of PTEN is critical for its tumor supressor function. *Proc Natl Acad Sci U S A* 95 (23):13513-8.

Nazarian, Ramin, Hubing Shi, Qi Wang, Xiangju Kong, Richard C. Koya, Hane Lee, Zugen Chen, Mi-Kyung Lee, Narsis Attar, Hooman Sazegar, Thinle Chodon, Stanley F. Nelson, Grant McArthur, Jeffrey A. Sosman, Antoni Ribas, and Roger S. Lo. 2010. Melanomas acquire resistance to B-RAF(V600E) inhibition by RTK or N-RAS upregulation. *Nature* 468 (7326):973-977.

Omholt, K., D. Krockel, U. Ringborg, and J. Hansson. 2006. Mutations of PIK3CA are rare in cutaneous melanoma. *Melanoma Res* 16 (2):197-200.

Onken, M. D., L. A. Worley, M. D. Long, S. Duan, M. L. Council, A. M. Bowcock, and J. W. Harbour. 2008. Oncogenic mutations in GNAQ occur early in uveal melanoma. *Invest Ophthalmol Vis Sci* 49 (12):5230-4.

Padua, R. A., N. C. Barrass, and G. A. Currie. 1985. Activation of N-ras in a human melanoma cell line. *Mol Cell Biol* 5 (3):582-5.

Paraiso, K. H., Y. Xiang, V. W. Rebecca, E. V. Abel, A. Chen, A. C. Munko, E. Wood, I. V. Fedorenko, V. K. Sondak, A. R. Anderson, A. Ribas, M. Dalla Palma, K. L. Nathanson, J. M. Koomen, J. L. Messina, and K. S. Smalley. 2011. PTEN loss confers BRAF inhibitor resistance to melanoma cells through the suppression of BIM expression. *Cancer Res*:In press.

Patton, E. E., H. R. Widlund, J. L. Kutok, K. R. Kopani, J. F. Amatruda, R. D. Murphey, S. Berghmans, E. A. Mayhall, D. Traver, C. D. Fletcher, J. C. Aster, S. R. Granter, A. T. Look, C. Lee, D. E. Fisher, and L. I. Zon. 2005. BRAF mutations are sufficient to promote nevi formation and cooperate with p53 in the genesis of melanoma. *Curr Biol* 15 (3):249-54.

Pleasance, Erin D., R. Keira Cheetham, Philip J. Stephens, David J. McBride, Sean J. Humphray, Chris D. Greenman, Ignacio Varela, Meng-Lay Lin, Gonzalo R. Ordonez, Graham R. Bignell, Kai Ye, Julie Alipaz, Markus J. Bauer, David Beare, Adam Butler, Richard J. Carter, Lina Chen, Anthony J. Cox, Sarah Edkins, Paula I. Kokko-Gonzales, Niall A. Gormley, Russell J. Grocock, Christian D. Haudenschild, Matthew M. Hims, Terena James, Mingming Jia, Zoya Kingsbury, Catherine Leroy, John Marshall, Andrew Menzies, Laura J. Mudie, Zemin Ning, Tom Royce, Ole B. Schulz-Trieglaff, Anastassia Spiridou, Lucy A. Stebbings, Lukasz Szajkowski, Jon Teague, David Williamson, Lynda Chin, Mark T. Ross, Peter J. Campbell, David R. Bentley, P. Andrew Futreal, and Michael R. Stratton. 2010. A comprehensive catalogue of somatic mutations from a human cancer genome. *Nature* 463 (7278):191-196.

Pomerantz, J., N. Schreiber-Agus, N. J. Liegeois, A. Silverman, L. Alland, L. Chin, J. Potes, K. Chen, I. Orlow, H. W. Lee, C. Cordon-Cardo, and R. A. DePinho. 1998. The Ink4a tumor suppressor gene product, p19Arf, interacts with MDM2 and neutralizes MDM2's inhibition of p53. *Cell* 92 (6):713-23.

Poulikakos, Poulikos I., Chao Zhang, Gideon Bollag, Kevan M. Shokat, and Neal Rosen. 2010. RAF inhibitors transactivate RAF dimers and ERK signalling in cells with wild-type BRAF. *Nature* 464 (7287):427-430.

Prickett, T. D., N. S. Agrawal, X. Wei, K. E. Yates, J. C. Lin, J. R. Wunderlich, J. C. Cronin, P. Cruz, S. A. Rosenberg, and Y. Samuels. 2009. Analysis of the tyrosine kinome in melanoma reveals recurrent mutations in ERBB4. *Nat Genet* 41 (10):1127-32.

Rakosy, Z., L. Vizkeleti, S. Ecsedi, A. Begany, G. Emri, R. Adany, and M. Balazs. 2008. Characterization of 9p21 copy number alterations in human melanoma by fluorescence in situ hybridization. *Cancer Genet Cytogenet* 182 (2):116-21.

Rimoldi, Donata, Suzanne Salvi, Danielle Lienard, Ferdy J. Lejeune, Daniel Speiser, Leonidas Zografos, and Jean-Charles Cerottini. 2003. Lack of BRAF Mutations in Uveal Melanoma. *Cancer Res* 63 (18):5712-5715.

Smalley, K. S., R. Contractor, T. K. Nguyen, M. Xiao, R. Edwards, V. Muthusamy, A. J. King, K. T. Flaherty, M. Bosenberg, M. Herlyn, and K. L. Nathanson. 2008. Identification of a novel subgroup of melanomas with KIT/cyclin-dependent kinase-4 overexpression. *Cancer Res* 68 (14):5743-52.

Soung, Y. H., J. W. Lee, S. Y. Kim, Y. P. Wang, K. H. Jo, S. W. Moon, W. S. Park, S. W. Nam, J. Y. Lee, N. J. Yoo, and S. H. Lee. 2006. Somatic mutations of the ERBB4 kinase domain in human cancers. *Int J Cancer* 118 (6):1426-9.

Stahl, J. M., A. Sharma, M. Cheung, M. Zimmerman, J. Q. Cheng, M. W. Bosenberg, M. Kester, L. Sandirasegarane, and G. P. Robertson. 2004. Deregulated Akt3 activity promotes development of malignant melanoma. *Cancer Res* 64 (19):7002-10.

Stott, F. J., S. Bates, M. C. James, B. B. McConnell, M. Starborg, S. Brookes, I. Palmero, K. Ryan, E. Hara, K. H. Vousden, and G. Peters. 1998. The alternative product from the human CDKN2A locus, p14(ARF), participates in a regulatory feedback loop with p53 and MDM2. *EMBO J* 17 (17):5001-14.

Strumberg, D. 2005. Preclinical and clinical development of the oral multikinase inhibitor sorafenib in cancer treatment. *Drugs Today (Barc)* 41 (12):773-84.

Tsai, J., J. T. Lee, W. Wang, J. Zhang, H. Cho, S. Mamo, R. Bremer, S. Gillette, J. Kong, N. K. Haass, K. Sproesser, L. Li, K. S. Smalley, D. Fong, Y. L. Zhu, A. Marimuthu, H. Nguyen, B. Lam, J. Liu, I. Cheung, J. Rice, Y. Suzuki, C. Luu, C. Settachatgul, R. Shellooe, J. Cantwell, S. H. Kim, J. Schlessinger, K. Y. Zhang, B. L. West, B. Powell, G. Habets, C. Zhang, P. N. Ibrahim, P. Hirth, D. R. Artis, M. Herlyn, and G. Bollag. 2008. Discovery of a selective inhibitor of oncogenic B-Raf kinase with potent antimelanoma activity. *Proc Natl Acad Sci U S A* 105 (8):3041-6.

Tsao, H., V. Goel, H. Wu, G. Yang, and F. G. Haluska. 2004. Genetic interaction between NRAS and BRAF mutations and PTEN/MMAC1 inactivation in melanoma. *J Invest Dermatol* 122 (2):337-41.

Tsao, H., M. C. Mihm, Jr., and C. Sheehan. 2003. PTEN expression in normal skin, acquired melanocytic nevi, and cutaneous melanoma. *J Am Acad Dermatol* 49 (5):865-72.

Tsao, H., X. Zhang, E. Benoit, and F. G. Haluska. 1998. Identification of PTEN/MMAC1 alterations in uncultured melanomas and melanoma cell lines. *Oncogene* 16 (26):3397-402.

Tsao, H., X. Zhang, K. Fowlkes, and F. G. Haluska. 2000. Relative reciprocity of NRAS and PTEN/MMAC1 alterations in cutaneous melanoma cell lines. *Cancer Res* 60 (7):1800-4.

Tsao, Hensin, Vikas Goel, Heng Wu, Guang Yang, and Frank G. Haluska. 2004. Genetic Interaction Between NRAS and BRAF Mutations and PTEN//MMAC1 Inactivation in Melanoma. *J Investig Dermatol* 122 (2):337-341.

Ugurel, S., R. Hildenbrand, A. Zimpfer, P. La Rosee, P. Paschka, A. Sucker, P. Keikavoussi, J. C. Becker, W. Rittgen, A. Hochhaus, and D. Schadendorf. 2005. Lack of clinical efficacy of imatinib in metastatic melanoma. *Br J Cancer* 92 (8):1398-405.

Van Raamsdonk, C. D., V. Bezrookove, G. Green, J. Bauer, L. Gaugler, J. M. O'Brien, E. M. Simpson, G. S. Barsh, and B. C. Bastian. 2009. Frequent somatic mutations of GNAQ in uveal melanoma and blue naevi. *Nature* 457 (7229):599-602.

Van Raamsdonk, C. D., K. R. Fitch, H. Fuchs, M. H. de Angelis, and G. S. Barsh. 2004. Effects of G-protein mutations on skin color. *Nat Genet* 36 (9):961-8.

Van Raamsdonk, C. D., K. G. Griewank, M. B. Crosby, M. C. Garrido, S. Vemula, T. Wiesner, A. C. Obenauf, W. Wackernagel, G. Green, N. Bouvier, M. M. Sozen, G. Baimukanova, R. Roy, A. Heguy, I. Dolgalev, R. Khanin, K. Busam, M. R. Speicher, J. O'Brien, and B. C. Bastian. 2010. Mutations in GNA11 in uveal melanoma. *N Engl J Med* 363 (23):2191-9.

Van Raamsdonk, Catherine D., Vladimir Bezrookove, Gary Green, Jurgen Bauer, Lona Gaugler, Joan M. O/'Brien, Elizabeth M. Simpson, Gregory S. Barsh, and Boris C. Bastian. 2009. Frequent somatic mutations of GNAQ in uveal melanoma and blue naevi. *Nature* 457 (7229):599-602.

Villanueva, Jessie, Adina Vultur, John T. Lee, Rajasekharan Somasundaram, Mizuho Fukunaga-Kalabis, Angela K. Cipolla, Bradley Wubbenhorst, Xiaowei Xu, Phyllis A. Gimotty, Damien Kee, Ademi E. Santiago-Walker, Richard Letrero, Kurt D'Andrea, Anitha Pushparajan, James E. Hayden, Kimberly Dahlman Brown, Sylvie Laquerre, Grant A. McArthur, Jeffrey A. Sosman, Katherine L. Nathanson, and Meenhard Herlyn. 2010. Acquired Resistance to BRAF Inhibitors Mediated by a RAF Kinase Switch in Melanoma Can Be Overcome by Cotargeting MEK and IGF-1R/PI3K. *Cancer Cell* 18 (6):683-695.

Wagle, N., C. Emery, M. F. Berger, M. J. Davis, A. Sawyer, P. Pochanard, S. M. Kehoe, C. M. Johannessen, L. E. Macconaill, W. C. Hahn, M. Meyerson, and L. A. Garraway. Dissecting Therapeutic Resistance to RAF Inhibition in Melanoma by Tumor Genomic Profiling. *J Clin Oncol.*

Wan, P. T., M. J. Garnett, S. M. Roe, S. Lee, D. Niculescu-Duvaz, V. M. Good, C. M. Jones, C. J. Marshall, C. J. Springer, D. Barford, and R. Marais. 2004. Mechanism of activation of the RAF-ERK signaling pathway by oncogenic mutations of B-RAF. *Cell* 116 (6):855-67.

Woodman, S. E., J. C. Trent, K. Stemke-Hale, A. J. Lazar, S. Pricl, G. M. Pavan, M. Fermeglia, Y. N. Gopal, D. Yang, D. A. Podoloff, D. Ivan, K. B. Kim, N. Papadopoulos, P. Hwu, G. B. Mills, and M. A. Davies. 2009. Activity of dasatinib against L576P KIT mutant melanoma: molecular, cellular, and clinical correlates. *Mol Cancer Ther* 8 (8):2079-85.

Wyman, K., M. B. Atkins, V. Prieto, O. Eton, D. F. McDermott, F. Hubbard, C. Byrnes, K. Sanders, and J. A. Sosman. 2006. Multicenter Phase II trial of high-dose imatinib mesylate in metastatic melanoma: significant toxicity with no clinical efficacy. *Cancer* 106 (9):2005-11.

Yang, G., A. Rajadurai, and H. Tsao. 2005. Recurrent patterns of dual RB and p53 pathway inactivation in melanoma. *J Invest Dermatol* 125 (6):1242-51.

Yang, Hong, Brian Higgins, Kenneth Kolinsky, Kathryn Packman, Zenaida Go, Raman Iyer, Stanley Kolis, Sylvia Zhao, Richard Lee, Joseph F. Grippo, Kathleen Schostack,

Mary Ellen Simcox, David Heimbrook, Gideon Bollag, and Fei Su. 2010. RG7204 (PLX4032), a Selective BRAFV600E Inhibitor, Displays Potent Antitumor Activity in Preclinical Melanoma Models. *Cancer Research* 70 (13):5518-5527.

Zhang, Y., Y. Xiong, and W. G. Yarbrough. 1998. ARF promotes MDM2 degradation and stabilizes p53: ARF-INK4a locus deletion impairs both the Rb and p53 tumor suppression pathways. *Cell* 92 (6):725-34.

9

BRAF V600E Mutated Gene Variant as a Circulating Molecular Marker in Metastatic Melanoma Patients

Viviana Vallacchi, Licia Rivoltini and Monica Rodolfo
Fondazione IRCCS Istituto Nazionale Tumori
Italy

1. Introduction

Cutaneous metastatic melanoma management has recently approached the age of individualized therapy (Romano et al., 2011). The discovery that the 1799T>A point mutation in the BRAF oncogene (BRAFV600E) occurs in ~50% of melanoma lesions and that melanoma cells bearing the mutation are oncogene addicted, i.e., strictly dependent upon BRAFV600E activity for growth and survival, have pointed to BRAFV600E as a promising target for therapy. Drugs targeting BRAF have been developed, and several clinical trials are currently ongoing. Phase I-II results recently reported remarkable tumor regression in the great majority of patients bearing disseminated BRAFV600E mutated melanoma disease after treatment with BRAFV600E-specific inhibitors.

In these trials, BRAF mutational status is determined to select patients who may benefit from therapy. However, melanoma specimens are not always available to perform this analysis; moreover, a negative result in a single tumor biopsy may cover the presence of mutation-positive tumor lesions. Because blood has been proven to represent a valuable alternative source of tumor-derived cells as well as of tumor-derived DNA, several technical approaches have been studied to detect BRAFV600E in RNA/DNA extracted from blood-derived circulating tumor cells and in circulating free DNA isolated from plasma or serum. For these reasons, circulating BRAFV600E has the potential as both a specific melanoma molecular marker and a monitoring factor to be used to evaluate clinical response.

In this chapter, we summarize the clinical and biological features of BRAF mutation in melanoma. Furthermore, we report a new BRAFV600E detection assay developed in our lab that shows high sensitivity and specificity.

2. BRAFV600E mutation in melanoma

Among the genetic lesions that frequently occur in melanoma, BRAF gene mutation is the most common and is detected in about 50% of melanoma (Davies et al., 2002). The BRAF gene encodes a serine-threonine kinase belonging to the MAPK kinase pathway, also known as the RAS/RAF/MEK/ERK pathway. This signaling pathway regulates important cellular processes, including cell growth, proliferation and migration; in physiological conditions, the signaling is triggered by activated growth factor receptors, which act as binding sites for adapter proteins that subsequently activate a cascade of kinases, including NRAS, BRAF, MEK and ERK, via phosphorylation. Activated ERK translocates to the cell nucleus, where it phosphorylates and activates many different substrates (Held et al., 2010; Poulikakos & Rosen, 2011; Young et al., 2009).

BRAF mutations identified in melanoma are in the kinase domain, which is encoded by exons 11 and 15, and are somatic. Somatic BRAF point mutations have been also detected in approximately 8% of other tumor types, including 30-70% of papillary thyroid cancers and 10% of colorectal cancers, and ovarian, breast and lung cancers (Cantwell-Dorris et al., 2011; Davies et al., 2002; Puzanov et al., 2011). No BRAF germline mutations have been found in familial or sporadic melanoma patients (Lang et al., 2003; Laud et al., 2003; Meyer et al., 2003a), although germline mutations have been shown to occur in Noonan, LEOPARD and cardio-facio-cutaneous syndromes, which are developmental disorders with overlapping features including distinctive facial dysmorphia, reduced growth, cardiac defects, skeletal and ectodermal anomalies and variable cognitive deficits (Sarkozy et al., 2009; Tidyman & Raouen, 2009). The relationship between BRAF germline polymorphisms and melanoma risk has also been investigated, and data obtained suggest that BRAF can be considered a low-risk susceptibility gene for melanoma (James et al., 2005; Meyer et al., 2003b).

It has been reported that melanocortin 1 receptor (MC1R) variants increase the risk of melanoma with BRAF mutations (Fargnoli et al., 2008; Landi et al., 2006; Scherer et al., 2010). The MC1R gene, which has been identified as a low-risk melanoma susceptibility gene (Williams et al., 2010), encodes a seven-pass transmembrane G-protein receptor that binds alpha-melanocyte stimulating hormone and plays a key role in the pigmentation process (Palmer et al., 2000; Rees, 2004; Valverde et al., 1995). The MC1R gene is highly polymorphic, and gene variants determine a partial or complete loss in the ability of the receptor to transduce signals, thus impairing the switch from pheomelanin to eumelanin production in response to UV radiation exposure (Healy et al., 2000). Further studies are needed to elucidate the mechanisms causing MC1R variants to select for BRAF somatic mutations (Hacker & Hayward, 2008).

BRAF mutations result in the constitutive activation of ERK, resulting in proliferation and growth advantage of melanoma cells. In 15-30% of melanoma, the RAS/RAF/MEK/ERK pathway is constitutively activated through NRAS mutation (Sekulic et al., 2008). As BRAF and NRAS mutations are mutually exclusive, hyperactivation of the MAPK pathway is very frequent in melanoma. Although the constitutive activation of the MAPK pathway is often required to promote the growth and proliferation of neoplastic cells, BRAF mutations are prevalent in melanoma, while mutations in tyrosine kinase receptors or in RAS genes are prevalent in other tumor types. Chromosomal rearrangements leading to the formation of BRAF fusion products, characterized by the lack of the BRAF auto-inhibitory domain and the aberrant activation of the MAPK pathway, have also been reported in pilocytic astrocytoma, thyroid, prostate and gastric cancer as well as melanoma (Ciampi et al., 2005; Cin et al., 2011; Dessars et al., 2007; Palanisamy et al., 2010).

The substitution of a valine (V) for glutamic acid (E) at position 600 (V600E) accounts for >90% of BRAF mutations identified in melanoma. BRAF mutations in melanoma are an early event as they can be detected in nevi and in primary melanoma (Figure 1) (Rodolfo et al., 2004; Thomas et al., 2006). Even if 60-70% of benign and dysplastic nevi show the BRAFV600E mutation, most of them do not progress to melanoma, suggesting that further alterations are necessary to promote malignant progression. In particular, it has been proposed that BRAF mutations may induce senescence and that abrogation of the mechanisms regulating this cellular process are required to induce tumor progression (Michaloglou et al., 2005). In primary melanoma, BRAFV600E mutation is rarely detected in lentigo maligna lesions which arise in chronically sun-exposed skin and show a high rate of RAS mutations, and in acral and mucosal melanoma that arise in non-exposed skin, which may show KIT gene mutation (Platz et al., 2008). Melanoma occurring in childhood and adolescence, as well as those occurring in patients with a family history of melanoma, show BRAFV600E mutation (Daniotti et al., 2009). Melanoma that arise in intermittently exposed body sites, in skin lacking signs of chronic sun-induced damage, and in younger people, show a >80% rate of BRAFV600E mutation (Curtin et al., 2005). BRAF mutation frequency appears higher in advanced lesions than primary tumors, and it does not seem to be related to the site of metastases. Moreover, different studies have reported that BRAF mutation is maintained during progression from primary tumor to metastatic lesions or is acquired during the development of metastases (Houben et al., 2004; Omholt et al., 2003; Shinozaki et al., 2004). These results suggested a possible direct link between mutated BRAF and the metastatic potential of melanoma cells.

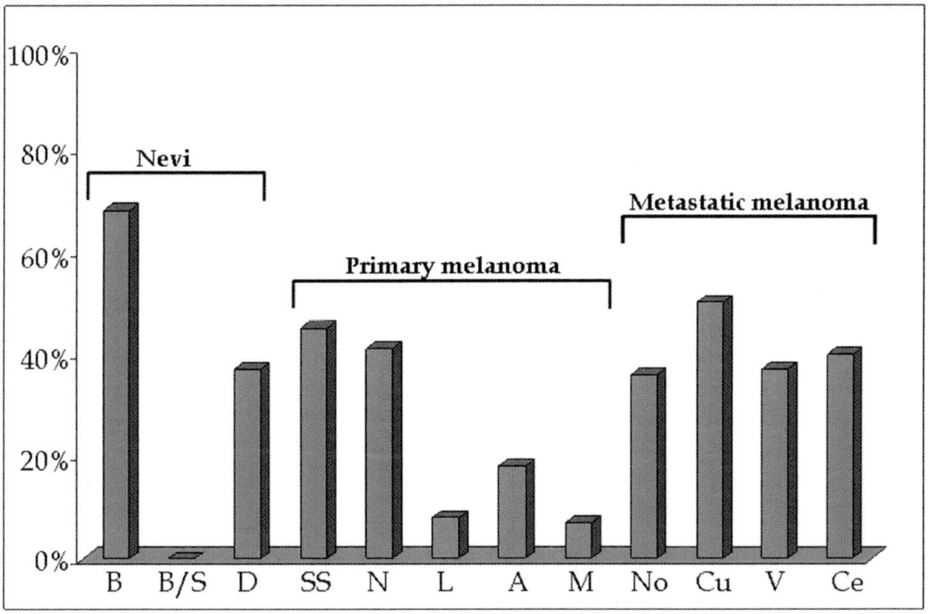

B: Benign nevi; B/S: Blue and Spitz nevi; D: Dysplastic nevi; SS: Superficial Spreading melanoma; N: Nodular melanoma; L: Lentigo maligna melanoma; A: Acral lentiginous melanoma; M: Mucosal melanoma; No: Nodal metastases; Cu: Cutaneous metastases; V: Visceral metastases; Ce: Cerebral metastases.

Fig. 1. Frequency of BRAFV600E mutation in nevi and melanoma lesions.

Several authors have studied the effects of BRAFV600E on global gene expression profiles of melanoma cells by microarray analysis and reported a BRAF mutation-associated gene expression signature (Pavey et al., 2004; Bloethner et al., 2005; Johansson et al., 2007). In particular, genes that encoded proteins involved in RAS/RAF/MEK/ERK signaling were identified among the genes differentially expressed between melanoma cell lines with or without BRAF mutation (Bloethner et al., 2005). In addition, a classifier able to discriminate between BRAF mutant and BRAF wild-type melanoma with high accuracy was built, including genes encoding phosphates and other genes biologically related to melanoma progression (Pavey et al., 2004). On the contrary, Hoek et al. failed to find a BRAF signature but identified three sample cohorts that represented melanoma groups characterized by different metastatic potential (Hoek et al., 2004). This discrepancy could be explained by considering the methods used to perform the analysis of array data; in fact, when the data by Hoek were re-analyzed with another statistical approach, a BRAF signature could be identified in these data (Johansson et al., 2007). Taken together, these results support the presence of a gene expression profile associated with BRAF mutation in melanoma and point to the genes that are potentially novel therapeutic targets.

3. BRAFV600E as a therapeutic target

The frequency and specificity of BRAFV600E mutation, together with the strict dependence of melanoma cell growth and survival on BRAFV600E activity (a phenomenon called oncogene addiction), have pointed to BRAFV600E as a promising therapeutic target.

Several BRAF inhibitors have been produced in the last years that have been or are currently being clinically tested (Sheperd et al., 2010). The first compound tested in clinical trials was Sorafenib (BAY43-9006), a multi-kinase inhibitor that targeted both wild-type and mutated BRAF, CRAF and other protein kinases, such as VEGFR2 and -3, PDGF, p38 MAPK, cKIT, FMS and RET (Wellbrock & Hurlstone, 2010). Sorafenib showed poor clinical activity when tested as a single agent, and in phase III trials in both front- and second-line therapies in combination with carboplatin and paclitaxol (Eisen et al., 2006; Hauschild et al., 2009). Other multi-kinase inhibitors that show a higher selectivity for BRAF than Sorafenib are currently under investigation in clinical trials (Dienstmann & Tabernero, 2011).

Several compounds that selectively inhibit BRAF have also been developed. Among them, GSK2118436 (SB-590885) has been tested in a phase I-II clinical trial and shows clinical responses in 60% of melanoma patients with BRAFV600 tumors, including patients having BRAFV600K and BRAFV600G mutations, with good tolerability (Kefford et al., 2010). Moreover, treatment with GSK2118436 induced a 20-100% reduction in the size of central nervous system lesions in patients with previously untreated brain metastases (Long et al., 2010).

Recently, the results of a phase I-II study that tested a specific BRAFV600E inhibitor, PLX4032 (RO5185426), were reported. Treatment with PLX4032 induced a complete or partial tumor regression in 81% of patients who had melanoma with BRAFV600E mutation, including progression-free survival for more than 7 months and manageable side effects, while patients with BRAF wild-type tumors showed no evidence of tumor regression (Flaherty et al., 2010). As a side effect, 31% of patients treated with PLX4032 developed low-grade squamous cell carcinomas, which were reported to occur also in patients treated with Sorafenib (Arnault et al., 2009). This side effect is possibly due to the selective mechanism of action of PLX4032 that shuts down only the activity of BRAFV600E while inducing the formation of BRAF-RAF1 heterodimers and RAF1-RAF1 homodimers, thus inducing hyper-activation of the MAPK pathway in both tumor cells and normal skin cells with wild-type BRAF (Hatzivassiliou et al., 2010; Heidorn et al., 2010; Poulikakos et al., 2010).

4. Mechanisms of resistance to BRAF inhibitors

Even if BRAFV600E tumors initially respond to PLX4032 treatment, the majority of patients relapsed within 2-18 months and developed resistance to the treatment. Furthermore, a subset of BRAFV600E tumors showed primary resistance as about 20% of patients did not respond to PLX4032 treatment (Flaherty et al., 2010). These findings indicate that the development of new therapeutic strategies using PLX4032 in combination with other targeted agents could be useful to prevent the acquisition of resistance. Several studies investigating the molecular mechanisms that promote resistance to RAF inhibitors have been recently reported. The restoration of MEK activity in BRAFV600E melanoma appears to be a crucial event in promoting the acquisition of resistance (Poulikakos & Rosen, 2011; Solit & Rosen, 2011; Solit & Sawyers, 2010; Tuma, 2011). In particular, MEK activity was restored by overexpressing other kinases such as RAF1 and COT/TPL2 (Johannessen et al., 2010) or by the de novo acquisition of a mutation in the NRAS gene (Nazarian et al., 2010). The COT gene was amplified in cell lines that showed intrinsic resistance to PLX4032 (Johannessen et al., 2010). Surprisingly, no secondary BRAF mutations were detected in tumors from patients with acquired resistance (Nazarian et al., 2010). Wagle et al. identified an activating mutation at codon 121 of MEK1 in the tumor from a patient who relapsed after developing resistance to PLX4032 treatment, thus demonstrating for the first time that resistance to PLX4032 is associated with the development of activating mutations in kinases downstream of BRAFV600E (Wagle et al., 2011). This discovery highlights the importance of establishing new combined therapies using MEK or ERK inhibitors with PLX4032 to overcome resistance. In fact, data obtained in preclinical studies demonstrated a synergism between BRAF and MEK inhibitors AZD6244 and GSK1120212 (Emery et al., 2009; Joseph et al., 2010; Paraiso et al., 2010). However, mechanisms that promote the acquisition of resistance independently of MEK activation have been described, including the increased activation of the receptor tyrosine kinases PDGFRβ (Nazarian et al., 2010) or IGF1R (Villaneuva et al., 2010), suggesting that the combination of receptor tyrosine kinase inhibitors with PLX4032 could be effective in the treatment of these patients. However in most patients, the mechanisms that promote the acquisition of resistance remain unclear (Nazarian et al., 2010).

5. BRAFV600E as a circulating disease biomarker

As blood has been proved to represent a valuable alternative source of tumor-derived cells and tumor-derived DNA/RNA, circulating BRAFV600E represents a potential circulating disease biomarker that could be useful when melanoma specimens are not available to test the BRAF mutational status for the selection of patients who will benefit from treatment with BRAF inhibitors. In addition, it could be used as a monitoring factor to evaluate clinical response.

Several studies reported that BRAFV600E is detectable in DNA/RNA extracted from circulating melanoma cells (CMC) (Kitago et al., 2009; Oldenburg et al., 2008). The assessment of CMC for monitoring the efficacy of therapeutic treatment and for predicting the disease outcome of melanoma patients has been proposed. Currently, RT-PCR and quantitative real-time RT-PCR are the methods most frequently used to detect CMC in melanoma. Both techniques are used to amplify genes expressed in melanoma cells, such as tyrosinase, MART-1, MAGE-3A and MITF (Koyanagi et al., 2010). Detection of the mutated

BRAF variant in blood samples requires the efficient isolation of CMC (Kitago et al., 2009) or the development of extremely sensitive techniques to detect the mutant sequence in a large excess of wild-type BRAF forms (Oldenburg et al., 2008).
Circulating free DNA (cfDNA) isolated from plasma or serum samples represents an alternative source of melanoma-derived DNA. Several studies reported the feasibility of detecting BRAFV600E mutation in the cfDNA from patients with melanoma (Board et al., 2009; Daniotti et al., 2007; De Giorgi et al., 2010; Pinzani et al., 2010; Yancovitz et al., 2007). Interestingly, Shinozaki and coworkers reported that the detection of circulating BRAV600E in the serum of patients treated with biochemotherapy correlates with poorer outcomes due to absence of response to the treatment (Shinozaky et al., 2007).
Some important limitations should be overcome to consider BRAFV600E as a reliable circulating disease biomarker. In fact, the studies previously mentioned demonstrated that BRAFV600E is detectable at stage IV and only in a few stage III melanoma patients, suggesting that it does not represent a marker for the detection of the disease in early-stage patients. Moreover, when matched plasma/serum and tumor samples from melanoma patients were tested for BRAFV600E, the concordance between the BRAF mutation rates of cfDNA and tumors showed some discrepancies, which could be due to a low sensitivity of the techniques used to perform the mutational analysis or to the heterogeneity of the tumor for the BRAFV600E mutation. For these reasons, different methods were developed to detect BRAFV600E mutation in high levels of BRAF wild-type DNA by increasing the specificity and sensitivity of the assays, as shown in Table 1, mainly through enriching the sample for the mutant variant or by selectively inhibiting the amplification of the BRAF wild-type form (Kitago et al., 2009; Oldenburg et al., 2008; Pinzani et al., 2011; Shinozaki et al., 2007; Yancovitz et al., 2007)

Method	Detection limit	Samples	Reference
Allele-Specific PCR	1:400 mut allele in wt alleles	Plasma	Daniotti et al., 2007
Mutant-specific PCR	0.1 ng of mut DNA in 100 ng of wt DNA	Plasma	Yancovitz et al., 2007
PNA/LNA clamp Real Time PCR	$1X10^{-4}$ U mut DNA in 10 U of wt DNA	Serum	Shinozaki et al., 2007
PBAS-PCR	10 melanoma cells in 1ml of blood	CMC	Oldenburg et al., 2008
Real Time PCR	1-5 melanoma cells in $5X10^{6}$ PBC	CMC	Kitago et al., 2009
ARMS allele-specific Real Time PCR	5 copies of mut DNA in 5000 copies of wt DNA	Serum	Board et al., 2009
LNA/allele-specific Real Time PCR	0.3% of mut alleles in wt alleles	Plasma	Pinzani et al., 2010
COLD PCR	3.1% of mut alleles in wt DNA	FFPE tissue	Pinzani et al., 2011

PNA: Peptide Nucleic Acid; LNA: Locked Nucleic Acid; PBAS: Primer-Blocking Allele-Specific; ARMS: Amplification Refractory Mutation System; COLD: CO-amplification at Lower Denaturation temperature; mut: mutated; wt: wild-type; 1U: amount of target DNA contained in 1 μg/ml of genomic DNA; PBC: Peripheral Blood Cells; FFPE: Formalin Fixed Paraffin Embedded

Table 1. Methods developed to detect BRAFV600E.

5.1 Other melanoma circulating biomarkers

Melanoma serum markers that have significant potential both as prognostic indicators and for monitoring the treatment response include lactate dehydrogenases (LDH), S100 calcium binding protein B (S100B), and melanoma inhibitory activity (MIA) molecule.

LDH are cytochrome c- or NAD(P)-dependent enzymes that act on either D- or L-lactate. Serum LDH is the only circulating biomarker shown to have a prognostic relevance in melanoma. Several studies have shown that high levels of circulating LDH correlate with a poor prognosis in stage IV melanoma patients and in other neoplastic diseases (Balch et al., 2009; Bedikian et al., 2008; Keilholz et al., 2002). For this reason, LDH was included in the current AJCC staging system, and its level is currently determined in melanoma patients having distant metastasis because patients with elevated LDH are assigned directly to the M1C category without considering the site of distant metastasis (Dickson & Gershenwald, 2011).

S100B is a protein that belongs to the S100 protein family and is mainly expressed by astrocytes, where it acts as a neurotrophic factor to promote neuronal survival. S100B is a well-characterized melanoma marker, and it is used as a diagnostic marker of melanocytic skin lesions in immunohistochemical staining. Several studies pointed out S100B as a prognostic marker of disease progression (Gogas et al., 2009; Jury et al., 2000) as increased serum levels in melanoma patients were predictive of disease progression. Even if not included in the AJCC staging system, Swiss and German guidelines recommend the determination of S100B serum levels in patients with Breslow thickness >1 mm every 3-6 months (Dummer et al., 2005; Garbe et al., 2007; Garbe et al., 2008).

MIA is a small protein secreted by malignant melanoma cells that exhibits an inhibitory effect on cell growth in vitro (Blesch et al., 1994). Even if a correlation between high MIA serum levels and metastatic melanoma progression has been reported (Bosserhoff et al., 1997; Stahlecker et al., 2000), MIA was shown to have lower sensitivity and specificity as a melanoma marker than S100B and LDH (Krahn et al., 2001).

Recently, microRNAs (miRNAs) have been proposed as a new class of potential circulating biomarkers that are detectable in various body fluids. miRNAs are non-coding RNAs consisting of 18-24 nucleotides that regulate mRNA and protein levels mainly by inducing mRNA degradation or by inhibiting translation (Ambros, 2004; Bartel, 2004). Recently, deregulation of a group of miRNAs was found in melanoma lesions in association with BRAF mutational status (Caramuta et al., 2010). miRNAs are also released into the extracellular space, where they can be found free or contained within vesicles such as microvesicles, exosomes, apoptotic vesicles and senescent bodies. The functional role of extracellular miRNAs as an intercellular communication system is poorly characterized (Reid et al., 2010). Extracellular miRNAs have been identified as ideal tumor circulating biomarkers because of their stability and easy quantification (Etheridge et al., 2010). For these reasons, circulating miRNAs have been investigated in many tumor types, including lung, colorectal, ovarian and pancreatic cancers, to evaluate their prognostic and diagnostic value (Reid et al., 2010). Few studies have assessed circulating miRNAs in the context of melanoma. Kanemaru et al. demonstrated that miRNA-221 serum levels are higher in melanoma patients than in healthy controls; in addition, miRNA-221 levels directly correlate with tumor thickness, staging and disease course (Kanemaru et al., 2011). In another study, 16 miRNAs were identified deregulated in blood cells of melanoma patients by comparison of miRNA expression profiles in blood cells of healthy donors; moreover, they were sufficient to distinguish melanoma patients from healthy individuals with high accuracy (Leidinger et al., 2010). Taken together, these studies suggest that miRNAs potentially could be prognostic and diagnostic circulating markers in melanoma, although larger studies and the standardization of isolation and detection techniques are needed to confirm these results.

6. Allele-specific real-time PCR-based detection of circulating BRAFV600E

It is possible to selectively eliminate the BRAF wild-type sequence and thus improve the sensitivity of the PCR performed to detect mutated circulating BRAF by taking advantage of the presence of a TspRI enzyme restriction site located at codon 600 of the BRAF wild-type sequence (Rimoldi et al., 2003). This restriction site is abrogated by BRAFV600E, and therefore it is possible to enrich for the BRAV600E allele by selectively eliminating wild-type sequences by performing TspRI digestion. We modified the experimental conditions described by Rimoldi et al. to improve sensitivity and specificity of an allele-specific TaqMan-based real-time method to detect BRAFV600E in colorectal cancer tissues (Benlloch et al., 2006). Figure 2 summarizes the steps of the assay developed to screen for BRAV600E mutation plasma or melanoma tissue biopsies.

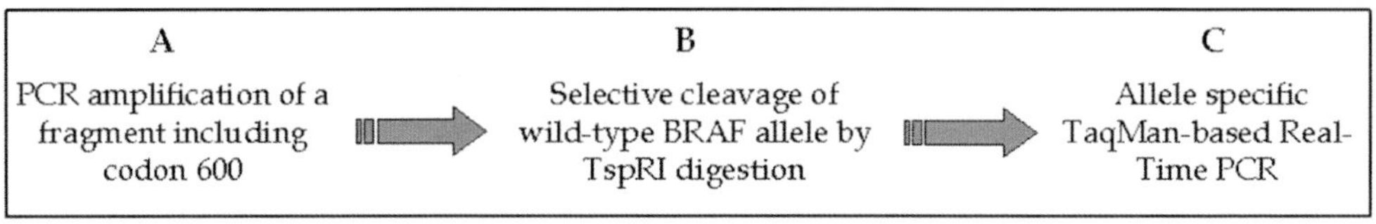

Fig. 2. Schematic representation of TaqMan-based Real-Time PCR method developed to detect few copies of BRAFV600E in a large amount of wild-type DNA.

Experimental conditions of each step are reported in paragraph 6.1.

6.1 Overview of the protocol

A 224-bp fragment that includes codon 600 of the BRAF gene is amplified from 5 ng DNA in a final reaction volume of 50 µl (Figure 2A). Amplification was performed with a pre-cycling hold at 95°C for 7 min followed by 37 cycles of PCR (95°C for 1 min, 55°C for 1 min and 72°C for 1 min) and a final extension at 72°C for 7 min using primers for exon 15 amplification reported by Davies (Davies et al., 2002). Twenty microliters of the PCR product were mixed with 1X NEB Buffer 4 supplemented with 100 µg/ml BSA (New England Biolabs) and then subjected to restriction digestion at 65°C overnight with 15 U TspRI (New England Biolabs) in a final digestion mix volume of 50 µl to enrich samples for the BRAFV600E mutant allelic variant (Figure 2B). Two microliters of the digestion product were used to perform an allele-specific TaqMan-based real-time PCR analysis (Figure 2C). The final reaction volume of 20 µl contained 10 µl 2X of TaqMan Genotyping Master Mix (Applied Biosystems), 18 pmol of each primer (BRAF-51F and BRAF-176R) and 5 pmol of each probe (BRAFmut and BRAFwt). The primer and probe sequences were reported previously by Benlloch (Benlloch et al., 2006). Amplification and detection were performed with an ABI PRISM 7900HT (Applied Biosystems) using the standard thermal profile conditions of the Absolute Quantification protocol. Data analysis was performed using the SDS (Sequence Detection System) version 2.2.2 software. Each experiment was performed in duplicate.

6.2 Results

Specificity of the technique was tested by assaying dilutions of BRAF mutated DNA (5 ng/µl) in wild-type DNA (5 ng/µl). The mutated DNA was obtained from a heterozygous melanoma cell line showing 2 copies of BRAF gene. Therefore, the allelic ratio was calculated considering one mutated allele out of 4 total alleles. Results obtained show that 1 copy of V600E allele can be detected when diluted in $8X10^5$ copies of wild-type alleles. Sensitivity of the technique was assayed by testing progressive dilutions in water of the BRAF mutated DNA. Results obtained show that BRAFV600E mutation can be detected starting from $6.25X10^{-5}$ ng of DNA.

This method showed an increase in both sensitivity and specificity when compared to the assays previously used in our lab to detect BRAFV600E (Daniotti et al., 2007). As shown in Figures 3 and 4, the selective elimination of the BRAF wild-type allele is a critical step required to increase both parameters. In fact, the BRAF mutated allele became detectable only when the wild-type allele was greatly reduced (Figure 3) or eliminated (Figure 4) after digestion with TsprRI.

Taken together, these results indicate that the new assay has an improved sensitivity and specificity for detecting BRAFV600E when tested on genomic DNA from melanoma when diluted in an excess of wild-type DNA or when present in a few copies as in water dilutions. Preliminary results obtained by testing matched plasma and tissues samples indicate that more samples test positive for BRAFV600E compared to the previously described technique (Daniotti et al., 2007) and suggest a potential clinical application of this technique.

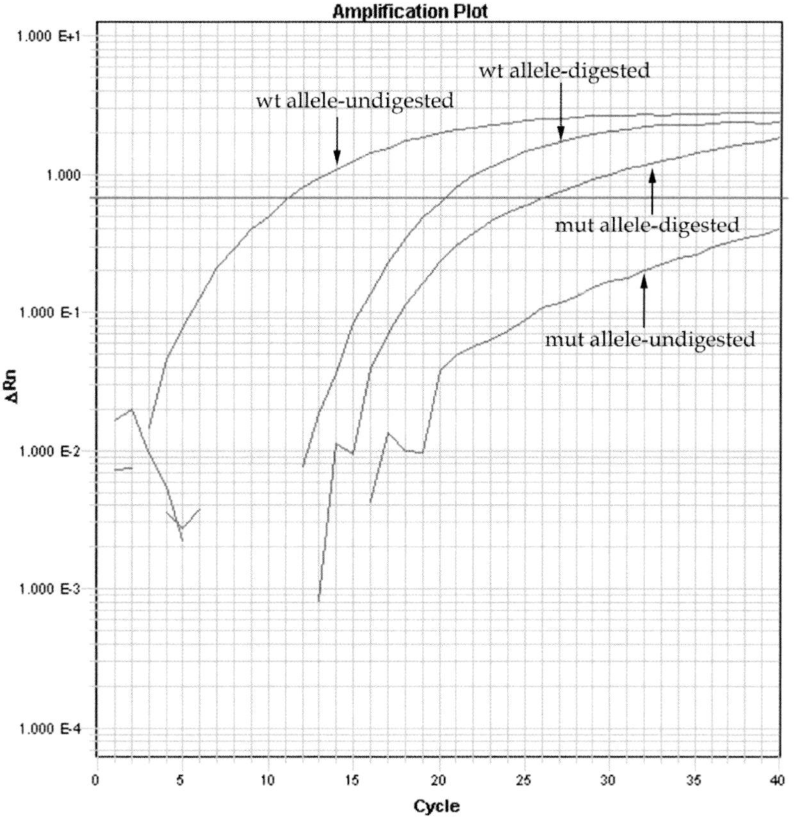

Fig. 3. TspRI digestion increases the specificity of BRAFV600E allele-specific real-time PCR.

TspRI digestion reduces the excess of the wild-type allele that is detected 9 cycles later compared to the undigested sample and allows the detection of the BRAFV600E allele. The red line represents the threshold line. wt: wild-type. mut: mutated.

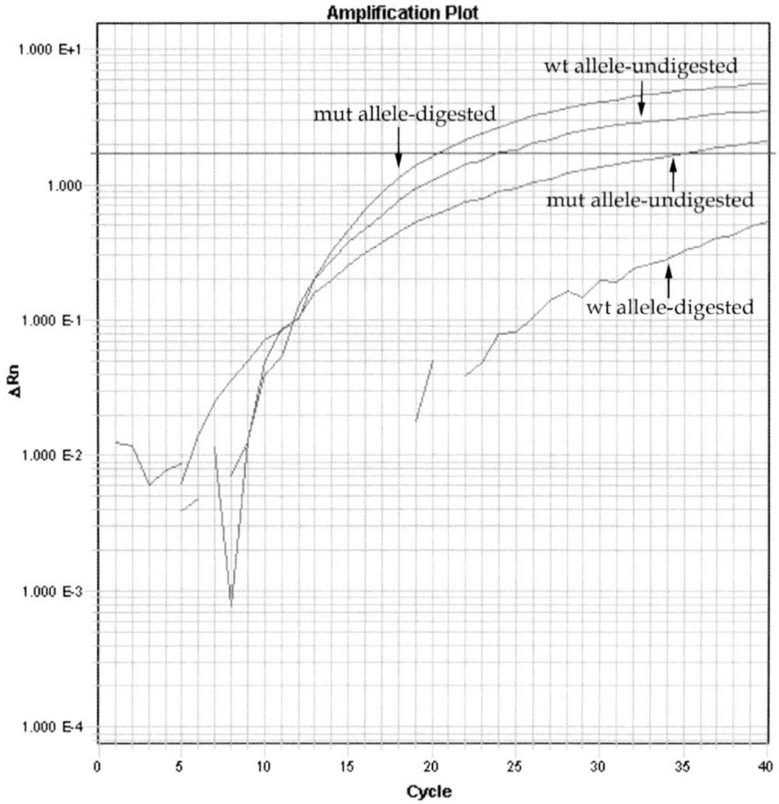

Fig. 4. TspRI digestion increases the sensitivity of the BRAFV600E allele-specific real-time PCR.

The amplification plot shows that the complete elimination of the BRAF wild-type template by TspRI digestion improves the sensitivity of mutated allele-specific PCR, anticipating its detection of about 14 cycles compared to undigested samples. The red line represents the threshold line. wt: wild-type. mut: mutated.

7. Conclusion

BRAFV600E currently represents the most specific circulating tumor marker available for cutaneous melanoma, although it will only detect about 50% of melanoma. Circulating BRAFV600E can be used to select patients to be treated with BRAF inhibitors when the tissue samples are not available for the analysis. In addition, detection methods for circulating BRAFV600E can be used to monitor the treatment response and evaluate disease relapse during follow-up. However, to use BRAFV600E as a blood marker, more sensitive technologies must be designed and validated to improve the sensitivity and specificity of the assays used to detect this mutation.

8. Acknowledgment

VV is recipient of a fellowship by the Italian Health Ministry, Grant RFPS 2006-4-341458.

9. References

Ambros, V. (2004). The functions of animal microRNAs. *Nature*, Vol. 431, No. 7006, (Sep 2004), pp. 350–355

Arnault, JP.; Wechsler, J., & Robert, C. (2009). Keratoacanthomas and squamous cell carcinomas in patients receiving sorafenib. *J Clin Oncol*, Vol. 27, No. 23, (Aug 2009). pp. 59-61.

Balch, CM; Gershenwald, JE., & Sondak VK. (2009). Final version of 2009 AJCC melanoma staging and classification. *J Clin Oncol*, Vol. 27, No. 36, (Dec 2009), pp. 6199-6206

Bartel, DP. (2004). MicroRNAs: genomics, biogenesis, mechanism, and function. *Cell*, Vol. 116, No. 2, (Jan 2004), pp. 281–297

Bedikian, AY.; Johnson, MM., & Hwu, P. (2008). Prognostic factors that determine the long-term survival of patients with unresecTable metastatic melanoma. *Cancer Invest*, Vol. 26, No. 6, (Jul 2008), pp. 624-633

Benlloch, S.; Payá, A., & Massutí, B. (2006). Detection of BRAF V600E mutation in colorectal cancer: comparison of automatic sequencing and real-time chemistry methodology. *J Mol Diagn*, Vol. 8, No. 5, (Nov 2006), pp.540-543

Blesch, A.; Bosserhoff, AK., & Bogdahn, U. (1994). Cloning of a novel malignant melanoma-derived growth-regulatory protein, MIA. *Cancer Res*, Vol. 54, No. 21, (Nov 1994), pp. 5695-5701

Bloethner, S.; Snellman, E., & Kumar, R. (2007). Differential gene expression in melanocytic nevi with the V600E BRAF mutation. *Genes Chromosomes Cancer*, Vol. 46, No. 11, (Nov 2007), pp. 1019-1027

Board, RE.; Ellison, G., & Hughes, A. (2009). Detection of BRAF mutations in the tumour and serum of patients enrolled in the AZD6244 (ARRY-142886) advanced melanoma phase II study. *Br J Cancer*, Vol. 101, No. 10, (Nov 2009), pp. 1724-1730

Bosserhoff, AK.; Kaufmann, M., & Buettner, R. (1997). Melanoma-inhibiting activity, a novel serum marker for progression of malignant melanoma. *Cancer Res*, Vol. 57, No. 15, (Aug 1997), pp. 3149-3153

Cantwell-Dorris, ER., O'Leary, JJ., & Sheils, OM. (2011). BRAFV600E: Implications for Carcinogenesis and Molecular Therapy. *Mol Cancer Ther*, Vol. 10, No. 3, (Mar 2011), pp. 385-394

Caramuta, S.; Egyházi, S., & Lui, WO. (2010). MicroRNA expression profiles associated with mutational status and survival in malignant melanoma. *J Invest Dermatol*, Vol. 130, No. 8, (Aug 2010), pp. 2062-2070

Ciampi, R., Knauf, JA., & Nikiforov, YE. (2005). Oncogenic AKAP9-BRAF fusion is a novel mechanism of MAPK pathway activation in thyroid cancer. *J Clin Invest*, Vol. 115, No. 9, (Jan 2005), pp. 94-101

Cin, H., Meyer, C., & Pfister, SM. (2011). Oncogenic FAM131B-BRAF fusion resulting from 7q34 deletion comprises an alternative mechanism of MAPK pathway activation in pilocytic astrocytoma. *Acta Neuropathol*, (2011)

Curtin, JA.; Fridlyand, J., & Bastian, BC. (2005). Distinct sets of genetic alterations in melanoma. *N Engl J Med*, Vol. 353, No. 20, (Nov 2005), pp. 2135-2147

Daniotti, M.; Vallacchi, V., & Rodolfo, M. (2007). Detection of mutated BRAFV600E variant in circulating DNA of stage III-IV melanoma patients. *Int J Cancer*, Vol. 120, No. 11, (Jun 2007), pp. 12439-12444

Daniotti, M.; Ferrari, A., & Rodolfo, M. (2009). Cutaneous melanoma in childhood and adolescence shows frequent loss of INK4A and gain of KIT. *J Invest Dermatol*, Vol. 129, No. 7, (Jul 2009), pp. 1759-1768

Davies, H.; Bignell, GR., & Futreal, PA. (2002). Mutations of the BRAF gene in human cancer. *Nature*, Vol. 417, No. 6892, (Jun 2002), pp. 949-954

De Giorgi, V.; Pinzani, P., & Massi, D. (2010). Circulating benign nevus cells detected by ISET technique: Warning for melanoma molecular diagnosis. *Arch Dermatol, Vol.* 146, No. 10, (Oct 2010), pp. 1120-1124

Dessars, B., De Raeve, LE., & Heimann, P. (2007). Chromosomal translocations as a mechanism of BRAF activation in two cases of large congenital melanocytic nevi. *J Invest Dermatol*, Vol. 127, No. 6, (Jun 2007), pp. 1468-1470

Dickson, PV. & Gershenwald, JE. (2011). Staging and prognosis of cutaneous melanoma. *Surg Oncol Clin N Am*, Vol. 20, No. 1, (Jan 2011), pp. 1-17

Dienstmann, R. & Tabernero, J. (2011). BRAF as a Target for Cancer Therapy. *Anticancer Agents Med Chem*, 2011

Dummer, R.; Panizzon, R., & Burg, G. (2005). Updated Swiss guidelines for the treatment and follow-up of cutaneous melanoma. *Dermatology*, Vol. 210, No. 1, 2005, pp. 39-44

Eisen, T., Ahmad, T., & Ratain, MJ. (2006). Sorafenib in advanced melanoma: a Phase II randomised discontinuation trial analysis. *Br J Cancer*, Vol. 95, No. 5, (Sep 2006), pp. 581-586

Emery, CM.; Vijayendran, KG., & Garraway LA. (2009). MEK1 mutations confer resistance to MEK and B-RAF inhibition. *Proc Natl Acad Sci U S A*, Vol. 106, No. 48, (Dec 2009), pp. 20411-20416

Etheridge, A.; Lee ,I., & Wang K. (2011). Extracellular microRNA: a new source of biomarkers. *Mutat Res*, 2011

Fargnoli, MC.; Pike, K., & Landi, MT. (2008). MC1R variants increase risk of melanoma harboring BRAF mutations. *J Invest Dermatol*, Vol. 128, No. 10, (Oct 2008), pp. 2485-2490

Flaherty, KT.; Puzanov, I., & Chapman, PB. (2010). Inhibition of mutated, activated BRAF in metastatic melanoma. *N Engl J Med*, Vol. 363, No. 9, (Aug 2010), pp. 809-819

Garbe, C.; Hauschild, A., & Kaufmann, R. (2007). Evidence and interdisciplinary consense-based German guidelines: diagnosis and surveillance of melanoma. *Melanoma Res*, Vol. 17, No. 6, (Dec 2007), pp. 393-399

Garbe, C.; Schadendorf, D., & Hauschild, A. (2008). Short German guidelines: malignant melanoma. *J Dtsch Dermatol Ges*, Vol. 6, Suppl 1, (May 2008), pp. S9-S14

Gogas, H.; Eggermont, AM., & Dummer R. (2009). Biomarkers in melanoma. *Ann Oncol*, Vol. 20, No. 6, (Aug 2009), pp. vi8-13

Hacker, E. & Hayward, NK. (2008). Germline MC1R variants and BRAF mutant melanoma. *J Invest Dermatol*, Vol. 128, No. 10, (Oct 2008), pp. 2354-2356

Hatzivassiliou, G.; Song, K., & Malek S. (2010). RAF inhibitors prime wild-type RAF to activate the MAPK pathway and enhance growth. *Nature*, Vol. 464, No. 7287, (Mar 2010, pp. 431-435

Hauschild, A., Agarwala, SS., & Keilholz, U. (2009). Results of a phase III, randomized, placebo-controlled study of sorafenib in combination with carboplatin and paclitaxel as second-line treatment in patients with unresecTable stage III or stage IV melanoma. *J Clin Oncol*, Vol. 27, No. 17, (Jun 2009), pp. 2823-2830

Healy, E.; Flannagan, N., & Rees, JL. (2000). Melanocortin-1-receptor gene and sun sensitivity in individuals without red hair. *Lancet*, Vol. 355, No. 9209, (Mar 2000), pp. 1072-1073

Heidorn, SJ.; Milagre, C., & Marais, R. (2010). Kinase-dead BRAF and oncogenic RAS cooperate to drive tumor progression through CRAF. *Cell*, Vol. 140, No. 2, (Jan 2010), pp. 209-21

Held, L.; Eigentler, TK., & Bauer, J. (2011). Oncogenetics of melanoma: basis for molecular diagnostics and therapy. *J Dtsch Dermatol Ges*, (2011)

Hoek, KS.; Schlegel, NC., & Dummer, R. (2006). Metastatic potential of melanoma defined by specific gene expression profiles with no BRAF signature. *Pigment Cell Res*, Vol. 19, No. 4, (Aug 2006), pp. 290-302

Houben, R.; Becker, JC., & Rapp UR. (2004). Constitutive activation of the Ras-Raf signaling pathway in metastatic melanoma is associated with poor prognosis. *J Carcinog*, Vol. 3, No. 1, (Mar 2004), pp. 6.

James, MR.; Roth, RB., & Duffy, DL. (2005). BRAF polymorphisms and risk of melanocytic neoplasia. *J Invest Dermatol*, Vol. 125, No. 6, (Dec 2005), pp. 1252-1258

Johannessen, CM.; Boehm, JS., & Garraway, LA. (2010). COT drives resistance to RAF inhibition through MAP kinase pathway reactivation. *Nature*, Vol. 468, No. 7326, (Dec 2010), pp. 968-972

Johansson, P.; Pavey, S., & Hayward, N. (2007). Confirmation of a BRAF mutation-associated gene expression signature in melanoma. *Pigment Cell Res*, Vol. 20, No. 3, (Jun 2007), pp. 216-221

Joseph, EW.; Pratilas, CA., & Rosen N. (2010). The RAF inhibitor PLX4032 inhibits ERK signaling and tumor cell proliferation in a V600E BRAF-selective manner. *Proc Natl Acad Sci U S A*, Vol. 107, No. 33, (Aug 2010), pp. 14903-14908

Jury, CS.; McAllister, EJ., & MacKie, RM. (2000). Rising levels of serum S100 protein precede other evidence of disease progression in patients with malignant melanoma. *Br J Dermatol*, Vol. 143, No. 2, (Aug 2000), pp. 269-274

Kanemaru, H.; Fukushima, S., & Ihn, H. (2011). The circulating microRNA-221 level in patients with malignant melanoma as a new tumor marker. *J Dermatol Sci*, Vol. 61, No. 3, (Mar 2011), pp. 187-193

Kefford, R., Arkenau, H., & Lebowitz, PF. Phase I/II study of GSK2118436, a selective inhibitor of oncogenic mutant BRAF kinase, in patients with metastatic melanoma and other solid tumors. *J Clin Oncol*, 2010, 28(15s), abstract 8503

Keilholz, U.; Martus, P., & Eggermont, AM. (2002). Prognostic factors for survival and factors associated with long-term remission in patients with advanced melanoma receiving cytokine-based treatments: second analysis of a randomised EORTC Melanoma Group trial comparing interferon-alpha2a (IFNalpha) and interleukin 2 (IL-2) with or without cisplatin. *Eur J Cancer*, Vol. 38, No. 11, (Jul 2002), pp. 1501-1511

Kitago, M.; Koyanagi, K., & Hoon, DS. (2009). mRNA expression and BRAF mutation in circulating melanoma cells isolated from peripheral blood with high molecular weight melanoma-associated antigen-specific monoclonal antibody beads. *Clin Chem*, Vol. 55, No. 4, (Apr 2009), pp. 757-764

Koyanagi, K.; O'Day, SJ., & Hoon, DS. (2010). Serial monitoring of circulating tumor cells predicts outcome of induction biochemotherapy plus maintenance biotherapy for metastatic melanoma. *Clin Cancer Res*, Vol. 16, No. 8, (Apr 2010), pp. 2402-2408

Krähn, G.; Kaskel, P., & Peter, RU. (2001). S100 beta is a more reliable tumor marker in peripheral blood for patients with newly occurred melanoma metastases compared with MIA, albumin and lactate-dehydrogenase. *Anticancer Res*, Vol. 21, No. 2B, (Mar-Apr 2001), pp. 1311-1316

Landi, MT.; Bauer, J., & Bastian, BC. (2006). MC1R germline variants confer risk for BRAF-mutant melanoma. *Science*, Vol. 313, No. 5786, (Jul 2006), pp. 521-522

Lang, J.; Boxer, M., & MacKie, R. (2003). Absence of exon 15 BRAF germline mutations in familial melanoma. *Hum Mutat*, Vol. 21, No. 3, (Mar 2003), pp. 327-330

Laud, K.; Kannengiesser, C., & Bressac-de Paillerets, B. (2003). BRAF as a melanoma susceptibility candidate gene? *Cancer Res*, Vol. 63, No. 12, (Jun 2003), pp. 3061-3065

Leidinger, P.; Keller, A., & Meese, E. (2010). High-throughput miRNA profiling of human melanoma blood samples. *BMC Cancer*, Vol. 10, (Jun 2010), pp. 262

Long, GV., Kefford, RF., & Falchook, G. Phase ½ study of GSK2118436, a selective inhibitor of V600 mutant BRAf kinase: evidence of activity in melanoma brain metastases. *Annals Oncol*, 2010, 21 (Suppl. 8), abstract LBA 27

Meyer, P.; Klaes, R., & Garbe C. (2003). Exclusion of BRAFV599E as a melanoma susceptibility mutation. *Int J Cancer*, Vol. 106, No. 1, (Aug 2003), pp. 78-80 (a)

Meyer, P.; Sergi, C., & Garbe, C. (2003). Polymorphisms of the BRAF gene predispose males to malignant melanoma.*J Carcinog*, Vol. 2, No. 1, (Nov 2003), pp. 7 (b)

Michaloglou, C.; Vredeveld, LC., & Peeper, DS. (2005). BRAFE600-associated senescence-like cell cycle arrest of human naevi. *Nature*, Vol. 436, no. 7051, (Aug 2005), pp. 720-724

Nazarian, R.; Shi, H., & Lo, RS. (2010). Melanoma acquire resistance to B-RAF(V600E) inhibition by RTK or NRAS upregulation. *Nature*, Vol. 468, No. 7326, (Dec 2010), pp. 973-977

Oldenburg, RP.; Liu, MS., & Kolodney, MS. (2008). Selective amplification of rare mutations using locked nucleic acid oligonucleotides that competitively inhibit primer binding to wild-type DNA. *J Invest Dermatol*, Vol. 128, No. 2, (Feb 2008), pp. 398-402

Omholt, K.; Platz, A., & Hansson, J. (2003). NRAS and BRAF mutations arise early during melanoma pathogenesis and are preserved throughout tumor progression. *Clin Cancer Res*, Vol. 9, No. 17, (Dec 2003), pp. 6483-6488

Palanisamy, N., Ateeq, B., & Chinnaiyan, AM. (2010). Rearrangements of the RAF kinase pathway in prostate cancer, gastric cancer and melanoma. *Nat Med.*, Vol. 16, No. 7, (Jul 2010), pp. 793-798.

Palmer, JS.; Duffy, DL., & Sturm, RA. (2000). Melanocortin-1 receptor polymorphisms and risk of melanoma: is the association explained solely by pigmentation phenotype? *Am J Hum Genet*, Vol. 66, No. 1, (Jan 2000), pp. 176-186

Paraiso, KH.; Fedorenko, IV., & Smalley, KS. (2010). Recovery of phospho-ERK activity allows melanoma cells to escape from BRAF inhibitor therapy. *Br J Cancer*, Vol. 102, No. 12, (Jun 2010), pp. 1724-1730

Pavey, S.; Johansson, P., & Hayward NK. (2004). Microarray expression profiling in melanoma reveals a BRAF mutation signature. *Oncogene*, Vol. 23, No. 23, (May 2004), pp. 4060-4067

Pinzani, P.; Salvianti, F., & Orlando, C. (2010). Allele specific taqman-based real-time PCR assay to quantify circulating BRAFV600E mutated DNA in plasma of melanoma patients. *Clin Chim Acta*, Vol. 411, No. 17-18, (Sep 2010), pp. 1319-1324

Pinzani, P.; Santucci, C., & Orlando, C. (2011). BRAF(V600E) detection in melanoma is highly improved by COLD-PCR. *Clin Chim Acta*, 2011

Platz, A.; Egyhazi, S., & Hansson, J. (2008). Human cutaneous melanoma; a review of NRAS and BRAF mutation frequencies in relation to histogenetic subclass and body site. *Mol Oncol*, Vol. 1, No. 4, (Apr 2008), pp. 395-405

Poulikakos, PI.; Zhang, C., & Rosen, N. (2010). RAF inhibitors transactivate RAF dimers and ERK signalling in cells with wild-type BRAF. *Nature*, Vol.464, No. 7287, (Mar 2010), pp. 427-30

Poulikakos, PI. & Rosen, N. (2011). Mutant BRAF melanoma--dependence and resistance. *Cancer Cell*, Vol. 19, No. 1, (Jan 2011), pp. 11-15

Puzanov, I., Burnett, P., & Flaherty, KT. (2011). The cardiofaciocutaneous syndrome. *Mol Oncol*, (2011)

Rees JL. (2004). The genetics of sun sensitivity in humans. *Am J Hum Genet*, Vol. 75, No. 5, (Nov 2004), pp. 739-751

Reid, G.; Kirschner, MB., & van Zandwijk, N. (2010). Circulating microRNAs: Association with disease and potential use as biomarkers. *Crit Rev Oncol Hematol*, (2010)

Rimoldi, D.; Salvi, S., & Cerottini JC. (2003). Lack of BRAF mutations in uveal melanoma. *Cancer Res*, Vol. 63, No. 18, pp. 5712-5715

Rodolfo, M.; Daniotti, M., & Vallacchi, V. (2004). Genetic progression of metastatic melanoma. *Cancer Lett*, Vol. 214, No. 2, (Oct 2004), pp.133-147

Romano, E.; Schwartz, GK., & Carvajal, RD. (2011). Treatment implications of the emerging molecular classification system for melanoma. *Lancet Oncol*

Sarkozy, A., Carta, C., & Tartaglia, M. (2009). Germline BRAF mutations in Noonan, LEOPARD, and cardiofaciocutaneous syndromes: molecular diversity and associated phenotypic spectrum. *Hum Mutat*, Vol. 30, No. 4, (Apr 2009), pp. 695-702

Scherer, D.; Rachakonda, PS., & Kumar, R. (2010). Association between the germline MC1R variants and somatic BRAF/NRAS mutations in melanoma tumors. *J Invest Dermatol*, Vol. 130, No. 12, (Dec 2010), pp. 2844-2848

Sekulic, A.; Haluska, P Jr., & Markovic SN; Melanoma Study Group of Mayo Clinic Cancer Center. (2008). Malignant melanoma in the 21st century: the emerging molecular landscape. *Mayo Clin Proc*, Vol. 83, No. 7, (Jul 2008), pp. 825-846

Shepherd, C.; Puzanov, I., & Sosman, JA. (2010). B-RAF inhibitors: an evolving role in the therapy of malignant melanoma. *Curr Oncol Rep*, Vol. 12, No. 3, (May 2010), pp. 3146-3152

Shinozaki, M.; Fujimoto, A., & Hoon, DS. (2004). Incidence of BRAF oncogene mutation and clinical relevance for primary cutaneous melanoma. *Clin Cancer Res*, Vol. 10, No. 5, (Mar 2004), pp. 1753-1757

Shinozaki, M.; O'Day, SJ., & Hoon, DS. (2007). Utility of circulating B-RAF DNA mutation in serum for monitoring melanoma patients receiving biochemotherapy. *Clin Cancer Res*, Vol. 13, No. 7, (Apr 2007), pp. 2068-2074

Solit, D. & Sawyers, CL. (2010). Drug discovery: How melanoma bypass new therapy. *Nature*, Vol. 468, No. 7326, (Dec 2010), pp. 902-903

Solit, DB. & Rosen, N. (2011). Resistance to BRAF inhibition in melanoma. *N Engl J Med*, Vol. 364, No. 8, (Feb 2011), pp. 772-774

Stahlecker, J.; Gauger, A., & Hein, R. (2000). MIA as a reliable tumor marker in the serum of patients with malignant melanoma. *Anticancer Res*, Vol. 20, No. 6D, (Nov-Dec 2000), pp. 5041-5044

Thomas, NE. (2006). BRAF somatic mutations in malignant melanoma and melanocytic naevi. *Melanoma Res*, Vol. 16, No. 2, (Apr 2006), pp. 97-103.

Tidyman, WE. & Rauen, KA. (2009). The RASopathies: developmental syndromes of Ras/MAPK pathway dysregulation. *Curr Opin Genet Dev*, Vol. 19, No. 3, (Jun 2009), pp. 230-236

Tuma, RS. (2011). Getting around PLX4032: studies turn up unusual mechanisms of resistance to melanoma drug. *J Natl Cancer Inst*, Vol. 103, No. 3, (Feb 2011), pp. 170-171, 177

Valverde, P.; Healy, E., & Thody, AJ. (1995). Variants of the melanocyte-stimulating hormone receptor gene are associated with red hair and fair skin in humans. *Nat Genet*, Vol. 11, No. 3, pp. 328-330

Villanueva, J.; Vultur, A., & Herlyn, M. (2010). Acquired resistance to BRAF inhibitors mediated by a RAF kinase switch in melanoma can be overcome by cotargeting MEK and IGF-1R/PI3K. *Cancer Cell*, Vol. 18, No. 6, (Dec 2010), pp. 683-695

Wagle, N.; Emery, C., & Garraway, LA. (2011). Dissecting Therapeutic Resistance to RAF Inhibition in Melanoma by Tumor Genomic Profiling. *J Clin Oncol*, (Mar 2011)

Wellbrock, C. & Hurlstone, A. (2010). BRAF as therapeutic target in melanoma. *Biochem Pharmacol*, Vol. 80, No. 5, (Sep 2010), pp. 561-567

Williams, PF.; Olsen, CM., & Whiteman, DC. (2010). Melanocortin- 1-receptor and risk of cutaneous melanoma: A meta-analysis and estimates of population burden. *Int J Cancer*, (2010)

Yancovitz, M.; Yoon, J., & Polsky, D. (2007). Detection of mutant BRAF alleles in the plasma of patients with metastatic melanoma. *J Mol Diagn*, Vol. 9, No. 2, (Apr 2007), pp. 178-183

Young, A.; Lyons, J., & McCormick, F. (2009). Ras signaling and therapies. *Adv Cancer Res*, Vol. 102, (2009), pp. 1-17

10

Ultraviolet Light as a Modulator of Melanoma Development

Graeme Walker[1] and Elke Hacker[2]
[1]*Skin Carcinogenesis Laboratory, Queensland Institute of Medical Research, Herston, Qld,*
[2]*AusSun Laboratory, Queensland University of Technology, Kelvin Grove, Qld, Australia*

1. Introduction

Epidemiological evidence is overwhelming that exposure of the skin to ultraviolet radiation (UVR) can increase one's risk of developing malignant melanoma. However the situation is complex, as melanoma development is associated with "intermittent" sun exposure, whereas epidermal keratinocyte-based skin cancers like squamous cell carcinoma (SCC) are associated with chronic UVR exposure. Thus it is difficult to talk in terms of a classical UVR carcinogenic mechanism for melanoma in general. Melanoma risk seems intricately associated with pigmentation characteristics. Genome wide association studies identify variants in genes involved in pigmentation as risk factors, generally the strongest signal being for the melanocortin receptor 1 gene (*MC1R*). One reason postulated to explain the odd relationship between UVR exposure and tumorigenesis is that there may be a unique carcinogenic mechanisms at play involving UVA, that is a weak carcinogen for skin cancer in general. Evidence for UVA causality in melanoma comes from some epidemiological studies, and to some extent from work with animal models. On the other hand, one can argue that there may not be a unique carcinogenic mechanism for melanoma, and that there are several factors that may help explain the apparent difference from typical mechanism of UVR mutagenesis involving classical UVR mutations. Firstly, in terms of normal cellular function, melanocytes principal function is to produce melanin pigment while epidermal keratinocytes are programmed to proliferate and then die as they generate and maintain the epidermis, a barrier for internal tissues and organs. Secondly, there may be genetic differences between individuals developing particular subtypes of melanoma and/or form of sun exposure. Thus particularly relates to susceptibility to naevus development, a critical factor associated melanoma development on the trunk, a site presumably receiving mainly "intermittent" sun exposure.

2. Epidemiology of melanoma

Major risk factors for cutaneous melanoma are shown below - approximate relative risk (RR) and 95% confidence intervals (CI) are shown in brackets (Gandini et al., 2005a; Gandini et al., 2005b):

1. One atypical naevus (RR 1.60, CI 1.4-1.8)

2. Five or more atypical naevus (RR 10.5, CI 5.1-21.5).
3. Multiple banal melanocytic naevi - 100 vs <15 (RR-6.9, CI 4.6-10.3).
4. Red versus dark hair (RR 3.6, CI 2.5-5.4).
5. Sunburns in childhood (RR 2.2, CI 1.73-2.89
6. Sunburns in adulthood (RR 1.9, CI 1.6-2.7)
7. Chronic sun exposure (RR 1.0, CI 0.8-1.1)

Apart from familial predisposition, the strongest risk factor for the development of cancer generally, the presence of naevi, especially dysplastic naevi, is the innate, or phenotypic factor that most increases the probability of developing a melanoma. Sunlight is the only environmental factor that has been consistently implicated as a cause of melanoma, leading to a melanoma incidence 10- to 20- fold higher among fair-skinned than dark-skinned peoples (Armstrong & Kricker, 1993). Among fair-skinned people, melanoma incidence increases with proximity to the equator and several studies have shown that fair-skinned migrants moving from high (e.g. UK) to low latitude countries (e.g. Australia, South Africa) have lower melanoma rates than native-born residents (Whiteman and Green, 1999; Khlat et al., 1992; McCredie et al., 1990; McMichael and Giles, 1988). Individuals with xeroderma pigmentosum (XP), a disorder in which sufferers have a gene mutation that diminishes their ability to repair UVR-induced DNA damage, have much higher risk of melanoma than the population average (Kraemer et al., 1994; Cleaver, 2006). Those with a past history of non-melanoma skin cancer (caused by high exposures to solar UVR) have a 3-fold higher risk of melanoma than the general population (Green et al., 1993).

3. Genetic basis of melanoma

3.1 Genes involved in familial melanoma susceptibility

Although many different genes can be somatically mutated in melanoma, as yet there are only two confirmed familial melanoma susceptibility loci, *CDKN2A* and *CDK4*. *CDKN2A* encodes INK4A and ARF, which regulate cell cycle progression via the INK4A/CDK4/pRB and ARF/MDM2/p53 pathways respectively, although undoubtedly there is significant cross talk between these two pathways, and with other pathways. The overwhelming majority of *CDKN2A* mutations in melanoma-prone kindreds affect only the *INK4A* transcript, or both transcripts, but *ARF*-specific mutations also predispose to melanoma (e.g. Randerson-Moor et al., 2001; Rizos et al., 2001). As *INK4A* mutations generally prevent CDK4 from being bound and inhibited by p16INK4A, the mechanism of tumorigenesis with *INK4A* or *CDK4* mutations is presumed to be equivalent (via pRB deregulation). Families carrying *CDKN2A* mutations usually, although not always, exhibit a naevus-prone phenotype (Goldstein et al., 2000) indicating that relaxation of melanocyte proliferation control induced by INK4A (or ARF) loss may be important in naevogenesis. However a recent study comparing the influence of sun exposure on melanoma risk in *CDKN2A* mutations carriers in Australia and the United Kingdom (Cust et al., 2011) suggests that they have to have the same cumulative risk of melanoma irrespective of the ambient UV irradiance in the region in which they live.

3.2 Genes associated with melanoma in genome wide association studies

Genome wide association (GWA) studies have been used to discover genes that confer risk for skin cancer development (Table 1). Some genes are associated both melanoma and non-melanoma skin cancer, especially basal cell carcinoma (BCC). Five genes associated with melanoma, *SLC45A2, TYRP1, TYR, MC1R,* and *ASIP*, encode proteins that are involved in various ways in regulating pigmentation. Little is known about how most of these may effect melanoma genesis and we are left to assume that the risk alleles may encode variants in these genes that simply result in lower levels of protective pigmentation. Notably, in respect to *MC1R* and *ASIP* (agouti signaling protein, an MC1R antagonist), there may be other explanations, which will be discussed below. The genes that confer the strongest risk for the development of naevi, *MTAP/CDKN2A* and *PLA2G6*, are not involved in the regulation of pigmentation.

Chromosome	Candidate gene	Pigmentation	Naevus count	Melanoma	BCC	SCC
1p36	*PAD15*	-		-	++	-
1q42	*RHOU*	-		-	++	-
5p13.3	*SLC45A2*	++		++	++	++
5p13.33	*TERT*	-		++	++	-
6q25	*IRF4*	++	+?	+?	-	-
7q32	*KLF14*	-		-	++	-
9p21	*CDKN2A*	-		-	++	-
9p21	*MTAP*		++	++		
9q23	*TYRP1*	++		++	-	-
11q13.2	*TPCN2*	++		-	-	
11q14	*TYR*	++		++	++	-
12q13	*KRT5*	-		-	++	-
12q21	*KITG*	++		-	-	
14q23	*SLC2A4*	++		-	-	
15q11	*OCA2*	++		-	-	-
15q13.1	*HERC2*	++		-	-	
15q21	*SLC24A5*	+		-	-	-
16q24.3	*MC1R*	++		++	++	
20q11	*ASIP*	++		++	++	-
22q13	*PLA2G6*		++	++		

Table 1. Adapted from Gerstenblith et al. (2010). A double plus sign (++) indicates a significant association ($P < 10^{-7}$) in GWAS. A single plus sign (+) indicates an association (P between 0.01 and 10^{-7}). A minus sign (-) indicates a null association ($P > 0.01$). A blank cell indicates that the locus in the left column has not been not tested. BCC=basal cell carcinoma. SCC =squamous cell carcinoma.

3.3 *MC1R*, melanoma risk and sun exposure

MC1R, the receptor for α–melanocyte stimulating hormone, is the most thoroughly studied melanoma risk gene. It functions largely to control the switch between red/yellow pheomelanin and black/brown eumelanin, hence it is sometimes referred to as the "red haired" gene. This gene is highly polymorphic in human populations with >65 variants documented. Variants have been classed into two groups based on the strength of their association with red hair (Sturm et al., 2003). The R variants (i.e. Asp84Glu, Arg151Cys, Arg160Trp, and Asp294His) are most highly correlated with red hair (mean OR 63.3, range 50.5-118.3) although the r variants are still associated to a lesser degree (mean OR 5.1, range

2.4-6.4). *MC1R* variants are not the sole determinant of hair colour, twin studies have observed discordant hair colour but identical *MC1R* haplotypes (Box et al., 1997). The molecular consequences of UVR upon melanocytes with variant melanocortin-1 receptors are variable. This has lead to debate over MC1R classification and which variants to include in assessing the impact of impaired *MC1R* function in melanoma (Hacker & Hayward, 2008). Beaumont et al. (2007) used *in vitro* studies to examine the functional impact of nine common *MC1R* variants and found that the V60L, D84E, R151C, I155T, R160W and R163Q variants showed impairment in cAMP coupling. Normal receptor expression was found for R142H and D294H variants, but reduced functional responses were observed, indicating that altered G-protein coupling may be responsible for this loss of function. The V92M isoform shows similar activity to the wild-type receptor, and along with V60L, is not associated with melanoma (Raimondi et al., 2008). Interestingly, melanoma risk due to the carriage of *MC1R* variants is stronger in individuals with dark hair and eyes, who do not have freckles, and tan well (Kanetsky et al., 2010). Thus the risk due to *MC1R* variation is certainly not limited to red heads.

The mechanism by which the carriage of *MC1R* variants increases melanoma risk is an area of intense investigation. The simplest explanation is simply the lower photo-protection afforded by red/yellow pheomelanin than brown/black eumelanin. Notably, *MC1R* variants are also associated with increased risk of non-melanoma skin cancer (table 1). In addition, pheomelanin is more likely than eumelanin to generate potentially damaging reactive oxygen species following UVR exposure (Hill, 1992; Takeuchi et al., 2004; Baldea et al., 2009). A popular explanation for the protective role of MC1R comes from cell culture experiments showing that melanocytes carrying melanoma-associated *MC1R* variants have less effective repair of both UVR-induced pyrimidine dimers and oxidative damage than wild-type cells and are more sensitive to UVR-induced cell death (Kadekaro et al., 2005; Bohm et al., 2005; Hauser et al., 2006; Song et al., 2009). Functional MC1R appears to be necessary to prevent UV-induced genomic instability within melanocytes.

4. The epidemiological association between sunlight and melanoma is complex

Despite the persuasive descriptive evidence linking sunlight with melanoma, several observations make clear that the association is complex and does not accord with a simple model in which the risk of melanoma increases directly with increasing levels of exposure to the sun. Melanoma occurs more commonly among indoor than outdoor workers (Beral & Robinson, 1981). Even in sunny countries most melanomas develop on sites that are habitually covered by clothing (such as the back), as opposed to sites more frequently exposed to the sun such as the face (Green et al., 1993). Many case-control studies of melanoma incidence report stronger associations with intermittent (short periods of intense sun exposure to untanned skin) rather than chronic patterns of sun exposure (Elwood & Jopson, 1997). Recreational sun exposure is a risk factor for melanoma on the trunk and limbs but not on the head and neck (Chang et al., 2009).

Chronic sun exposure and a "classical" UVR carcinogenic mechanism involving UVB-induced DNA damage is accepted to be responsible for the development of SCC. One reason frequently proposed for the lack of association of melanoma with chronic sun exposure is that there may be a different carcinogenic mechanism for melanoma, possibly involving UVA exposure. The potential role of UVA in the induction of melanoma has been reviewed elsewhere (e.g. Wang et al., 2001; Moan et al., 2008; Godar et al. 2009). Sunlight at different latitudes contains vastly different rations of UVA/UVB, with a greater proportion of UVB nearer the equator, and less closer to the poles. Because the change in melanoma incidence with latitude is much smaller than that for SCC (which is dependent upon cumulative UVB exposure) it is hypothesized that UVA play a role at least in exacerbating the development of melanoma (Godar et al., 2009; Wang et al., 2010). Other ideas revolve around the notion that office workers are at higher relative risk possibly due excessive UVA that can penetrate glass (Godar et al., 2009). Further, recreational exposure, generally agreed to increase melanoma risk, can include solarium use. Depending on the lamp type used, artificial tanning devices (sunbeds or solariums) emit higher UVA/UVB ratios and possibly higher UVA doses than found in sunlight (Miller et al., 1998; Gerber et al., 2002). A meta-analysis of nineteen studies has shown that exposure to sunbeds at a young age is the most damaging, with a relative risk for "first exposure under the age of 35" of 1.75 (95% CI, 1.35, 2.26) (International Agency for Research on Cancer Working group on artificial UV light and skin cancer, 2007). A large prospective cohort study of 106,366 women in Sweden and Norway showed that solarium use at ages 30-39 linked to a relative risk of 1.49 (95% CI, 1.11-2.00)(Veierod et al., 2011). Thus epidemiological evidence suggests that sunbeds are health hazards in terms of melanoma risk and that UVA has a plausible role in the development of this neoplasm. Hence epidemiological data is somewhat supportive of the view that the full UVR spectrum may be carcinogenic in melanoma. It should be noted that at any point on the earth it is difficult to precisely predict the UVA/UVB ratio in sunlight as it can greatly vary with time of day, altitude, latitude and climate factors (De Fabo et al., 2004).

5. Naevus and melanoma subtypes

From the point of view of basic biology differences between melanoma and non-melanoma skin cancer in terms of their relationship with UVR exposure is not surprising. Melanocytes are long living cells, resistant to apoptosis, whose principal function is to produce melanin. In contrast, the primary function of keratinocytes is to provide a protective barrier, the epidermis, which is in a continual state of regeneration, supplied by proliferation of epidermal basal layer keratinocytes that initiates a programmed process of differentiation and apoptosis as needed. Melanocytes can undergo a form of proliferation, where they form senescent groups, or nests, which are termed naevi. Such lesions are negative for proliferation markers, but can progress to malignancy, albeit at an extremely low frequency (Grichnik, 2008). There are multiple subtypes of naevi. These include dermal (blue naevi), compound (common acquired, spitz and congenital naevi) and epidermal (e.g. reed naevi) lesions (Grichnik, 2008). These subtypes may be influenced differently by UVR exposure, and there may be differences in their propensities for transformation (e.g. which is probably much less for dermal naevi). Hence the subtype of naevus can be a confounding factor when studying environmental and genetic factors influencing naevo genesis. For instance the positive association between naevus count and *IRF4* gene variation (Duffy et al., 2010) varies greatly for different subtypes (dermal versus compound naevi).

Likewise there are several major melanoma subtypes, and then subtle forms within each group. Superficial spreading melanoma (SSM) is the most common form in Caucasians (around 70% of all melanomas). It follows a radial growth phase with atypical melanocytes, either as single cells or nests at all levels of the epidermis (Smoller, 2006), followed by an invasive vertical growth phase. Nodular melanoma (NM) are primary dermal lesions characterized by growth through the dermis, generally lack epidermal involvement, and a very sharply circumscribed with virtual lack of radial spread (Smoller, 2006). Lentigo maligna melanoma (LMM) is the only subtype unequivocally associated with chronic sun exposure. Lesions display confluent spread of melanocytes along the epidermal basal layer and in the upper portion of the hair follicle and are invariably associated with solar elastosis in adjacent skin (Smoller, 2006). SMM and NM, but not LMM, sometimes have naeval remnants present on histopathology. Acral lentiginous and mucosal melanomas are epidermal lesions that occur on palmoplantar and mucosal surfaces respectively, and are assumed not to be influenced by UVR exposure. Clearly, any discussion of the effects of chronic versus intermittent sun exposure has to consider melanoma subtype.

6. The divergent pathway model of melanoma

To assess the effects of chronic versus intermittent sun exposure melanomas have been stratified into chronic sun damage (CSD) or non-chronic sun damage (non-CSD) melanomas, either histologically by assessing solar elastosis, a measure of chronic exposure (e.g. Curtin et al., 2005), or by comparing melanomas developing on the head and neck (an anatomical region of high cumulative sun exposure), and the trunk (a region of intermittent exposure). While these two methods of classification may create some confounding differences, overall the use of either system supports the conclusion of a complex relationship between melanoma and sun exposure that has lead to the proposal of a "divergent pathway" model (Whiteman et al., 2003). According to this model (Figure 1) the pathways diverge after an initial insult that stabilizes the melanocyte. This may be early life exposure to UVR given that childhood sunburns are a risk factor for melanoma (Whiteman et al., 2001). What happens thereafter depends upon a combination of host characteristics and subsequent patterns and doses of UVR exposure. Melanomas that develop on the head and neck are associated with solar elastosis (a marker of CSD), low naevus count, and relatively late age of onset. In contrast, melanomas developing on the trunk via the intermittent UVR (non-CSD) pathway tend to have relatively earlier age of onset and are associated with higher naevus count.

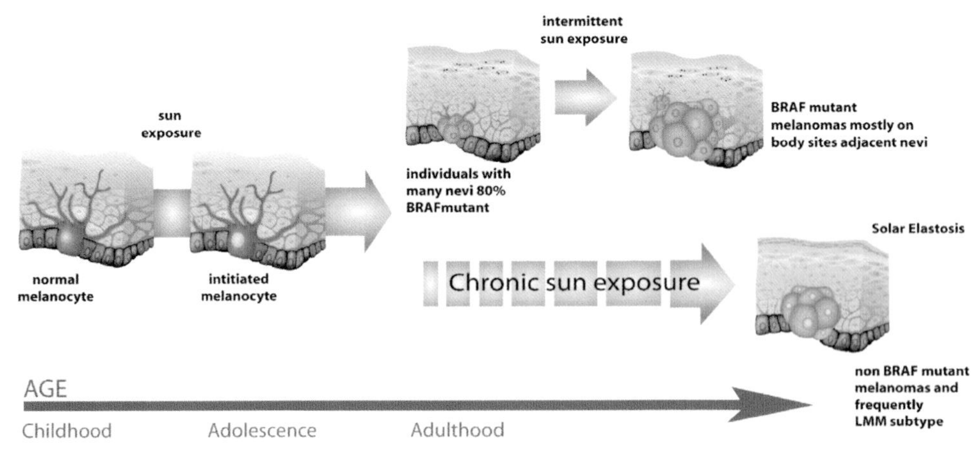

Fig. 1. Schematic depiction of the divergent pathways model for melanoma development.

Several studies have published findings concordant with the divergent pathway hypothesis (Carli and Palli, 2003; Chang et al., 2009; Bataille et al., 1998). Given the strong association between truncal (non-CSD) melanomas and naevus development, and the fact that most naevi carry *BRAF* mutations (Pollock et al., 2003), it is not surprising that the non-CSD melanomas also tend to carry *BRAF* mutations (reviewed in Platz et al., 2008). A greater tendency for melanocytes to proliferate in this branch of the model has been proposed (Whiteman et al., 2001). This may manifest as innate propensity for "proliferation" (a tendency to form nests, i.e. naevi), or proliferation in response to UVR exposure. To our knowledge inter-individual variation in the latter has only been reported once. Stierner et al. (1989) exposed buttock skin (seven UVB exposures with dose gradually increased to give slight erythema), and collected biopsies three weeks after last exposure. They found variation in the melanocyte proliferative response to UVR. Individuals that showed the biggest increase had the lowest pre-existing density. There was no association between melanocyte number increase, minimal erythemal dose, or skin type (the presence, or not, of naevi was not mentioned). Hence, although the sample size was small, this study does indicate different proliferative potential of melanocytes between individuals. We cannot know how these responses influence melanoma development except in prospective studies, but we can begin to look at genes and other phenotypic measures that may stratify the two pathways and allow better predication of risk. There are some suggestions that not only naevus risk may be important, but also the propensity of individuals with less naevi to be prone to developing solar elastosis (Thomas et al., 2010). Arguing against this, individuals with DNA repair defects (e.g. XP patients) frequently develop lentigo melanomas without solar elastosis (Spatz et al., 2001), indicating that repeated or unrepaired UVR-induced DNA damage in the skin may be more important than the presence of solar elastosis *per se*. To sum up, the divergent pathway hypothesis provides some basis for explaining why melanoma as a whole is most associated with intermittent sun exposure.

7. Stratification of CSD and non-CSD melanomas by innate phenotypic and genetic variation

7.1 MC1R variants

Landi et al. (2006) reported that individuals in Italian and U.S. cohorts that developed *BRAF*-mutant melanomas via the "naevus" (non-CSD) pathway tended to carry *MC1R* variants more frequently than those developing CSD melanomas. However studies undertaken in cohorts from Australia and North Carolina found no association between germline *MC1R* status and somatic *BRAF* mutations in melanomas (Thomas et al., 2007; Hacker et al., 2010a). More recently, the Italian sample population originally reported in Landi et al. (2006) has been expanded to include another 92 melanomas and they reported that germline *MC1R* variants were associated with melanomas carrying *BRAF*-mutations independent of solar elastosis measures (Fargnoli et al., 2008). Conflicting data has continued to appear, with results from a German sample of 173 melanoma patients showing the opposite effect, with individuals carrying *MC1R* variants less likely to acquire somatic *BRAF* mutations in tumours (Scherer et al., 2010). *MC1R* is considered the most important of the "moderate" risk genes for melanoma. However its relationship to CSD versus non-CSD associated melanoma is a matter of debate. It is possible that the discordant study findings reflect that fact that *MC1R* is extremely polymorphic within and between ethnic populations, and that the small sample sizes for each study means that chance association with the non-CSD melanoma pathway cannot be excluded.

7.2 Genes controlling the development of naevi

Given that the "intermittent" exposure arm of the divergent pathway is associated with the presence of naevi, we should be able to obtain clues about how to differentiate the pathways based on genes that confer naevus risk. Naevi are benign proliferations of melanocytes, and the number of naevi individuals tend to develop is under strong genetic control (English & Armstrong, 1994; Harrison et al., 1994). Monozygotic, or identical twin pairs, share all genes and have extremely highly correlated naevus counts (twin1 vs twin2, r=0.94), whereas dizygotic twin pairs share on average only half of their genes, and their naevus counts are considerably less correlated (r=0.60) (Zhu et al., 1999). The great majority naevi carry the *BRAF*^{V600E} which seems to be an early event in melanoma development but not sufficient to transform naevocytes (Pollock et al., 2003). Instead, the expression of the mutant form in melanocytes leads to growth arrest characteristic of senescence (Michaloglou et al., 2005). However the presence of *BRAF*^{V600E} does not inform in terms of how naevi might develop. Here we must look to genetic studies that might provide some hints to the molecular mechanisms involved. GWAS have also identified variants associated with development of naevi at chromosomal regions 9p21 and 22q13 (Falchi et al., 2009; Zhu et al., 2007). The strongest signal on 9p21 was located in the *MTAP* gene, which encodes methylthioadenosine phosphorylase, an enzyme involved in nucleoside metabolism. On 22q13 the SNP with the highest association lies within *PLA2G6*, a gene belonging to the phospholipase A2 superfamily. Notably, the 9p21 locus accounted for 3.0% of nevus count variance, whereas the 22q13 locus accounted for only 0.7%. Thus the *MTAP/CDKN2A* locus is the strongest candidate region for naevus susceptibility. Clearly *MTAP* is an excellent candidate, but so is *CDKN2A* given its historical involvement in melanoma and the fact that individuals in families carrying *CDKN2A* mutations commonly have many naevi. It is thought that SNPs in the *MTAP* gene may confer long-range regulation of the *CDKN2A* locus. The various lines of evidence for long distance regulation of the *CDKN2A* locus are reviewed in Peters (2008). This would be an analogous situation to the *OCA2* gene, whose influence on eye colour is not due to *OCA2* coding variants, but to remote regulation by a SNP in the adjacent gene (Sturm et al., 2008). Another study on twins (Duffy et al., 2010) has revealed another association, this time with *IRF4* (Interferon regulatory factor-4). Here the effect is somewhat weaker, and associated only with naevus development in an age-specific context (stronger effect in younger individuals). It will be very important to understand the mechanisms by which these genes confer naevus susceptibility given that the potential to develop naevi is the critical stratifying factor for the divergent pathways.

The number of naevi an individual develops does not appear to just an innate trait, it may also be associated with levels of sun exposure, especially in children (reviewed in Gallagher et al., 1995; Bauer et al., 2003). Recent studies examining the association of holidays overseas among young white English women found an increased in naevus count, particularly on anatomical sites intermittently exposed to sunlight, supporting the hypothesis that intermittent sun exposure is of relevance in the aetiology of naevi (Silva Idos, et al., 2009).

7.3 UVR-induced proliferation of melanocytes

Of possible relevance is how the branches of the divergent pathways differ in terms of the propensity of melanocytes in the skin to proliferate after UVR. Early studies in humans demonstrated that melanocyte density was correlated with sun exposure (Mitchell, 1963; Staricco & Pinkus, 1957; Stierner et al., 1989). Work by Quevedo and Colleagues (1965) reported that in mice melanocyte density increased up to 4-fold following repeated UVR exposure, possibly due to increased mitotic activity of melanocytes (Rosdahl, 1978). More recent experiments have shown that melanocyte proliferation is greater following exposure to UVB than UVA, and that a single dose has a substantially greater effect than the same dose fractionated over several days (An et al., 2001; van Schanke et al., 2005). The generation of melanoma in mouse models using neonatal UVR is usually, although not always, accompanied by a strong proliferative response of melanocytes and their migration to the burnt area of the skin (Walker et al., 2009; Ferguson et al., 2010). Melanocyte proliferation would seem to be linked to the tanning response, which increases the amount of pigment in the skin, and is driven by UVB-induced damage to the skin. This is akin to "delayed tanning", that can occur 1-5 d after exposure, and is primarily due to increased melanin production, although multiple exposures induce proliferation of melanocytes resulting in increased numbers in human skin (Yamaguchi et al., 2008). This is a long lasting protective pigmentation, unlike UVA-induced intermediate pigment darkening (IPD), which results from oxidation of pre-existing melanin, fades quickly, and is not protective against subsequent exposures. Interestingly, the induction of active melanocytes in mouse skin is also produced by chemical carcinogens, and the more carcinogenic the compound the greater the tanning response (Iwata et al., 1981). Liver carcinogens that are not metabolically activated in skin are ineffective. The compound most effective in inducing melanocyte proliferation was 7,12-dimethylbenz[a]anthracene (DMBA), a very potent skin carcinogen. Thus the response of melanocytes is driven either by UVR or compounds that induce adducts within the DNA of skin cells.

Melanocyte proliferation after UVR is thought to be driven by cytokines released by the microenvironment (Figure 2). UVR exposure modulates the production by keratinocytes (and probably other cells) of endothelins, Kit ligand (KITL), fibroblast growth factors (FGFs), and many others, which are all regulate melanocyte function (Hirobe, 2005; Lin & Fisher, 2007; Imokawa, 2004). These include α-MSH (alpha melanocyte stimulating hormone), ACTH and a range of other growth factors. α-MSH and ACTH both bind to the MC1R on the surface of melanocytes, which activates the cyclic-AMP dependent kinase pathway, and the production of melanin pigments and possibly melanocyte proliferation. Most of these signaling molecules are known to enhance pigmentation, but little is known about how they might influence melanocyte proliferation *in vivo*. Mutations in mice that cause disruption keratinocyte function (resulting in epidermal thickening), for instance by germline activating keratin 4a or epidermal growth factor mutation (Fitch et al., 2003), or keratinocyte-specific ablation of β1-Integrin (López-Rovira et al., 2005), result in increased melanocyte numbers in the epidermis. This can also occur without epidermal hyperplasia by keratinocyte-specific overexpression of p53 (McGowan et al., 2008), Kit ligand (Kunisada et al., 1998), or, surprisingly, deletion of Fgf2 (Weiner et al., 2007). Treating human skin xenografted on to mice with exogenous FGF2, endothelin 3, and KITL resulted in the development of pigmented lesions, which only required UVB exposures repeatedly for one month for progression to melanoma (Berking et al., 2004). Hence signals from DNA damaged keratinocytes may play a role in inducing melanocytes to proliferate. To quote Lin and Fisher (2007), "*could it be that keratinocytes are the primary UV responding population, and melanoma formation is largely a consequence of reactive secondary stimulation?*" In fact the injection of highly active αMSH analogues may be naevis promoting (Cardones et al., 2009; Langan et al., 2009). However the notion of UVR-induced melanocyte proliferation being melanomagenic is at odds with findings that stimulation of melanocytes with factor such as a-MSH (e.g. Bohm et al., 2005; Hauser et al., 2006; Abdel-Malek et al., 2009), Endothelin 1, (Kadekaro et al., 2005) and KITL

(Serre et al., 2011) improve DNA repair efficiency after UVR and are thus proposed to be protective for melanoma. Clearly we are only at the beginning of understanding how melanocyte UVR responses influence melanoma development. Whether genetic variation in humans that augment the proliferative response of an individual's melanocytes to UVR could increase susceptibility to a particular pathway of melanoma development (as suggested by Whiteman et al., 2003, and Rivers, 2004) remains to be determined.

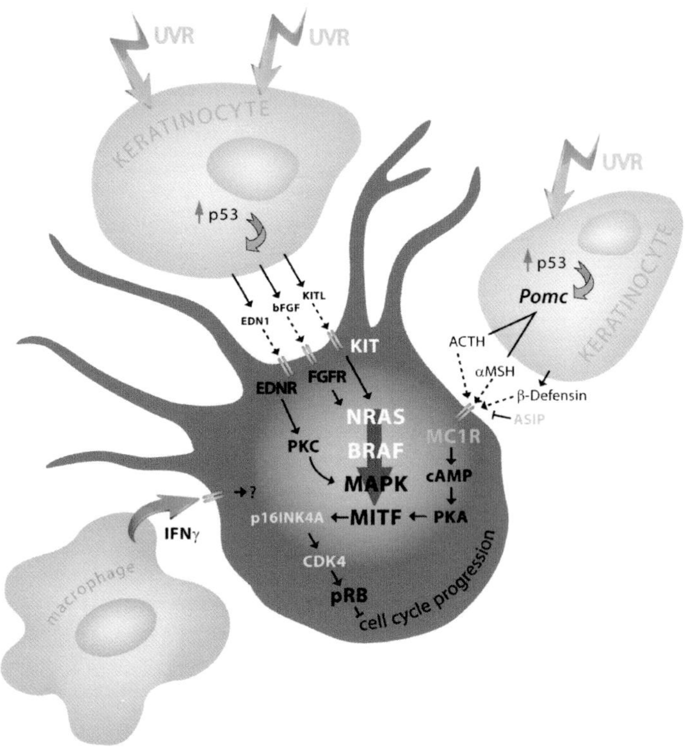

Fig. 2. Pathways regulating melanocyte function.
Keratinocytes expresses various growth factors that bind to melanocyte receptors that regulate critical intracellular pathways. Expression of these factors is increased after damage to the skin such as after UVR exposure. Germline mutations in *p16INK4A* and *CDK4* (light blue) confer susceptibility to familial melanoma. *KIT*, *NRAS* and *BRAF* (white) are mutated somatically in melanomas. *MC1R* and *ASIP* variants (yellow) confer increased risk for melanoma development. In addition, macrophages that infiltrate the skin after UVR may stimulate melanocytes. Activation of the pathways depicted result in increased pigment production and distribution to adjacent keratinocytes, and increased survival, DNA repair, and proliferation of the melanocyte.

7.4 Stratification of CSD and non-CSD by somatic mutations signatures

Examination of melanomas of various subtypes by array comparative genome hybridization (CGH) has detected significant differences at specific genomic locations such that DNA copy number differences could stratify melanomas into CSD, non-CSD, acral and mucosal melanomas (the latter two assumed not associated with sun exposure)(Curtin et al., 2005). Subsequently the same group detected activating mutations of KIT in 28% (n=18) of CSD melanomas versus 0% (n=18). This raised hopes that KIT mutation status may differentiate CSD and non-CSD melanomas, but a subsequent Australian publication (Handolias et al., 2010) showed that the frequency of *KIT* receptor gene mutations in CSD melanomas is very low. Thus *KIT* mutation may not a good discriminator of CSD and non-CSD melanomas. In contrast, it has consistently been shown that mutation of *KIT* is much more common in acral and mucosal lesions (Curtin et al., 2005; Smalley et al., 2009). As described above we are left with fact that *BRAF* mutations are more common in melanomas arising in the non-CSD group, and a tendency for *NRAS* mutations to be more often present CSD melanomas. Notably the frequency of *NRAS* mutants in this group is relatively low, hence it would be only a signature for a small proportion of CSD melanomas. Nonetheless a recent meta-analysis of all published studies showed that *NRAS* mutation is found in 24% of CSD melanomas and 17% of non-CSD melanomas and calculated that *NRAS* mutation is significantly associated with CSD melanoma (OR 1.9, 95% CI 1.11-3.20)(Lee et al., 2010). Despite the significant difference, *NRAS* mutation appears to be a weak discriminator of the CSD and non-CSD pathways. *BRAF* mutation is a better discriminator, having been found in 30% of CSD melanomas and 49% of non-CSD melanoma. *BRAF* mutation is significantly associated with non-CSD melanoma (OR 2.4, 95% CI 1.35-3.10). Unlike SSM and NM, few LMs (10-20%) harbor $BRAF^{V600E}$, (Hocker & Tsao, 2007). Hence there does not seem to be a strong mutations signature for the non-CSD pathway except for *BRAF*, which is mutated in over 80% of naevi. The stratification of CSD and non-CSD pathways in terms of *BRAF* mutation may have more to do with their differential association with naevus development than the forms of UVR exposure.

8. Vitamin D and potential protective effects of chronic sun exposure on melanoma?

Vitamin D has been shown to inhibit proliferation and induce differentiation in some melanoma cells, although melanoma cell lines have demonstrated resistance to vitamin D growth arrest (Danielsson et al., 1998,1999; Reichrath et al., 2007). A population-based study of 528 melanoma cases found that the presence of solar elastosis (dermal sun damage) was associated with a better prognosis for melanoma patients (Berwick et al., 2005). These findings have provoked speculation that as chronic sun damage induces a less aggressive form of melanoma (LMM), perhaps vitamin D levels might somehow slow melanoma growth and/or improve prognosis. To further determine if the anti-proliferative effect of vitamin D is modifying outcome for melanoma patients, Downing and colleagues, (2008) carried out a study to compare two populations with similar ethnic background but potentially different environmental influences. Patients diagnosed with invasive melanoma between 1993 and 2003 in Yorkshire (n= 4170) and New South Wales (NSW, n= 30,520) were identified from cancer registry databases and prognostic information (age, sex, socioeconomic background, tumour site and Breslow thickness) was examined. Five-year relative survival was 86.9% (95% CI, 85.2-88.5) in Yorkshire and 88.6% (95% CI, 88.1-89.1) in NSW. There was a suggestion of reduced risk for death in Australia, but differences in tumour thickness appeared to be the most important factor. The difference in survival may be due to the strong health promotion message for screening of skin cancer in Australia resulting in increased detection of early thin lesions with better outcomes. A recent follow-up study of 872 patients from the Leeds cohort (median follow-up, 4.7 years) has shown that higher 25-hydroxyvitamin D3 levels, at diagnosis, were associated with both thinner tumours and better survival from melanoma, independent of Breslow thickness (Newton-Bishop et al., 2009). This data needs to be validated in additional sample sets and the level of vitamin D in the follow up period examined. Understanding the balance between optimal sun exposure to limit skin cancer risk while maintaining adequate vitamin D levels has been further complicated by work from Damian et al. (2010), which found that vitamin D had a presumably undesirable immunosuppressive effect when vitamin D analogues were applied topically to irradiated skin. On the other hand, Mason et al. (2010) reported that increased vitamin D levels reduced DNA damage *in vitro* following UVR and subsequently reduced UVR-induced immunosuppression in mouse and human skin. Currently data do not allow us to predict with any accuracy whether there may be a true causal influence of low Vitamin D levels on melanoma outcome. Although there is no solid evidence as such, we cannot discount that CSD melanomas may have an innately better prognosis because they are not associated with naevus susceptibility (certainly this would be the case for LMM which are well known to have better outcomes than SSM and NM).

9. Animals as model systems for melanoma

To mechanistically link sun exposure and melanoma is very difficult because individual sun exposure, especially based on recall, is difficult to assess, and the ratio of UVB/UVA varies greatly with geographical location, season, and time of day. This leads to great uncertainty in inferences about how different wavelengths influence melanoma development, hence sometimes model experimental systems can be useful, and animal models for carcinogenesis can provide complementary information when epidemiological studies have difficulty avoiding confounding factors. Grey horses and certain strains of pig are models for genetic susceptibility to melanoma, although there is no evidence for any effects of UVR exposure (Rosengren Pielberg et al., 2008; Seltenhammer et al., 2004). Opossom, guinea pigs and Angora goats have also been used as models for melanocytic lesion development (Chan et al., 2001; Menzies et al., 2004; Green et al., 1996). However except for goats, UVR exposure is not known to play any role in melanoma development in these animals. All of these species are very expensive to maintain, and generally limited in terms of the availability of reagents such as antibodies, and resources for genetic analyses. Various strains of fish including zebrafish (reviewed by Patton et al., 2010) and other fish species such as *Xiphophorus* (discussed in more detail below) are tractable models where UVR exposure can exacerbate the development of melanoma.

9.1 Modeling chronic-induced melanoma in mice

In contrast to the ability to induce SCC in wild type mice using chronic treatment regimens, a pre-existing genetically engineered mutation, and exposure of neonates, is necessary for inducing murine melanoma (Noonan et al., 2001). There are three reasons proposed to explain why mice develop melanoma after neonatal UVR, but not after chronic exposures to adult animals. First, neonatal mice have epidermal melanocytes that are likely to be damaged by UVR, whereas adult mice do not. Second, the heightened sensitivity of neonatal melanocytes to proliferation following UVR may be destabilizing (Walker et al., 2009), and third, the lack of inflammatory response to UVR in neonates may create a tolerant environment for melanocyte transformation (Wolnicka-Glubisz et al., 2007; McGee et al., 2011). It is thought that murine neonatal UVR may be somewhat analogous to childhood sunburn (Noonan et al., 2001). Despite it being a somewhat specialized system, there is much we can learn using the neonatal UVR about how UVR results in melanocyte transformation. For instance using the *Mt-Hgf* model (with overexpression hepatocyte growth factor throughout the skin) it has been shown that UVB, and not UVA, induces melanoma (de Fabo et al., 2004), and that use of sunscreen can attenuate its development (Klug et al., 2010).

The skin of hairless mice contains some epidermal melanocytes, hence the animals represent a murine system amenable to chronic UVR exposures. Van Schanke et al. (2006) have carried out extensive UVR carcinogenesis studies on such animals carrying *Ink4a/Arf* deletion, with some cohorts also with co-deletion of the nucleotide excision repair gene *Xpa*. The mice developed naevi at a low rate spontaneously which was greatly increased by UVB treatment (how much depended upon the protocol and genotype). The naevi occasionally progressed to melanoma. Naevus development was dramatically increased by *Xpa* deletion, implicating UVB-induced pyrimidine dimer-type mutations in the pathogenesis of the lesions. Consistent with human melanoma, where intermittent exposures are most important, a single high dose erythemal exposure was much more effective at inducing naevi than the same dose delivered daily in a fractionated regimen (van Schanke et al., 2006).

In terms of using adult mice for UVR studies, a major problem is that they do not have epidermal melanocytes (and murine melanomas that develop are mostly dermal). Mice overexpressing Kitl in their keratinocytes (*K14-Kitl*) have epidermal melanocytes throughout life (Kunisada et al., 1998). They do not develop melanoma after chronic UVR exposures (Yamazaki et al., 2005). Even when crossed onto a DNA repair defective background (Xpa-null) no lesions were detected using a standard chronic UVB exposure protocol. But when the total UVB dose was increased over one half of the *K14-Kitlg::Xpa*$^{-/-}$ animals developed epidermal lesions reminiscent of lentigo and nodular melanomas (Yamazaki et al., 2005). Thus very high (almost physiological irrelevant) doses of UVB, plus a DNA repair defect, is need to induce transformation of the epidermal melanocytes in these mice. Interestingly, the animals developed very few SCCs, which both the high and low dose regimens do very effectively in wild type mice, hence it is thought that the extreme hyperpigmentation may be somewhat protective for both forms of skin cancer in this model. Nonetheless, murine epidermal melanocytes are apparently not totally resistant to transformation by UVR *per se*. It is possible that albino versions of the *K14-Kitl* model may have potential as a mouse model for chronic UVR-induced melanoma. Chronic UVR is somewhat effective in inducing melanomas in *Tyr-Hras*^{G12V} transgenic mice on an albino, but not pigmented strain background (Broome Powell, et al., 1999). However in *Mt-Hgf* transgenics chronic adult exposures do not exacerbate the development of melanoma (Noonan et al., 2001).

10. Mechanisms of UVR carcinogenesis in melanoma

10.1 Evidence of UVB causality in melanoma

The ultraviolet spectrum that plays a physiological role in skin cancer development is arbitrarily divided into UVB (280-315 nm) and UVA 315-400 nm). Non-melanoma skin cancer (especially SCC) is undeniably associated with chronic UVR exposure, and tumours carry "classical" UVB signature mutations resulting from mis-repaired cyclobutane pyrimidine dimer (CPD) or pyrimidine (6-4) pyrimidone photoproducts (6-4 PPs) adducts. The action spectrum for SCC induction in mice, and the inferred action spectrum for SCC in humans, peaks at 293 nm, firmly within the UVB range (de Gruijl et al., 1993). This overlaps with the action spectrum for CPD formation and sunburn. UVB, but not UVA, very effectively induces non-melanoma and melanoma skin cancer in mice (De Gruijl et al., 1993; De Fabo et al., 2004). Evidence of a critical role for UVB in melanoma induction comes from humans (van Steeg & Kramer, 1999) and mice (Yang et al., 2007) carrying nucleotide excision repair (NER) enzyme mutations (in *XP* genes) where melanoma incidence is dramatically increased after UVR exposure. XP patients have extreme sun sensitivity and burn very easily (van Steeg & Kramer, 1999). Melanomas from these individuals frequently carry *TP53* and *PTEN* gene mutations that show classic C-T or CC-TT UVB signatures and lesions are similar in body site distribution associated with chronic UVR exposure (Spatz et al., 2001; Wang et al., 2009). Further, the majority of melanomas in these individuals appear to be of the lentigo type, but they do not exhibit the solar elastosis that is invariably present in the same melanoma subtypes developing in DNA repair-proficient individuals (Spatz et al., 2001).

More information about the melanoma UVR mutation signature comes from the first melanoma genome sequence (Pleasance et al., 2010). Of 33,000 single point mutations detected, nearly 70% were C-T transitions. The only other nucleotide change above levels expected by chance were G-T transitions (9%) that can be a marker for UVA-induced damage (Agar et al., 2004). Notwithstanding the fact that only one melanoma, a secondary with undetected primary, was sequenced (Pleasance et al., 2010), and that some mutations could have been acquired by sun exposure during tumour development, these results suggest that CPD adducts may be critical driver of melanoma genesis. This is remarkably similar to the results of a recent review of all known *CDKN2A* and *TP53* point mutations in melanoma (Hocker & Tsao, 2007) which found that the frequency of UVB-signature mutations (65 and 55 % respectively) in these two genes in melanoma is similar to that found in SCC, a skin cancer with well-characterized UVB causality. Despite the presence of these UVR signature mutations, the overall mutation rate of these two genes in primary cutaneous melanomas is very low (7.9% and 11.8% respectively) (Hocker & Tsao, 2007), accounting for only about 10% of all melanomas. By comparison, *BRAF* or *NRAS* are mutated in more than 70% of all cutaneous melanomas (Hocker & Tsao, 2007).

Although we usually concentrate on CPDs as the mutagenic adduct, UVB also induces 6-4PPs, which are larger the CPDs, hence recognized and removed much more rapidly by nucleotide excision repair (NER). It has been hypothesized that 6-4PPs may be involved in melanoma induction, not via a mutagenic mechanism, rather via their deregulation of genome surveillance and transcription mechanisms leading to downstream changes that may deregulate the melanocyte (Mitchell et al., 2010). It is known that the two forms of UVB-induced photoproduct induce differential effects within cells (Lo et al., 2005). 6-4PP lesions are much more important in triggering cell death, whereas the response of the cell to CPD lesions mainly involves cell cycle arrest. An important role for 6-4PPs in melanoma is a speculative but interesting potential alternate aetiogy. Of note, 6-4PPs play no role in the generation of SCC in mice, CPD adducts are necessary and sufficient (Jans et al., 2005).

10.2 Evidence of UVA causality in melanoma

In contrast to UVB, UVA is generally extremely inefficient at inducing CPDs, oxidative damage, erythema, and non-melanoma skin cancer in mice (De Gruijl et al., 1993; Besaratinia & Pfeifer, 2008; Runger & Kappes, 2008). However UVA can induce 8-oxo-guanine (8-oxoG) oxidative adducts that can results in the formation of G-T transversions

(Agar et al., 2004). Results of another study suggest that T-G transversion is a UVA "signature" (Drobetsky et al., 1995). UVA-specific lesions in the p53 gene have been detected in skin constructs and squamous tumours (Agar et al., 2004; Huang et al., 2009). In contrast, *in vivo* studies using "Big Blue" mice, and *in vitro* data, suggests that UVA-induced mutations are mainly of the pyrimidine dimer type (Mouret et al., 2006; Besaratinia & Pfeifer, 2008; Runger & Kappes, 2008). An interesting idea regarding the role of UVA in melanoma is that UVA and UVB generate a similar DNA mutation spectrum (although UVA is much less effective at inducing CPDs), but that UVA-induced cellular stress and repair response is not as great, thus lesions may not be as effectively removed (Runger & Kappes, 2008). Possibly this would only apply after relatively pure UVA exposures, for instance from solaria, or through glass.

Notably, most of the studies mentioned above have used keratinocytes and fibroblasts, and not melanocytes to assess the mutagenicity of UVA. A recent study suggests that UVA is much more effective than UVB in inducing reactive oxygen species in melanocytes than in the other cell types (Wang et al., 2010). In addition, melanocytes are less efficient in removing CPDs and oxidative DNA damage. As discussed by Runger, (2011), these findings are at odds with some other studies, but nonetheless are indicative of potential differences between the responses of melanocytes and other skin cells to UVR. Runger, (2011) also raises the question of why if there is so much oxidative damage induced by UVA why are lesions typical for such stress vastly underrepresented in melanoma (e.g. Pleasance et al., 2010)? He suggests that this could relate to the low mutagenicity of 8-oxoG adducts.

The ability of UVA to generate melanoma in *Xiphophorus* backcross fish is suggestive of a role for UVA in melanoma development (Setlow et al., 1989; Setlow, 1999). This has long been interpreted to infer UVA causality for melanoma, probably based on melanin photosensitization and subsequent oxidative damage to DNA. UVA is about 1000-fold less effective than UVB in inducing erythema and SCC, whereas in fish melanoma induction there is only about a 10-fold difference between the effects of UVB and UVA. Given the overwhelming preponderance of UVA in natural sunlight, if the fish action spectrum held up in humans, UVA would dominate melanoma causality. *Xiphophorus* are a complicated model. They carry photolyase, a light-inducible system that very rapidly and specifically repairs specific DNA adducts (e.g.. CPD-photolyase removes CDPs). Such repair systems are present in most of the plant and animal kingdom except for rodents and primates. Thus the fish experiments are carried out in the dark, and activation (by light) of the photolyase reduces melanoma incidence to background levels. Recently Timmins and colleagues used electron paramagnetic resonance assays to show that the action spectrum for melanoma and melanin radical production overlap (Wood et al., 2006), further evidence for melanin radical causation. However the notion that UVA is more effective than UVB in inducing melanoma in fish has been questioned by Mitchell et al., (2010), after similar experiments using apparently the same strain of fish. This conflicting result from the original study (Setlow et al., 1989) may be largely explained by the fact that latest study used more animals to make the results more statistically significant, and followed the fish for a longer time, allowing for later age of onset of some melanomas. Further, the fish also carry nucleotide excision repair activity, and melanoma development is exacerbated in fish with defective NER (Mitchell et al., 2007). The authors point out that UVA exposure is still potentially very important in the induction of melanoma in humans, but it may not be via a melanin radical-based mechanism.

One would expect that if melanin sensitization were an important mechanism, we would not see the huge increase in melanoma risk for patients with XP, unless they also lacked a defence against the melanin radicals.However there remains an anomaly that Africans with albinism (i.e. no melanin, or low levels), who practice poor sun protection, have been consistently shown to only very rarely develop melanoma (reviewed in Wood et al., 2006). In 164 such patients in Tanzania actinic keratoses were found in 100%, and SCC in 34%, of albino individuals over 30 years old, but no melanomas were found (Lookingbill et al., 1995). In these cases childhood sunburns do not seem to drive subsequent melanoma development.

The only other model used as evidence for UVA causality in melanoma is the South American opossum, *Monodelphis Domestica*, although the effect is weak (Mitchell et al., 2007). A study on focal pigmented hyperplasia developing in the opossum after UVA (Ley, 2001) showed that the action spectrum for the development of these lesions was much closer to the SCC action spectrum rather than the fish action spectrum. Nonetheless pure UVA does seem able to induce melanocyte proliferations in these animals, albeit not melanomas. Another interesting model is the guinea pig. These animals develop naevi after chronic UVB but not after chronic UVA exposures (Menzies et al., 2004). Neonatal UVB and not UVA induces melanoma in albino *Mt-Hgf* mice (De Fabo et al., 2004). In short, the fish is the only published model for UVA-induced melanoma and the conclusions have been questioned. However there is some evidence using pigmented *Mt-Hgf* mice that UVA can increase melanoma penetrance after neonatal exposure (Fisher et al., 2009, meeting report from the 6th international melanoma congress), but it does not induce melanoma in albino *Mt-Hgf* mice. UVB effectively induces melanoma on both pigmented and non-pigmented backgrounds. Because the UVA effect is only seen in pigmented mice, the carcinogenic mechanism may involve increased oxidative stress induced by photosensitized melanin. Application of inhibitors of melanin synthesis before and after UVR exposure of appropriate animal models may provide an avenue to test the melanin radical hypothesis. It appears that the debate about the role of UVA in melanoma induction is not over.

It must be pointed out that the murine and fish studies cannot model cumulative lifetime exposure to UVA in sunlight. We cannot rule out a role for UVA given that although the genotoxicity (i.e. frequency of dimers) is much higher in the UVB, UVA is far more abundant in sunlight (at least 20-fold). Not only are there debates about the role of UVA, there are even studies suggesting a protective role for UVA. Here, with UVB dose kept constant, increasing UVA dose protects against epidermal apoptosis (Ibuki et al., 2007) and SCC induction in mice (Forbes et al., 1978). Which wavelengths are critical for melanoma formation? In some ways this is irrelevant, and the real question is what type of adducts are needed? The balance of evidence to date suggests that the susceptibility of a melanocytes to UVR-induced transformation depends mostly upon the presence of classical CPD type adducts that if not properly removed result in C-T or CC-TT mutations. However this has not been formally proven.

10.3 Role of UVR in generating *BRAF* and *NRAS* mutations

The DNA base changes causing activating mutations in *BRAF* and *NRAS* do not represent classical UVB signatures, thus other mechanisms have been proposed for their causation. $BRAF^{V600E}$ is found in several internal malignancies, arguing against a specific role for UVR, and more suggestive of a role for generalized oxidative damage, or another mechanism (Dhomen et al., 2007). The $BRAF^{V600E}$ mutation is generally caused by a T>A transversion, and one theory regarding the possibly role of UVR in the generation of this change relates to error prone repair at the V600 mutation site in *BRAF* caused by adjacent pyrimidine dimers (Thomas et al., 2006). On the other hand, Besaratinia, & Pfeifer, (2008) show that there are many types of lesions that can be induced by solar UVR, which although uncommon, could explain some of the mutations in detected in *BRAF*, particularly as there is selection pressure for the "required" the amino acid change. As discussed by Lund & Timmins, (2007) bulky adducts formed by reactive melanin species may be involved. None of these theories have been functionally tested. However in many melanomas the base change resulting in the *NRAS* codon 61 mutations is a G>T transversion (Hocker & Tsao, 2007). It has been experimentally confirmed *in vitro* using murine fibroblasts, that an 8-oxoG-mediated transcriptional mutagenesis mechanism greatly enhances the acquisition of such mutations (Saxowskya et al., 2008). Using a system that selected for clones carrying mutant *HRAS*^{Q61} mutations they showed that these were very rare in wild type murine fibroblasts but common in cells lacking the enzyme 8-oxoguanine DNA-glycosylase 1 (Ogg1), which repairs 8-oxoG lesions. The mutations were induced by G-T changes in the transcribed strand of the *HRAS* transcript. Thus while *NRAS* mutations may be induced in melanomas following UVB exposure, this mechanistic data best supports a role for oxidative adducts in their formation rather then CPDs. There is little mechanistic data to support the genesis of the *BRAF*^{V600E} mutation from oxidative stress, only the observation that it is sometimes found in mucosal and acral melanomas, not associated with sun exposure, and in internal cancers (thyroid and colorectal) (Dhomen et al., 2007).

It is difficult to glean much from murine melanoma models regarding the potential role of UVR in inducing *BRAF* or *NRAS* mutations. *Braf* mutations have not been detected in murine melanomas. One interesting finding comes from work with *Ink4a/Arf*$^{-/-}$*/Xpc*$^{+/-}$ mice. These mice, essentially the only example of mice developing melanoma due to UVR exposure without carrying an engineered oncogenic mutation, resulted in development of melanomas that frequently carried *Kras*^{Q61} mutations. Similarly, melanomas induced by UVB in *Ink4a/Arf*$^{-/-}$*/Xpa*$^{+/-}$ adult hairless mice occasionally carried an *Nras*^{Q61} mutation (van Schanke et al., 2006). The Ras^{Q61} mutations in the NER-deficient mice were mainly G-T changes, again reflective of mis-repaired 8-oxoG adducts rather than mis-repaired CPDs.

As suggested by Runger, (2011), oncogenes can only function as such due to very specific gain-of-function mutations that can only occur as certain amino acid changes, "*thus the DNA base change may rather indicate a constraint on the amino acid change than the identity of the mutagen*".

11. UVR, melanoma, and the immune system

11.1 Immunosuppression

There is undoubtedly an interplay between damaged melanocytes and immunocytes, whether just after UVR exposure or during tumour progression. It has long been known that the UVR exposure can suppress the immune system and create an environment tolerant to the growth of tumour cells that should be targeted for immunological destruction. Margaret Kripke and colleagues (Donawho et al., 1996) described how the growth of implanted tumours in mice is enhanced by local photoimmunosuppression. How much of a role it plays in melanoma development is unknown. Transplant patients taking immunosuppressive drugs are at a particularly heightened risk of skin cancer, particularly SCC, but it is a matter of debate whether they are at increased risk of melanoma. Out of nine studies recently reviewed (Bastiaannet et al., 2007), five reported between 2 and 4-fold increased risk, and four reported no increased risk. If immunosuppressed patients are at increased melanoma risk, it is low, and much less than the risk of developing SCC. Despite this, individuals taking immunosuppressive drugs sometimes develop eruptive naevi, and this form of melanocyte proliferation is proposed to be due to the effects of immunosuppression rather than the drugs that induce it (Zattra et al., 2009).

An important factor in the initiation of melanoma in mice by neonatal and not adult exposure is that neonates exhibit a defective inflammatory response to UVR compared to adults (Wolnicka-Glubisz et al., 2007; McGee et al., 2011). There may be ways to investigate the role that photoimmunosuppression plays in UVR-induced tumorigenesis. For example, (Jans et al. 2005) used mice carrying an inducible photolyase system that very rapidly removes CPDs from the skin after UVR exposure. Removal of CPDs from the whole skin significantly reduces both SCC development and immunosuppression. However, removal of CPDs specifically from the epidermal basal layer (using *K14-Photolyase* transgenics) similarly reduced tumorigenesis, but did not prevent photoimmunosuppression (Jans et al., 2006). Thus immunosuppression seems to depend upon damage throughout the epidermis and dermis, whereas SCC is driven largely by UVR damage to basal layer keratinocytes, suggesting that immunosuppression may be important but not essential for the initiation of this skin cancer in mice (at least in terms of UVR damage-driven SCCs). The relative contribution of direct DNA damage to melanocytes, and photoimmunosuppression, in melanoma needs to be clarified.

11.2 UVR-induced inflammation

One of the difficulties in studying UVR causality in melanoma is not only that multiple UVR response mechanisms such as DNA repair, proliferation and immune response play a role, but they are often not independent of each other. We can look at the normal response of melanocytes to UVR (Figure 2), in particular the multiple effects of cytokines that are released in the skin to activate melanocytes. Upon UVR-induced damage keratinocytes upregulate their expression of the pro-opiomelanocortin (Pomc) gene. Pomc encodes a pro-peptide that is cleaved to generate α-MSH, ACTH and β-endorphin (Cui et al., 2007). Together, these peptides have pleiotropic effects on endocrine and neuroendocrine signaling, and the immune system (Brzoska et al., 2008), in addition to the melanotropic function of αMSH. Another protein upregulated in the epidermis after UVR exposure, KITL, can drive proliferation and migration of both pro-inflammatory mast cells as well as melanocytes (Kunisada et al., 1998). Pro-inflammatory cytokines like interleukin 12 (Schwarz et al., 2002) and interleukin-18 (Schwarz et al., 2006) can increase DNA repair capability of melanocytes after UVR exposure. In the case of interleukin-18, this may be via upregulation of KITL (Hue et al., 2005). Another secreted protein, previously known only for its role in immune responses to infectious agents, β-Defensin, is upregulated over 50-fold in human epidermis after UVR exposure (Enk et al., 2006) and is possibly involved in melanocye response to UVR as another ligand for the MC1R (Candille et al., 2007). Thus the release of cytokines within the skin not only activates the immune system, but also induces protective responses in the melanocye itself (e.g. increased pigmentation, proliferation, and DNA repair).

The proliferative burst of melanocytes emanating from the upper portion of the hair follicle in neonatal mice presents an excellent opportunity to investigate how melanocytes are activated by UVR exposure. Zaidi et al. (2011) have cleverly utilized the power of the genetically modified mice to look into the mechanism of this melanocyte response. They used a genetically engineered mouse model inducibly expressing green fluorescent protein (GFP) in melanocytes. GFP was induced immediately after UVB exposure and melanocytes were isolated via fluorescence activated cell sorting at various time-points after neonatal UVR. Gene expression array analysis on these cells detected a strong signature of interferon-gamma (IFNγ)-induced genes that coincided with the appearance of melanocytes in the epidermis. It was subsequently shown that that the melanocyte response is largely driven by IFNγ released from infiltrating macrophages. Further experiments indicated that not only can macrophages influence melanocyte proliferation in the context of UVR exposure, but that they also contribute to the pro-tumorigenic inflammatory microenvironment of melanomas. This is possibly the first study to establish a direct link between the immune and melanocytic systems during the immediate skin response to UVR.

12. Conclusion

Because, measured on a population basis, melanoma induction by UVR appears to be via a very different mechanism (i.e. via intermittent exposure) than for keratinocyte-derived cancers (i.e. via chronic exposure), it has been postulated that there are different carcinogenic mechanisms at play (Setlow, 1999). Different mutagenic DNA adducts are proposed to be involved, including UVA-induced oxidative lesions, UVB-induced pyrimidine dimers and 6-4PPs. In studies of human populations individual sun exposure level, based on recall, can be difficult to assess, but also the ratio of UVB/UVA varies greatly with geographical location, season, and time of day. This leads to uncertainty in inferences about how much exposure and which wavelengths most influence melanoma development. However epidemiological work has lead to the proposal of the divergent pathway model for melanoma, where some melanomas develop as a result of intermittent exposure, others after chronic exposures (Whiteman et al., 2003). The major difference between the chronic and intermittent branches of the model is the presence of naevi, the great majority of which carry *BRAF* mutations, in the former. Naevi can develop spontaneously. Hence the presence of or propensity to develop naevi increases melanoma risk. Even limited sun exposure appears to increases this risk, whereas for individuals not prone to develop naevi a relatively high cumulative lifetime UVR damage may often be necessary. Nevus cells proliferate strongly, and move to a suprabasal (malignant-like) location if subjected to only a single UVB exposure *in vivo* (Carrera et al., 2008). Thus naevus cells, unlike normal melanocytes within the skin, are extremely sensitive to UVB-induced damage. It is not known if there is a mechanistic difference in UVR mutagenesis between the two CSD and non-CSD pathways. However, judging from the mutation spectrum in human melanoma, dominated by pyrimidine dimer type mutations, the most parsimonious conclusion may be that it is not necessary to invoke a different mutagenic mechanism *per se* to explain apparent differences in UVR causality between melanoma and non-melanoma skin cancer. In both cases pyrimidine dimer type DNA lesions are involved.

If multiple carcinogenic mechanisms are at play, this can be tested in a number of ways. The stratification of melanomas into CSD and non-CSD has been critical in enhancing our understanding of divergent mechanisms of melanoma genesis, but since the two major forms of melanoma, SSM and NM can be associated with either forms of exposure, further stratification may be necessary (Of note, LMM clearly has a different aetiology from NM and SSM). This may be in the form of the discovery of better somatic mutation signatures, as well as further innate genetic differences between the two groups. The development of further tests to differentiate between the two groups could help in terms of targeting particularly susceptible groups within the population for health education campaigns and more frequent screening. High throughput genome sequencing of large numbers of melanomas of various subtypes and association with CSD or non-CSD should clarify which type of DNA adducts are driving melanoma development, and in doing so might go some way towards clarifying the role of UVB versus UVA in the genesis of melanoma. Improved animals models should also be informative.

13. Acknowledgements

Of necessity we have had to be somewhat selective and we apologize to colleagues whose work we have not discussed. G.W. is funded by a Queensland Cancer Council Senior Research Fellowship. E.H is funded by a National Health and Medical Research Fellowship.

14. References

Abdel-Malek, Z. A., Ruwe, A., Kavanagh-Starner, R., Kadekaro, A. L., Swope, V., Haskell-Luevano, C., Koikov, L., Knittel, J. J. (2009). alpha-MSH tripeptide analogs activate the melanocortin 1 receptor and reduce UV-induced DNA damage in human melanocytes. *Pigment Cell Melanoma Res*, 22, 5, 635-44.

Agar, N. S, Halliday, G. M., Barnetson, R. S., Ananthaswamy, H. N., Wheeler, M., Jones, A. M. (2004). The basal layer in human squamous tumors harbors more UVA than UVB fingerprint mutations: a role for UVA in human skin carcinogenesis. *Proc Natl Acad Sci USA*, 101, 14, 4954-9.

An, H. T., Yoo, J. Y., Lee, M. K., Sin, M. H., Rhie, G. E., Seo, J. Y., Chung, J. H., Eun, H. C. & Cho, K. H. (2001). Single dose radiation is more effective for the UV-induced activation and proliferation of melanocytes than fractionated dose radiation. *Photodermatol Photoimmunol Photomed*, 17, 266-71.

Armstrong, B. K. & Kricker, A. (1993). How much melanoma is caused by sun exposure? *Melanoma Res*, 3, 395-401.

Baldea, I., Mocan, T., & Cosgarea, R. (2009). The role of ultraviolet radiation and tyrosine stimulated melanogenesis in the induction of oxidative stress alterations in fair skin melanocytes. *Exp Oncol*, 31, 4, 200-8.

Bataille, V., Grulich, A., Sasiseni , P., Swerdlow, A., Newton Bishop, J., McCarthy, W., Hersey , P. & Cuzick, J. (1998). The association between naevi and melanoma in populations with different levels of sun exposure: a joint case-control study of melanoma in the UK and Australia. *Br J Cancer*, 77, 505-10.

Bastiaannet, E., Homan-van der Heide, J. J., Ploeg, R.J., Hoekstra, H. J. (2007). No increase of melanoma after kidneytransplantation in the northern part of The Netherlands. *Melanoma Res*, 17, 6, 349-53.

Bauer, J. & Garbe, C. (2003). Acquired melanocytic nevi as risk factor for melanoma development. A comprehensive review of epidemiological data. *Pigment Cell Res*, 16, 3, 297-306.

Beaumont, K. A., Shecker, S. N., Newton, R. A., James, M. R., Stow, J. L., Duffy, D. L. & Sturm, R. A. (2007). Receptor function, dominant negative activity and phenotype correlations for MC1R variant alleles. *Hum Mol Genet*, 16, 2249-60.

Beral, V. & Robinson, N. (1981). The relationship of malignant melanoma, basal and squamous skin cancers to indoor and outdoor work. *Br J Cancer*, 44, 886-91.

Berking, C., Takemoto, R., Satyamoorthy, K., Shirakawa, T., Eskandarpour, M., Hansson, J., VanBelle, P.A., Elder, D.E., & Herlyn, M. (2004). Induction of melanoma phenotypes in human skin by growth factors and ultraviolet B. *Cancer Res,* 64, 3, 807-11.

Besaratinia, A., & Pfeifer, G. (2008). Sunlight ultraviolet radiation and BRAF V600 mutagenesis in human melanoma. *Hum Mut*, 29, 8, 993-991.

Berwick, M., Armstrong, B. K., Ben-Porat, L., Fine, J., Kricker, A., Eberle, C. & Barnhill, R. (2005). Sun exposure and mortality from melanoma. *J Natl Cancer Inst*, 97, 195-9.

Böhm, M., Wolff, I., Scholzen, T. E., Robinson, S. J., Healy, E., Luger, T. A., Schwarz, T., & Schwarz, A. (2005). alpha-Melanocyte-stimulating hormone protects from ultraviolet radiation-induced apoptosis and DNA damage. *J Biol Chem*, 280, 7, 5795-802.

Box, N. F., Wyeth, J. R., O'Gorman, L. E., Martin, N. G. & Sturm, R. A. (1997) Characterization of melanocyte stimulating hormone receptor variant alleles in twins with red hair. *Hum Mol Genet,* 6, 1891-7.

Brenner, M., Coelho, S. G., Beer, J. Z., Miller, S. A., Wolber, R., Smuda, C. & Hearing, V. J. (2009). Long-lasting molecular changes in human skin after repetitive in situ UV irradiation. *J Invest Dermatol*, 129, 1002-11.

Broome Powell, M., Gause, P. R, Hyman, P., Gregus, J., Lluria-Prevatt, M., Nagle, R., & Bowden, G. T. (1999). Induction of melanoma in TPras transgenic mice. *Carcinogenesis*, 20, 9, 1747-53.

Brzoska, T., Luger, T.A., Maaser, C., Abels, C., & Böhm, M. (2008). Alpha-melanocyte-stimulating hormone and related tripeptides: biochemistry, antiinflammatory and protective effects in vitro and in vivo, and future perspectives for the treatment of immune-mediated inflammatory diseases. *Endocr Rev*, 29, 5, 581-602.

Candille, S. I., Kaelin. C. B., Cattanach. B. M., Yu. B., Thompson. D. A., Nix. M. A., Kerns. J. A., Schmutz. S. M., Millhauser. G. L., & Barsh. G. S. (2007). A β-defensin mutation causes black coat color in domestic dogs. *Science*, 318, 5855, 1418-23.

Cardones, A., & Grichnik, J. M. (2009). α-Melanocyte-Stimulating Hormone–Induced Eruptive Nevi. *Arch Dermatol,* 145, 4, 441-444.

Carli, P. & Palli, D. (2003) Re: Melanocytic nevi, solar keratoses, and divergent pathways to cutaneous melanoma. *J Natl Cancer Inst*, 95, 1801.

Carrera, C., Puig, S., Llambrich, A., Palou, J., Lecha, M., Massi, D., & Malvehy J. (2008). Development of a human in vivo method to study the effect of ultraviolet radiation and sunscreens in melanocytic nevi. *Dermatology*, 217, 2, 124-36.

Chan, J., Robinson, E. S., Atencio, J., Wang, Z., Kazianis, S., Coletta, L. D., Nairn, R. S., & McCarrey, J. R. (2001). Characterization of the CDKN2A and ARF genes in UV-induced melanocytic hyperplasias and melanomas of an opossum (Monodelphis domestica). *Mol Carcinog*, 31, 1, 16-26.

Chang, Y. M., Barrett, J. H., Bishop, D. T., Armstrong, B. K., Bataille, V., Bergman, W., Berwick, M., Bracci, P. M., Elwood, J. M., Ernstoff, M. S., Gallagher, R. P., Green, A. C., Gruis, N. A., Holly, E. A., Ingvar, C., Kanetsky, P. A., Karagas, M. R., Lee, T. K., Le Marchand, L., Mackie, R.M., Olsson, H., Østerlind, A., Rebbeck, T. R., Sasieni, P., Siskind, V., Swerdlow, A. J., Titus-Ernstoff, L., Zens, M.S., & Newton-Bishop. J. A. (2009). Sun exposure and melanoma risk at different latitudes: a pooled analysis of 5700 cases and 7216 controls. *Int J Epidemiol*, 38, 814-30.

Cleaver, J. E. (2006). The biology of xeroderma pigmentosum. In Hearing, V. (Ed.) From *melanocytes to melanoma: The progression to malignancy*. pp.291-310. Totowa, N.J, Humana Press.

Cohen, C., Zavala-Pompa, A., Sequeira, J. H., Shoji, M., Sexton, D. G., Cotsonis, G., Cerimele, F., Govindarajan, B., Macaron, N. & Arbiser, J. L. (2002). Mitogen-actived protein kinase activation is an early event in melanoma progression. *Clin Cancer Res*, 8, 3728-33.

Costin, G. E., & Hearing, V. J. (2007). Human skin pigmentation: melanocytes modulate skin color in response to stress. *FASEB J*, 21, 4, 976-94.

Cui, R., Widlund, H. R., Feige, E., Lin, J. Y., Wilensky, D. L., Igras, V. E., D'Orazio, J., Fung, C. Y., Schanbacher, C. F., Granter, S. R., & Fisher, D. E. (2007). Central role of p53 in the suntan response and pathologic hyperpigmentation. *Cell*, 128, 5, 853-64.

Curtin, J. A., Busam, K., Pinkel , D. & Bastian, B. C. (2006). Somatic activation of KIT in distinct subtypes of melanoma. *J Clin Oncol*, 24, 4340-6.

Curtin, J. A., Fridlyand, J., Kageshita, T., Patel, H. N., Busam, K. J., Kutzner, H., Cho, K. H., Aiba, S., Brocker, E. B., Leboit, P. E., Pinkel, D. & Bastian, B.C. (2005). Distinct sets of genetic alterations in melanoma. *N Engl J Med*, 353, 2135-47.

Cust, A. E., Harland, M., Makalic, E., Schmidt, D., Dowty, J. G., Aitken, J. F., Agha-Hamilton, C., Armstrong, B. K., Barrett, J. H., Chan, M., Chang, Y. M., Gascoyne, J., Giles, G. G., Holland, E. A., Kefford, R .F., Kukalizch, K., Lowery, J., Randerson-Moor, J. A., Schmid, H., Taylor, C. F., Whitaker, L., Hopper, J. L., Newton-Bishop, J. A., Mann, G. J., Bishop, D. T., & Jenkins, M. A. (2010). Melanoma risk for CDKN2A mutation carriers who are relatives of population-based case carriers in Australia and the UK. *J Med Genet*, [Epub ahead of print].

Damian, D. L., Kim, Y. J., Dixon, K. M., Halliday, G. M., Javeri, A. & Mason, R. S. (2010). Topical calcitriol protects from UV-induced genetic damage but suppresses cutaneous immunity in humans. *Exp Dermatol*, 19, e23-30.

Danielsson, C., Fehsel, K., Polly, P. & Carlberg, C. (1998). Differential apoptotic response of human melanoma cells to 1 alpha,25-dihydroxyvitamin D3 and its analogues. *Cell Death Differ*, 5, 946-52.

Danielsson, C., Torma, H., Vahlquist, A. & Carlberg, C. (1999) Positive and negative interaction of 1,25-dihydroxyvitamin D3 and the retinoid CD437 in the induction of human melanoma cell apoptosis. *Int J Cancer*, 81, 467-70.

De Fabo, E. C., Noonan, F. P., Fears, T., & Merlino, G. (2004). Ultraviolet B but not ultraviolet A radiation initiates melanoma. *Cancer Res*, 64, 18, 6372-6.

de Gruijl F. R, Sterenborg H. J., Forbes, P. D., Davies, R. E., Cole, C., Kelfkens, G., van Weelden, H., Slaper, H., & van der Leun J. C. (1993). Wavelength dependence of skin cancer induction by ultraviolet irradiation of albino hairless mice. *Cancer Res*, 53, 1, 53-60.

Domen, N., & Marais, R. (2007). New insights into BRAF mutations in cancer. *Curr Opin Genet Dev*, 17, 1, 31-39.

Donawho, C. K., Muller, H .K., Bucana, C. D., & Kripke, M. L. (1996). Enhanced growth of murine melanoma in ultraviolet-irradiated skin is associated with local inhibition of immune effector mechanisms. *J Immunol*, 157, 2, 781-6.

Downing, A., Yu, X. Q., Newton-Bishop, J. & Forman, D. (2008). Trends in prognostic factors and survival from cutaneous melanoma in Yorkshire, UK and New South Wales, Australia between 1993 and 2003. *Int J Cancer*, 123, 861-6.

Duffy, D. L., Iles, M. M., Glass, D., Zhu, G., Barrett, J. H., Höiom, V., Zhao, Z.Z., Sturm, R.A., Soranzo, N., Hammond, C., Kvaskoff, M., Whiteman, D. C., Mangino, M., Hansson, J., Newton-Bishop, J.A.; GenoMEL, Bataille, V., Hayward, N. K., Martin, N. G., Bishop, D. T., Spector, T .D., & Montgomery, G. W. (2010). *IRF4* variants have age-specific effects on nevus count and predispose to melanoma. *Am J Hum Genet* 87, 1, 6-16.

Drobetsky, E.A., Turcotte, J., & Châteauneuf, A. (1995). A role for ultraviolet A in solar mutagenesis. *Proc Natl Acad Sci USA*, 92, 6, 2350-4.

Edlundh-Rose, E., Egyhazi, S., Omholt, K., Mansson-Brahme, E., Platz , A., Hansson, J. & Lundberg, J. (2006). NRAS and BRAF mutations in melanoma tumours in relation to clinical characteristics: a study based on mutation screening by pyrosequencing. *Melanoma Res*, 16, 471-8.

Elwood, J. M. & Jopson, J. (1997). Melanoma and sun exposure: an overview of published studies. *Int J Cancer*, 73, 198-203.

English, D. R. & Armstrong, B. K. (1994). Melanocytic nevi in children. I. Anatomic sites and demographic and host factors. *Am J Epidemiol*, 139, 390-401.

Enk, C. D., Jacob-Hirsch, J., Gal, H., Verbovetski, I., Amariglio, N., Mevorach, D., Ingber, A., Givol, D., Rechavi, G., Hochberg, M. (2006). The UVB-induced gene expression profile of human epidermis in vivo is different from that of cultured keratinocytes. *Oncogene*, 25, 18, 2601-14.

Falchi, M., Bataille, V., Hayward, N. K., Duffy, D. L., Bishop, J. A., Pastinen, T., Cervino, A., Zhao, Z. Z., Deloukis, P., Soranzo, N., Elder, D. E., Barrett, J. H., Martin, N. G., Bishop, D. T., Montgomery, G. W. & Spector, T. D. (2009). Genome-wide association study identifies variants at 9p21 and 22q13 associated with development of cutaneous nevi. *Nat Genet*, 41, 915-9.

Fargnoli, M. C., Pike K., Pfeiffer, R. M., Tsang, S., Rozenblum, E., Munroe, D. J., Golubeva, Y., Calista, D., Seidenari, S., Massi, D., Carli, P., Bauer, J., Elder, D. E., Bastian, B. C., Peris, K. & Landi, M. T. (2008). MC1R variants increase risk of melanomas harboring BRAF mutations. *J Invest Dermatol*, 128, 2485-90.

Ferguson, B., Muller, H. K, Handoko, H. Y., Khosrotehrani, K., Beermann, F., Hacker, E., Soyer, H. P., Bosenberg, M., Walker, G. J. (2010). Differential roles of the pRb and Arf/p53 pathways in murine naevus and melanoma genesis. *Pigment Cell Melanoma Res*, 23, 6, 771-80.

Fitch, K. R., McGowan, K. A., van Raamsdonk, C. D., Fuchs, H., Lee, D., Puech, A., Hérault, Y., Threadgill, D. W., Hrabé de Angelis, M., Barsh, G.S. (2003). Genetics of dark skin in mice. Genes Dev, 17(2), 214-28.

Fisher D., Barnhill, R., Hodi, F. S., Herlyn, M., Merlino, G., Medrano, E., Bastian, B., Landi, T.M. & Sosman, J. (2009). Melanoma from bench to bedside: meeting report from the 6th international melanoma congress. *Pigment Cell Melanoma Res*, 23, 14–26.

Fisher, D., Barnhill, R. Hodi, F., Herlyn, M., Merlino, G., Medrano, E., Bastian, B., Landi, T., & Sosman, J. (2009). Melanoma from bench to bedside: meeting report from the 6th international melanoma congress. *Pigment Cell Melanoma Res,* 23, 1, 14-26.

Forbes, P. D., Davies, R. E., & Urbach, F. (1978). Experimental ultraviolet photocarcinogenesis: wavelength interactions and time-dose relationships. *Natl Cancer Inst Monogr*, 50, 31-8.

Gallagher, R. P., & McLean, D. I. (1995). The epidemiology of acquired melanocytic nevi. A brief review. *Dermatol Clin* 13, 3, 595-603.

Gandini, S., Sera, F., Cattaruzza, M. S., Pasquini, P., Picconi, O., Boyle, P., Melchi, C. F. (2005a). Meta-analysis of risk factors for cutaneous melanoma: II. Sun exposure. *Eur J Cancer*.41, 1, 45-60.

Gandini, S., Sera, F., Cattaruzza, M. S., Pasquini, P., Abeni, D., Boyle, P., Melchi, C. F. (2005b). Meta-analysis of risk factors for cutaneous melanoma: I. Common and atypical naevi. *Eur J Cancer,* 41, 1, 28-44.

Gerber, B., Mathys, P., Moser, M., Bressoud, D., Braun-Fahrlander, C. (2002). Ultraviolet emission spectra of sunbeds. *Photochem Photobiol*, 76,664–668

Gerstenblith, M. R., Shi, J., & Landi, M. T. (2010). Genome-wide association studies of pigmentation and skin cancer: a review and meta-analysis. *Pigment Cell Melanoma Res*, 23, 5, 587-606.

Godar, D. E., Landry, R. J., & Lucas, A. D. (2009). Increased UVA exposures and decreased cutaneous Vitamin D3 levels may be responsible for the increasing incidence of melanoma. *Med Hypoth*, 72, 434-443.

Goldstein, A. M., Struewing, J. P., Chidambaram, A., Fraser, M. C., & Tucker, M. A. (2000). Genotype-phenotype relationships in U.S. melanoma-prone families with CDKN2A and CDK4 mutations. *J Natl Cancer Inst*, 92, 12, 1006-10.

Green, A., Maclennan, R., Youl, P. & Martin, N. (1993). Site distribution of cutaneous melanoma in Queensland. *Int J Cancer*, 53, 232-6.

Green, A., Neale, R., Kelly, R., Smith, I., Ablett, E., Meyers, B., & Parsons, P. (1996). An animal model for human melanoma. *Photochem Photobiol*, 64, 3, 577-80.

Grichnik, J. M. (2008). Melanoma, nevogenesis, and stem cell biology.J Invest Dermatol, 128(10), 2365-80.

Hacker, E., & Hayward, N. K. (2008). Germline MC1R variants and BRAF mutant melanoma. *J Invest Dermatol*, 128, 2354-6.

Hacker, E., Hayward, N. K., Dumenil, T., James, M. R. & Whiteman, D. C. (2010a). The association between MC1R genotype and BRAF mutation status in cutaneous melanoma: findings from an Australian population. *J Invest Dermatol*, 130, 241-8.

Handolias, D., Salemi, R., Murray, W., Tan, A., Liu, W., Viros, A., Dobrovic, A., Kelly, J., & McArthur, G.A. (2010). Mutations in KIT occur at low frequency in melanomas arising from anatomical sites associated with chronic and intermittent sun exposure. *Pigment Cell Melanoma Res,* 23, 2, 210-5.

Harrison, S. L., Maclennan, R., Speare, R. & Wronski, I. (1994). Sun exposure and melanocytic naevi in young Australian children. *Lancet*, 344, 1529-32.

Hauser, J. E., Kadekaro, A. L., Kavanagh, R. J., Wakamatsu, K., Terzieva, S., Schwemberger, S., Babcock, G., Rao, M. B., Ito, S., & Abdel-Malek Z. A. (2006). Melanin content and

MC1R function independently affect UVR-induced DNA damage in cultured human melanocytes. *Pigment Cell Res*, 19, 4, 303-14.

Hill, H. Z. (1992). The function of melanin or six blind people examine an elephant. *Bioessays* 14, 1, 49-56.

Hirobe, T. (2005). Role of keratinocyte-derived factors involved in regulating the proliferation and differentiation of mammalian epidermal melanocytes. *Pigment Cell Res*, 18, 1, 2-12.

Hocker, T., & Tsao, H. (2007). Ultraviolet radiation and melanoma: a systematic review and analysis of reported sequence variants. *Hum Mutat*, 28, 6, 578-88.

Huang, X. X., Bernerd, F., Halliday, G .M. (2009). Ultraviolet A within sunlight induces mutations in the epidermal basal layer of engineered human skin. *Am J Pathol*, 174, 4, 1534-43.

Hue, J., Kim, A., Song, H., Choi, I., Park, H., Kim, T., Lee, W.J., Kang, H., Cho, D. (2005). IL-18 enhances SCF production of melanoma cells by regulating ROI and p38 MAPK activity. *Immunol Lett*, 96, 2, 211-7.

Ibuki, Y., Allanson, M., Dixon, K. M., & Reeve, V.E. (2007). Radiation sources providing increased UVA/UVB ratios attenuate the apoptotic effects of the UVB waveband UVA-dose-dependently in hairless mouse skin. *J Invest Dermatol*, 127, 9, 2236-44.

Imokawa, G. (2004). Autocrine and paracrine regulation of melanocytes in human skin and in pigmentary disorders. *Pigment Cell Res*. 17, 2, 96-110.

International Agency for Research on Cancer Working Group on artificial ultraviolet (UV) light and skin cancer. (2007). The association of use of sunbeds with cutaneous malignant melanoma and other skin cancers: A systematic review. *Int J Cancer*, 120, 5, 1116-22.

Iwata, K., Inui, N., & Takeuchi, T. (1981). Induction of active melanocytes in mouse skin by carcinogens: a new method for detection of skin carcinogens. *Carcinogenesis*, 2, 7, 589-93.

Jans, J., Schul, W., Sert, Y.G., Rijksen, Y., Rebel, H., Eker, A. P., Nakajima, S., van Steeg, H., de Gruijl, F. R., Yasui, A., Hoeijmakers, J. H., & van der Horst, G. T. (2005). Powerful skin cancer protection by a CPD-photolyase transgene. *Curr Biol*, 15, 2, 105-15.

Kadekaro, A. L., Kavanagh, R., Kanto, H., Terzieva, S., Hauser, J., Kobayashi, N., Schwemberger, S., Cornelius, J., Babcock, G., Shertzer, H. G., Scott, G., & Abdel-Malek, Z. A. (2005). α-Melanocortin and endothelin-1 activate antiapoptotic pathways and reduce DNA damage in human melanocytes. *Cancer Res*, 65, 10, 4292-9.

Kanetsky, P.A., Panossian, S., Elder, D. E., Guerry, D., Ming, M.E., Schuchter, L., & Rebbeck, T. R. (2010). Does MC1R genotype convey information about melanoma risk beyond risk phenotypes? *Cancer*, 116, 10, 2416-28.

Khlat, M., Vail, A., Parkin, M. & Green, A. (1992). Mortality from melanoma in migrants to Australia: variation by age at arrival and duration of stay. *Am J Epidemiol*, 135, 1103-13.

Kielbassa, C., Roza, L., & Epe B. (1997). Wavelength dependence of oxidative DNA damage induced by UV and visible light. *Carcinogenesis*, 18, 4, 811-6.

Klug, H., Tooze, J. A., Graff-Cherry, C., Anver, M., Noonan, F., Fears, T. R., Tucker, M., De Fabo, E., & Merlino, G. (2010). Sunscreen prevention of melanoma in man and mouse. *Pigment Cell Melanoma Res*, 23, 6, 835-7.

Kraemer, K. H., Lee, M. M., Andrews, A. D. & Lambert, W. C. (1994). The role of sunlight and DNA repair in melanoma and nonmelanoma skin cancer. The xeroderma pigmentosum paradigm. *Arch Dermatol*, 130, 1018-21.

Kunisada, T., Lu, S.Z., Yoshida, H., Nishikawa, S., Nishikawa, S., Mizoguchi, M., Hayashi, S., Tyrrell, L., Williams, D.A., Wang, X., & Longley, B.J. (1998). Murine cutaneous mastocytosis and epidermal melanocytosis induced by keratinocyte expression of transgenic stem cell factor. *J Exp Med*, 187, 10, 1565-73.

Landi, M. T., Bauer, J., Pteiffer, R. M., Elder, D. E., Hulley, B., Minghetti, P., Calista, D., Kanetsky, P. A., Pinkel, D. & Bastian, B. C. (2006). MC1R germline variants confer risk for BRAF-mutant melanoma. *Science*, 313, 521-2.

Langan, E. A. Ramlogan, D., Jamieson, L. A., Rhodes, L. E. (2009). Change in moles linked to use of unlicensed "sun tan jab". *BMJ*, 338, b277.

Lee, J. H., Choi, J.W., & Kim, Y. S. (2010). Frequencies of BRAF and NRAS mutations are different in histological types and sites of origin of cutaneous melanoma: a meta-analysis. *Br J Dermatol*, [Epub ahead of print].

Ley, R. D. (2001). Dose response for ultraviolet radiation A-induced focal melanocytic hyperplasia and nonmelanoma skin tumors in Monodelphis domestica. *Photochem Photobiol*, 73, 1, 20-3.

Lin, J. Y. & Fisher, D. E. (2007). Melanocyte biology and skin pigmentation. *Nature*, 445, 843-50.

Lo, H. L., Nakajima, S., Ma, L., Walter, B., Yasui, A., Ethell, D. W., & Owen, L. B. (2005). Differential biologic effects of CPD and 6-4PP UV-induced DNA damage on the induction of apoptosis and cell-cycle arrest. *BMC Cancer*, 19, 5, 135.

López-Rovira, T., Silva-Vargas, V., & Watt, F. M. (2005). Different consequences of beta1 integrin deletion in neonatal and adult mouse epidermis reveal a context-dependent role of integrins in regulating proliferation, differentiation, and intercellular communication. *J Invest Dermatol*, 125, 6, 1215-27.

Lookingbill, D. P., Lookingbill, G. L., & Leppard, B. (1995). Actinic damage and skin cancer in albinos in northern Tanzania: findings in 164 patients enrolled in an outreach skin care program. *J Am Acad Dermatol*, 32, 4, 653-8.

Lund, L.P., & Timmins, G.S. (2007). Melanoma, long wavelength ultraviolet and sunscreens: controversies and potential resolutions. *Pharmacol Ther*, 114, 2, 198-207.

Mason, R. S. (2010). Vitamin D: a hormone for all seasons. *Climacteric*, 14, 197-203.

Mattei, S., Colombo, M. P., Melani, C., Silvani, A., Parmiani, G. & Herlyn, M. (1994). Expression of cytokine/growth factors and their receptors in human melanoma and melanocytes. *Int J Cancer*, 56, 853-7.

McCredie, M., Coates, M. S. & Ford, J. M. (1990). Cancer incidence in migrants to New South Wales from England, Wales, Scotland and Ireland. *Br J Cancer*, 62, 992-5.

McGee, H. M., Malley, R. C., Muller, H. K., & Woods, G. M. (2011). Neonatal exposure to UVR alters skin immune system development, and suppresses immunity in adulthood. *Immunol Cell Biol*, [Epub ahead of print].

McGowan, K. A., Li, J. Z., Park, C. Y., Beaudry, V., Tabor, H. K., Sabnis, A. J., Zhang, W., Fuchs, H., de Angelis, M. H., Myers, R. M., Attardi, L. D., & Barsh, G. S. (2008). Ribosomal mutations cause p53-mediated dark skin and pleiotropic effects. *Nat Genet*, 40, 8, 963-70.

McMichael, A. J. & Giles, G. G. (1988). Cancer in migrants to Australia: extending the descriptive epidemiological data. *Cancer Res*, 48, 751-6.

Menzies, S. W., Greenoak, G. E., Abeywardana, C. M., Crotty, K. A., & O'Neill, M. E. (2004). UV light from 290 to 325 nm, but not broad-band UVA or visible light, augments the formation of melanocytic nevi in a guinea-pig model for human nevi. *J Invest Dermatol*, 123, 2, 354-60.

Michaloglou, C., Vredeveld, L. C., Soengas, M. S., Denoyelle, C., Kuilman, T., Van Der Horst, C. M., Majoor, D. M., Shay, J. W., Mooi, W. J. & Peeper, D. S. (2005). BRAFE600-associated senescence-like cell cycle arrest of human naevi. *Nature*, 436, 720-4.

Mitchell, R. E. (1963). The Effect of Prolonged Solar Radiation on Melanocytes of the Human Epidermis. *J Invest Dermatol*, 41, 199-212.

Mitchell, D., Paniker, L., Sanchez, G., Trono, D., & Nairn, R. (2007). The etiology of sunlight-induced melanoma in Xiphophorus hybrid fish. *Mol. Carcinogen*, 46, 8, 679-84.

Mitchell, D. L., Fernandez, A. A., Nairn, R. S., Garcia, R., Paniker, L., Trono, D., Thames, H.D., & Gimenez-Conti, I. (2010). Ultraviolet A does not induce melanomas in a Xiphophorus hybrid fish model. *Proc Natl Acad Sci USA*, 107, 20, 9329-34.

Mitchell, D. L., Fernandez, A. A. (2011). Different types of DNA damage play different roles in the etiology of sunlight-induced melanoma. *Pigment Cell Melanoma Res*, 24, 1, 119-24.

Miller, S. A., Hamilton, .S. L, Wester, U. G., Cyr, W. H. (1998). An analysis of UVA emissions from sunlamps and the potential importance for melanoma. Photochem Photobiol, 68(1), 63-70.

Moan, J., Porojnicu, A. C., Dahlback, A. (2008). Ultraviolet radiation and malignant melanoma. *Adv Exp Med Biol, 624*, 104-16.

Mouret, S., Baudouin, C., Charveron, M., Favier, A., Cadet, J., Douki, T. (2006). Cyclobutane pyrimidine dimers are predominant DNA lesions in whole human skin exposed to UVA radiation. *Proc Natl Acad Sci USA*, 103, 37, 13765-70.

Newton-Bishop, J. A., Beswick, S., Randerson-Moor, J., Chang, Y. M., Affleck, P., Elliot, F., Chan, M., Leake, S., Karpavicius, B., Haynes, S., Kukalizch, K., Whitaker, L., Jackson, S., Gerry, E., Nolan, C., Bertram, C., Marsden, J., Elder, D. E., Barrett, J. H. & Bishop, D. T. (2009) Serum 25-hydroxyvitamin D3 levels are associated with breslow thickness at presentation and survival from melanoma. *J Clin Oncol*, 27, 5439-44.

Noonan, F. P., Recaio, J. A., Takayama, H., Duray, P., Anver, M. R., Rush, W. L., De Fabo, E. C. & Merlino, G. (2001). Neonatal sunburn and melanoma in mice. *Nature*, 413, 271-2.

Patton, E. E., Mitchell, D. L. & Nairn, R. S. (2010). Genetic and environmental melanoma models in fish. *Pigment Cell Melanoma Res*, 23, 3, 314-37.

Platz, A., Egyhazi, S., Ringborg, U., & Hansson, J. (2008). Human cutaneous melanoma; a review of NRAS and BRAF mutation frequencies in relation to histogenetic subclass and body site. *Mol Oncol*, 1, 4, 395-405.

Pleasance, E. D., Cheetham, R. K., Stephens, P. J., McBride, D. J., Humphray, S. J., Greenman, C. D., Varela, I., Lin, M. L., Ordóñez, G. R., Bignell, G. R., Ye, K., Alipaz, J., Bauer, M. J., Beare, D., Butler, A., Carter, R. J., Chen, L., Cox, A. J., Edkins, S., Kokko-Gonzales, P. I., Gormley, N. A., Grocock, R. J., Haudenschild, C. D., Hims, M. M., James, T., Jia, M., Kingsbury, Z., Leroy, C., Marshall, J., Menzies, A., Mudie, L. J., Ning, Z., Royce, T., Schulz-Trieglaff, O. B., Spiridou, A., Stebbings, L. A., Szajkowski, L., Teague, J., Williamson, D., Chin, L., Ross, M.T., Campbell, P.J., Bentley, .D.R, Futreal, P.A., & Stratton, M. R. (2010). A comprehensive catalogue of somatic mutations from a human cancer genome. *Nature*, 463, 7278, 191-6.

Peters, G. (2008). Tumor suppression for ARFicionados: the relative contributions of p16INK4a and p14ARF in melanoma. *J Natl Cancer Inst* 100, 11, 784-95.

Platz A, Egyhazi S, Ringborg U, Hansson J. (2008). Human cutaneous melanoma; a review of *NRAS* and *BRAF* mutation frequencies in relation to histogenetic subclass and body site. *Mol Oncol*, 1, 4, 395-405.

Pollock, P. M., Harper, U. L., Hansen, K. S., Yudt, L. M., Stark, M., Robbins, C. M., Moses, T. Y., Hostetter, G., Wagner, U., Kakareka, J., Salem, G., Pohida, T., Heenan, P., Duray, P., Kallioniemi, O., Hayward, N. K., Trent, J. M., & Meltzer, P. S. (2003). High frequency of BRAF mutations in nevi. *Nat Genet*, 33, 19-20.

Quevado, W. C., Jr., Szabo, G., Virks, J. & Sinesi, S. J. (1965). Melanocyte populations in UV-irradiated human skin. *J Invest Dermatol*, 45, 295-8.

Raimondi, S., Sera, F., Gandini, S., Iodice, S., Caini, S., Maisonneuve, P. & Fargnoli, M. C. (2008). MC1R variants, melanoma and red hair color phenotype: a meta-analysis. *Int J Cancer*, 122, 2753-60.

Randerson-Moor, J. A., Harland, M., Williams, S., Cuthbert-Heavens, D., Sheridan, E., Aveyard, J., Sibley, K., Whitaker, L., Knowles, M., Bishop, J. N., & Bishop, D. T. (2001). A germline deletion of p14(ARF) but not CDKN2A in a melanoma-neural system tumour syndrome family. *Hum Mol Genet*, 10, 1, 55-62.

Reichrach, J., Rech, M., Moeini, M., Meese, E., Tilgen, W. & Seifert, M. (2007). In vitro comparison of the vitamin D endocrine system in 1,25(OH)2D3-responsive and -resistant melanoma cells. *Cancer Biol Ther*, 6, 48-55

Rivers, J.K. (2004). Is there more than one road to melanoma? *Lancet*, 363, 9410, 728-30.

Rizos, H., Puig, S., Badenas, C., Malvehy, J., Darmanian, A. P., Jiménez, L., Milà, M., & Kefford, R. F. (2001). A melanoma-associated germline mutation in exon 1beta inactivates p14ARF. *Oncogene*, 20, 39, 5543-7.

Rosdahl, I. K. (1978). Melanocyte mitosis in UVB-irradiated mouse skin. *Acta Derm Venereol*, 58, 217-21.

Rosengren Pielberg, G., Golovko, A., Sundström, E., Curik, I., Lennartsson, J., Seltenhammer, M. H., Druml, T., Binns, M., Fitzsimmons, C., Lindgren, G., Sandberg, K., Baumung, R., Vetterlein, M., Strömberg, S., Grabherr, M., Wade, C., Lindblad-Toh, K., Pontén, F., Heldin, C. H., Sölkner, J., & Andersson, L. (2008). A cis-acting regulatory mutation causes premature hair graying and susceptibility to melanoma in the horse. *Nat Genet*, 40, 8, 1004-9.

Runger, T., Kappes, U. (2008). Mechanisms of mutation formation with long-wave ultraviolet radiation (UVA). *Photoderm Photommunol Photomed*, 24, 2-10.

Rünger, T. M. (2011). Is UV-induced mutation formation in melanocytes different from other skin cells? *Pigment Cell Melanoma Res*, 24, 1, 10-12.

Saxowskya, T., Meadowsa, K., Klunglandb, A., & Doetscha, W. (2008). 8-Oxoguanine-mediated transcriptional mutagenesis causes Ras activation in mammalian cells. *Proc Natl Acad Sci USA*, 105, 18877-18882.

Scherer, D., Rachakonda, P.S., Angelini, S., Mehnert, F., Sucker, A., Egberts, F., Hauschild, A., Hemminki, K., Schadendorf, D., & Kumar, R. (2010). Association between the germline MC1R variants and somatic BRAF/NRAS mutations in melanoma tumors. *J Invest Dermatol*, 130, 12, 2844-8.

Schwarz, A., Ständer, S., Berneburg, M., Böhm, M., Kulms, D., van Steeg, H., Grosse-Heitmeyer, K., Krutmann, J., & Schwarz, T. (2002). Interleukin-12 suppresses ultraviolet radiation-induced apoptosis by inducing DNA repair. *Nat Cell Biol*, 4, 1, 26-31.

Schwarz, A., Maeda, A., Stander, S., van Steeg, H., & Schwarz T. (2006). IL-18 reduces ultraviolet radiation-induced DNA damage and thereby affects photoimmunosuppression. *J Immunol*, 176, 5, 2896-2901.

Seltenhammer, M. H., Heere-Ress, E., Brandt, S., Druml, T., Jansen, B., Pehamberger, H., Niebauer, G. W. (2004). Comparative histopathology of grey-horse-melanoma and human malignant melanoma. Pigment Cell Res, 17(6), 674-81.

Serre, C., Lebleu, A., Bergeron, L., Plantivaux, A., Botto, J. M., Dal Farra, C., & Domloge, N. (2011). Microarray profiling of gene expression in human keratinocytes suggests a new protective activity against UV-induced DNA damage for a compound previously known to interact with SCF-KIT signalling pathway. *Int J Cosmet Sci*, [Epub ahead of print].

Setlow, R. B., Woodhead, A. D., & Grist, E. (1989). Animal model for ultraviolet radiation-induced melanoma: platyfish-swordtail hybrid. *Proc Natl Acad Sci USA*, 86, 22, 8922-6.

Setlow, R. B. (1999). Spectral regions contributing to melanoma: a personal view. *J Investig Dermatol Symp Proc*, 4, 1, 46-9.

Silva Idos, S., Higgins, C. D., Abramsky, T., Swanwick, M. A., Frazer, J., Whitaker, L. M., Blanshard, M. E., Bradshaw, J., Apps, J. M., Bishop, D. T., Newton-Bishop, J. A., & Swerdlow, A. J. (2009). Overseas sun exposure, nevus counts, and premature skin aging in young English women: a population-based survey. *J Invest Dermatol*, 129, 1, 50-9.

Smalley, K. S., Sondak, V. K., & Weber, J. S. (2009). c-KIT signaling as the driving oncogenic event in sub-groups of melanomas. *Histol Histopathol*, 24, 5, 643-50. Review.

Smoller, B. R. (2006). Histologic criteria for diagnosing primary cutaneous malignant melanoma. *Mod Pathol*, 19, Suppl 2, S34-40.

Song, X., Mosby, N., Yang, J., Xu, A., Abdel-Malek, Z., & Kadekaro, A. L. (2009). α-MSH activates immediate defense responses to UV-induced oxidative stress in human melanocytes. *Pigment Cell Melanoma Res*, 22, 6, 809-18.

Spatz, A., Giglia-Mari, G., Benhamou, S., & Sarasin, A. (2001). Association between DNA repair-deficiency and high level of p53 mutations in melanoma of Xeroderma pigmentosum. *Cancer Res*, 61, 6, 2480-6.

Staricco, R. J. & Pinkus, H. (1957). Quantitative and qualitative data on the pigment cells of adult human epidermis. *J Invest Dermatol*, 28, 33-45.

Stierner, U., Rosdahl, I., Augustsson, A., & Kagedal, B. (1989). UVB irradiation induces melanocyte increase in both exposed and shielded human skin. *J Invest Dermatol*, 92, 561-564.

Sturm, R. A., Duffy, D. L., Box, N. F., Newton, R. A., Shepherd, A. G., Chen, W., Marks, L. H., Leonard, J. H. & Martin, N. G. (2003). Genetic association and cellular function of MC1R variant alleles in human pigmentation. *Ann N Y Acad Sci*, 994, 348-58.

Sturm, R. A., Duffy, D. L., Zhao, Z .Z., Leite, F. P., Stark, M. S., Hayward, N. K., Martin, N. G., Montgomery, G. W. (2008). A single SNP in an evolutionary conserved region within intron 86 of the HERC2 gene determines human blue-brown eye color. Am J Hum Genet, 82(2), 424-31.

Tadokoro, T., Kobayashi, N., Zmuzka, B. Z., Ito, S., Wakamatsu, K., Yamaguchi, Y., Korossy, K. S., Miller, S. A., Beer, J. Z. & Hearing, V. J. (2003). UV-induced DNA damage and melanin content in human skin differing in racial/ethnic origin. *FASEB J*, 17, 1177-9.

TadokoroA, T., Yamaguchi, Y., Batzer, J., Coelho, S. G., Zmudzak, B. Z., Miller, S. A., Wolber, R., Beer, J. Z. & Hearing, V. J. (2005). Mechanisms of skin tanning in different racial/ethnic groups in response to ultraviolet radiation. *J Invest Dermatol*, 124, 1326-32.

Takeuchi, S., Zhang, W., Wakamatsu, K., Ito, S., Hearing, V. J., Kraemer, K. H., & Brash, D.E. (2004). Melanin acts as a potent UVB photosensitizer to cause an atypical mode of cell death in murine skin. *Proc Nat Acad Sci USA*, 101, 42, 15076-81.

Thomas, N. E., Edmiston, S. N., Alexander, A., Millikan, R. C., Groben, .P. A, Hao, H., Tolbert, D., Berwick, M., Busam, K., Begg, C. B., Mattingly, D., Ollila, D.W., Tse, C. K., Hummer, A., Lee-Taylor, J., & Conway, K. (2007). Number of nevi and early-life ambient UV exposure are associated with BRAF-mutant melanoma. *Cancer Epidemiol Biomarkers Prev*, 16, 991-7.

Thomas, N. E., Kricker, A., From, L., Busam, K., Millikan, R. C., Ritchey, M. E, Armstrong, B. K., Lee-Taylor, J., Marrett, L. D., Anton-Culver, H., Zanetti, R., Rosso, S., Gallagher, R. P., Dwyer, T., Goumas, C., Kanetsky, P. A., Begg, C. B., Orlow, I., Wilcox, H., Paine, S., & Berwick, M. (2001). Associations of cumulative sun exposure and phenotypic characteristics with histologic solar elastosis. Genes, Environment, and Melanoma Study Group. *Cancer Epidemiol Biomarkers Prev*, 19, 11, 2932-41.

Thomas, N., Berwick, M., & Cordeiro, M. (2006). Could *BRAF* mutations in melanocytic lesions arise from DNA damage induced by ultraviolet radiation. *J Invest Dermatol*, 126, 1693-1696.

van Schanke, A., Jongsma, M. J., Bisschop, R., van Venrooij, G. M., Rebel, H., & de Gruijl, F. R. (2005). Single UVB overexposure stimulates melanocyte proliferation in murine skin, in contrast to fractionated or UVA-1 exposure. *J Invest Dermatol*, 124, 241-7.

van Schanke, A., van Venrooij, G. M., Jongsma, M. J., Banus, H. A., Mullenders, L. H., van Kranen, H. J., & de Gruijl F. R. (2006). Induction of nevi and skin tumors in Ink4a/Arf Xpa knockout mice by neonatal, intermittent, or chronic UVB exposures. *Cancer Res*, 66, 5, 2608-15.

van Steeg, H., & Kraemer, K. H. (1999). Xeroderma pigmentosum and the role of UV-induced DNA damage in skin cancer. *Mol Med Today*, 5, 2 86-94.

Veierod, M. B., Adami, H. O., Lund, E., Armstrong, B. K. & Weiderpass, E. (2011). Sun and solarium exposure and melanoma risk: effects of age, pigmentary characteristics, and nevi. *Cancer Epidemiol Biomarkers Prev*, 19, 111-20.

Wachsmuth, R. C., Gaut, R. M., Barrett, J. H., Saunders, C. L., Randerson-Moor, J. A., Eldridge, A., Martin, N. G., Bishop, T. D. & Newton-Bishop, J. A. (2001). Heritability and gene-environment interactions for melanocytic nevus density examined in a U.K. adolescent twin study. *J Invest Dermatol*, 117, 348-52.

Walker, G. J., Kimlin, M.G., Hacker, E., Ravishankar, S., Muller, H. K., Beermann, F., Hayward, N. K. (2009). Murine neonatal melanocytes exhibit a heightened proliferative response to ultraviolet radiation and migrate to the epidermal basal layer. *J Invest Dermatol*, 129, 1, 184-9

Wang, Y., Digiovanna, J. J., Stern, J. B., Hornyak, T. J., Raffeld, M., Khan, S. G., Oh, K. S., Hollander, M. C., Dennis, P. A., & Kraemer, K. H. (2009). Evidence of ultraviolet type mutations in xeroderma pigmentosum melanomas. *Proc Natl Acad Sci USA*, 106, 15, 6279-84.

Wang, H. T., Choi, B., Tang, M. S. (2010). Melanocytes are deficient in repair of oxidative DNA damage and UV-induced photoproducts. *Proc Natl Acad Sci USA*, 107, 27, 12180-5.

Weiner, L., Han, R., Scicchitano, B. M., Li, J., Hasegawa, K., Grossi, M., Lee, D., & Brissette, J. L. (2007). Dedicated epithelial recipient cells determine pigmentation patterns. *Cell* 130, 5, 932-42.

Whiteman, D. & Green, A. (1999). The pathogenesis of melanoma induced by ultraviolet radiation. *N Engl J Med*, 341, 766-7.

Whiteman, D. C., Whiteman, C. A. & Green, A. C. (2001). Childhood sun exposure as a risk factor for melanoma: a systematic review of epidemiologic studies. *Cancer Causes Control*, 12, 69-82.

Whiteman, D. C., Watt, P., Purdue, D. M., Hughes, M. C., Hayward, N. K. & Green, A. C. (2003) Melanocytic nevi, solar keratoses, and divergent pathways to cutaneous melanoma. *J Natl Cancer Inst*, 95, 806-12.

Wolnicka-Glubisz, A., Damsker, J., Constant, S., Corn, S., De Fabo, E., Noonan, F. (2007). Deficient inflammatory response to UV radiation in neonatal mice. *J Leukoc Biol*, 81, 6, 1352-61.

Wood, S. R., Berwick, M., Ley, R. D., Walter, R. B., Setlow, R. B., Timmins, G. S. (2006). UV causation of melanoma in Xiphophorus is dominated by melanin photosensitized oxidant production. *Proc Natl Acad Sci USA*, 103, 11, 4111-5.

Yamaguchi, Y., Coelho, S. G., Zmudzka, B. Z., Takahashi, K., Beer, J. Z., Hearing, V. J., & Miller, S. A. (2008). Cyclobutane pyrimidine dimer formation and p53 production in human skin after repeated UV irradiation. *Exp Dermatol*, [Epub ahead of print].

Yamazaki, F., Okamoto, H., Miyauchi-Hashimoto, H., Matsumura, Y., Itoh, T., Tanaka, K., Kunisada, T., & Horio, T. (2004). XPA gene-deficient, SCF-transgenic mice with epidermal melanin are resistant to UV-induced carcinogenesis. *J Invest Dermatol*, 123, 1, 220-8.

Yamazaki, F., Okamoto, H., Matsumura, Y., Tanaka, K., Kunisada, T., & Horio, T. (2005). Development of a new mouse model (xeroderma pigmentosum a-deficient, stem cell factor-transgenic) of ultraviolet B-induced melanoma. *J Invest Dermatol*, 125, 3, 521-5.

Yang, G., Curley, D., Bosenberg, M., & Tsao, H. (2007). Loss of xeroderma pigmentosum C (Xpc) enhances melanoma photocarcinogenesis in Ink4a-Arf-nudeficient mice. *Cancer Res*, 67, 12, 5649-5657.

Zaidi, M. R., Davis, S., Noonan, F. P., Graff-Cherry, C., Hawley, T. S., Walker, R. L., Feigenbaum, L., Fuchs, E., Lyakh, L., Young, H. A., Hornyak, T. J., Arnheiter, H., Trinchieri, G., Meltzer, P. S., De Fabo, E. C., & Merlino, G. (2011). Interferon-γ links ultraviolet radiation to melanomagenesis in mice. *Nature*, 469, 7331, 548-53.

Zattra, E., Fortina, A.B., Bordignon, M., Piaserico, S., & Alaibac, M. (2009). Immunosuppression and melanocyte proliferation. *Melanoma Res*, 19, 2, 63-8.

Zhu, G., Duffy, D. L., Eldridge, A., Grace, M., Mayne, C., O'Gorman, L., Aitken, J. F., Neale, M. C., Hayward, N. K., Green, A. C. & Martin, N. G. (1999). A major quantitative-trait locus for mole density is linked to the familial melanoma gene CDKN2A: a maximum-likelihood combined linkage and association analysis in twins and their sibs. *Am J Hum Genet*, 65, 483-92.

Zhu, G., Montgomery, G. W., James, M. R., Trent, J. M., Hayward, N. K., Martin, N. G. & Duffy, D. L. (2007). A genome-wide scan for naevus count: linkage to CDKN2A and to other chromosome regions. *Eur J Hum Genet*, 15, 94-102.

11

Dual Roles of the Melanoma CAM (MelCAM/METCAM) in Malignant Progression of Melanoma

Guang-Jer Wu
Department of Microbiology and Immunology and The Emory Winship Cancer Institute, Emory University School of Medicine, Atlanta, USA

1. Introduction

1.1 General properties and functions of METCAM/MUC18

Human *METCAM* (*huMETCAM*), a *CAM* in the immunoglobulin-like gene superfamily, is an integral membrane glycoprotein. Alternative names for *METCAM* are *MUC18* [1], *CD146* [2], *MCAM* [3], *MelCAM* [4], *A32* [5], and *S-endo 1* [6]. To avoid confusion with mucins and to reflect its biological functions, we have renamed *MUC18* as *METCAM* (*met*astasis *CAM*), which means an immunoglobulin-like *CAM* that affects or regulates metastasis [7]. The *huMETCAM* has 646 amino acids that include a N-terminal extra-cellular domain of 558 amino acids, which has 28 amino acids characteristic of a signal peptide sequence at its N-terminus, a transmembrane domain of 24 amino acids (amino acid #559-583), and a cytoplasmic domain of 64 amino acids at the C-terminus. *HuMETCAM* has eight putative N-glycosylation sites (*Asn-X-Ser/Thr*), of which six are conserved, and are heavily glycosylated and sialylated resulting in an apparent molecular weight of 113,000-150,000. The extra-cellular domain of the protein comprises five immunoglobulin-like domains (V-V-C2-C2-C2) [1, 7] and an X domain [7]. The cytoplasmic tail contains peptide sequences that will potentially be phosphorylated by protein kinase A (*PKA*), protein kinase C (*PKC*), and casein kinase 2 (*CK 2*) [1, 7-8]. My lab has also cloned and sequenced the mouse *METCAM* (*moMETCAM*) cDNA, which contains 648 amino acids with a 76.2% identity with *huMETCAM*, suggesting that *moMETCAM* is likely to have biochemical properties and biological functions similar to the human counter part [9]. The structure of the *huMETCAM* protein is depicted in Fig. 1, suggesting that *METCAM*, similar to most *CAMs*, plays an active role in mediating cell-cell and cell-extracellular interactions, crosstalk with many intracellular signaling pathways, and modulating the social behaviors of cells [7].

It is now well documented that although tissue specific signatures exist in different cancer types, cancers from different tissues also express some common genes [10-12]. One group of them is cell adhesion molecules (*CAMs*). *CAMs* do not merely act as a molecular glue to hold together homotypic cells in a specific tissue or to facilitate interactions of heterotypic cells; *CAMs* also actively govern the social behaviors of cells by affecting the adhesion status of cells and modulating cell signaling [13]. They control cell motility and invasiveness by

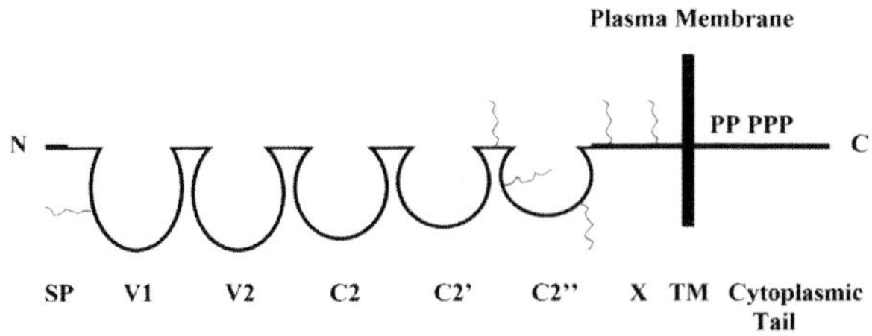

Fig. 1. **HuMETCAM protein structure.** SP stands for signal peptide sequence, V1, V2, C2, C2′, C2″ for five Ig-like domains (each held by a disulfide bond) and X for one domain (without any disulfide bond) in the extracellular region, and TM for transmembrane domain. P stands for five potential phosphorylation sites (one for PKA, three for PKC, and one for CK2) in the cytoplasmic tail. The six conserved N-glycosylation sites are shown as wiggled lines in the extracellular domains of V1, between C2′ and C2″, C2″, and X.

mediating the remodeling of cytoskeleton [13]. They also actively mediate the cell-to-cell and cell-to-extracellular matrix interactions to allow cells to constantly respond to physiological fluctuations and to alter/remodel the surrounding microenvironment for survival [14]. They do so by crosstalk with cellular surface growth factor receptors, which interact with growth factors that may be secreted from stromal cells or released from circulation and embedded in the extracellular matrix [13-14]. Thus an altered expression of *CAMs* affects the motility and invasiveness of many tumor cells *in vitro* and metastasis *in vivo* [13-14]. *CAMs* also play an important role in the favorable soil that provides a proper microenvironment at a suitable period to awaken the dormant metastatic tumor cells to enter into an aggressive growth phase. Actually, the metastatic potential of a tumor cell, as documented in many carcinomas, is the consequence of a complex participation of many over- and under-expressed *CAMs* [13-14]. Based on the above information, aberrant expression of *huMETCAM* may also affect the motility and invasiveness of many tumor cells *in vitro* and metastasis *in vivo*. It is logical to hypothesize that *HuMETCAM* should play an important role in regulating the malignant progression of many cancer types [7, 13]. Nevertheless, in this chapter we will only review its positive or negative roles in the tumorigenesis and metastasis of human and mouse melanoma cells.

HuMETCAM is expressed in a limited number of normal tissues, such as hair follicular cells, smooth muscle cells, endothelial cells, cerebellum, normal mammary epithelial cells, basal cells of the lung, activated T cells, intermediate trophoblast, [15] and normal nasopharyngeal epithelial cells [16]. The protein is not expressed in melanocyte, but it is overly expressed in most (67%) malignant melanoma cells [1]. Thus it was postulated to play a role in the progression of human melanoma. Likewise, the expression of mouse METCAM (moMETCAM) was positively correlated with the metastatic ability of several mouse melanoma cell lines [9]. Since then, it has been proven that METCAM is not just correlative with the progression of melanoma, but also is capable of inducing non-metastatic melanoma cell lines to metastasize in various mouse models. First, it was shown that the stable ectopic expression of the huMETCAM cDNA gene in three non-metastatic human cutaneous melanoma cell lines increases the metastatic abilities of these cell lines in immune-deficient xenograft mouse models [3,17]. Second, it was shown that the stable ectopic expression of moMETCAM cDNA in two low-tumorigenic and low-metastatic mouse melanoma cell lines, K10 ($tumor^-/met^{low}$) and K3 ($tumor^+/met^{low}$), increases their metastatic abilities in immune-competent syngeneic C3H brown mice [18].

However, METCAM enables both human and mouse melanoma cells to metastasize only under an experimental metastasis assay (tail vein injection), not under a spontaneous metastasis assay (subcutaneous injection). In addition, the ectopic expression of METCAM in METCAM-minus melanoma cell lines has no effect or a slight suppressive effect on the tumorigenesis. Taken together, this suggests that METCAM promotes the metastasis of melanoma cells only at later stages of progression (it has been found that fibroblast growth factor-2 initiates the metastatic process) [19].

Recently, we further investigated the effect of moMETCAM expression on tumorigenesis and metastasis of a different mouse melanoma subline #9 of K1735 (K1735-9 or K9), which is also METCAM-minus and lowly metastatic, but has a highly tumorigenic phenotype (tumor^{+++}/met^{low}), in the syngeneic C3H mouse model. We tested the effect of ectopic expression of moMETCAM on *in vitro* growth rate, motility, and invasiveness and *in vivo* subcutaneous tumor growth and pulmonary metastasis. Similar to the two isogenic K10 and K3 sublines, ectopic expression of METCAM did not significantly affect *in vitro* growth rate, but greatly increased *in vitro* motility and invasiveness. Surprisingly, unlike K10 and K3 sublines, ectopic expression of METCAM in K9 cells decreased tumorigenicity and suppressed their ability to establish pulmonary nodules. The suppressive effect of METCAM is not limited to the K9 mouse melanoma cell line, but is also observed in two human ovarian cancer cell lines (our unpublished results).

We suggest that METCAM-mediated tumorigenesis and metastasis of melanoma cells and other cancer cells is dependent on intrinsic co-factors of different K1735 sublines and cancer types. The establishment of an immune-competent syngeneic mouse model for the METCAM-mediated progression is physiologically more relevant to and should provide knowledge more applicable to clinical melanoma than immune-deficient xenograft mouse models. The putative mechanisms of METCAM-mediated promotion/suppression of melanoma progression will also be discussed.

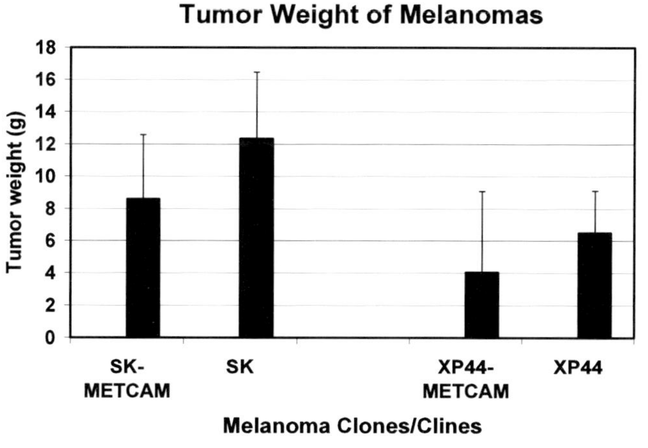

Fig. 2. Effect of over-expression of huMETCAM on tumor formation of two human melanoma cell lines, SK and XP-44 [17]. SK-METCAM and XP44-METCAM were two clones of human melanoma cell lines, SK and XP44, respectively, which were transfected with huMETCAM and expressed a high level of huMETCAM. Statistical analysis was not possible because detailed data was not provided.

2. Metcam and melanoma tumorigenesis

Over-expression of *METCAM* had a slight tumor suppression effect on tumorigenesis of human melanoma cells in xenograft mice [17], as shown in Fig. 2, but it had no effect on tumorigenesis of two sublines, #3 (K3) and #10 (K10), of the mouse melanoma cell line K1735 in syngeneic mice [18]. Fig. 3 only shows the effect of *moMETCAM* on the tumorigenesis of K3.

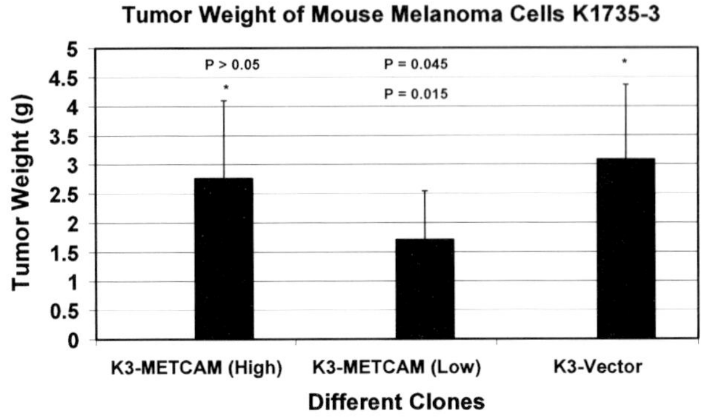

Fig. 3. Effect of over-expression of moMETCAM on tumor formation of a mouse melanoma cell line K1735 subline #3 (K3) [18]. K3-METCAM (High) and K3-METCAM (Low) were two K3 clones transfected with moMETCAM cDNA that expressed a high and a low level of moMETCAM, respectively. K3-Vector, as a negative control, was one clone transfected with an empty vector and did not express any moMETCAM. Asterisks show the results of the clone used as the references for the P-value calculation. The P-values should be compared with the reference (asterisk) on the same row.

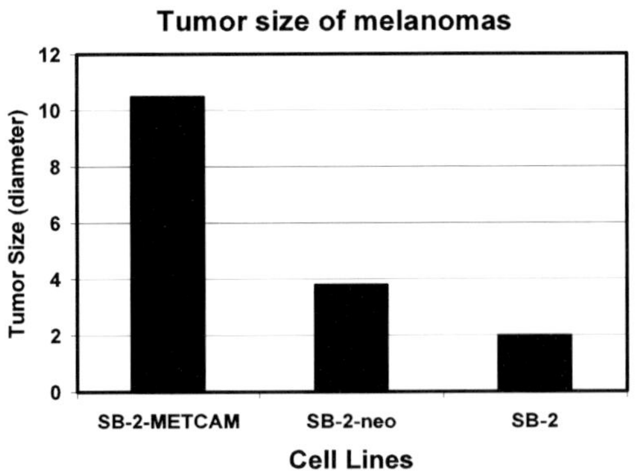

Fig. 4. Effect of over-expression of huMETCAM on tumor formation of a human melanoma cell line SB-2 [3]. SB-2 is a human melanoma cell line, which did not express any huMETCAM. SB-2-neo is the SB-2 cells transected with the empty vector, as a negative control. SB-2-METCAM is a clone of the SB-2 cells which were transfected with huMETCAM cDNA and expressed a high level of huMETCAM. Since tumor formation was only shown in one nude mouse for each clone, statistical analysis was not possible.

Only one group showed that over-expression of *METCAM* increased tumorigenesis of a human melanoma cell line in xenograft mice [3]; however the results were questionable because only the tumorigenicity of one mouse injected with *METCAM*-expressing clone and one mouse with control cells was shown and thus no standard deviations were indicated and no statistical analysis done, as shown in Fig. 4.

The most convincing evidence for its tumor suppressor effect is in the subline #9 of the mouse melanoma cell line *K1735* (*K1735-9 or K9*) in syngeneic *C3H* mice. Over-expression of *moMETCAM* in the *K9* cells significantly decreased subcutaneous tumorigenesis in immunocompetent syngeneic *C3H* mice [20-21], as shown in Fig. 5.

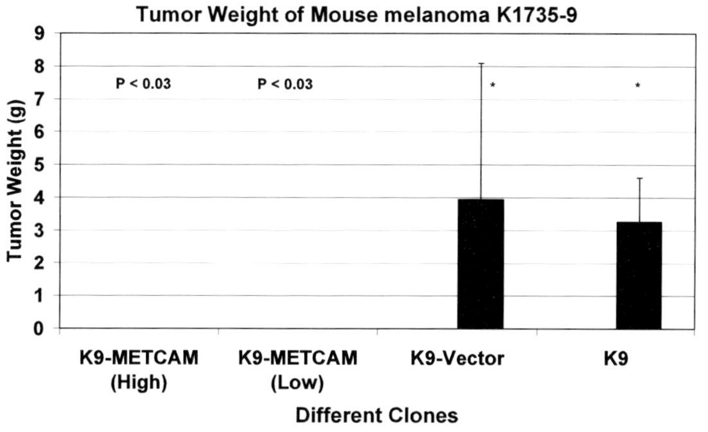

Fig. 5. Effect of over-expression of moMETCAM on tumor formation of a mouse melanoma K1735 subline #9 (K1735-9 or K9) in immune competent syngeneic C3H mice [20-21]. K9-METCAM (High) and K9-METCAM (Low) were two transfected clones, which expressed a high and a low level of moMETCAM, respectively. K9-Vector was one clone transfected with the empty vector, as a negative control. K9 was the K1735 subline #9 cells, also as a negative control. Both K9-Vector and K9 did not express any moMETCAM.

3. Metcam and melanoma metastasis

HuMETCAM/MUC18 was originally found to be abundantly expressed on the cellular surface of most malignant human melanomas; since then, it has been postulated to play a role in the progression of human melanoma [1]. This notion is also supported by the positive correlation of *moMETCAM* expression with the metastatic ability of several mouse melanoma cells lines [9]. Definitive proof comes from the results that the stable, ectopic expression of the *huMETCAM* cDNA gene in three non-metastatic human cutaneous melanoma cell lines increases the metastatic abilities of these cell lines in immune-deficient mouse models [3, 17]. Furthermore, the stable, ectopic expression of *moMETCAM* cDNA in two low-metastatic mouse melanoma cell lines increases the metastatic abilities of these cell lines in immune-competent syngeneic mice [18], as shown in Figs. 6 & 7.

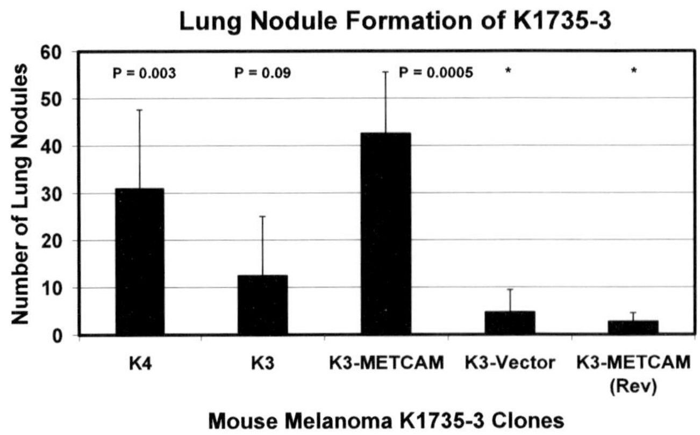

Fig. 6. Enforced expression of moMETCAM increased lung nodule formation of mouse melanoma K1735-3 (K3) cells in syngeneic C3H mice. K4, the highly tumorigenic and metastatic subline #4 of K1735 (Tumor+++/Methigh), was used as a positive control. K3-METCAM clone expressed a high level of moMETCAM. K3, K3-Vector, and K3-METCAM (Rev), in which the moMETCAM cDNA was inserted into the expression vector in anti-sense orientation, were the control clones that did not express any moMETCAM.

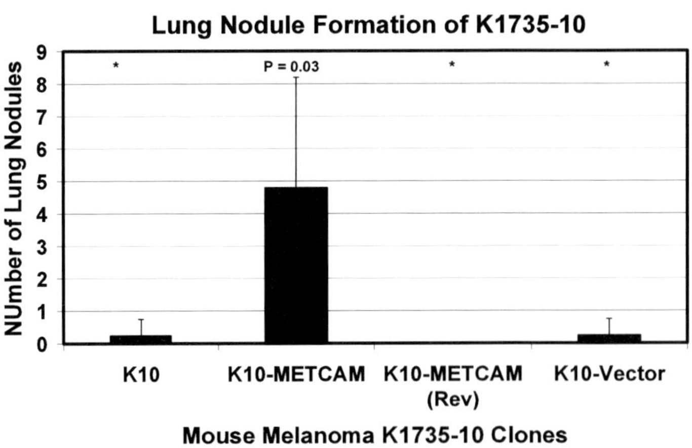

Fig. 7. Enforced expression of moMETCAM increased lung nodule formation of mouse melanoma K1735-10 (K10) cells in syngeneic C3H mice. The K10-METCAM clone expressed a high level of moMETCAM. K10, K10-Vector, and K10-METCAM (Rev), in which the moMETCAM cDNA was inserted into the expression vector in anti-sense orientation, were the control clones that did not express any moMETCAM.

However, *METCAM* enables melanoma cells to establish pulmonary metastasis only when the cells are injected into the tail vein (experimental metastasis assay) [3, 17-18], thus bypassing the initial stages of metastasis. No metastasis was found when *METCAM*-expressing melanoma cells were injected subcutaneously (spontaneous metastasis assay) either in immune-deficient mouse models [3, 17] or in immune-competent syngeneic mouse models [18]. Taken together, *METCAM* promotes the metastasis of melanoma cells, but at later stages [7]; thus over-expression of *METCAM* did not initiate the metastasis of melanoma cells. This result is consistent with the recent observation that fibroblast growth factor 2, but not *huMETCAM*, nor integrin, actually initiates the malignant progression of subcutaneous melanocyte into melanoma [19].

METCAM increases the progression of most melanoma cell lines with the exception of one mouse melanoma subline, K1735-9. We found over-expression of *moMETCAM* in one mouse melanoma *K1735* subline #9 (K1735-9 or *K9*) decreased pulmonary lung nodule formation when cells were injected into tail veins (experimental metastasis test) [20-21], as shown in Fig. 8.

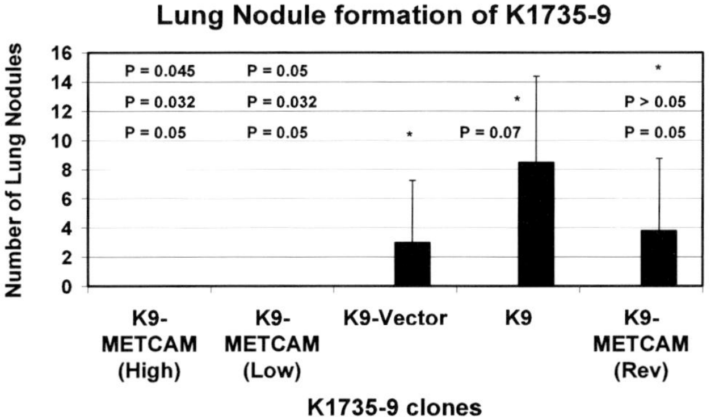

Fig. 8. Enforced expression of moMETCAM suppressed lung nodule formation of mouse melanoma K1735-9 (K9) cells in syngeneic C3H mice. Clones K9-METCAM (High) and K9-METCAM (Low) clones expressed high and low levels of moMETCAM, respectively. K9-Vector, K9, and K9-METCAM (Rev), in which the moMETCAM cDNA was inserted into the expression vector in anti-sense orientation, were the control clones that did not express any moMETCAM.

Summary

Table 1 summarizes the possible role of *METCAM* in the tumorigenesis and metastasis of various melanoma cells.

Melanoma cells	Tumorigenesis	Metastasis	References
Clinical melanoma and human melanoma cell lines	No effect	Increasing (effect is in the late stages)	3, 17
Mouse melanoma K1735 sublines #3 and #10	No effect or slight suppression	Increasing (effect is in the late stages)	9, 18
Mouse melanoma K1735 subline #9	Suppression	Suppression	20, 21

Table 1. The role of *METCAM* in the tumorigenesis and metastasis of melanoma cells.

As shown in Table 1, *huMETCAM* does not affect the tumorigenesis of most melanoma cell lines, but it increases metastasis, thus is a metastatic gene, for most melanoma cell lines. However, in one case it acts as a tumor suppressor and a metastasis suppressor for a mouse melanoma subline.

4. Mechanisms of metcam-mediated melanoma progression

How does *METCAM* mediate or regulate tumorigenesis and metastasis of melanoma cells? We may be able to find some common clues to begin understanding its mechanisms by deducing knowledge learned from the tumorigenesis of other tumors [10-14, 22] and the *huMETCAM*-mediated progression of melanoma [23-25] and tumor angiogenesis [2, 26-29].
First, the transcriptional expression of *METCAM* gene may be regulated by *PKA/CREB* (cAMP-responsive element binding protein), *AP-2α* [24-25] and other transcription factors, such as *SP-1, c-Myb, N-Oct2, ETs, CArG, Egr-1,* and transcription factors binding to insulin response elements [7]. Among these potential regulators, it is well documented that the *AP-2α* transcription factor plays a crucial tumor suppressor role in the progression of melanoma [25]. However, the roles of other transcription regulators, tissue specific enhancers and repressors, epigenetic control, and control at the level of chromatin remodeling of the gene have still yet to be investigated [7].
Second, since the cytoplasmic tail of *METCAM* contains consensus sequences potentially to be phosphorylated by *PKA, PKC,* and *CK2,* it may manifest its functions by cross-talk with various signaling pathways mediated by these protein kinases [7]. For example, *METCAM* expression in melanoma cells is reciprocally regulated by *AKT,* in which *AKT* up-regulates the level *METCAM* and over-expression of *METCAM* activates endogenous *AKT,* which in turn inhibits apoptosis and increases survival ability [23]. However the detailed mechanism of how *AKT* up-regulates the expression of *METCAM* has not been worked out. *PKA, PKC,* and *CK2* may phosphorylate the cytoplasmic tail of *METCAM,* which then facilitates its interaction with *FAK,* thus promoting cytoskeleton remodeling. Alternatively, after phosphorylation of its cytoplasmic tail by these protein kinases, *METCAM* may interact with the downstream effectors of *Ras,* activating *ERK* and *JNK,* which in turn may transcriptionally activate the expression of *AKT* or other genes that promote the proliferation and angiogenesis of tumor cells. Though *METCAM* has not been shown to be a substrate of *CK2,* which has been shown to phosphorylate other *CAMs,* such as *CD44, E-cadherin, L1-CAM,* and *vitronectin,* it is also likely that *CK2* may be able to phosphorylate *METCAM* and link it to *AKT* and affect the proliferation, survival and other tumorigenesis-related functions of tumor cells [30].
Third, after the engagement of *METCAM* with the ligand(s) or extracellular matrix, it may transmit the outside-in signals into tumor cells by activating *FAK* and the downstream signaling components, promoting cytoskeleton remodeling and increasing tumor cell motility and invasiveness [2, 7].
Fourth, from what we know about the roles of other *CAMs* in the progression of other tumors [10-14, 22], it is logical to postulate that *METCAM* may affect cancer cell progression by cross-talk with signaling pathways that affect apoptosis, survival and proliferation and angiogenesis of tumor cells [7, 13, 22]. Thus *METCAM* may affect tumorigenesis and metastasis by altering the expression of various indexes in apoptosis, survival signaling, proliferation signaling, and angiogenesis. To support this notion, we have found that *METCAM* promotes the progression of prostate cancer cells by increasing proliferative

ability (with elevated levels of *Ki67* and *PCNA*), by increasing survival ability (with an elevated level of phosphorylated *AKT*), and by increasing angiogenic ability (with elevated levels of *VEGF*, *VEGFR2*, and *CD31*) [31]; but it has no effect on the process of apoptosis. In fact, *METCAM* promotes the progression of melanoma cells differently by preventing the apoptosis of melanoma cells [32] and reciprocally affecting the expression of a survival index, phospho-*AKT* [23]. Further systematic studies by using specific RNAi's to knockdown the downstream effectors one by one in *METCAM*-expressing clones may be necessary to further understand this aspect of the mechanism.

Fifth, *METCAM* may mediate the hematogenous spreading of melanoma cells, which had been implicated by its expression in endothelial cells, as well as in malignant melanoma cells [26]. Furthermore it has been shown to be present in the junctions of endothelial cells [27-28] and essential for tumor angiogenesis in at least three tumor cell lines [29] and human prostate cancer *LNCaP* cells [31, 33]. It is highly likely that *METCAM* expression may promote the hematogenous spreading of melanoma cells. However, it is not known if *METCAM* plays a role in the lymphatic spread of cancer cells. Recent results from one group showed that *METCAM* is one of the lymphatic metastasis-associated genes, which is up-regulated in malignant mouse hepatocarcinoma [34]; suggesting that *METCAM* may also play a role in promoting lymphatic metastasis of melanoma cells. But the details of how *METCAM* mediates hematogenous or lymphatic spreading of melanoma cells have still yet to be investigated. Labeling the cells with viable dyes and following the process in real time by using a non-intruding, but highly photo-penetrating imaging method of photoacoustic tomography (PAT) [35-36] may be useful for monitoring each step in the *METCAM*-mediated progression. For the *METCAM*-mediated dynamic spreading of melanoma cells *in vivo*, the PAT imaging method coupled with using hairless syngeneic mouse animal models [37] should reveal the process more clearly and in real time.

Sixth, *METCAM* has been shown to express in normal mesenchymal cells (smooth muscle, endothelium, and Schwann cells) in the tissue stroma and to be a marker for the mesenchymal stem cells [38]. *METCAM* may play an important role in regulating melanoma dormancy or awakening, driving or preventing melanoma cells to pre-metastatic niche, and formatting a microenvironment for favorable or unfavorable melanoma growth in secondary sites.

Seventh, *METCAM* may affect the progression of cancer cells by interactions with the host immune system, which, however, has been shown to have a paradoxical role in tumor progression [39]. Recently one group has shown that a subset of host B lymphocytes may control melanoma metastasis through METCAM-dependent interaction [40]. On the other hand, it is highly likely that the tumor suppression effect of *METCAM* expression in melanoma *K1735-9* subline may be due to the interaction of *METCAM*-expressing cells with the host immune defense system in the immunocompetent syngeneic *C3H* brown mouse, since the intrinsic motility and invasiveness of mouse melanoma *K1735-9* was increased by *METCAM* expression [20-21]. For example, the surface *METCAM* expressed in this particular melanoma cell line may have a homophilic interaction with the *NK* cells, which also express *METCAM*, and enhance the cytotoxic functions of *NK* cells [41]. This hypothesis should be testable by studying the METCAM-mediated progression of METCAM-expressing K1735-9 cells in mice treated with antibodies against *CD4+T* cells, *CD8+T* cells, or *NK* cells, or mice with a combined treatment with the antibodies to impair the functions of these immune cells.

Eighth, malignant progression of cancer cells has been shown to associate with abnormal glycosylation, resulting in expression of altered carbohydrate determinants [42]. Thus, the glycosylated status of *METCAM* in different cancer types may be different from normal cells, thus manifesting positive or negative effect on the progression of melanoma cells. This aspect of the METCAM-mediate cancer progression has not been well studied, but is especially intriguing since METCAM possesses six conserved N-glycosylation sites in the extracellular domain [7-9].

We should always keep in mind that the mechanisms of *METCAM*-mediated melanoma progression may be slightly different in different melanoma cell lines due to their different intrinsic properties, which provide different co-factors and/or different ligand(s) that either positively or negatively regulate the *METCAM*-mediated tumorigenesis and metastasis. To further understand the role of *METCAM* in these processes, it is essential to identify the co-factors and the *METCAM*-cognate heterophilic ligand(s), which modulate the biological functions of *METCAM*. The endeavor in this direction appears to be promising: from our preliminary attempts we may have successfully found a possible candidate of METCAM's heterophilic ligand in *METCAM*-expressing human melanoma SK-Mel-28 cells [7].

Mechanisms of *METCAM*-mediated negative role in the progression of melanoma cells have not been studied at all. In some cancers does *METCAM* behave like E-cadherin, which always plays a negative role in the tumorigenesis and metastasis of melanoma as well as most epithelial cancer cells [13] But even *E-cadherin* may function differently in different cancer cells. For example, its expression is temporally different and correlates with different stages during the progression of ovarian cancer [43]: *E-cadherin* is not expressed in the ovarian surface epithelial cells, but is expressed in premalignant lesions and in well-differentiated tumors, and finally is not expressed in late-stage invasive tumors [43]. Alternatively, METCAM may behave differently from *E-cadherin* by being modulated by different cofactors or ligands, which are expressed at different stages of the cancer. The tumor suppressor role of *METCAM* is not restricted to the mouse melanoma K9 subline and it was first suggested in breast cancer cells [44]; however, the tumor suppression of METCAM in breast cancer cell lines could not be reproduced [45]. Recently we also found the tumor suppressor role of METCAM in two human ovarian cancer cell lines [46]. The tumor suppressor role of METCAM in ovarian cancer cells is different from mouse melanoma subline K9 in that the *METCAM* expression suppressed the intrinsic motility and invasiveness of human ovarian cancer cells [46]. Our preliminary results appear to suggest an alternative mechanism that a soluble form of *METCAM*, which is produced by *MMPs* in the METCAM-expressing cells, may mediate the suppressive effect in ovarian cancer cells, similar to the production of a soluble form of *P-cadherin* by the induced MMPs in breast cancer cells, which then dictates, instead of suppresses, the aggressive behavior of the breast cancer cells [47].

5. Conclusion and clinical applications

METCAM may have a key positive function in the progression of most melanoma cell lines. On the other hand, it may also have a key function in suppressing the progression of a few melanoma cell lines. To further understand its mechanisms in these processes, it is crucial to define its functional domains, identify its cognate ligand(s) and cofactor regulators, and study its cross-talk with members of various signaling pathways [7]. These model systems may be useful for real time observation of the dynamic process of cancer progression by using a non-intrusive and high photo-penetrating imaging system, such as the newly developed photoacoustic tomography (*PAT*), to further understanding the process in mouse models [35-36]. The knowledge gained would also be useful for designing effective means to decrease or even to block the metastatic potential of these cancers. Along these lines, preclinical trials using a fully humanized anti-*METCAM* antibody against melanoma growth and metastasis [48-49] and using a mouse anti-*METCAM* monoclonal antibody against angiogenesis and tumor growth of hepatocarcinoma, leiomyosarcoma, and pancreatic cancer [29] have been successfully demonstrated. Alternatively, small soluble peptides derived from *METCAM* may also be useful for blocking the tumor formation and tumor angiogenesis of melanoma cells [33, 50-51]. The attachment of these reagents to nanoparticles may be another alternative for therapeutic use [52].

6. Acknowledgement

I thank Mr. Jonathan C. - Y. Wu for critical reading of the manuscript and proof reading of the English.

7. References

[1] Lehmann, J. M., Reithmuller, G., Johnson, J. P. 1989, "MUC18, a marker of tumor progression in human melanoma." Proc. Natl. Acad. Sci. USA, 86, 9891-9895.

[2] Anfosso, F., Bardin, N., Vivier, E., Sabatier, F., Sampol, J., Dignat-George, F., 2001, "Outside-in signaling pathway linked to CD146 engagement in human endothelial cells." J. Biol. Chem., 276, 1564-1569.

[3] Xie, S., Luca, M., Huang, S., Gutman, M., Reich, R., Johnson, J. P., Bar-Eli, M. 1997, "Expression of MCAM/MCU18 by human melanoma cells leads to increased tumor growth and metastasis." Cancer Research, 57, 2295-2303.

[4] Shih, I. M., Elder, D. E., Hsu, M. Y., Herlyn, M. 1994, "Regulation of Mel-CAM/MUC18 expression on melanocytes of different stages of tumor progression by normal keratinocytes." Am. J. Pathol., 145, 837-845.

[5] Shih, I. M., Elder, D. E., Speicher, D., Johnson, J. P., and Herlyn, M. 1994, "Isolation and functional characterization of the A32 melanoma-associated antigen." Cancer Research, 54, 2514-2520.

[6] Bardin, N., George, F., Mutin, M., Brisson, C., Horschowski, N., Frances, V., Lesaule, G., Sampol, J. 1996, "S-endo1, a pan-endothelial monoclonal antibody recognizing a novel human endothelial antigen." Tissue Antigens, 48, 531-539.

[7] Wu, G. - J. 2005, "METCAM/MUC18 expression and cancer metastasis." Current Genomics, 6, 333-349.

[8] Wu, G. – J., Wu, M. - W. H., Wang, S. W., Liu, Z., Peng, Q., Qu, P., Yang, H., Varma, V. A., Sun, Q., Petros, J. A., Lim. S., and Amin, M. B. 2001, "Isolation and characterization of the major form of human MUC18 cDNA gene and correlation of MUC18 over-expression in prostate cancer cells and tissues with malignant progression." Gene, 279, 17-31.

[9] Yang, H. Wu, M. - W. H., Wang, S. W., Liu, Z., Wu, G. - J. 2001, "Isolation and characterization of murine MUC18 cDNA, and correlation of its expression in murine melanoma cell lines with their metastatic ability." Gene, 265, 133-145.

[10] Vogelstein, B., Kinzler, K. W. 2004, "Cancer genes and the pathways they control." Nature Medicine, 10, 789-799.
[11] Christofori, G. 2006, "New signals from the invasive front." Nature, 44, 444-450.
[12] Gupta, G. P. and Massague, J. 2006, "Cancer metastasis: building a frame work." Cell, 127, 679-695.
[13] Cavallaro, U., Christofori, G. 2005, "Cell adhesion and signaling by cadherins and Ig-CAMs in cancer." Nature Reviews/Cancer, 4, 118-132.
[14] Chambers, A., Groom, A. C. and MacDonald, I. C. 2002, "Dissemination and growth of cancer cells in metastatic sites." Nature Reviews/Cancer 2, 563-572.
[15] Shih, I. M. 1999, "The role of CD146 (MelCAM), in biology and pathology." Am. J. Pathol., 189, 4-11.
[16] Lin, J. C., Chiang, C. F., Wang, S. W., Wang, W. Y., Kwan, P. C., and Wu, G. - J. 2010, "Decreased expression of METCAM/MUC18 correlates with the appearance of, but its increased expression with metastasis of nasopharyngeal carcinoma." (Submitted).
[17] Schlagbauer-Wadl, H., Jansen, B., Muller, M., Polterauer, P., Wolff, K., Eichler, H.-G., Pehamberger, H, Konak, E., and Johnson, J. P. 1999, "Influence of MUC18/MCAM/CD146 expression on human melanoma growth and metastasis in SCID mice." Int. J. Cancer, 81, 951-955.
[18] Wu, G. - J., Fu, P., Wang, S. W., and Wu, M. - W. H. 2008, "Enforced expression of MCAM/MUC18 increases *in vitro* motility and invasiveness and *in vivo* metastasis of two mouse melanoma K1735 sublines in a syngeneic mouse model." Molecular Cancer Research, 6 (11), 1666-1677.
[19] Meier, F., Caroli, U., Satyamoorthy, K., Schittek, B., Bauer, J., Berking, C., Moller, H., Maczey, E., Rassner, G., Herlyn, M., Garbe, C. 2003, "Fibroblast growth factor-2 but not Mel-CAM and/or $\alpha3$ integrin promotes progression of melanocytes to melanoma." Expt. Dermatology, 12, 296-306.
[20] Wu, G. - J., Peng, Q., Wang, S. W., Yang, H., and Wu, M. - W. H. 2001, "Effect of MUC18 expression on the in vitro invasiveness and in vivo tumorigenesis and metastasis of mouse melanoma cell lines in a syngeneic mouse model", The proceedings of the 92nd Annual Meeting of American Association for the Cancer Research, 42, p.516 Abstract # 2776.
[21] Wu, G.-J., and Wu, M. - W. H. 2011, "Ectopic expression of MCAM/MUC18 increases in vitro motility and invasiveness, but decreases tumorigenesis and metastasis of a mouse melanoma K1735-9 subline in a syngeneic mouse model." (In preparation).
[22] Hanahan, D., and Weinberg, R. A. 2000, "The hallmarks of cancer." Cell, 100, 57-70.
[23] Li, G., Kalabis, J., Xu, X., Meier, F., Oka, M., Bogenrieder, T., and Herlyn, M. 2003, "Reciprocal regulation of MelCAM and AKT in human melanoma." Oncogene 22, 6891-6899.
[24] Melnikva, V. O., Balasubramanian, K., Villares, G. J., Debroff, A. S., Zigler, M., Wang, H., Petersson, F., Price, J. E., Schroit, A., Prieto, V. G., Hung, M. – C., and Bar-Eli, M. 2009, "Crosstalk between protease-activated receptor1 and platelet-activating factor receptor regulates melanoma cell adhesion molecule (MCAM/MUC18) expression and melanoma metastasis." J. Biol. Chem., 284(42), 28845-28855.

[25] Melnikova, V. O., Debroff, A. S., Zigler, M., Villares, G. J., Braeuer, R., Wang, H., Huang, L., and Bar-Eli, M. 2010, "CREB inhibits AP-2α expression to regulate the malignant phenotype of melanoma." PLoS One, 5, e12452.

[26] Sers, C., Riethmuller, G. and Johnson, J. P. 1994, "MUC18, a melanoma-progression associated molecule, and its potential role in tumor vascularization and hematogenous spread." Cancer Research, 54, 5689-5694.

[27] Bardin, N., Anfosso, F., Masse, J., Cramer, E., Sabatier, F., LeBivic, A., Sampol, J., Dignat-George, F. 2001, "Identification of CD146 as a component of the endothelial junction involved in the control of cell-cell adhesion." Blood, 98, 3677-3684.

[28] Kang, Y., Wang, F., Feng, J., Yang, D., Yang, X. and Yan, X. 2006, "Knockdown of CD146 reduces the migration and proliferation of human endothelial cells." Cell Research, 16, 313-318.

[29] Yan, X., Lin, Y., Tang, D., Shen, Y., Yuan, M., Zhang, Z., Li, P., Xia, H., Li, L., Luo, D., Liu, Q., Mann, K., and Bader, B. L. 2003, "A novel anti-CD146 monoclonal antibody, AA98, inhibits angiogenesis and tumor growth." Blood, 102, 184-191.

[30] Maggio, F., and Pinna, L. A. 2003, "One-thousand-and-one substrates of protein kinase CK2?" FASEB J., 17, 349-368.

[31] Wu, G. - J., Wu, M. – W. H, and Liu, Y. 2011, "Enforced expression of human METCAM/MUC18 increases the tumorigenesis of human prostate cancer cells in nude mice." J Urology 185, 1504-1512.

[32] Datta, S. R., Brunet, A., and Greenberg, M.E. 1999, "Cellular survival: a play in three AKTs." Genes and Development 13, 2905-2927.

[33] Wu, G. - J., and Son, E. L. 2006, "Soluble METCAM/MUC18 blocks angiogenesis during tumor formation of human prostate cancer cells." The proceedings of the 97th Annual Meeting of American Association for the Cancer Research, 47, #252.

[34] Song, B., Tang, J. - W., Wang, B., Cui, X.- N., Zhou, C.-H., and Hou, L. 2005, Screening for lymphatic metastasis-associated genes in mouse hepatocarcinoma cell lines Hca-F and Hca-P using gene chip." Chinese J. Cancer, 24(7), 774-780.

[35] Zhang, Q., Liu, Z., Carney, P. R., Yuan, Z., Chen. H., Roper, S. N. and Jiang, H. 2008, "Non-invasive imaging of epileptic seizures in vivo using photoacoustic tomography (PAT)." Phys. Med. Biol., 53, 1921-1931.

[36] Wang, L. V. 2008, "Prospects of photoacoustic tomography." Med. Phys., 35(12), 5758-5767.

[37] Schaffer, B. S., Grayson, M. H., Wortham, J. M. Kubicek, C. B., McCleish, A. T., Prajapati, S. I., Nelon, L. D., Brady, M. M., Jung, I, Hosoyama, T., Sarro, L. M., Hanes, M.A., Rubin, B. P., Michalek, J. E., Clifford, C. B., Infante, A. J., and Keller, C. 2010, "Immune competency of a hairless mouse strain for improved preclinical studies in genetically engineered mice." Mol. Cancer Therapy, 9(8), 2354-2364.

[38] Sorrentino, A. Ferracin, M., Castelli, G., Biffoni, M., Tomaselli, G., Baiocchi, M., Fatica, A., Negrini, M., Peschle, C., and Valtieri, M. 2008, "Isolation and characterization of CD146+ multipotent mesenchymal stromal cells." Exp. Hematol., 36, 1035-1046.

[39] deVisser, K. E., Eichten, A., and Coussens, L. M. 2006, "Paradoxical roles of the immune system during cancer development." Nature Review/Cancer 6, 24-37.

[40] Staquicini, F., Tandle, A., Libutti, S. K., Sun, J., Zigler, M., Bar-Eli, M., Aliperti, F., Perez, E. C., Gershenwald, J. E., Mariano, M., Pasqualini, R., Arap, W., and Lopes, J. D. 2008, "A subset of host B lymphocytes controls melanoma metastasis through a

melanoma cell adhesion molecule/MUC18-dependent interaction: evidence from mice and humans." Cancer Research, 68(20), 8419-8428.

[41] Despoix, N., Walzer, T. Jouve, N, Blot-Chabaud, M., Bardin, N., Paul, P., Lyonnet, L., Vivier, E., Dignat-George, F., and Vely, F. 2008, "Mouse CD146/MCAM is a marker of natural killer cell maturation." Eur. J. Immunol., 38, 2855-2864.

[42] Kannagi, R., Izawa, M., Koike, T., Miyazaki, K., and Kimura, N. 2004, "Carbohydrate-mediated cell adhesion in cancer metastasis and angiogenesis." Cancer Science 95(5), 377-384.

[43] Wu, C., Cipollone, J., Maines-Bandiera, S., Tan, C., Karsan, A., Auersperg, N., Roskelley, C. D. 2008, "The morphogenic function of E-cadherin-mediated adherens junctions in epithelial ovarian carcinoma formation and progression." Differentiation, 76, 193-205.

[44] Shih, I. M., Hsu, M. - Y. Palazzo, J. P., and Herlyn, M. 1997, "The cell-cell adhesion receptor MEL-CAM acts as a tumor suppressor in breast carcinoma." Am. J. Pathology, 151, 745-751.

[45] Zeng, G., Cai, S., and Wu, G. - J. 2011, "Up-regulation of METCAM/MUC18 promotes motility, invasion, and tumorigenesis of human breast cancer cells." BMC Cancer 2011, 11:113 (30 March 2011) doi: 10.1186/1471-2407-11-113.

[46] Zeng, G. and Wu, G. - J. 2011, "METCAM/MUC18 over-expression suppresses *in vitro* motility and invasiveness and *in vivo* progression of human ovarian cancer cells." (in preparation).

[47] Ribeiro, A. S., Albergaria, A., Sousa, B., Correia, A. L., Bracke, M., Seruca, R., Schmitt, F.C., and Paredes, J. 2010, "Extracellular cleavage and shedding of P-cadherin: a mechanism underlying the invasive behaviour of breast cancer cells." Oncogene, 29, 392-402.

[48] Mills, L., Ellez, C., Huang, S., Baker, C., McCarty, M., Green, L., Gudas, J. M., Feng, X., and Bar-Eli, M. 2002, "Fully human antibodies to MCAM/MUC18 inhibit tumor growth and metastasis of human melanoma." Cancer Research, 62, 5106-5114.

[49] Leslie, M. C., Zhao, Y. – J., Lachman, L. B., Hwu, P., Wu, G. - J., and Bar-Eli, M. (2007) "Immunization against MUC18/MCAM, a novel antigen that drives melanoma invasion and metastasis." Gene therapy, 14, 316-323.

[50] Satyamoothy, K., Muyrers, J., Meier, F., Patel, D. and Herlyn, M. 2001, "Mel-CAM-specific genetic suppressor elements inhibit melanoma growth and invasion through loss of gap junction communication." Oncogene, 20, 4676-4684.

[51] Hafner, C., Samwald, U., Wagner, S., Felici, F., Heere-Ress, E., Jensen-Jarolim, E., Wolff, K., Scheiner, O., Pehamberger, H., and Breiteneder, H. 2002, "Selection of mimotopes of the cell surface adhesion molecule of Mel-CAM from a random pVIII-28aa phage peptide library." J. Invest. Dermatol., 119, 865-869.

[52] Nie, S. 2006, "Nanotechnology for personalized and predictive medicine." Nanomedicine, 2(4), 305.

12

Dual Function of Wnts in Human Cutaneous Melanoma

Ksenia Kulikova, Alexey Kibardin, Nikolay Gnuchev,
Georgii Georgiev and Sergey Larin
Institute of Gene Biology, RAS
Russia

1. Introduction

The cellular signaling pathways that respond to Wnts control numerous processes ranging from gastrulation to aging and govern cell fate determination and patterning (Clevers, 2006). Wnt signaling abnormalities often lead to developmental disorders and lethal malignancies. In melanoma aberrant activation of Wnt signaling is often observed. Wnt signaling pathway is a very complex process. Its ligands, called Wnts, can signal via several pathways referred to as the canonical Wnt signaling and two noncanonical Wnt signaling pathways. According to the modern view, the canonical Wnt signaling branch is predominately involved in control of proliferation and differentiation acting at a transcriptional level, whereas the noncanonical ones affect cell motility and cytoskeletal rearrangements. In the case of melanoma, the canonical and the noncanonical Wnt pathways can play opposite roles. The noncanonical Wnt cascade promotes metastasis. Overexpression of Wnt5a correlates with a poor prognosis for patients. The canonical Wnt cascade has long been considered as fully oncogenic. However, a lot of data confirms that it can act as a tumor suppressor by promoting cell differentiation.

2. Wnt proteins and their interactions

Wnt genes were identified both in vertebrates and invertebrates whereas plants, unicellular eukaryotes and prokaryotes appear to lack them (Miller, 2001). In humans, the Wnt family encompasses 19 members. All of them are defined by sequence homology rather than by functional properties (Wnt homepage). *Wnt* genes encode highly modified glycoproteins of 38-43 kDa that have typical features of the secreted growth factors, including a hydrophobic signal sequence, lack of transmembrane domains, an *N*-glycosilation site and a sustained spacing of conserved cysteine residues (McMahon, 1992). It is considered that posttranslational lipid modifications are essential for the Wnt function. Treatment of Wnts with the acylprotein thioesterase that removes palmitates leads to both hydropathy and signaling activity reduction (Willert et al., 2003). Moreover, mutations that prevent palmitoylation of cysteine residues in Wnt1, Wnt3a, Wnt5a result in significant decrease of their biological activity, presumably due to inability to bind Frizzled (Fz) receptors. These mutations do not affect secretion. In contrast, a mutation of the conserved serine in Wnt3a abrogates palmitoleic acid addition and blocks secretion. Considering these observations, it is believed that the palmitoleic acid modification is required for secretion, whereas the palmitate modification is critical for receptor binding (Cadigan & Peifer, 2009).

Complexity of the Wnt signaling is greatly enhanced by abundance of potential receptors. There are several groups of receptor molecules that can bind Wnts. The first group found to transduce the Wnt signal is the Frizzled (Fz) receptor family. The Fz proteins were identified both in vertebrates and invertebrates. In human and mice, the Fz family includes ten members (Wnt homepage). It is believed that Fz proteins are the real G-protein-coupled receptors that can activate the heterotrimeric G-protein to transmit signal from Wnts. Like typical GPCR, they have seven hydrophobic transmembrane domains, glycosylation and phosphorylation sites for cyclic AMP-dependent protein kinase (PKA), protein kinase C (PKC) and casein kinase 2 (CK2), and are able to form homomeric and heteromeric complexes with other members of the Fz family. However, there are several differences between the Fz receptors and other GPCRs. The Fz receptors lack two conserved motifs, Asp-Arg-Tyr and Asn-Pro-X-X-Tyr. The Asp-Arg-Tyr motif is located in the second intracellular loop of several GPCRs and is crucial for G protein coupling. The Asn-Pro-X-X-Tyr motif is present at the end of the seventh transmembrane segment of GPCRs (Angers & Moon, 2009). The classical Fz receptor consists of a long highly glycosilated *N*-terminal extension, that is positioned outside of the cell, seven transmembrane domains and a short cytoplasmic tail. An amino terminal region called a cysteine-rich domain (CRD) is intended for the direct Wnt binding. The carboxyl terminus contains a consensus PDZ domain-binding motif (S/T-X-V) that is important for interaction with cytoplasmic proteins (Miller, 2001). Wnt/Fz combination at the surface of the cell determinates the type of G-protein subunits to be utilized and the kind of cellular response to occur (Liu et al., 1999; Malbon et al., 2001).

In addition to the Fz receptors, Wnt can bind to molecules of the low density lipoprotein (LDL) receptor-related protein (LRP) family. The Wnt-LRP coupling is considered to induce or stabilize the formation of the Fz-LRP-Wnt ternary complex. Wnts have a low affinity to LRP, as compared to Fz, so there is an idea that the coupling occurs between LRP and the Wnt–Fz complex (Tamai et al., 2000). Two members of the vertebrate LRP family, LRP5 and LRP6, are able to bind Wnts. The LRP6 mutant mice phenotype resembles defects caused by several individual *Wnt* genes deficiency (Pinson et al., 2000). LRP overexpression in *Xenopus* leads to activation of the Wnt signaling (Tamai et al., 2000). Moreover, binding of some extracellular inhibitors to LRP leads to abrogation of the Wnt signaling transduction (Itasaki et al., 2003; Glinka et al., 1998). Unlike to the Fz receptors, LRP6 is a single-pass transmembrane protein. It has a highly modular structure consisting of the extracellular domain (ECD) that mediates LRP6-ligand interactions, and the intracellular domain (ICD) that transduces extracellular signals to cytoplasmic effectors. ECD contains the extracellular proteins binding YWTD domains, EGF-like repeats, and LDL repeats. ECD is supposed to act as an autoinhibitory signal, since LRP6 lacking the ECD can constitutively activate the Wnt pathway. In contrast, the ICD domain is sufficient for the activation of the Wnt signalling pathway. The overexpression of the isolated ICD induces constitutive activation of the canonical Wnt signaling. The ICD domain is rich in proline, serine, and threonine and has a conserved PPSPXS motif critical for its function (Niehrs & Shen, 2010).

Repertoire of the Wnt receptor molecules is broader than that of the Fz and LRP proteins. The Wnt ligands can also signal through alternative receptors, structurally related homologs Ror1 and Ror2 that belong to the receptor tyrosine kinase (RTK) superfamily, and Ryk that is an atypical tyrosine kinase receptor. Transgenic mice with the Ror2 loss-of-function mutations demonstrate very similar phenotype to mice with the Wnt5a depletion (Oishi et al., 1999). Ror2 contains extracellular Fz-like cysteine-rich domains (CRDs), membrane-proximal Kringle domains and immunoglobulin (Ig)-like domains. While CRDs and the Ig-like domains participate in ligand binding, function of the Kringle domains is still unclear. However, it is assumed that the Kringle domains in Ror act as recognition modules for binding of the Wnt regulatory proteins (Minami et al., 2010). Another receptor molecule Ryk is thought to mediate the Wnt signaling. Unlike to Ror2, Ryk is an atypical Tyr kinase receptor. It lacks kinase activity due to amino acid substitutions in the evolutionarily conserved residues of the intracellular kinase domains (Halford et al., 1999; Hovens et al., 1992). In addition to the intracellular kinase domain, Ryk contains a single transmembrane domain and an extracellular Wnt inhibitory factor (WIF) domain. The last one mediates binding of various Wnt ligands (Halford & Stacker, 2001). The choice of a ligand for interaction is rather controversial. According to different data, Ryk can bind both canonical and noncanonical Wnts. The physical interaction between Ryk and Wnt1 and Wnt3a with subsequent activation of the canonical Wnt signaling was demonstrated in the HEK293T cells (Lu et al., 2004). On the contrary, the noncanonical Wnt5a serves as a binding partner for Ryk in the Wnt5a-mediated axon guidance (Keeble et al., 2006).

To complete the description of the Wnt-interacting partners, a special group of proteins that can bind Wnt ligands but unable to participate in signal transduction should be mentioned. These proteins act as inhibitors blocking the Wnt functional activity. The soluble Frizzled-Related Proteins (sFRPs) represent a typical example of the extracellular Wnt inhibitors. They bind to Wnt proteins preventing them from coupling with their receptors. sFRPs are able to block both canonical and noncanonical Wnt signaling pathway. Another soluble Wnt inhibitor is called WIF-1 (Wnt inhibitory factor). Unlike to sFRPs, it does not contain a CRD domain. However, it can bind to Wnts through a unique domain that is similar to extracellular region of the Ryk receptors (Patthy, 2000).

Another group of the Wnt signaling inhibitors consists of secreted Wnt antagonists. The Dickkopf (Dkk) family of the Wnt antagonists inhibits the Wnt signaling by direct binding to LRP5/6 (Glinka et al.,1998). It is considered that Dkk can form a ternary complex with LRP5/6 and a single-pass transmembrane receptor Kremen-1 in order to promote LRP5/6 internalization with subsequent inactivation of the Wnt signaling (Mao et al., 2002). Binding of LRP by soluble Wnt signaling inhibitors is not a unique feature of Dkk. Some other secreted Wnt inhibitors (Wise and SOST) use the same mechanism (Itasaki et al., 2003; Semenov et al., 2005).

Availability of different receptors, co-receptors and inhibitors create cellular context. An effect of the Wnt signaling pathway depends not on the Wnt ligand itself, but on the Wnt ligand in the cellular context. The same Wnt ligand can activate different Wnt signaling branches, and classification of Wnt ligands based on a type of Wnt signaling activated seems artificial.

2.1 Different branches of the Wnt signaling

The Wnt signaling is commonly considered as a combination of at least three different signaling branches: the β-catenin pathway, the Wnt/Ca^{2+} pathway and the planar cell polarity (PCP) pathway. There is evidence of significant crosstalk between them.

2.1.1 The canonical Wnt signaling pathway

The canonical Wnt signaling pathway, or the β-catenin pathway, was the first Wnt signaling discovered. It participates in multiple biological processes including embryogenesis, cell proliferation and differentiation in adults, stem cell renewal in multiple tissues (hematopoietic, epidermal, and intestinal) and tumorigenesis (Clevers, 2006). A lot of growth genes (*c-myc, cyclin D1, PPARδ*) are under control of this signaling (He et al., 1998, 1999; Tetsu & McCormick, 1999). Other target genes include the matrix metalloproteinase, fibronectin and the transcription factors AP-1, c-jun and fra1 (Brabletz et al., 1999; Gradl et al., 1999; Mann et al., 1999). The canonical Wnt signaling pathway can be activated by Wnts, such as Wnt1, Wn3a and Wnt8. In the absence of Wnts, concentration of the cytoplasmic β-catenin is maintained at a low level by a special destruction complex. The destruction complex consists of the scaffolding proteins Axin and APC (adenomatous polyposis coli), GSK3β (glycogen synthase kinase 3β), CKI (casein kinase I), PP2A (protein phosphatase 2A) and, probably, ubiquitin ligase β-TrCP. When the destruction complex is active, β-catenin is phosphorylated by GSK3β. The phosphorylated β-catenin in turn is recognized by the ubiquitin ligase β-TrCP, which targets it for ubiquitin-mediated proteosomal degradation (Weeraratna, 2005). The canonical Wnt signaling is initiated by simultaneous binding of the Wnt ligand both to Fz receptor and LRP-5/6 coreceptor (Tamai et al., 2000). The ternary complex formation recruits a group of proteins including Disheveled (Dvl), Axin and GSK3β to the plasma membrane, where they form the Lrp6 signalosomes (Bilic et al., 2007). Aggregation causes CK1γ and GSK3β-mediated LRP6 phosphorylation. According to the modern view, the cytoplasmic scaffolding protein Dvl is required for the LRP6 aggregation and phosphorylation (Niehrs & Shen, 2010). Wnt-stimulated Dvl becomes hyper-phosphorylated and forms polymers that are recruited to the plasma membrane, providing a platform for the Axin-GSK3β relocation (Cliffe et al., 2003). This relocation in turn results in inhibition of the β-catenin phosphorylation and further signaling transduction (Mao et al., 2001). The β-catenin stabilization is a key event in activation of the canonical Wnt signaling. The stabilized β-catenin accumulates in the cytoplasm, translocates into the nucleus and participates in target gene regulation. β-catenin by itself is unable to bind DNA, but it can induce transcriptional activity of Tcf/Lef1 (Behrens et al., 1996). In the absence of β-catenin, Tcf/Lef1 acts as a transcriptional repressor. It can bind to the consensus motif (A/T)(A/T)CAA(A/T)G on DNA but has no trans-activation domain to induce transcription. In the β-catenin/Tcf/Lef1 complex, Tcf/Lef1 facilitates DNA-binding whereas β-catenin provides transactivation domains (Brantjes et al., 2002).

2.1.2 The noncanonical Wnt signaling pathways

At least two additional signaling pathways activated by Wnt ligands have been identified: the Wnt/Ca^{2+} pathway and the PCP pathway. Both of them are β-catenin-independent and are referred to as the noncanonical signaling pathways. Similar to the β-catenin signaling, the noncanonical pathways are essential for embryogenesis. They regulate multiple morphogenetic processes including gastrulation and neural tube closure (Jenny & Mlodzik, 2006; Kohn & Moon, 2005).

2.1.2.1 The Wnt/Ca^{2+} pathway

The Wnt/Ca^{2+} pathway includes calcium release from the intracellular stores and induction of enzymatic activity of Ca^{2+}-dependent protein kinases like calmodulin kinases, protein kinase C (PKC) and calcineurin (Kohn & Moon, 2005). The first ligand identified to induce transient spikes of the intracellular calcium is Wnt5a. In *Xenopus* embryos, it was shown that Wnt5a expression blocked the ability of the canonical Wnt8 to induce axis duplication. These data confirmed an idea of existence of multiple Wnt signaling pathways. The more precise data came from studies in *Xenopus* and zebrafish models. It was revealed that Wnt5a overexpression phenocopied overexpression of a serpentine receptor that stimulates the intracellular calcium release in a G-protein-dependent manner. Later, an appropriate Fz receptor Rfz-2 was identified (Kuhl et al., 2000). The Wnt coupling to receptor (Fz, Rfz2) leads to dissociation of the Gα and Gβ/γ subunits. Gβ/γ activates phospholipase C (PLC), which translocates to the membrane and hydrolyzes phosphotidylinositol 4,5- biphosphate (PIP2) into inositol 1,4,5- triphosphate (IP3) and di-acyl glycerol (DAG). DAG activates PKC, while IP3 induces Ca^{2+} release from the intracellular stores. Elevation of the intracellular calcium level in turn stimulates the Ca^{2+}-dependent effector molecules. Reminiscent of the canonical Wnt signaling-mediated Dvl translocation, Wnt5a expression results in PKC translocation to the plasma membrane where it is able to interact with its target proteins (Weeraratna, 2005). There is a positive feedback loop between PKC and Wnt5a. Inhibition of PKC can result in decrease of Wnt5a expression, whereas PKC activation leads to Wnt5a upregulation (Jonsson et al., 1998). Signaling cascades activated by PKC affect cytoskeletal organization and cell motility.

2.1.2.2 The Planar Cell Polarity pathway

Another noncanonical Wnt signaling pathway is the Planar Cell Polarity, or PCP, pathway. It was initially discovered in *Drosophila melanogaster*, but later found to control some critical biological processes in vertebrates (Mlodzik, 2002; Wang & Nathans, 2007). Polarity is an important feature in living organisms, underlying the proper performance of many functions. There are several kinds of polarity. Epithelial cells are polarized in two different manners. Besides apical-basal polarity, they also display polarization along the plane of the epithelial layer orthogonal to the apical-basal axis. This kind of polarization is called tissue polarity, or planar cell polarity (PCP). It is notable that, besides the epithelial cell polarity, the PCP proteins also provide mesenchymal cell intercalation during axis elongation process in vertebrates (*Xenopus* and zebrafish). The principal mechanism for tissue elongation is an insertion of mesenchymal cells between their neighbors along one axis. In this case, the mesenchymal cells have no apical-basal polarity but are able to extend polarized protrusions in the same direction. Thus, these cells are oriented with respect to direction of movement (Zallen, 2007). The transmembrane PCP proteins Frizzled, Strabismus, and Flamingo and the cytoplasmic PCP proteins Dvl and Prickle are critical for proper intercalation (Keller, 2002; Myers et al., 2002; Wallingford et al., 2002). Reestablishing of cell polarity after a mitotic cell division is also dependent on the PCP pathway (Nechiporuk & Vasioukhin, 2006). The Wnt/PCP pathway controls activity of the small GTPases Rho and Rac. The Rho signaling branch requires activation of the Dvl-Daam-1 (Dishevelled-associated activator of morphogenesis 1) complex and results in the Rho-associated kinase (ROCK) and myosin activation (Habas et al., 2001; Marlow et al., 2002; Weiser et al., 2007). Daam-1 is a member of the Formin protein family. It mediates an assembly of the Dvl-RhoA complex acting as a scaffolding protein (Habas et al., 2001). The Rac branch of signaling is Daam-1-independent. It requires another domain of Dvl to induce activity of small Rac GTPase. Activated Rac in turn stimulates Jun kinase (JNK) (Habas et al., 2003; Li et al., 1999). The PCP pathway regulates modifications of actin cytoskeleton structures and, as a consequence, provides cytoskeletal rearrangements and directed migration. In addition, it is considered that, unlike to the above mentioned pathways, the PCP cascade appears to function independently of transcription.

Actually, the majority of molecular cascades connected with Rho/Rac GTPases and PKC mostly affect cell motility. This observation allows to suggest that the noncanonical Wnt signaling branches are implicated exactly in these processes. Contrariwise, the canonical Wnt signaling controls predominately proliferation and differentiation acting at a transcriptional level.

2.2 Wnt signaling in skin biology

In embryogenesis, components of the Wnt cascade are involved in multiple processes including neural crest induction, specification and differentiation (Dorsky et al., 1998). Neural crest cells arise from a region called neural folds at the border of the neural plate and non-neural ectoderm. During neurulation, neural folds converge at the dorsal midline of an embryo to form the neural tube. According to the conventional view, this process is mediated by molecular signals emanating from the ectoderm and receiving by the neuroepithelium. Numerous experiments in amphibian, zebrafish, avian and murine embryos revealed Wnt signaling as a driving force in this process (Garćia-Castro et al., 2002; Huang & Saint-Jeannet, 2004; Lewis et al., 2004). Depletion of the main effector component of the canonical Wnt signaling, β-catenin, abrogates the neural crest induction (Wu et al., 2005), and the promoter region of neural crest-specific gene *Slug* contains a binding site for Lef/β-catenin complex (Vallin et al., 2001).

The fate of the neural crest cells is also under control of the Wnt signaling pathway. Some reports confirm that Wnt6 and Wnt8 are required both for the neural crest induction and its expansion (Labonne & Bronner-Fraser, 1998; Sakai et al., 2005). After neurulation, neural crest cells from the roof plate of the neural tube undergo an epithelial-to-mesenchymal transition and migrate to the peripheral sites. This migration is an elaborate process, tightly controlled on a molecular level. It is believed that, unlike to the neural crest induction controlled by the canonical Wnt signaling, migration of neural crest cells mostly depends on another kind of the Wnt signaling called the noncanonical or the Planar Cell Polarity (PCP). Inhibition of the PCP factors like Wnt11, Frizzled7 (Fz7) and Dishevelled (Dvl) results in a failure of the neural crest cells migration, indicating that the noncanonical Wnt signaling is essential for the neural crest migration *in vivo* (De Calisto et al., 2005).

The neural crest cells give rise to diverse cell types, including neurons, glia and melanocytes. Neurogenic and melanogenic populations of the neural crest cells have distinct migratory specificities governed by expression of different surface receptors and signaling moleculars, including Wnts (Thomas & Erickson, 2008). The Wnt signaling is supposed to be important for the neural crest cells specification. Neuroblasts and glioblasts show strong expression of the Wnt signaling inhibitor protein called Frzb-1. Conversely, the Frzb-1 expression level in melanoblasts is decreased (Jin et al., 2001). Other evidence of the Wnt signaling participation in the neural crest cells specification comes from knockout studies. The Wnt1 and Wnt3a double-knockout mice exhibit defects in the neural crest cell derivatives, including melanocytes (Ikeya et al., 1997). The β-catenin knockout in the neural crest cells leads to loss of both melanocytes and sensory neurons (Hari et al., 2002). In the presence of Wnt3a in conditioned medium, the cultured quail neural crest cells evolve into melanoblasts (Jin et al., 2001). Injection of mRNA encoding cytoplasmic β-catenin into the neural crest cells of a zebrafish embryo targets them to a pigment cell fate at the expense of neurons and glia (Dorsky et al., 1998). In melanocytes, the canonical ligand Wnt3a promotes up-regulation of the microphthalmia-associated transcription factor (MITF), the master regulator of melanogenesis. The MITF expression starts in melanoblasts soon after their migration from the neural tube, and loss of MITF results in the absence of melanocytes

(Thomas & Erickson, 2009). Interestingly, the MITF expression is abolished in the fibroblasts derived from skin treated with the Wnt signaling inhibitor Dkk-1. Along with the MITF inhibition, these samples also show the decreased β-catenin expression level. Dkk-1 is supposed to be a key molecular determinant for a regional specificity in human skin pigmentation. Hands and feet express Dkk-1 at a higher level comparing to a trunk, and are less pigmented due to a lower melanocyte density. It is believed that in epidermis Dkk-1 inhibits both melanocyte differentiation and melanin production (Yamaguchi et al., 2007).

The terminal cell differentiation can be inhibited in a β-catenin-independent manner. A way to keep cells in a precursor state is provided by a member of the Tcf/Lef family, Tcf-3, that acts as a repressor of the Wnt-mediated transcription. Tcf-3 is normally expressed in the hair follicle bulge and basal layer of the outer root sheath. Ectopic expression of Tcf-3 in interfollicular epidermis inhibits terminal keratinocytes differentiation and induces a shift to progenitor-like molecular phenotype (Nguyen et al., 2006). The noncanonical Wnt signaling activated by Wnt5a also can antagonize the canonical signaling and inhibit expression of melanogenic antigens (Dissanayake et al., 2008). This observation leads to an idea that, whereas the canonical Wnt signaling is important for melanoblasts positioning and differentiation, the other Wnt signaling type serves for maintenance of the de-differentiated cell state. The idea is supported by data from the hematopoetic stem cells (HSCs). These cells are maintained in a quiescent state by Wnt5a, and the canonical Wnt signaling, contrariwise, makes them differentiate (Nemeth et al., 2007). The melanocyte stem cells express receptors for the Wnt signaling pathway on their surfaces (Yamada et al., 2010). Taking into account these data and the data from melanocytes regulation, it was speculated that Wnt5a could be involved in the quiescence maintenance of the melanocyte stem cells (MSCs), keeping them in their niche environment (Nishikawa & Osawa, 2007; O'Connell & Weeraratna, 2009). Stem cells committed to the melanocyte lineage reside in the bulge area of hair follicles (Nishimura et al., 2002). Being a source of melanoblasts and melanocytes, in adults they are most likely to be related to hyperpigmentation and age-associated hair graying (Yamada et al., 2010).

Mammalian skin serves many critical biological functions to maintain homeostasis. Evidence indicates that the Wnt signaling is implicated in this process. The protective function of skin can be disturbed by wounding. The only way to restore skin integrity and, as a result, its protective function is healing of the wound. Unfortunately, wound healing and true regeneration are not the same. Cutaneous repair after the loss of full-thickness skin usually leads to scarring. The healed tissue contains a collagen-rich dermal matrix with a stratified epithelial covering. It is less elastic, has a lower tensile strength level and unable to form skin appendages. Interestingly, skin actually has a potential to regenerate, since it contains the multipotent epidermal stem cells in hair follicles and the undifferentiated mesenchymal cells in the dermis. Thus, it is postulated that scar repairing is more favorable than regeneration due to molecular context in the affected area. It is considered that the Wnt signaling pathway contributes significantly to this molecular context. To elucidate the role of the Wnt signaling in wound healing, the Wnt expression is examined at various times after wounding. Wnt-4 is expressed early in the process, while Wnt-5a and Wnt-11 expression peaks are at the time of wound remodeling. The "TOPGAL" mice experiments reveal that the canonical Wnt signaling activity is increased in the hair follicles adjacent to the lesion, but not within the wound or overlying epithelium. Furthermore, the stabilized β-catenin expression results in epithelial appendages formation like hair follicles and sebaceous glands within the wound (Fathke et al., 2006). The rate of wound closure is not affected by the β-catenin expression. Interestingly, the TGFβ-induced wound healing is partially regulated by β-catenin. Expression of *Mmp-3* and *Mmp-14* stimulated by TGFβ requires the β-catenin expression (Cheon et al., 2005). The noncanonical Wnt signaling is also able to direct adult skin progenitor cells toward regeneration. Wound transduction with the retrovirus expressing the typical noncanonical Wnt ligand Wnt-5a leads to even more abundant epithelial appendage formation in the wound, as compared with the stabilized β-catenin expression. Moreover, the authors report that the noncanonical Wnt signaling activation in epidermis is not associated with epithelial tumors, in contrast to the β-catenin-dependent signaling whose activation sometimes results in tumor formation (Fathke et al., 2006).

Skin development and homeostasis are considerably dependent on regulation by the Wnt signaling. It is implicated in the neural crest induction and specification, determining of epidermal and melanocyte stem cells fate, hair follicle establishment and entry of its cells into the active growth phase and wound healing. Considering significance of the Wnt signaling in skin biology, it is not surprising that its malfunctions are often seen in different pathological conditions. Expression pattern of many Wnts is affected in malignant melanoma.

2.3 Wnt signaling in melanoma

Aberrant activation of the Wnt signaling pathways is often observed in melanoma. The cutaneous melanoma is considered as a neural crest-derived malignancy. It originates from the melanocyte progenitor cells or from the pigment-producing melanocytes. Taking into account that the Wnt signaling cascades play a crucial role in the neural crest induction, specification and melanocyte differentiation, implication of the different Wnt signaling branches in melanoma pathogenesis seems quite natural.

The cutaneous melanoma is a common skin cancer characterized by high aggressiveness, morbidity and mortality. The melanoma development is a multistep process. It includes a congenital or acquired nevus, a dysplastic atypical nevus, a radial growth phase (RGP) melanoma, a vertical growth phase (VGP) melanoma and a metastatic melanoma (Larue & Beermann, 2007). Uncontrolled cell proliferation leads to the mole formation. It is considered that further immortalization is required for melanoma induction (Larue et al., 2009). A fraction of atypical nevi undergoes malignant transformation into a RGP melanoma with low probability to metastasize. Unlike to RGP, a VGP melanoma has high invasive and metastatic capabilities. A metastatic melanoma is usually resistant to chemotherapy and radiation (Govindarajan et al., 2007). It is believed that components of the Wnt signaling cascades can contribute to all stages of melanoma progression. There are several hypotheses describing potential roles of the canonical and noncanonical Wnt signaling branches in melanomagenesis. Thus, according to one of them, aberrations in the canonical signaling lead to melanoma formation, whereas the noncanonical Wnt signaling malfunctions are associated with metastatic progression. Furthermore, during melanoma progression, the β-catenin signaling serves as a negative regulator of tumor growth. Numerous data confirms this idea. However, it is worth mentioning that some researchers argue against this conception. They consider the canonical Wnt signaling as a fully oncogenic. Anyway, the Wnt signaling is somehow implicated in melanoma progression. In the case of melanoma, Wnt1, Wnt3a and Wnt5a are best described. Wnt1 and Wnt3a are considered as the canonical ligands and Wnt5a as an activator of the Wnt/Ca^{2+} pathway.

2.3.1 Implication of the canonical Wnt signaling in melanoma cell fate

In normal skin, melanocytes are interspersed among keratinocytes at the epidermal-dermal border. Physical and functional interaction with keratinocytes provides control of melanocyte proliferation and differentiation. In the absence of this control, melanocytes tend to rapid proliferation and expression of cell surface molecules normally associated with melanoma (McGary et al., 2002). A transmembrane protein E-cadherin is considered as the major mediator of human melanocyte adhesion to keratinocytes. Loss of E-cadherin is often associated with tumorigenesis including melanoma (Haass et al., 2005). Interestingly, E-cadherin does not only act as a cell-cell adhesion molecule, but also mediates intracellular signaling through β-catenin. Indeed, β-catenin was originally identified as an interlink between E-cadherin and α-catenin in the adherens junctions (Cowin, 1994; Gumbiner & Neuron, 1993; Nagafuchi & Takeichi, 1989; Ozawa et al., 1989). Downregulation of E-cadherin leads to release of β-catenin from the membrane-associated pool and to increase of its transcriptional activity. The activated canonical Wnt signaling is found in approximately one third of melanomas (Larue et al., 2009). Keeping in mind that the β-catenin signaling promotes expression of many "growth" genes, including *cyclin D* and *c-myc*, constitutive activation of this cascade can potentially stimulate tumor formation. For example, *c-myc* is a well-known oncogene. Its overexpression is found in a variety of human cancers including colorectal cancer, breast cancer, leukemia and melanoma (Dang, 1999). Inhibition of *c-myc* is supposed to be an important step in tumor growth restriction. Supporting this idea, the *c-myc* antisense oligonucleotides have been shown to decrease proliferation of different cancer cells (Iversen et al., 2003).

Expression of the canonical Wnt signaling negative regulators is often reduced in melanoma. Thus, Dkk-1, -2 and -3 are downregulated or lost both in melanoma cell lines and tumor samples (Kuphal et al., 2006). Dkk-1 and Dkk-2 inhibit the β-catenin signaling by binding to LRP5/6 coreceptor. It has been shown that Dkk-1 can suppress melanocyte growth and melanogenesis (Yamaguchi et al., 2004). Activation of the Dkk-1 expression results in inhibition of tumorigenicity and induction of apoptosis in melanoma cells during *in vivo* growth in the athymic nude mice (Mikheev et al., 2007). Another Wnt signaling inhibitor repressed in melanoma is WIF-1 (Wnt inhibitory factor-1) (Haqq et al., 2005). Unlike to Dkk, WIF-1 binds directly to the Wnt ligand blocking its signaling activity. Unfortunately, it remains unknown, which type of the Wnt signaling is inhibited by WIF-1. Anyway, the WIF-1 silencing may be a critical event in constitutive activation of the canonical Wnt pathway in melanoma cells. It is reported that melanoma cell growth is suppressed by WIF-1 overexpression, and the suppression is related to transcriptional and translational inhibition of the canonical Wnt signaling components, including β-catenin, Dvl-3, and cyclin D1 (Lin et al., 2007).

Besides extracellular inhibitors of the canonical Wnt signaling, like Dkk and WIF-1, expression of the cytoplasmic CK1α in melanoma is frequently decreased or completely lost. CK1α is responsible for initial phosphorylation of β-catenin that is required for the GSK3β-mediated β-catenin degradation (Liu et al., 2002). CK1α expression in invasive melanoma cells decreases growth rate and induces cell cycle arrest and apoptosis, whereas suppression of CK1α in primary melanomas has an opposite effect. Evidence confirming β-catenin implication in this effect comes from the β-catenin downregulation experiments. Inhibition of the β-catenin expression in the nonmetastatic melanoma cell lines results in inhibition of invasive growth (Sinnberg et al., 2010).

As mentioned above, β-catenin is a multifunctional protein, and its function is supposed to depend on cellular localization. At the membrane, β-catenin is a component of the cadherin adherens junctions and in the nucleus it acts as a transcriptional activator of the canonical Wnt signaling target genes. There are several reports that β-catenin is accumulated in the cytoplasm or nucleus of human melanoma cell lines and original tumors (Rubinfeld et al., 1997). But unlike to other cancers, the elevated level of β-catenin in melanoma is rarely associated with mutations (Giles et al., 2003). Melanoma is very heterogeneous. The activity and regulation of the canonical Wnt signaling vary significantly among different patients. Nuclear β-catenin localization is not always sufficient for the canonical Wnt signaling activation. Several cell lines with high nuclear β-catenin level are unable to activate this signaling (Kulikova et al., in press).

According to some notions, β-catenin can induce melanocyte immortalization by bypassing the senescence barrier (Delmas et al., 2007). A growth arrest after a limited number of divisions represents a good way to protect cells from oncogenic transformation (Campisi, 2005). Uncontrolled proliferation and delayed senescence are considered to be enough for melanoma transformation. Activating mutations in N-Ras and B-Raf (the MAP-kinase signaling pathway) can provide signals for proliferation, whereas β-catenin is believed to contribute to senescence escape (Delmas et al., 2007; Gray-Schopfer et al., 2005; Tsao et al., 2000). Senescence is associated with the G_0/G_1-like cell cycle arrest induced by the tumor suppressor Rb1 that in turn is controlled by $p16_{INK4a}$ (Narita et al., 2003). In melanoma, the $p16_{INK4a}$ expression is often silenced by genetic and epigenetic mechanisms. It has been shown that in transgenic mice, the stabilized β-catenin decreases a number of melanoblasts and stimulates immortalization of primary skin melanocytes by silencing the $p16_{INK4a}$ promoter (Delmas et al., 2007). Transgenic animals expressing the stabilized form of β-catenin demonstrate an elevated β-catenin level in the nucleus of target cells that mimics the constitutively active β-catenin in melanomas. Moreover, in human melanoma cells, this activated β-catenin represses $p16_{INK4a}$ directly in a TCF4-dependent manner. It should be noted that β-catenin by itself is unable to induce either melanocyte proliferation or melanoma formation. However, the double transgenic animals carrying both N-Ras and β-catenin mutations show a high rate of melanoma incidences. Moreover, these double mutants are more subject to melanomagenesis than the single N-Ras transgenic mice. Thus, it has been postulated that the constitutively activated canonical Wnt signaling acts synergistically with the MAP kinase pathways in order to induce melanoma in the absence of the $p16_{INK4a}$ mutation (Delmas et al., 2007).

The MAP kinase and β-catenin signaling cascades regulate activity of the master regulator of melanogenesis, MITF-M. In melanoma characterized by simultaneous activation of N-Ras and β-catenin, the MITF level is higher than in N-Ras-driven tumors (Larue et al., 2009). MITF-M regulates a wide range of biological processes including cell proliferation and differentiation (Palmieri et al., 2009). According to the current hypothesis, the β-catenin capacity to activate MITF-M underlies its ability to regulate the melanocyte number (Widlund et al., 2002; Larue & Delmas, 2006; Schepsky et al., 2006). A high level of MITF activity restricts cell division, whereas a low level is associated with proliferation (Carreira et al., 2005, 2006; Loercher et al., 2005; Wellbrock & Marais, 2005). Thus, β-catenin, being a direct regulator of the MITF-M expression, can affect melanocyte proliferation. In case of the β-catenin transgenic mice, the overactivated canonical Wnt signaling can lead to MITF activation and restriction of melanoblast proliferation.

In spite of numerous studies confirming the β-catenin implication in malignant transformation of melanocytes, the exact role of the Wnt/β-catenin signaling in melanoma and especially in melanoma metastasis remains quite controversial. Whereas a lot of papers claim that β-catenin is not associated with melanoma progression (not transformation), there is a report revealing a form of β-catenin that does correlate to the disease stage. Surprisingly, this phosphorylated form of β-catenin in human melanoma bioptic samples is accumulated in nucleus. However, as far as we know, the phosphorylated β-catenin is usually targeted for degradation in the cytoplasm (Kielhorn et al., 2003). Moreover, in contrast to the results from transgenic mice revealing no activation of proliferation in response to the stabilized β-catenin, in human melanoma cell lines β-catenin induced melanoma growth mediated by the MITF upregulation (Widlund et al., 2002). On the other hand, a lot of data demonstrate that the β-catenin signaling actually acts as a negative regulator of melanoma progression. Almost all benign nevi are positive for the nuclear β-catenin, but the rate of nevi transformation into melanoma is very low (Tsao et al., 2003). Metastatic melanoma progression is associated with a loss of the nuclear β-catenin. Contrariwise, the nuclear accumulation of β-catenin is a good sign for patients (Bachmann et al., 2005; Chien et al., 2009; Kageshita et al., 2001; Maelandsmo et al., 2003). The canonical Wnt signaling plays a crucial role in the pigment cell biology (Fang D et al., 2006). Wnt3a and Wnt1 are factors required for differentiation of pluripotent stem cells into functional melanocytes (Dorsky et al., 1998). Treatment of melanoma cells with Wnt3a results in increased pigmentation, transcriptional upregulation of melanogenic antigens and decreased metastatic ability (Chien et al., 2009). The Wnt3a-upregulated melanogenic antigens, including Trpm1, Kit, Met, and Mlana, are normally associated with melanocyte differentiation. They are frequently lost during metastatic tumor progression (Ryu et al., 2007). Transfection of the B16 melanoma cells with Wnt3a leads to decreased proliferation and induces differentiation (Chien et al., 2009). Moreover, silencing of β-catenin in this cell line actually promotes metastasis (Takahashi et al., 2008). Inhibition of negative regulators of the canonical Wnt signaling has a similar effect. The GSK3β suppression increases melanogenesis both in the B16 cells and melanocytes and decreases proliferation of the cultured B16 and human melanoma cells (Bellei et al., 2008; Chien et al., 2009).

Thus, the canonical Wnt signaling pathway seems to play a dual role in melanomagenesis, depending on the context. On the one hand, it can somehow contribute to melanocyte transformation, and on the other, it can restrain tumor progression. Taking into consideration all these observations, it is possible that the Wnt/β-catenin signaling may be required to maintain a homeostasis (Lucero et al., 2010). The dysregulation of specific transcriptional programs in melanocytes or nevi can lead to early melanoma transformation.

2.3.2 Contribution of the noncanonical Wnt signaling to melanoma metastasis

Regarding the noncanonical Wnt cascades in melanoma, almost all data available at the moment is related to the Wnt5a and Wnt/Ca^{2+}-signaling pathway. It is likely that Wnt/Ca^{2+}-pathway is not implicated in melanocyte transformation, but rather contributes to melanoma progression. The Wnt5a overexpression is frequently observed in highly aggressive melanomas (Bittner et al., 2000; Dissanayake et al., 2007; Weeraratna et al., 2002). There is a positive correlation between its expression and a tumour stage (Weeraratna et al., 2002). Moreover, Wnt5a was identified as a good criterion for melanoma division into highly aggressive tumors and less invasive counterparts (Bittner et al., 2000). Transfection of less aggressive melanoma cells with Wnt5a converts them into more metastatic derivates. Moreover, in melanoma, Wnt5a is predominantly presented at the leading edge of invasion. It is considered that the conversion is connected with the PKC activation (Weeraratna et al., 2002). The PKC signaling is often associated with alterations in cell motility, invasion and metastasis. Wnt5a can promote melanoma progression via the PKC-mediated mechanisms (Mapelli et al., 1994; Weeraratna et al., 2002). Another possible mechanism that can underlie the Wnt5a-dependent metastasis is the PCP pathway. Wnt5a, as well as Wnt1 and Wnt11, has been shown to activate the PCP pathway. Key components of this cascade, Rac, Rho and Cdc42, participate in melanoma metastasis (Choi & Han, 2002; Clark et al., 2000; Nakahara et al., 2003). But, unfortunately, there is no direct evidence supporting this idea.

The Wnt5a signaling can antagonize the β-catenin signaling (Topol et al., 2003). As it was discussed before, silencing of the β-catenin signaling in melanoma cells actually promotes metastasis (Takahashi et al., 2008). Taken together, these observations provide a model where melanoma metastasis is at least partially associated with the Wnt5a-mediated repression of the β-catenin signaling. Notably, treatment of melanocytes with Wnt5a can induce their apoptosis but not transformation (O'Connell & Weeraratna, 2009). However, in melanoma, the Wnt5a-mediated increase in CamKII phosphorylation has been shown to protect cells against the Trail-induced apoptosis (Dissanayake et al., 2007; Xiao et al., 2005). Considering the tumor suppressor role of Wnt5a in other cancers, it is easy to speculate that a cellular context may be very important for the Wnt5a response determination. Moreover, balance between the canonical and noncanonical Wnt signaling pathways may be crucial for homeostasis maintenance (O'Connell & Weeraratna, 2009). In benign nevi, Wnt5a may prevent the β-catenin-dependent melanocyte transformation; in melanoma progression, the canonical Wnt signaling may inhibit the Wnt5a-driven metastasis. The opposite is true for melanomagenesis. The aberrantly activated canonical Wnt signaling is important for melanoma establishment, and, during cancer progression, it should be inhibited by the Wnt5a signaling in order to keep melanoma cells undifferentiated.

Expression of Wnt5a in the nevi is quite controversial. While some researchers argue against the Wnt5a expression in the majority of benign nevi, others report the relatively strong Wnt5a expression (Da Forno et al., 2008; Mapelli et al., 1994; Pham et al., 2003). However, this disagreement can be explained by different sensitivity of methods used for Wnt5a detection. Considering high motility of the nevus cells and association of Wnt5a with decreased proliferation, the observation of a high Wnt5a level in the nevi is quite conforming to the behavior of these cells.

Multiple data confirms that Wnt5a mediates its effects via the PKC activation (Dissanayake et al., 2007). In order to activate the noncanonical Wnt signaling in melanoma cells, Wnt5a must bind to a specific cohort of receptors, including Fz2, Fz5 and Ror2 (Billiard et al., 2005; Weeraratna et al., 2002). Treatment of melanoma cells with an antibody against Fz5 leads to inhibition of the PKC activation, reduced motility and invasion of melanoma cells (Sen et al., 2001, Weeraratna et al., 2002). But the major Wnt5a receptor implicated in melanoma metastasis is supposed to be Ror2 (O'Connell et al., 2010). Like Wnt5a, it is upregulated predominantly in metastatic melanomas and has a negative correlation with melanoma patients survival (O'Connell et al., 2010). A knockdown of this receptor abrogates ability of Wnt5a to signal and mediate metastasis. Interestingly, overexpression or silencing of Wnt5a increases or decreases level of Ror2, respectively. However, downregulation of Ror2 has no effect on the Wnt5a expression (O'Connell et al., 2010).

Wnt5a can promote melanoma metastasis via different cellular mechanisms. First of all, it can induce morphological changes of melanoma cells. There is a report showing that transfection of melanoma cells (derived from an axillary lymph node) with the low endogenous Wnt5a expression with the Wnt5a-coding plasmid leads to shift from compact and roughly triangular cell shape into thin and spreading morphology. Cell shape changes were accompanied by increase in a number of contacts with the substrate (increased adhesion), actin cytoskeleton reorganization and PKC activation. Moreover, the transfected cells were more motile, as compared with the parent cells. Interestingly, the most affected PKC isoforms in the Wnt5a-transfected cells were PKC_{μ} and $PKC_{\beta II}$, that are considered to participate in cytoskeletal organization and invasion, respectively (Weeraratna et al., 2002).

Morphological changes induced by the Wnt5a overexpression remind characteristics of the mesenchymal phenotype. Actually, cells with similar features are observed in many cancers. Mesenchymal motility is characterized by polarized and elongated cell morphology. It requires degradation of extracellular matrix (ECM) components in order to generate a "path" for moving cells (Parri et al., 2009). Wnt5a is considered to promote exactly this form of invasion. Thus, the Wnt5a overexpression stimulates production of matrix metalloproteinases like MMP-2 and MMP7 that degrade ECM (O'Connell et al., 2008; Pukrop et al., 2006). It also induces a shift in expression of cadherins, from E-cadherins to N-cadherins (Hsu et al., 2002). This shift decreases cell-to-cell contacts and facilitates cell-to-ECM interactions. Notably, Wnt5a also increases a level of an intermediate filament protein called vimentin and up-regulates expression of the transcriptional factor Snail, which are typical components of the mesenchymal cells. Wnt5a mediates its action on vimentin and Snail levels via the PKC activation (Dissanayake et al., 2007). Snail is a transcription factor capable of reducing the E-cadherin expression by binding to E-box elements in the cadherin promoter (Batlle et al., 2000). There is a positive feedback between Wnt5a and PKC. Wnt5a induces production of PKC, and vice versa (Jonsson et al., 1998). Thus, on the one hand, Wnt5a is able to support its own expression level, and on the other, it can affect cell motility through induction of the Snail-mediated E-cadherin repression.

Besides the N-cadherin and vimentin expression, Wnt5a also stimulates expression of the glycosaminoglycan hyaluronan receptor CD44, a tumor cell homing and metastasis-associated gene, and inhibits expression of the metastasis suppressor of melanoma KISS-1 (Dissanayake et al., 2007). CD44 is a promigratory factor. *In vitro* study reveals its ability to enhance melanoma cell invasion in collagen gel (Albini, 1998). Inhibition of the Wnt5a-induced PKC activation significantly reduces the CD44 expression (Dissanayake et al., 2007).

Recently it has been shown that Wnt5a can increase the calpain protease-mediated cleavage of the cytoskeletal protein filamin. In the migratory osteoblast cells, filamin can induce filopodia formation. Overexpression of filamin is frequently observed in highly metastatic melanomas. In these cells filamin is distributed in a diffuse manner. Its cleavage is associated with enhanced cell motility (Nomachi et al., 2008; O'Connell et al., 2009). Inhibition of filamin in melanoma decreases cell migration. Calpain is a Ca^{2+}-sensitive protein. Thus, Wnt5a promotes melanoma metastasis by induction of Ca^{2+} release and subsequent activation of calpain and calpain-mediated filamin cleavage (O'Connell et al., 2009).

Another mechanism underlying melanoma metastasis is associated with alterations in cell adhesion. In the case of melanoma, adhesion predicts a less favorable outcome for patients. Many cell adhesion molecules are upregulated during tumor progression (O'Connell & Weeraratna, 2009). There is a notion explaining a positive correlation between enhanced adhesion and invasion. It is considered that for efficient tumor dissemination cancer cells

must bind to endothelial cells (Albini, 1998; Cardones et al., 2003). Activated endothelial cells expose numerous adhesion molecules (VCAM-1, ICAM-1, E-selectin) on their surfaces (Chirivi et al., 1996). These adhesion molecules present good binding partners for cancer cell receptors. Cancer cells can both promote endothelial cells activation by production of IL-1α and enhance expression of its receptors for interaction with endothelial cells (Albini, 1998). Thus, melanoma is pushed towards invasion by enhanced adhesion. β1 integrins promote the CXCR4-mediated interaction between tumor and endothelial cells (Cardones et al., 2003). And α3β1 integrin has been shown to provide migration and invasion of several melanoma cell lines (Melchiori et al., 1995). Wnt5a overexpression can lead to increase in substrate adhesion (Weeraratna et al., 2002). Moreover, melanoma cells exposed to the CXCL12 chemokine gradient demonstrate redistribution of the melanoma cell adhesion molecules (MCAM) into a polarized structure. And this process is controlled by the Wnt5a signaling (Witze et al., 2008).
At last, the Wnt5a signaling has been shown to modulate immunogenicity of melanoma cells. The melanoma-associated antigens important for the cytotoxic T lymphocyte (CTL) response include MART-1, DCT, TYRP-1 (GP75) and GP100 (SILV). All of them are regulated by the transcription factors Sox10, Pax3 and MITF. Wnt5a can decrease melanosomal antigen expression by activation of PKC and STAT3 (Dissanayake et al., 2008) It is believed that PKC stimulated by Wnt5a is implicated in the STAT3 phosphorylation (Gartsbein et al., 2006; Sheldahl et al., 1999). Phosphorylated STAT3 is active and can reduce the Pax3 expression (Kamaraju et al., 2002). Inhibition of the Pax3 expression in turn results in the MITF repression and subsequent MART-1 silencing. Treatment of melanoma cells with phorbol ester has the same effect as the Wnt5a stimulation, and in the presence of STAT3 or PKC inhibitors, Wnt5a loses its ability to decrease the MART-1 expression (Dissanayake et al., 2008). Ratio of the Wnt5a-positive to the MART-1-negative tumors is increasing dramatically in metastasis (Dissanayake et al., 2008). Initially, it was demonstrated that melanoma patients could be separated into several cohorts according to their Wnt5a and MITF status (Hoek et al., 2006). A cohort with the high Wnt5a and low MITF expression has a weak proliferative, but a high metastatic potential. And cohort with the low Wnt5a and high MITF demonstrates opposite features: a high ability to proliferate and a low ability to metastasize. It is useful to remember that MITF is considered as a target of the Wnt/β-catenin signaling. And loss of the nuclear transcriptionally active β-catenin is frequently observed at the advanced stages of melanoma. Thus, an opposite correlation between the canonical and noncanonical Wnt signaling functions in melanomas can be revealed. During metastasis, melanoma cells prefer to downregulate their antigen expression in order to escape from immune surveillance of the tumors. The evidence for the notion comes from the experiment with MART-1 positive/negative cells presented to cytotoxic T-cells. The cytotoxic T-lymphocytes could be activated by melanoma cells expressing MART-1. Treatment of these cells with the recombinant Wnt5a abrogates their ability to activate the cytotoxic T-cells and makes them more resistant to cytolysis. The opposite is also true. Silencing of Wnt5a by siRNA in Wnt5a high-leveled cells enhances the MART-1 expression and susceptibility to the T-cells-mediated cytolysis (Dissanayake et al., 2008).

3. Conclusion

The Wnt signaling pathways compose a really complex network both in melanocytes and in melanoma. Multiple receptors, coreceptors, inhibitors and agonists create a cellular context that can vary significantly in benign nevi and tumors. The context determines a kind of a response to the Wnt ligand stimulation and gives a key to understanding why the canonical and noncanonical Wnt signaling cascades can act both as oncogenic and tumor suppressor factors. The Wnt5a and β-catenin signaling cascades play opposite roles in melanomagenesis. The canonical Wnt signaling is critical at the early stages of tumor development, but in advanced melanoma it serves as a tumor suppressor by promoting more differentiated phenotype. The Wnt5a signaling pathway does not participate in melanoma formation. On the contrary, it can control the canonical signaling preventing its aberrant activation. However, overexpression of Wnt5a is often associated with aggressive melanoma phenotype and is believed to promote metastasis. Thus, normally melanocyte homeostasis is maintained by tightly regulated system, and aberrations in the system regulation result in melanomagenesis.

4. Acknowledgment

This work was supported by a grant from Russian Foundation for Basic Research (11-04-01863-a), (http://www.rfbr.ru) and by the Molecular and Cell Biology Program of the Russian Academy of Sciences.

5. References

Albini, A. (1998). Tumor and endothelial cell invasion of basement membranes. *Pathol Oncol Res*, Vol. 4, No. 3, (n.d.), pp. (230-241), ISSN 1532-2807

Angers, S., & Moon, R.T. (2009). Proximal events in Wnt signal transduction. *Nature*, Vol. 10, No. 7, (July 2009), pp. (468-477), ISSN 0028-0836

Bachmann, I.M., Straume, O., Puntervoll, H.E., Kalvenes, M.B., & Akslen, L.A. (2005). Importance of P-cadherin, beta-catenin, and Wnt5a/frizzled for progression of melanocytic tumors and prognosis in cutaneous melanoma. *Clin Cancer Res*, Vol. 11, No. 24, (December 2005), pp. (8606–8614), ISSN 1557-3265

Batlle, E., Sancho, E., Francí, C., Domínguez, D., Monfar, M., Baulida, J., & García De Herreros, A. (2000). The transcription factor Snail is a repressor of E-cadherin gene expression in epithelial tumour cells. *Nat Cell Biol*, Vol. 2, No. 2, (Febraury 2000), pp. (84-89), ISSN 1465-7392

Behrens, J., von Kries, J. P., Kuhl, M., Bruhn, L., Wedlich, D., Grosschedl, R., & Birchmeier, W. (1996). Functional interaction of beta-catenin with the transcription factor LEF-1. *Nature*, Vol. 382, No. 6592, (August 1996), pp. (638–642), ISSN 0028-0836

Bellei, B., Flori, E., Izzo, E., Maresca, V., & Picardo, M. (2008). GSK3beta inhibition promotes melanogenesis in mouse B16 melanoma cells and normal human melanocytes. *Cell Signal*, Vol. 20, No. 10, (October 2008), pp. (1750–1761), ISSN 1873-3913

Bilic, J., Huang, Y.L., Davidson, G., Zimmermann, T., Cruciat, C.M., Bienz, M., & Niehrs, C. (2007). Wnt induces LRP6 signalosomes and promotes dishevelled-dependent LRP6 phosphorylation. *Science*, Vol. 316, No. 5831, (June 2007), pp. (1619–1622), ISSN 0036-8075

Billiard, J., Way, D.S., Seestaller-Wehr, L.M., Moran, R.A., Mangine, A., & Bodine, P.V. (2005). The orphan receptor tyrosine kinase Ror2 modulates canonical Wnt signaling in osteoblastic cells. *Mol Endocrinol*, Vol. 19, No. 1, (January 2005), pp. (90–101), ISSN 0888-8809

Bittner, M., Meltzer, P., Chen, Y., Jiang, Y., Seftor, E., Hendrix, M., Radmacher, M., Simon, R., Yakhini, Z., Ben-Dor, A., Sampas, N., Dougherty, E., Wang, E., Marincola, F., Gooden, C., Lueders, J., Glatfelter, A., Pollock, P., Carpten, J., Gillanders, E., Leja, D., Dietrich, K., Beaudry, C., Berens, M., Alberts, D., & Sondak, V. (2000). Molecular classification of cutaneous malignant melanoma by gene expression profiling. *Nature*, Vol. 406, No. 6795, (August 2000), pp. (536–540), ISSN 0028-0836

Brabletz, T., Jung, A., Dag, S., Hlubek, F., & Kirchner, T. (1999). β-catenin regulates the expression of the matrix metalloproteinase-7 in human colorectal cancer, *Am J Pathol*, Vol. 155, No. 4, (October 1999), pp. (1033–1038), ISSN 1525-2191

Brantjes, H., Barker, N., van Es, J., & Clevers, H. (2002). TCF: Lady Justice casting the final verdict on the outcome of Wnt signalling. *Biol Chem*, Vol. 383, No. 2, (Febrary 2002), pp. (255–261), ISSN 0021-9258

Cadigan, K.M., & Peifer, M. (2009). Wnt signaling from development to disease: insights from model systems. *Cold Spring Harb Perspect Biol*, Vol. 1, No. 2, (August 2009), a002881, ISSN 1943-0264

Campisi, J. (2005). Senescent cells, tumor suppression, and organismal aging: good citizens, bad neighbors. *Cell*, Vol.120, No. 4, (February 2005), pp. (513–522), ISSN 0092-8674

Cardones, A.R., Murakami, T., & Hwang, S.T. (2003). CXCR4 enhances adhesion of B16 tumor cells to endothelial cells in vitro and in vivo via beta(1) integrin. *Cancer Res*, Vol. 63,No. 20, (October 2003), pp. (6751–6757)

Carreira, S., Goodall, J., Aksan, I., La Rocca, S.A., Galibert, M.D., Denat, L., Larue, L., & Goding, C.R. (2005). Mitf cooperates with Rb1 and activates p21Cip1 expression to regulate cell cycle progression. *Nature*, Vol. 433, No. 7027, (February 2005), pp. (764–769), ISSN 0028-0836

Carreira, S., Goodall, J., Denat, L., Rodriguez, M., Nuciforo, P., Hoek, K.S., Testori, A., Larue, L., & Goding, C.R. (2006). Mitf regulation of Dia1 controls melanoma proliferation and invasiveness. *Genes & Dev*, Vol. 20, No. 24, (December 2006), pp. (3426–3439), ISSN 0890-9369

Cheon, S., Poon, R., Yu, C., Khoury, M., Shenker, R., Fish, J., & Alman, B.A. (2005). Prolonged beta-catenin stabilization and tcf-dependent transcriptional activation in hyperplastic cutaneous wounds. *Lab Invest*, Vol. 85, No. 3, (March 2005), pp. (416-425), ISSN 0023-6837

Chien, A.J., Moore, E.C., Lonsdorf, A.S., Kulikauskas, R.M., Rothberg, B.G., Berger, A.J., Major, M.B., Hwang, S.T., Rimm, D.L., & Moon, R.T. (2009). Activated Wnt/beta-catenin signaling in melanoma is associated with decreased proliferation in patient tumors and a murine melanoma model. *Proc Natl Acad Sci USA*, Vol. 106, No. 4, (January 2009), pp. (1193–1198)

Chirivi, R.G., Chiodoni, C., Musiani, P., Garofalo, A., Bernasconi, S., Colombo, M.P., & Giavazzi, R. (1996). IL-lalpha genetransfected human melanoma cells increase tmnor-cell adhesion to endothelial cells and their retention in the lung of nude mice, *lnt J Cancer*, Vol. 67, No. 6, (September), pp. (856-863), ISSN 0020-7136

Choi, S.C., & Han, J.K. (2002). Xenopus Cdc42 regulates convergent extension movements during gastrulation through Wnt/Ca2+ -signaling pathway. *Dev Biol*, Vol. 244, No. 2, (April 2002), pp. (342-357), ISSN 0012-1606

Clark, E.A., Golub, T.R., Lander, E.S., & Hynes, R.O. (2000). Genomic analysis of metastasis reveals an essential role for RhoC. *Nature*, Vol. 406, No. 6795, (August 2000), pp. (532–535), ISSN 0028-0836

Clevers, H. (2006). Wnt/β-catenin signaling in development and disease. *Cell*, Vol. 127, No. 3, (November 2006), pp. (469–480), ISSN 0092-8674

Cliffe, A., Hamada, F., & Bienz, M. (2003). A role of Dishevelled in relocating Axin to the plasma membrane during wingless signaling. *Curr Biol*, Vol. 13, No. 11, (May 2003), pp. (960-966), ISSN 0960-9822

Cowin, P. (1994). Unraveling the cytoplasmic interactions of the cadherin superfamily. *Proc. Natl Acad Sci USA*, Vol. 91, No. 23, (November 1994), pp. (10759–10761)

Da Forno, P.D., Pringle, J.H., Hutchinson, P., Osborn, J., Huang, Q., Potter, L., Hancox, R.A., Fletcher, A., & Saldanha, G.S. (2008). WNT5A expression increases during melanoma progression and correlates with outcome. *Clin Cancer Res*, Vol. 14, No. 18, (September 2008), pp. (5825-5832), ISSN 1557-3265

Dang, C.V. (1999). c-Myc target genes involved in cell growth, apoptosis, and metabolism. *Mol Cell Biol*, Vol. 19, No. 1, (January 1999), pp. (1–11), ISSN 0270-7306

De Calisto, J., Araya, C., Marchant, L., Riaz, C.F., & Mayor, R. (2005). Essential role of non-canonical Wnt signalling in neural crest migration. *Development*, Vol. 132, No. 11, (June 2005), pp. (2587-2597), ISSN 0950-1991

Delmas. V., Beermann, F., Martinozzi, S., Carreira, S., Ackermann, J., Kumasaka, M., Denat, L., Goodall, J., Luciani, F., Viros, A., Demirkan, N., Bastian, B.C., Goding, C.R., & Larue, L. (2007). Beta-catenin induces immortalization of melanocytes by suppressing p16INK4a expression and cooperates with N-Ras in melanoma development. *Genes Dev*, Vol. 21, No. 22, (November 2007), pp. (2923–2935), ISSN 0890-9369

Dissanayake, S.K., Olkhanud, P.B., O'Connell, M.P., Carter, A., French, A.D., Camilli, T.C., Emeche, C.D., Hewitt, K.J., Rosenthal, D.T., Leotlela, P.D., Wade, M.S., Yang, S.W., Brant, L., Nickoloff, B.J., Messina, J.L., Biragyn, A., Hoek, K.S., Taub, D.D., Longo, D.L., Sondak, V.K., Hewitt, S.M., & Weeraratna, A.T. (2008). Wnt5A regulates expression of tumor-associated antigens in melanoma via changes in signal transducers and activators of transcription 3 phosphorylation. *Cancer Res*, Vol. 68, No. 24, (December 2008), pp. (10205-10214)

Dissanayake, S.K., Wade, M., Johnson, C.E., O'Connell, M.P., Leotlela, P.D., French, A.D., Shah, K.V., Hewitt, K.J., Rosenthal, D.T., Indig, F.E., Jiang, Y., Nickoloff, B.J., Taub, D.D., Trent, J.M., Moon, R.T., Bittner, M., & Weeraratna, A.T. (2007). The Wnt5A/protein kinase C pathway mediates motility in melanoma cells via the inhibition of metastasis suppressors and initiation of an epithelial to mesenchymal transition. *J Biol Chem*, Vol. 282, No. 23, (June 2007), pp. (17259–17271), ISSN 0021-9258

Dorsky, R., Moon, R., & Raible, D. (1998). Control of neural crest cell fate by the Wnt signalling pathway. *Nature*, Vol. 396, No. 6709, (November 1998), pp. (370-373), 9845073

Fang, D., Leishear, K., Nguyen, T.K., Finko, R., Cai, K., Fukunaga, M., Li, L., Brafford, P.A., Kulp, A.N., Xu, X., Smalley, K.S., & Herlyn, M. (2006). Defining the conditions for the generation of melanocytes from human embryonic stem cells. *Stem Cells*, Vol. 24, No. 7,(July 2006), pp. (1668–1677)

Fathke, C., Wilson, L., Shah, K., Kim, B., Hocking, A., Moon, R., & Isik, F. (2006). Wnt signaling induces epithelial differentiation during cutaneous wound healing. *BMC Cell Biology*, 7:4, (January 2006), ISSN 1471-2121

García-Castro, M.I., Marcelle, C., & Bronner-Fraser, M. (2002). Ectodermal Wnt function as a neural crest inducer. *Science*, Vol. 297, No. 5582, (August 2002), pp. (848-851), ISSN 0036-8075

Gartsbein, M., Alt, A., Hashimoto, K., Nakajima, K., Kuroki, T., & Tennenbaum, T. (2006). The role of protein kinase C delta activation and STAT3 Ser727 phosphorylation in insulin-induced keratinocyte proliferation. *J Cell Sci*, Vol. 119, No. Pt3, (Febrary 2006), pp. (470–481), ISSN 0021-9533

Giles, R.H., van Es, J.H., & Clevers, H. (2003). Caught up in a Wnt storm: Wnt signaling in cancer. *Biochim Biophys Acta*, Vol. 1653, No. 1, (June 2003), pp. (1-24)

Glinka, A., Wu, W., Delius, H., Monaghan, A.P., Blumenstock, C., & Niehrs, C. (1998). Dickkopf-1 is a member of a new family of secreted proteins and functions in head induction. *Nature*, Vol. 391, No. 6665, (January 1998), pp. (357–362), ISSN 0028-0836

Govindarajan, B., Sligh, J.E., Vincent, B.J., Li, M., Canter, J.A., Nickoloff, B.J., Rodenburg, R.J., Smeitink, J.A., Oberley, L., Zhang, Y., Slingerland, J., Arnold, R.S., Lambeth, J.D., Cohen, C., Hilenski, L., Griendling, K., Martínez-Diez, M., Cuezva, J.M., & Arbiser, J.L. (2007). Overexpression of Akt converts radial growth melanoma to vertical growth melanoma. *Clin Invest*, Vol. 117, No, 3, (March 2007), pp. (719–729), ISSN 0021-9738

Gradl, D., Kühl, M. & Wedlich, D. (1999). The Wnt/Wg signal transducer beta-catenin controls fibronectin expression. *Mol Cell Biol*, Vol. 19, No. 8, (August 1999), pp. (5576–5587), ISSN 0270-7306

Gray-Schopfer, V.C., da Rocha Dias, S., & Marais, R.. (2005). The role of B-RAF in melanoma. *Cancer Metastasis Rev*, Vol. 24, No. 1, (January 2005), pp. (165–183), ISSN 0167-7659

Gumbiner, B.M. (1993). Proteins associated with the cytoplasmic surface of adhesion molecules. *Neuron*, Vol. 11, No. 4, (October 1993), pp. (551–564), ISSN 0896-6273

Haass, N.K., Smalley, K.S., Li, L., & Herlyn, M. (2005). Adhesion, migration and communication in melanocytes and melanoma. *Pigment Cell Res*, Vol. 18, No. 3, (June 2005), pp. (150–159), ISSN 0893-5785

Habas, R., Dawid, I.B., & He, X. (2003). Coactivation of Rac and Rho by Wnt/Frizzled signaling is required for vertebrate gastrulation. *Genes Dev*, Vol. 17, No. 2, (January 2003), pp. (295-309), ISSN 0890-9369

Habas, R., Kato, Y., & He, X. (2001). Wnt/Frizzled activation of Rho regulates vertebrate gastrulation and requires a novel Formin homology protein Daam1. *Cell*, Vol. 107, No. 7, (December 2001), pp. (843-854), ISSN 0092-8674

Halford, M.M., & S.A. Stacker. (2001). Revelations of the RYK receptor. *Bioessays*, Vol. 23, No. 1, (January 2001), pp. (34–45), ISSN 0265-9247

Halford, M.M., Oates, A.C., Hibbs, M.L., Wilks, A.F. & Stacker, S.A. (1999). Genomic structure and expression of the mouse growth factor receptor related to tyrosine kinases (Ryk). *J Biol Chem*, Vol. 274, No. 11, (March 1999), pp. (7379-7390), ISSN 0021-9258

Haqq, C., Nosrati, M., Sudilovsky, D., Crothers, J., Khodabakhsh, D., Pulliam, B.L., Federman, S., Miller, J.R. 3rd, Allen, R.E., Singer, M.I., Leong, S.P., Ljung, B.M., Sagebiel, R.W., & Kashani-Sabet, M. (2005). The gene expression signatures of melanoma progression. *Proc Natl Acad Sci USA*, Vol. 102, No. 17, (April 2005), pp. (6092–6097)

Hari, L., Brault, V., Kleber, M., Lee, H.Y., Ille, F., Leimeroth, R., Paratore, C., Suter, U., Kemler, R., & Sommer, L. (2002). Lineage-specific requirements of beta-catenin in neural crest development. *J Cell Biol*, Vol. 159, No. 5, (December 2002), pp. (867–880), ISSN 0021-9525

He, T.C., Chan, T.A., Vogelstein, B., & Kinzler, K.W. (1999). PPARdelta is an APC-regulated target of nonsteroidal anti-inflammatory drugs. *Cell*, Vol. 99, No. 3,(October 1999), pp. (335–345), ISSN 0092-8674

Hoek, K.S., Schlegel, N.C., Brafford, P., Sucker, A., Ugurel, S., Kumar, R., Weber, B.L., Nathanson, K.L., Phillips, D.J., Herlyn, M., Schadendorf, D., & Dummer, R. (2006). Metastatic potential of melanomas defined by specific gene expression profiles with no BRAF signature. *Pigment Cell Res*, Vol. 19, No. 4, (August 2006), pp. (290–302), ISSN 0893-5785

Hovens, C.M., Stacker, S.A., Andres, A.C., Harpur, A.G., Ziemiecki, A. & Wilks, A. F. (1992). RYK, a receptor tyrosine kinase-related molecule with unusual kinase domain motifs. *Proc Natl Acad Sci USA*, Vol. 89, No, 24, (December 1992), pp. (11818-11822)

Hsu, M.Y., Meier, F., & Herlyn, M. (2002). Melanoma development and progression: a conspiracy between tumor and host. *Differentiation*, Vol. 70, No. 9-10, (December 2002), pp. (522–536), ISSN 0301-4681

Huang, X., & Saint-Jeannet, J.P. (2004). Induction of the neural crest and the opportunities of life on the edge. *Dev Biol*, Vol. 275, No. 1, (November 2004), pp. (1–11), ISSN 0012-1606

Ikeya, M., Lee, S.M., Johnson, J.E., McMahon, A.P., & Takada, S. (1997). Wnt signalling required for expansion of neural crest and CNS progenitors. *Nature*, Vol. 389, No. 6654, (October 1997), pp. (966–970), ISSN 0028-0836

Itasaki, N., Jones, C.M., Mercurio, S., Rowe, A., Domingos, P.M., Smith, J.C., & Krumlauf, R. (2003). Wise, a context-dependent activator and inhibitor of Wnt signaling. *Development*, Vol. 130, No. 18, (September 2003), pp. (4295–4305), ISSN 0950-1991

Iversen, P.L., Arora, V., Acker, A.J., Mason, D.H., & Devi, G.R. (2003). Efficacy of antisense morpholino oligomer targeted to c-myc in prostate cancer xenograft murine model and a Phase I safety study in humans. *Clin Cancer Res*, Vol. 9, No. 7, (July 2003), pp. (2510–2519), ISSN 1557-3265

Jenny, A., & Mlodzik, M. (2006). Planar cell polarity signaling: a common mechanism for cellular polarization. *Mt Sinai J Med*, Vol. 73, No. 5, (September 2006), pp. (738–750)

Jin, E.J., Erickson, C.A., Takada, S., & Burrus, L.W. (2001). Wnt and BMP signaling govern lineage segregation of melanocytes in the avian embryo. *Dev Biol*, Vol. 233, No. 1, (May 2001), pp. (22-37), ISSN 0012-1606

Jönsson, M., Smith, K., & Harris, A.L. (1998). Regulation of Wnt5a expression in human mammary cells by protein kinase C activity and the cytoskeleton. *Br J Cancer*, Vol. 78, No. 4, (August 1998), pp. (430- 438), ISSN 0007-0920

Kageshita, T., Hamby, C.V., Ishihara, T., Matsumoto, K., Saida, T., & Ono, T. (2001). Loss of beta-catenin expression associated with disease progression in malignant melanoma. *Br J Dermatol*, Vol. 145, No. 2, (August 2001), pp. (210–216), ISSN 0007-0963

Kamaraju, A.K., Bertolotto, C., Chebath, J., & Revel, M. (2002). Pax3 down-regulation and shutoff of melanogenesis in melanoma B16/F10.9 by interleukin-6 receptor signaling. *J Biol Chem*, Vol. 277, No. 17, (April 2002), pp. (15132–15141), ISSN 0021-9258

Keeble, T.R., Halford, M.M., Seaman, C., Kee, N., Macheda, M., Anderson, R.B., Stacker, S.A., & Cooper, H.M. (2006). The Wnt receptor Ryk is required for Wnt5a-mediated axon guidance on the contralateral side of the corpus callosum. *J Neurosci*, Vol. 26, No. 21, (May 2006), pp. (5840-5848), ISSN 0270-6474

Keller, R. (2002). Shaping the vertebrate body plan by polarized embryonic cell movements. *Science*, Vol. 298, No. 5600, (December 2002), pp. (1950–1954), ISSN 0036-8075

Kielhorn, E., Provost, E., Olsen, D., D'Aquila, T.G., Smith, B.L., Camp, R.L., & Rimm, D.L: (2003). Tissue microarray-based analysis shows phospho-beta-catenin expression in malignant melanoma is associated with poor outcome. *Int J Cancer*, Vol. 103, No. 5, (February 2003), pp. (652–656)

Kohn, A.D., & Moon, R.T. (2005). Wnt and calcium signaling: beta-catenin- independent pathways. *Cell Calcium*, Vol. 38, No. 3-4, (September-October 2005), pp. (439– 446), 16099039

Kühl, M., Sheldahl, L.C., Park, M., Miller, J.R., & Moon, R.T. (2000). The Wnt/Ca2+-pathway: a new vertebrate Wnt signaling pathway takes shape. *Trends Genet*, Vol. 16, No. 7, (June 2000), pp. (279–283), ISSN 0168-9525

Kulikova, K., Posvyatenko, A., Gnuchev, N., Georgiev, G., Kibardin, & Larin, S. Nuclear β-catenin localization is not sufficient for canonical Wnt signaling activation in human melanoma cell lines. *Molecular Biology,* in press., ISSN 0026-8933

Kuphal, S., Lodermeyer, S., Bataille, F., Schuierer, M., Hoang, B.H., & Bosserhoff, A.K. (2006). Expression of Dickkopf genes is strongly reduced in malignant melanoma. *Oncogene*, Vol. 25, No. 36, (August 2006), pp. (5027–5036), ISSN 0950-9232

LaBonne, C., & Bronner-Fraser, M. (1998). Neural crest induction in Xenopus: evidence for a two-signal model. *Development*, Vol.125, No. 13, (July 1998), pp. (2403–2414), ISSN 0950-1991

Larue, L. & Delmas, V. (2006). The WNT/β-catenin pathway in melanoma. *Front. Biosci*, Vol. 11, (January 2006), pp. (733–742), ISSN 1945-0516

Larue, L., & Beermann, F. (2007). Cutaneous melanoma in genetically modified animals. *Pigment Cell Res*, Vol. 20, No. 6, (December 2007), pp. (485–497), ISSN 0893-5785

Larue, L., Luciani, F., Kumasaka, M., Champeval, D., Demirkan, N., Bonaventure, J., & Delmas, V. (2009). Bypassing melanocyte senescence by β-catenin: A novel way to promote melanoma. *Pathol Biol (Paris)*, Vol. 57, No.7-8, (November-December 2009), pp. (543–547)

Lewis, J.L., Bonner, J., Modrell, M., Ragland, J.W., Moon, R.T., Dorsky, R.I., & Raible, D.W. (2004). Reiterated Wnt signaling during zebrafish neural crest development. *Development*, Vol. 131, No. 6, (March 2004), pp. (1299-1308), ISSN 0950-1991

Li, L., Yuan, H., Xie, W., Mao, J., Caruso, A.M., McMahon, A., Sussman, D.J., & Wu, D. (1999) Dishevelled proteins lead to two signaling pathways. Regulation of LEF-1 and c-Jun N-terminal kinase in mammalian cells. *J Biol Chem*, Vol. 274, No. 1, (January 1999), pp. (129-134), ISSN 0021-9258

Lin, Y.C., You, L., Xu, Z., He, B., Yang, C.T., Chen, J.K., Mikami, I., Clément, G., Shi, Y., Kuchenbecker, K., Okamoto, J., Kashani-Sabet, M., & Jablons, D.M. (2007). Wnt inhibitory factor-1 gene transfer inhibits melanoma cell growth. *Hum Gene Ther*, Vol. 18, No. 4, (April 2007), pp. (379–386), ISSN 1043-0342

Liu, C., Li, Y., Semenov, M., Han, C., Baeg, G.H., Tan, Y., Zhang, Z., Lin, X., & He, X. (2002). Control of β-catenin phosphorylation/degradation by a dual-kinase mechanism. *Cell*, Vol. 108, No. 6, (March 2002), pp. (837–847), ISSN 0092-8674

Liu, T., Liu, X., Wang, H., Moon, R.T., & Malbon, C.C. (1999). Activation of rat frizzled-1 promotes Wnt signaling and differentiation of mouse F9 teratocarcinoma cells via pathways that require Galpha(q) and Galpha(o) function, *J Biol Chem*, Vol. 274, No. 47, (November 1999), pp. (33539–33544), ISSN 0021-9258

Loercher, A.E., Tank, E.M., Delston, R.B., & Harbour, J.W. (2005). MITF links differentiation with cell cycle arrest in melanocytes by transcriptional activation of INK4A. *J Cell Biol*, Vol. 168, No. 1, (January 2005), pp.(35–40), ISSN 0021-9525.

Lu, W., Yamamoto, V., Ortega, B. & Baltimore, D. (2004). Mammalian Ryk is a Wnt coreceptor required for stimulation of neurite outgrowth. *Cell*, Vol. 119, No. 1, (October 2004), pp. (97–108), ISSN 0092-8674

Lucero, O.M., Dawson, D.W., Moon, R.T., & Chien, A.J. (2010). A re-evaluation of the "oncogenic" nature of Wnt/beta-catenin signaling in melanoma and other cancers. *Curr Oncol Rep*, Vol. 12, No. 5, (September 2010), pp. (314–318), ISSN 1534-6269

Maelandsmo, G.M., Holm, R., Nesland, J.M., Fodstad, O., & Florenes, V.A. (2003). Reduced betacatenin expression in the cytoplasm of advanced-stage superficial spreading malignant melanoma. *Clin Cancer Res*, Vol. 9, No. 9, (August 2003), pp. (3383–3388), ISSN 1557-3265

Malbon, C.C., Wang, H., & Moon, R.T. (2001). Wnt signaling and heterotrimeric G-proteins: strange bedfellows or a classic romance? Biochem Biophys Res Commun, Vol. 287, No. 3, (September 2001), pp. (589–593), 11563835 Mann, B., Gelos, M., Siedow, A., Hanski, M.L., Gratchev, A., Ilyas, M., Bodmer, W.F., Moyer, M.P., Riecken, E.O., Buhr, H.J., & Hanski, C. (1999). Target genes of beta-catenin-T cell-factor/lymphoid-enhancer-factor signaling in human colorectal carcinomas. *Proc Natl Acad Sci USA*, Vol. 96, No. 4, (February 1999), pp. (1603–1608)

Mao, B., Wu, W., Davidson, G., Marhold, J., Li, M., Mechler, B.M., Delius, H., Hoppe, D., Stannek, P., Walter, C., Glinka, A., & Niehrs, C. (2002). Kremen proteins are Dickkopf receptors that regulate Wnt/beta-catenin signalling. *Nature*, Vol. 417, No. 6889, (June 2002), pp. (664–667), ISSN 0028-0836

Mao, B., Wu, W., Li, Y., Hoppe, D., Stannek, P., Glinka, A. & Niehrs, C. (2001). LDL-receptor-related protein 6 is a receptor for Dickkopf proteins. *Nature*, Vol. 411, No. 6835, (May 2001), pp. (321-325), ISSN 0028-0836

Mapelli, E., Banfi, P., Sala, E., Sensi, M., Supino, R., Zunino, F., & Gambetta, R.A. (1994). Effect of protein kinase C inhibitors on invasiveness of human melanoma clones expressing different levels of protein kinase C isoenzymes. *Int J Cancer*, Vol. 57, No. 2, (April 1994), pp. (281–286), ISSN 0020-7136

Marlow, F., Topczewski, J., Sepich, D., & Solnica-Krezel, L. (2002). Zebrafish Rho kinase 2 acts downstream of Wnt11 to mediate cell polarity and effective convergence and extension movements. *Curr Biol*, Vol. 12, No. 11, (June 2002), pp. (876-884), ISSN 0960-9822

McGary, E.C., Lev, D.C., & Bar-Eli, M. (2002). Cellular adhesion pathways and metastatic potential of human melanoma.. *Cancer Biol Ther*, Vol. 1, No. 5, (September-October 2002), pp. (459-465), ISSN 1538-4047

McMahon, A.P. (1992). The Wnt family of developmental regulators, *Trends Genet*, Vol. 8, No. 7, (July 1992), pp. (236-242), ISSN 0168-9525

Melchiori A., Mortarini R., Carlone S. et al. (1995), The α3β1 integrin is involved in melanoma cell migration and invasion, *Exp Cell Res*, Vol. 218, No. 1, (July 1995), pp. (233-242), ISSN 0014-4827

Mikheev, A.M., Mikheeva, S.A., Rostomily, R., & Zarbl, H. (2007). Dickkopf-1 activates cell death in MDA-MB435 melanoma cells. *Biochem Biophys Res Commun*, Vol. 352, No. 3, (January 2007), pp. (675–680), ISSN 0006-291X

Miller, J.R. (2001). The Wnts. *Genome Biol*, Vol. 3, No. 1, (n. d.), ISSN 474-7596

Minami, Y., Oishi, I., Endo, M., & Nishita, M. (2010). Ror-family receptor tyrosine kinases in noncanonical Wnt signaling: their implications in developmental morphogenesis and human diseases. *Dev Dyn*, Vol. 239, No. 1, (January 2010), pp. (1–15), ISSN 1058-8388

Mlodzik, M. (2002). Planar cell polarization: do the same mechanisms regulate *Drosophila* tissue polarity and vertebrate gastrulation? *Trends Genet*, Vol. 18, No. 11, (Novemver 2002), pp. (564-571), ISSN 0168-9525

Myers, D.C., Sepich, D.S., & Solnica-Krezel, L. (2002). Convergence and extension in vertebrate gastrulae: cell movements according to or in search of identity? *Trends Genet*, Vol. 18, No. 9, (September 2002), pp. (447–455), ISSN 0168-9525

Nagafuchi, A., & Takeichi, M., (1989). Transmembrane control of cadherin-mediated cell adhesion: a 94 kDa protein functionally associated with a specific region of the cytoplasmic domain of E-cadherin. *Cell Regul*, Vol. 1, No. 1, (November 1989), pp. (37–44), ISSN 1044-2030

Nakahara, H., Otani, T., Sasaki, T., Miura, Y., Takai, Y., & Kogo, M. (2003). Involvement of Cdc42 and Rac small G proteins in invadopodia formation of RPMI7951 cells. *Genes Cells*, Vol. 8, No. 12, (December 2003), pp. (1019–1027), ISSN 1356-9597

Narita, M., Nũnez, S., Heard, E., Narita, M., Lin, A.W., Hearn, S.A., Spector, D.L., Hannon, G.J., & Lowe, S.W. (2003). Rb-mediated heterochromatin formation and silencing of E2F target genes during cellular senescence. *Cell*; Vol. 113, No. 6, (June 2003), pp. (703–716), ISSN 0092-8674

Nechiporuk, T. & Vasioukhin, V. (2006). Planar cell polarity planes the inconveniences of cell division into a smooth morphogenetic process. *Dev Cell*, Vol. 10, No. 2, (February 2006), pp. (153-154), ISSN 1534-5807

Nemeth, M.J., Topol, L., Anderson, S.M., Yang, Y., & Bodine, D.M. (2007). Wnt5a inhibits canonical Wnt signaling in hematopoietic stem cells and enhances repopulation. *Proc Natl Acad Sci USA*, Vol. 104, No. 39, (September 2007), pp. (15436–15441)

Niehrs, C., & Shen, J. (2010). Regulation of Lrp6 phosphorylation. *Cell Mol Life Sci*, Vol. 67, No. 15, (August 2010), pp. (2551–2562), ISSN 1420-682X

Nishikawa, S., & Osawa, M. (2007). Generating quiescent stem cells. *Pigment Cell Res*, Vol. 20, No. 4, (August 2007), pp. (263–270), ISSN 0893-5785

Nishimura, E.K., Jordan, S.A., Oshima, H., Yoshida, H., Osawa, M., Moriyama, M., Jackson, I.J., Barrandon, Y., Miyachi, Y., & Nishikawa, S. (2002). Dominant role of the niche in melanocyte stem-cell fate determination, *Nature*, Vol. 416, No. 6883, (April 2002), pp. (854–860), ISSN 0028-0836

Nomachi, A., Nishita, M., Inaba, D., Enomoto, M., Hamasaki, M., & Minami, Y. (2008). Receptor tyrosine kinase Ror2 mediates Wnt5a-induced polarized cell migration by activating c-Jun N-terminal kinase via actin-binding protein Filamin A, *J Biol Chem*, Vol. 283, No. 41, (October 2008), pp. (27973–27981), ISSN 0021-9258

O'Connell, M.P., French, A.D., Leotlela, P.D., & Weeraratna, A.T. (2008). Assaying Wnt5A-mediated invasion in melanoma cells. *Methods Mol Biol*, Vol. 468, (n.d.), pp. (243–253), ISSN 1064-3745

O'Connell, M.P., & Weeraratna, A.T. (2009). Hear the Wnt Ror: how melanoma cells adjust to changes in Wnt. *Pigment Cell Melanoma Res*, Vol. 22, No. 6, (December 2009), pp. (724–739), ISSN 1755-1471

O'Connell, M.P., Fiori, J.L., Baugher, K.M., Indig, F.E., French, A.D., Camilli, T.C., Frank, B.P., Earley, R., Hoek, K.S., Hasskamp, J.H., Elias, E.G., Taub, D.D., Bernier, M., & Weeraratna, A.T. (2009). Wnt5A activates the calpain-mediated cleavage of Filamin A. *J Invest Dermatol*, Vol. 129, No. 7, (July 2009), pp. (1782–1789), ISSN 0022-202X

O'Connell, M.P., Fiori, J.L., Xu, M., Carter, A.D., Frank, B.P., Camilli, T.C., French, A.D., Dissanayake, S.K., Indig, F.E., Bernier, M., Taub, D.D., Hewitt, S.M., & Weeraratna, A.T. (2010). The orphan tyrosine kinase receptor, ROR2, mediates Wnt5A signaling in metastatic melanoma. *Oncogene*, Vol. 29, No. 1, (October 2009), pp. (34-44), ISSN 0950-9232

Oishi, I., Takeuchi, S., Hashimoto, R., Nagabukuro, A., Ueda, T., Liu, Z.J., Hatta, T., Akira, S., Matsuda, Y., Yamamura, H., Otani, H., & Minami, Y. (1999). Spatio-temporally regulated expression of receptor tyrosine kinases, mRor1, mRor2, during mouse development: implications in development and function of the nervous system. *Genes Cells*, Vol. 4, No. 1, (January 1999), pp. (41–56), ISSN 1356-9597

Ozawa, M., Baribault, H., & Kemler, R. (1989), The cytoplasmic domain of the cell adhesion molecule uvomorulin associates with three independent proteins structurally related in different species. *EMBO J*, Vol. 8, No. 6, (June 1989), pp. (1711 -1717)

Palmieri, G., Capone, M., Ascierto, M.L., Gentilcore, G., Stroncek, D.F., Casula, M., Sini, M.C., Palla, M., Mozzillo, N., & Ascierto, P.A. (2009). Main roads to melanoma *J Transl Med*, Vol. 7:86, (October 2009), ISSN 1479-5876

Parri, M., Taddei, M.L., Bianchini, F., Calorini, L., & Chiarugi, P. (2009). EphA2 reexpression prompts invasion of melanoma cells shifting from mesenchymal to amoeboid-like motility style. *Cancer Res*, Vol. 69, No. 5, (March 2009), pp. (2072-2081)

Patthy, L (2000). The WIF module. *Trends Biochem Sci*, Vol. 25, No. 1, (January 2000), pp. (12–3), ISSN 0968-0004

Pham, K., Milovanovic, T., Barr, R.J., Truong, T., & Holcombe, R.F. (2003). Wnt ligand expression in malignant melanoma: Pilot study indicating correlation with histopathological features. *Mol Pathol*, Vol. 56, No. 5, (October 2003), pp. (280–285)

Pinson, K.I., Brennan, J., Monkley, S., Avery, B.J., & Skarnes, W.C. (2000). An LDL-receptor-related protein mediates Wnt signalling in mice. *Nature*, Vol. 407, No. 6803, (September 2000), pp. 535-538), ISSN 0028-0836

Pukrop, T., Klemm, F., Hagemann, T., Gradl, D., Schulz, M., Siemes, S., Trümper, L., & Binder, C. (2006). Wnt 5a signaling is critical for macrophage-induced invasion of breast cancer cell lines. *Proc Natl Acad Sci USA,* Vol. 103, No. 14, (April 2006), pp. (5454–5459)

Rubinfeld, B., Robbins, P., El-Gamil, M., Albert, I., Porfiri, E., & Polakis, P. (1997). Stabilization of beta-catenin by genetic defects in melanoma cell lines. *Science*, Vol. 275, No, 5307, (March 1997), pp. (1790-1792), ISSN 0036-8075

Ryu, B., Kim, D.S., Deluca, A.M., & Alani, R.M. (2007). Comprehensive expression profiling of tumor cell lines identifies molecular signatures of melanoma progression. *PLoS ONE,* Vol. 2, No. 7, (July 2007), pp. (e594)

Sakai, D., Tanaka, Y., Endo, Y., Osumi, N., Okamoto, H., & Wakamatsu, Y. (2005). Regulation of *Slug* transcription in embryonic ectoderm by β-catenin-Lef/Tcf and BMP-Smad signaling. *Dev Growth Differ,* Vol. 47, No. 7, (September 2005), pp. (471–482)

Schepsky, A., Bruser, K., Gunnarsson, G.J., Goodall, J., Hallsson, J.H., Goding, C.R., Steingrimsson, E., & Hecht, A. (2006). The microphthalmia-associated transcription factor Mitf interacts with β-catenin to determine target gene expression. *Mol Cell Biol,* Vol. 26, No. 23, (December 2006), pp. (8914–8927), ISSN 0270-7306

Semenov, M., Tamai, K., & He, X. (2005). SOST is a ligand for LRP5/LRP6 and a Wnt signaling inhibitor. *J Biol Chem,* Vol. *280,* No. 29, (July 2005), pp. (26770–26775), ISSN 0021-9258

Sen, M., Chamorro, M., Reifert, J., Corr, M., & Carson, D.A. (2001). Blockade of Wnt-5A/frizzled 5 signaling inhibits rheumatoid synoviocyte activation. *Arthritis Rheum*, Vol. 44, No. 4, (April 2001), pp. (772–781)

Sheldahl, L.C., Park, M., Malbon, C.C., & Moon, R.T. (1999). Protein kinase C is differentially stimulated by Wnt and Frizzled homologs in a G-protein-dependent manner. *Curr Biol*, Vol. 9, No. 13, (July 1999), pp. (695–698), ISSN 0960-9822

Sinnberg, T., Menzel, M., Kaesler, S., Biedermann, T., Sauer, B., Nahnsen, S., Schwarz, M., Garbe, C., & Schittek, B. (2010). Suppression of casein kinase 1alpha in melanoma cells induces a switch in beta-catenin signaling to promote metastasis. *Cancer Res*, Vol. 70, No. 17, (September 2010), pp. (6999–7009)

Takahashi, Y., Nishikawa, M., Suehara, T., Takiguchi, N., & Takakura, Y. (2008). Gene silencing of b-catenin in melanoma cells retards their growth but promotes the formation of pulmonary metastasis in mice. *Int J Cancer*, Vol. 123, No. 10, (Novemver 2008), pp. (2315–2320)

Tamai, K., Semenov, M., Kato, Y., Spokony, R., Liu, C., Katsuyama, Y., Hess, F., Saint-Jeannet, J.P., & He, X. (2000). LDL-receptor-related proteins in Wnt signal transduction. *Nature*, Vol. 407, No. 6803, (September 2000), pp. (530-535), ISSN 0028-0836

Tetsu, O., & McCormick, F. (1999). Beta-catenin regulates expression of cyclin D1 in colon carcinoma cells. *Nature*, Vol. 398, No. 6726, (April 1999), pp. (422–426), ISSN 0028-0836

Thomas, A.J., & Erickson, C.A. (2009). FOXD3 regulates the lineage switch between neural crest-derived glial cells and pigment cells by repressing MITF through a non-canonical mechanism. *Development*, Vol. 136, No. 11, (June 2009), pp. (1849-1858), ISSN 0950-1991

Topol, L., Jiang, X., Choi, H., Garrett-Beal, L., Carolan, P.J., & Yang, Y. (2003). Wnt-5a inhibits the canonical Wnt pathway by promoting GSK-3-independent b-catenin degradation. *J Cell Biol*, Vol. 162, No. 5, (September 2003), pp. (899–908), ISSN 0021-9525

Tsao, H., Bevona, C., Goggins, W., & Quinn, T. (2003), The transformation rate of moles (melanocytic nevi) into cutaneous melanoma: a population-based estimate. *Arch Dermatol*, Vol. 139, No. 3, (March 2003), pp. (282–288)

Tsao, H., Zhang, X., Fowlkes, K., & Haluska, F.G. (2000). Relative reciprocity of NRAS and PTEN/MMAC1 alterations in cutaneous melanoma cell lines. *Cancer Res*, Vol. 60, No. 7, (April 2000), pp. (1800–1804)

Vallin, J., Thuret, R., Giacomello, E., Faraldo, M.M., Thiery, J.P., & Broders, F. (2001). Cloning and characterization of three *Xenopus* slug promoters reveal direct regulation by Lef/β-catenin signaling. *J Biol Chem*, Vol. 276, No. 32, (August 2001), pp. (30350-30358), ISSN 0021-9258

Wallingford, J.B., Fraser, S.E., & Harland, R.M. (2002). Convergent extension: the molecular control of polarized cell movement during embryonic development. *Dev Cell*, Vol. 2, No. 6, (June 2002), pp. (695–706), ISSN 1534-5807

Wang, Y., & Nathans, J. (2007). Tissue/planar cell polarity in vertebrates: new insights and new questions. *Development*, Vol. 134, No. 4, (February 2007), pp. (647-658), ISSN 0950-1991

Weeraratna, A.T. (2005). A Wnt-er Wonderland - The complexity of Wnt signaling in melanoma. *Cancer and Metastasis Rev*, Vol. 24, No. 2, (June 2005), pp. (237–250), ISSN 0167-7659

Weeraratna, A.T., Jiang, Y., Hostetter, G., Rosenblatt, K., Duray, P., Bittner, M., & Trent, J.M. (2002). Wnt5a signaling directly affects cell motility and invasion of metastatic melanoma. *Cancer Cell*, Vol. 1, No. 3, (April 2002), pp. (279–288)

Weiser, D.C., Pyati, U.J., & Kimelman, D. (2007). Gravin regulates mesodermal cell behavior changes required for axis elongation during zebrafish gastrulation. *Genes Dev*, Vol. 21, No. 12, (June 2007), pp. (1559-1571), ISSN 0890-9369

Wellbrock, C. & Marais, R. (2005). Elevated expression of MITF counteracts B-RAF-stimulated melanocyte and melanoma cell proliferation. *J Cell Biol*, Vol. 170, No. 5, (August 2005), pp. (703–708), ISSN 0021-9525

Widlund, H.R., Horstmann, M.A., Price, E.R., Cui, J., Lessnick, S.L., Wu, M., He, X., & Fisher, D.E. (2002). Beta-catenin-induced melanoma growth requires the downstream target Microphthalmia-associated transcription factor. *J Cell Biol*, Vol. 158, No. 6, (September 2002), pp. (1079–1087), ISSN 0021-9525

Willert, K., Brown, J.D., Danenberg, E., Duncan, A.W., Weissman, I.L., Reya, T., Yates, J.R. 3rd, & Nusse, R. (2003). Wnt proteins are lipid modified and can act as stem cell growth factors. *Nature*, Vol. 423, No. 6938, (May 2003), pp. (448-452), ISSN 0028-0836

Witze, E.S., Litman, E.S., Argast, G.M., Moon, R.T., & Ahn, N.G. (2008). Wnt5a control of cell polarity and directional movement by polarized redistribution of adhesion receptors. *Science*, Vol. 320, No. 5874, (April 2008), pp, (365–369), ISSN 0036-8075

Wnt homepage: http://www.stanford.edu/group/nusselab/cgi-bin/wnt

Wu, J., Yang, J., & Klein, P.S. (2005). Neural crest induction by the canonical Wnt pathway can be dissociated from anterior-posterior neural patterning in *Xenopus*. *Dev Biol*, Vol. 279, No. 1, (March 2005), pp. (220–232)

Xiao, C., Yang, B.F., Song, J.H., Schulman, H., Li, L., & Hao, C. (2005). Inhibition of CaMKII-mediated c-FLIP expression sensitizes malignant melanoma cells to TRAIL-induced apoptosis. *Exp Cell Res*, Vol. 304, No. 1, (March 2005), pp. (244–255), ISSN 0014-4827

Yamada, T., Akamatsu, H., Hasegawa, S., Inoue, Y., Date, Y., Mizutani, H., Yamamoto, N., Matsunaga, K., & Nakata, S. (2010). Melanocyte stem cells express receptors for canonical Wnt-signaling pathway on their surface. *Biochem Biophys Res Commun*, Vol. 396, No. 4, (June 2010), pp. (837–842), ISSN 0006-291X

Yamaguchi, Y., Brenner, M., & Hearing, V.J. (2007). The regulation of skin pigmentation. *J Biol Chem*, Vol. 282, No. 38, (September 2007), pp. (27557-27561), ISSN 0021-9258

Yamaguchi, Y., Morita, A., Maeda, A., & Hearing, V.J. (2009). Regulation of skin pigmentation and thickness by Dickkopf 1 (DKK1). *J Investig Dermatol Symp Proc*, Vol. 14, No. 1, (August 2009), pp. (73–75), 19675559

Zallen, J.A. (2007). Planar Polarity and Tissue Morphogenesis. *Cell*, Vol. *129*, No. 6, (June 2007), pp. (1051-1063), ISSN 0092-8674

13

A POU3F2-MITF-SHC4 Axis in Phenotype Switching of Melanoma Cells

Thomas Strub, Dominique Kobi,
Dana Koludrovic and Irwin Davidson
Institut de Génétique et de Biologie Moléculaire et Cellulaire
CNRS; INSERM; Université de Strasbourg
France

1. Introduction

Malignant melanoma is one of the most aggressive human cancers. Metastatic melanoma is highly resistant to genotoxic radiotherapy and chemotherapeutic treatments and patients have a median survival of under a year from diagnosis. As primary melanoma tumours can metastasise very early in tumour development (Chin et al., 2006), rapid diagnosis and curative surgery remain the best hopes for control of the disease. Early surgery that removes radial growth phase tumours that have not yet initiated vertical growth phase can be very effective and prevent further development. However, once the primary tumour has begun to invade the local epidermal and dermal environment treatment becomes much more complicated

Why melanoma has such a high propensity to invade and metastasize is not well understood, but may be related to the developmental characteristics of the melanocyte lineage. Melanocytes derive from pluripotent neural crest cells as non-pigmented melanoblasts (Dupin et al., 2007; Dupin et al., 2006; Thomas and Erickson, 2008). During embryogenesis melanoblasts migrate via the dorso-lateral pathway to populate the basal layer of the epidermis and hair follicles, as well as a number of other sites including the inner ear and the heart (Yajima and Larue, 2008). The ability of transformed melanoma cells to rapidly invade and migrate away from the primary tumour perhaps reflects an inherent characteristic inherited from their embryonic state.

Neural crest-derived cells are specified as melanoblasts by expression of MIcrophthalmia-associated Transcription Factor (MITF), a basic helix-loop-helix transcription factor belonging to the MYC superfamily (Goding, 2000a; Goding, 2000b; Hemesath et al., 1994). The *MITF* locus encodes multiple isoforms generated by alternate splicing and use of internal promoters (Steingrimsson, 2008). The MITF-M isoform (hereafter designated simply as MITF) is produced specifically in the melanocyte lineage from an intronic promoter. MITF is required for melanoblast survival and differentiation of the retinal pigment epithelium (RPE) (Hou and Pavan, 2008; McGill et al., 2002). Consequently, MITF-null mice exhibit a white coat colour due to the loss of the melanocyte lineage and a small (microphthalmic) eye phenotype due to loss of the RPE (Hodgkinson et al., 1993; Hughes et al., 1993; Moore, 1995; Steingrimsson et al., 1994). In humans, mutation of the *MITF* gene is responsible for Waardenburg syndrome type 2 (WS2) ((Tassabehji et al., 1994), a syndrome characterised by pigmentary defects and hearing loss highlighting the important role of the melanocytes located in the inner ear. MITF is thus the master regulator specifying the identify and properties of the melanocyte lineage.

It is now commonly accepted that exposure to solar UV irradiation and consequent DNA damage and mutation, especially during childhood, is the primary cause of most forms of melanoma (Bennett, 2008b). Melanoma can arise spontaneously, but often result from a stepwise process via accumulations of genetic changes leading first to formation of a benign naevus (mole) which can remain stable throughout the individual's life. If one of the cells in the naevus then acquires additional mutations it can go on and form the malignant tumour.

In contrast to many other tumours where a diversity of mutations can be found, melanoma formation is tightly associated with specific genetic changes. Activating mutations in BRAF especially the *BRAF^{V600E}* mutation or mutations in NRAS are found in more than 60% of primary melanomas. (Bennett, 2008a). The resulting constitutive activation of the MAP kinase pathway promotes melanocyte proliferation, but cells with activated BRAF or NRAS eventually arrest proliferation in what is assumed to be a senescent state in the form of benign nevi. Escape from this arrested state involves additional mutations one of the most frequent of which is inactivation of the CDKN2A locus encoding the cyclin dependent kinase inhibitor p16INK4 (Larue and Beermann, 2007). This inactivation can occur through genetic lesions (Bennett, 2008a) or DNA hypermethylation and epigenetic silencing (Richards and Medrano, 2009; Rothhammer and Bosserhoff, 2007), or repression via activation of Wnt/beta-catenin signalling (Delmas et al., 2007). The accumulation of these genetic and epigentic changes allows normal melanocytes to become immortal, escape senescence and go on to form malignant tumours.

2. Phenotype switching versus genetic changes in tumour formation

Following the genetic and epigentic changes described above, transformed melanoma cells enter the radial then the vertical growth phase where they acquire invasive properties. This is a critical event in tumour formation and two models have been put forward to account for how cells acquire the ability to invade neighbouring tissues, the lymphatic system and eventually form distant metastasis. Cells in the primary tumour may acquire further genetic changes that promote invasion and metastasis. This would be an essentially irreversible genetic event that, unless additional mutations arise, would fix the properties of these cells. An alternate model that has been put forward in the case of melanoma is 'phentoype switching' which postulates that cells can reversibly switch from proliferative to invasive states (Hoek and Goding, 2010). This process involves a specific set of changes in gene expression and hence altered transcription factor activity and can take place dynamically within a population of cells in response to signals from the tumour microenvironment.

The 'phentoype switching' model is based on two sets of observations. Firstly, analysis of 86 cultured melanoma cell lines showed that they could be divided into two classes ; highly proliferative cells with low invasive potential and slowly dividing cells with much higher migratory and invasive potential (Hoek et al., 2008; Hoek et al., 2006). Gene expression profiling of these different cell types defined two distinct expression signatures in which a collection of 105 genes show the highest differential expression. The invasive signature is characterised by up regulation of genes such as INHBA, COL5A1, and SERPINE1 that are involved in modifying the extracellular environment and are often known targets of TGFb signalling. In contrast, many of the proliferative signature genes are targets of Wnt signaling. Importantly however, a key feature of the two profiles revealed that invasive phenotype cells exhibited low levels of MITF, while proliferative phenotype cells expressed high levels of MITF (Hoek et al., 2008; Hoek et al., 2006). These observations define at least two cell populations that differ in proliferative and invasive properties and are defined by distinct gene expression profiles including differential MITF expression.

The second set of observations supporting this model are derived from experiments showing that when MITF high and MITF low cells are used to make xenografts, the resulting tumours comprise cell expressing both high and low MITF expression levels (Hoek et al., 2008). Hence, while the original cells were rather homogenous with respect to MITF expression, the resulting tumours are heterogenous. The tumour microenvironment may therefore modify the gene expression profile allowing cells to switch from one state to the other in a dynamic way.

This model is complicated by the observation that a low abundance subpopulation of cells that have strongly reduced MITF expression arise spontaneously in *in vitro* cultures of high-MITF expressing cell lines (Cheli et al., 2011). Depletion of these cells from the population leads to a strong reduction in tumour formation, whereas the purified low-MITF expressing population has high tumour formation potential and rapidly recovers higher MITF expression after subcutaneous injection. These observations confirm that cells can dynamically and even spontaneously switch their MITF expression and that low-MITF expressing cells have much higher tumour initiating capacity.

These observations made from xenografted tumour cell lines have been confirmed in primary human tumours. Staining of primary tumours with antibodies against MITF showed a heterogenous pattern with cells that exhibited high levels of MITF and others that showed lower levels or were completely negative (Goodall et al., 2008). These results highlight the heterogeneity of cell populations within human tumours. This idea is reinforced by the observation that cells in human tumours with no MITF staining expressed high levels of a second transcription factor POU3F2 (also known as N-OCT3 or BRN2), while cells expressing high MITF showed low levels of POU3F2 (Goodall et al., 2008). Thus, these two transcription factors can act as markers for different cell populations within tumours. In an elegant approach, Pinner et al, (Pinner et al., 2009) used intravital imaging to follow the fate of xenografted human melanoma cells engineered to express green fluorescent protein under the control of the POU3F2 promoter. They were clearly able to show that the POU3F2 promoter was upregulated in motile cells and that these cells exhibited a de-differentiated phenotype with diminished pigmentation.

Together the above results are consistent with the idea that cells expressing high levels of MITF are proliferative, but poorly motile and invasive, while those expressing low levels of MITF, but high levels of POU3F2 are highy motile and invasive and that this phenotype is acquired in a dynamic and reversible fashion in tumours. Spontaneous switching can also take place to a certain extent in cell culture, however, the low frequency of this event makes it a difficult process to follow. More recently however, Thurber et al (Thurber et al., 2011), showed that growth of high MITF expressing cells as non-adherent 'melanospheres' dramatically enhanced the frequency of low MITF/high POU3F2 expressing cells. Similarly, when we grew 501Mel cells expressing high levels of MITF in human embryonic stem cell medium under non-adherent conditions they readily form melanospheres, where we observe the appearance of a significant fraction of low MITF expressing cells in the spheres (Fig. 1). Thus, the change from monolayer to 3 dimensional culture in stem cells medium strongly influences MITF expression. Thurber et al, (Thurber et al., 2011) also showed using siRNA silencing that POU3F2 was an activator and MITF a repressor of the Notch pathway. Loss of POU3F2-MITF signaling resulted in decreased capacity to form melanospheres and invasion through a collagen matrix. This *in vitro* model appears to recapitulate some of the characteristics of MITF and POU3F2 signaling seen in tumours and may therefore facilitate the identification of the signals and mechanisms that regulate melanoma cell heterogeneity in tumours.

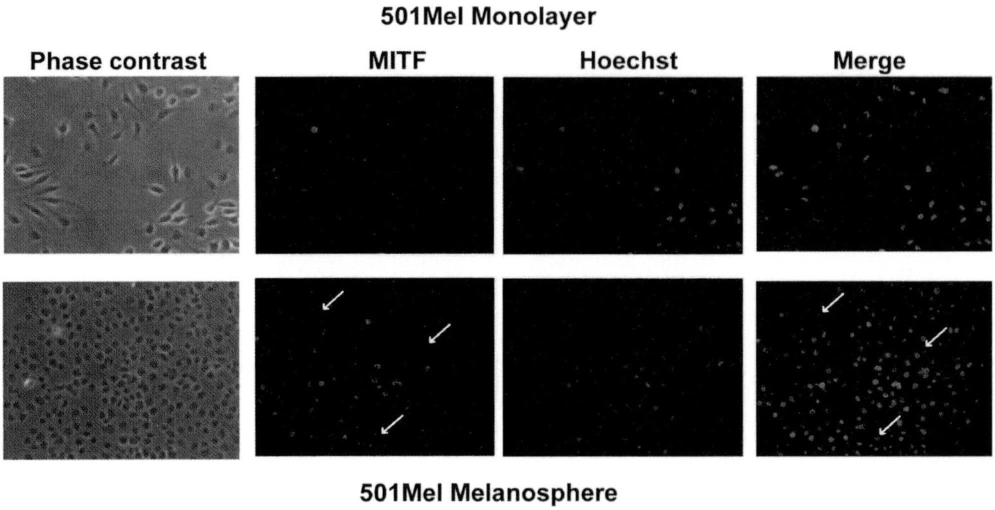

Fig. 1. Heterogenous MITF expression in 501Mel cells grown as melanospheres. The upper panels show phase contrast, MITF-labelling, nuclear Hoechst staining and the merge between the MITF and Hoechst signals of 501Mel cells grown as adherent monolayers under standard conditions. Almost all nuclei are stongly stained with MITF antibody. In the lower panels, the cells were grown as melanospheres in human stem cell medium and a significant number of low-MITF expressing cells can now be seen. Representative low-MITF expressing cells are indicated by arrows.

3. The MITF-POU3F2 axis in melanoma

The results described above show that high levels of MITF promote melanoma cell proliferation and that MITF and POU3F2 show reciprocal levels of expression. Key questions are therefore how does MITF promote proliferation and how does POU3F2 regulate MITF expression, proliferation and motility.

i. POU3F2 an activator and a repressor of critical target genes in melanoma.

POU (Pit, Oct1, Unc86) domain transcription factors play diverse functions in many physiological processes. The POU family factors have a bipartite DNA binding domain formed by the conserved POU-specific domain (POUs) and the POU homeodomain (POUh) that are joined by a linker region of variable length (Phillips and Luisi, 2000; Ryan and Rosenfeld, 1997). The POUs and POUh domains each comprise a helix-turn-helix structure of which the third helix recognises the DNA and provides sequence specificity (Cook and Sturm, 2008; Klemm et al., 1994).

POU3F2 and POU4F1 (BRN3) are involved in development of the central nervous system (Schonemann et al., 1998). Genetic studies in mice have demonstrated that POU3F2 is required for generation of specific neuronal lineages in the endocrine hypothalamus and the posterior pituitary gland (Nakai et al., 1995; Schonemann et al., 1995). POU3F2 also plays a role in the production and positioning of neocortical neurons (Sugitani et al., 2002). In addition to the nervous system, several studies have reported that POU3F2 is expressed in normal melanocytes and is upregulated in malignant melanoma cells where its expression is regulated by the Wnt/β-catenin and activated BRAF signalling pathways (Cook et al., 2003; Eisen et al., 1995; Goodall et al., 2004a; Goodall et al., 2004b; Thomson et al., 1995). However, POU3F2 has not yet been selectively inactivated in the melanocyte lineage and genetic dissection of its role in normal melanocyte physiology and in melanoma will be a welcome and important addition to the field.

POU3F2 directly represses MITF in melanoma cells through binding directly to the proximal internal promoter driving expression of the MITF-M isoform (Goodall et al., 2008). At least 3 POU3F2 binding sites have been identified at the MITF-M locus, two in the proximal promoter region upstream of the transcription start site (TSS) and a third intronic site downstream of the TSS (Kobi et al., 2010). Wellbrock et al., (Wellbrock et al., 2008) have shown that in some melanoma cell types POU3F2 mediates the regulatory effect of the $BRAF^{V600E}$ mutation and induces MITF expression. As discussed above, this suggestion is at odds with what is observed in tumours and melanospheres. To reconcile what may appear to be contradictory observations, we have suggested that the POU3F2 binding to the site closest to the TATA element may repress *MITF-M* transcription through steric hindrance of the basal transcription machinery, for example TFIID, while POU3F2 may activate *MITF-M* transcription via binding to the other sites in the proximal promoter and downstream intron (Kobi et al., 2010). The ability to activate or repress may then be modulated by POU3F2 concentration being able to efficiently compete with TFIID binding and repress MITF expression only at high concentrations. This model would reconcile the observation that POU3F2 is a transcription activator with the reciprocal MITF/POU3F2 expression seen in melanoma tumours (Goodall et al., 2008; Pinner et al., 2009).

Another means by which POU3F2 and MITF may regulate each others expression is through control by miR-211. Boyle et al., (Boyle et al., 2011) have compared miRNA expression profiles and identified miR-211 as down-regulated in melanoma cell lines compared to normal melanocytes. MiR-211 is derived from the TRPM1 gene whose expression is directly regulated by MITF and it targets POU3F2 expression. Thus MITF driven expression of TRPM1/miR-211 provides a mechanism by which high MITF levels maintain low POU3F2 levels. MiR-211 may also have other targets in melanoma. Levy et al., (Levy et al., 2010) have shown that expression of miR-211 reduced migration and invasion in human melanomas with low miR-211 levels. They propose IGF2R, TGFBR2, and NFAT5 as miR-211 targets that mediate the phenotypic effects of its overexpression. In contrast, Mazar et al., (Mazar et al., 2010) identified KCNMA1, encoding a calcium ion-regulated potassium channel protein, as a miR-211 target that influences melanoma cell aggressivity. MiR-211 has therefore many potential targets that influence melanoma cell properties.

Can all of the effects of POU3F2 in melanoma be ascribed to its ability to repress MITF or does it regulate other target genes involved in melanoma development? Genome wide chromatin immunoprecipitation (ChIP) coupled to array hybridisation (ChIP-chip) profiling of POU3F2 promoter occupancy identified target genes that may be involved in modulating the properties of melanoma cells (Kobi et al., 2010). For example, siRNA-mediated knockdown and transfection of reporter genes indicates that POU3F2 regulates expression of stem cell factor (Kit ligand, *Kitl* or *Steel)* via a cluster of 4 closely spaced binding sites located in the proximal promoter. Amplification and/or activating mutations of the KIT gene, encoding the KITL receptor, have been frequently found in mucosal, acral, and chronic sun-damaged melanomas (Garrido and Bastian, 2009), where it appears to promote melanoma development. The KITL/KIT pathway is also critical for promoting melanocyte migration during embryogenesis and hence may also be important in regulating the migratory/invasive properties of melanoma cells (Wehrle-Haller, 2003). POU3F2 may therefore modulate the properties of melanoma cells via autocrine KITL signalling.

A second mechanism by which POU3F2 may enhance the motile and malignant properties of melanoma cells is through regulation of the cGMP-specific phosphodiesterase PDE5A. Arozarena et al (Arozarena et al., 2011) have shown that POU3F2 binds to two sites in the PDE5A proximal promoter upstream of the TSS to repress its expression. PDE5A down-regulation has only a minor effect on proliferation, but potently increases melanoma cell invasion. Diminished PDE5A levels lead to an increase in cGMP and in cytosolic Ca2+, stimulating contractility and inducing invasion. In agreement with this idea, PDE5A levels are also down-regulated in human melanoma tumours. Hence, this model postulates that in melanoma cells, oncogenic BRAF promotes invasion through POU3F2-mediated repression of PDE5A. The ability of POU3F2 to act as a repressor at the PDE5A promoter is nevertheless surprising considering that it acts as a potent transcriptional activator in many other promoter contexts (Kobi et al., 2010).

ii. MITF activates genes required for proliferation and represses genes involved in invasion.

As described above, evidence from cell based models and human tumours suggest that MITF is a major regulator of melanoma cell proliferation. SiRNA-mediated silencing of MITF in proliferative melanoma cells leads to a rapid growth arrest confirming that it is indeed a critical regulator of proliferation (Carreira et al., 2006). Acute loss of MITF through siRNA mediated silencing has been reported to arrest cells at the G1/S phase transition through indirect regulation of CDKN1B ($p27^{Kip1}$) via direct regulation of Diaphanous related formin *DIAPH1*. DIAPH1 promotes actin polymerization and coordinates the actin cytoskeleton and microtubule networks at the cell periphery (Carreira et al., 2006). MITF directly regulates DIAPH1 expression leading to reorganization of the actin cytoskeleton, accounting at least in part for the dramatic change in cell morphology seen upon MITF silencing, and increased ROCK-dependent invasiveness. MITF regulation of DIAPH1 also indirectly controls CDNK1B degradation leading to a G1 cell cycle arrest.

While the above model accounts for many of the changes seen upon MITF silencing, it has been shown more recently that loss of MITF also leads to defects in mitosis and induces cell senescence (Giuliano et al., 2010; Strub et al., 2011). MITF silenced cells exhibit many characteristics of senescence such as enlarged and flattened cell morphology and senescence-associated β-galactosidase staining and heterochromatin foci. Giuliano et al (Giuliano et al., 2010) showed that acute MITF silencing induced the DNA damage response leading to activation of ATM and CHK2 resulting in p53 phosphorylation and stabilization. SiRNA depletion and pharmacologic inhibition showed that the DNA-damage response is required for entry into senescence.

How does MITF regulate both the proliferative and invasive properties of melanoma cells, and why does loss of MITF result in DNA damage? To answer these questions, Strub et al (Strub et al., 2011) used ChIP coupled to high throughput seqencing (ChIP-seq) to profile genomic MITF occupancy and RNA-seq following MITF silencing to identify MITF regulated genes. As currently available antibodies do not efficiently ChIP MITF, 501Mel cells expressing 3HA-tagged MITF were used. ChIP-seq was perfomed not only for tagged MITF, but also for RNA polymerase II (Pol II) and trimethylation of lysine 4 of histone H3 (H3K4me3), a covalent histone modification found at the 5′-end of transcribed genes (Ruthenburg et al., 2007). An example of MITF occupancy of the highly expressed Tyrosinase locus is shown in Fig. 2, where at least 5 MITF-occupied sites can be detected both upstream and downstream of the TSS along with transcribing RNA Pol II. Overall, 12139 MITF occupied loci were identified, 9447 of which could be annotated to more than 5000 potential target genes.

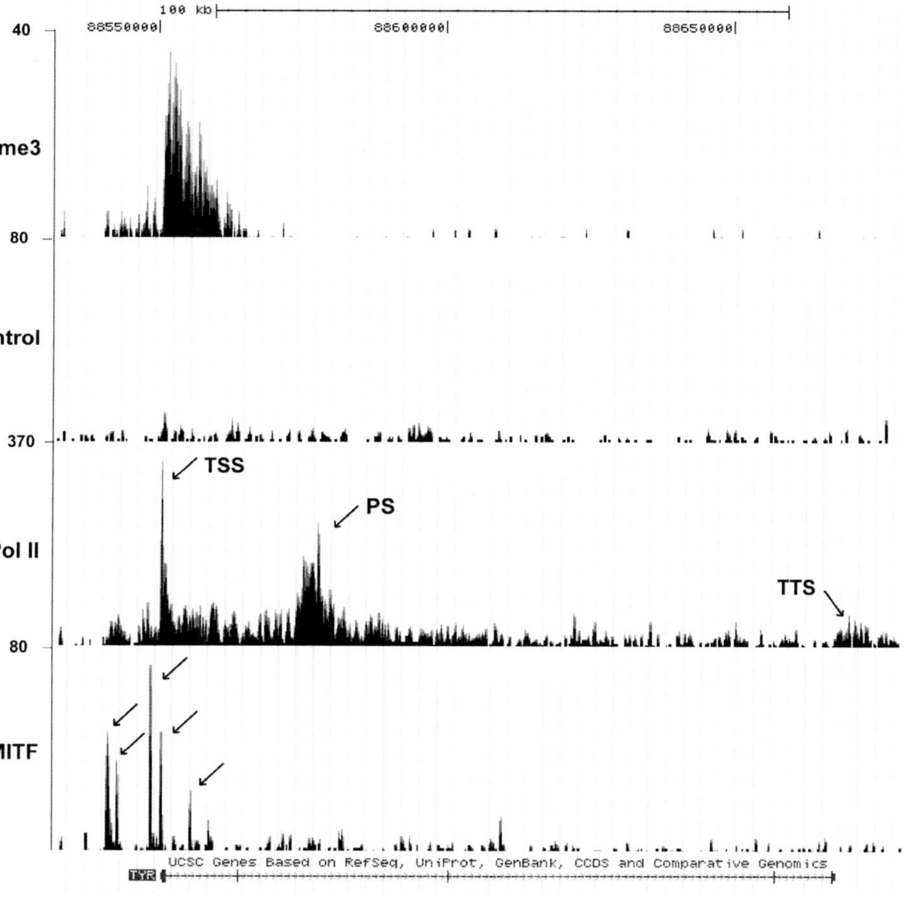

Fig. 2. Example of MITF-occupancy at the Tyrosinase locus. UCSC genome browser view of MITF and Pol II-occupancy and H3K4me3 at the *TYR* locus. The principal MITF occupied sites are indicated by arrows. TSS shows the engaged Pol II at the transcription start site, PS, enhanced Pol II occupany at an intronic pause site, and TTS, the transcription termination site downstream of the *TYR* polyadenylation site. The data are adapted from the data set of Strub et al, (Strub et al., 2011).

To determine which of these potential targets are regulated by MITF in 501Mel cells, RNA-seq was performed following MITF silencing identifying a large collection of both up and down-regulated genes (Strub et al., 2011). Amongst the genes that appear positively regulated by MITF are at least 31 genes involved in DNA replication, recombination and repair including *LIG1* encoding DNA ligase 1, involved in the religation of Okazaki fragments during DNA replication, as well as religation during DNA repair and maintenance of genome stability (Bentley et al., 2002; Tomkinson and Mackey, 1998), and *TERT* (Telomerase reverse transcriptase) required for the proper replication of telomeres and frequently expressed in human tumours, (Artandi and DePinho, 2000; Artandi and DePinho, ; Kim et al., 1994; Rudolph et al., 1999). In addition, MITF regulates a set of 39 genes involved in centromere organisation and mitosis including the G2-specific cyclins B1 and F (*CCNB1, CCNF*) that promote entry into mitosis, as well as polo-like kinase 1 (*PLK1*) (Schmit et al., 2009), the CENPA-nucleosome associated and CENPA-nucleosome distal complexes and the chromosomal passenger complex. Consequently, siMITF silencing leads to mitotic defects with a high frequency of binucleate and micronuclei containing cells.

Together these results provide a more comprehensive picture of how MITF promotes proliferation by activating genes involved in DNA replication and repair as well as mitosis. Loss of expression of genes like *LIG1* and *TERT* leads to incomplete DNA replication and telomere exposition activating the DNA damage and the senescence responses. We propose that, acute siMITF silencing in rapidly proliferating cells induces replication and mitotic defects too severe to be repaired and cells enter in senescence. However, the existence of senescent cells in human melanoma tumours has not yet been investigated and our results do not exclude the possibility that *in vivo*, decreased MITF expression could be offset by up-regulation of other pathways that suppress senescence to produce slow-cycling invasive cells. Alternatively, a more gradual reduction of MITF expression such as may take place in tumours would allow cells to adapt progressively to slower growth due to diminished levels of replication and mitosis factors and not accumulate the high levels of DNA damage that trigger the senescence response.

In contrast to the above, genomic profiling of MITF occupancy revealed genes that appear to be directly repressed by MITF. Amongst these are genes influencing metastasis such as *MCAM* (Ouhtit et al., 2009), *SHC4* (Fagiani et al., 2007). Comparison of the ChIP-seq and mRNA-seq data shows the presence of at least 3 upstream and two intronic MITF occupied sites at the SHC4 locus and enhanced mRNA expression upon MITF knockdown (Figs. 3A and B). Increased SHC4 protein expression can also be seen upon MITF silencing (Fig 3C). SHC4 therefore appears to be directly repressed by MITF suggesting that MITF both activates and represses transcription in a promoter context-dependent manner similar to POU3F2 discussed above.

SHC4 (also known as SHCD (Hawley et al., 2011), or RaLP, retinoic acid-like inducible like protein) belongs to the family of SRC homology and collagen (Shc) signal transduction adaptor proteins. These proteins share a common organisation with an N-terminal phosphotyrosine-binding (PTB) domain, a central region rich in proline and glycine residues (CH1) and a C-terminal SRC homologue 2 (SH2) domain (Pasini et al., 2009). A second N-terminal collagen homology (CH2) region is present in the longest isoform of SHC4. SHC4 is of particular interest in melanoma as its expression is tightly correlated with tumour stage. SHC4 expression is low or undetectable in benign nevi and in early radial growth phase tumours, but is strongly expressed in the vertical growth phase and in metastases. SHC4 functions as a substrate of activated IGF-1 and EGF receptors to enhance MAPK signaling and cell migration (Fagiani et al., 2007; Pasini et al., 2009). In contrast, SHC4 silencing in metastatic cells reduces their migration *in vitro* and inhibits tumour growth *in vivo*.

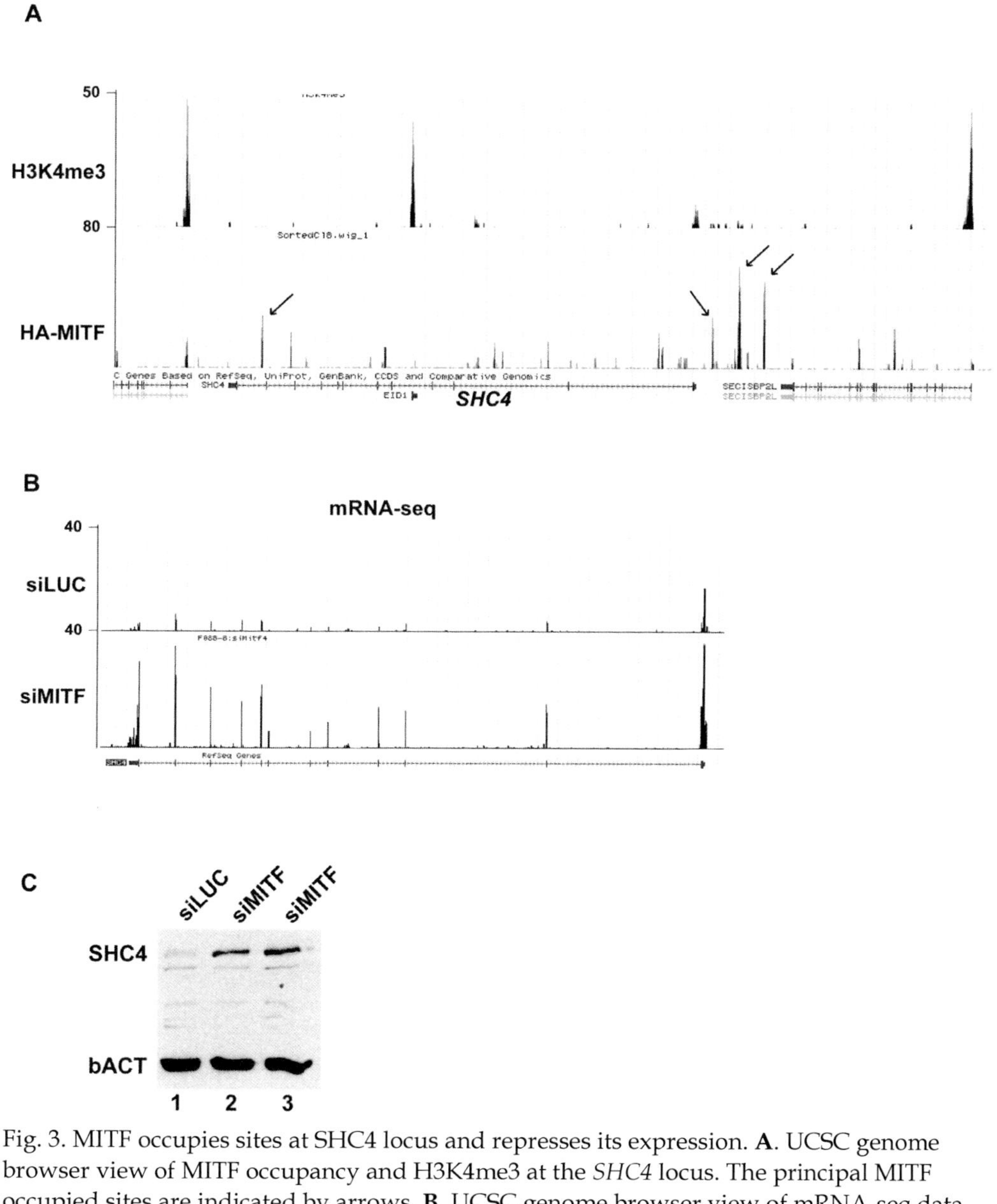

Fig. 3. MITF occupies sites at SHC4 locus and represses its expression. **A**. UCSC genome browser view of MITF occupancy and H3K4me3 at the *SHC4* locus. The principal MITF occupied sites are indicated by arrows. **B**. UCSC genome browser view of mRNA-seq data from 501Mel cells treated with control Luciferase or MITF siRNAs. Increased expression of the SHC4 gene can be clearly observed in the siMITF cells. **C.** Immunoblot showing increased SHC4 protein expression in total extracts from 501Mel cells following MITF silencing with 20 or 50 nM of siRNA (lanes 2 and 3, respectively). ChIP- and mRNA-seq data are adapted from Strub et al, (Strub et al., 2011).

Together with the results of the ChIP- and RNA-seq, these observations suggest a novel MITF-SHC4 axis in the control of melanoma cell invasion. Proliferating cells express high levels of MITF that repress SHC4 expression, but the loss of MITF that takes place during phenotype switching de-represses SHC4 expression to promote migration and metastasis (summarised in Fig. 4).

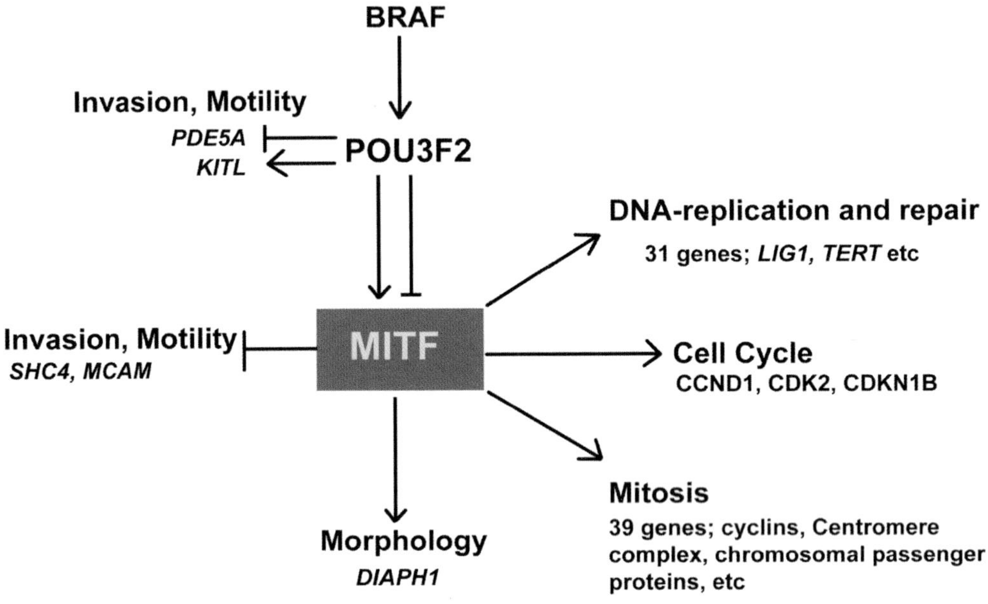

Fig. 4. Summary of regulatory interactions. in the POU3F2-MITF-SHC4 axis. As described in the main text, activated BRAF induces POU3F2 expression which in turn has been described to either activate or repress MITF expression. POU3F2 also activates *KITL* expression but represses *PDE5A* to promote motility and migration. MITF activates a series of genes involved in DNA replication and repair, mitosis and critical cyclin genes, but represses expression of SHC4 and MCAM that promote invasion and metastasis.

4. Future perspectives

In this review, we have limited our discussion to the hypothesis that POU3F2, MITF and SHC4 form a regulatory axis that controls the proliferative and invasive properties of melanoma cells. These are of course not the only transcription factors that regulate the properties of melanoma cells. For example, recent studies have shown that GLI2 and ATF2 modulate the invasive properties of melanoma cells. GLI2 is a transcription factor normally associated with Sonic Hedgehog (SHH) signaling is present in melanoma cells where its expression is rather controlled by TGFbeta and SMAD signaling (Alexaki et al., 2010; Dennler et al., 2009; Santiago-Walker and Herlyn, 2010). GLI2 is overexpressed in subpopulations of cells and these GLI2-high cells metastasise to bone more readily than GLI2-low cells. GLI2 appears to promote invasion and metastasis through suppression of E-cadherin expression leading to a mesenchymal-like phenotype. Also, the transcription factor ATF2 has been shown to attenuate melanoma susceptibility to apoptosis and to promote its ability to form tumors in xenografts (Bhoumik and Ronai, 2008; Shah et al., 2011). In mouse melanoma models, expression of mutant ATF2 in melanocytes strongly attenuated tumour formation. ATF2 appears to modulate MITF expression through ATF2-JunB-dependent suppression of expression of SOX10 a factor that binds to and activates the MITF-M promoter. Morevover, on melanoma tissue microarrays, a high nuclear ATF2 to MITF ratio was associated with metastatic disease and poor prognosis. In the future it will important to develop more complex mouse melanoma models in which POU3F2 and/or MITF, GLI2 and ATF2 are (in)activated or mutated to study combinatorial control by multiple transcription factors in melanoma. This will be a challenging, but important task.

We have discussed the proposition that the regulatory interactions between POU3F2-MITF-SHC4 explain in part the phenotype switching of melanoma cells. However, one important and outstanding question concerns the signal(s) in the tumour microenvironment responsible for modulating the expression of POU3F2 and MITF. Are these diffusable signals emanating from cells within or outside the tumour or are cell-cell contacts between the tumour cells and the stroma or amongst tumour cells involved ? An alternative possibility is that phenotype switching may take place spontaneously through transient stochastic changes in the expression of POU3F2 or MITF in single cells that set up a reinforcing positive feedback loop to establish a novel stable state. For example, down-regulation of MITF leads to up-regulation of POU3F2 (Strub et al., 2011), but elevated levels of POU3F2 repress MITF. Given this situation, a transient reduction in MITF could set up a reinforcing loop of POU3F2-mediated MITF repression. This would explain the spontaneous appearance of cells low-MITF expressing cells in *in vitro* cultures of otherwise high-MITF expressing cell types. It remains possible that in the tumour environment, extracellular signals may influence the expression of MITF or POU3F2, but the important point is that the effect of these signals can be amplified by the positive and negative feedback loops between these factors. The role that stochastic changes in transcriptional 'noise' may play in biological processes is only just beginning to be considered (Kashyap et al., 2009; Leisner et al., 2008). Whatever the mechanism involved, key features of melanoma cells are their plasticity and heterogeneity. As discussed above, Cheli et al (Cheli et al., 2011) identified low-MITF expression as a criteria for selecting cells with enhanced tumour initiating properties. This fits with the previously proposed 'rheostat' model of MITF expression where high levels of MITF drive a G1/S arrest and differentiation, while low levels are associated with slow cycling tumour initiating cells, and intermediate levels are optimum for proliferation (Carreira et al., 2006; Hoek and Goding, 2010).

However, MITF is not the only biomarker that has been used to select slow cycling tumour initiating cells. Roesch et al., (Roesch et al., 2010) have used the JARID1B histone demethylase as a marker to identify a population of slow cycling cells within the tumour population. Similar to purified low-MITF cells, purified JARID1B-positive cells give rise to a highly proliferative progeny showing the dynamics of their expression. Moreover, JARID1B silencing promotes a transient acceleration of tumor growth that is followed by exhaustion.

This observation suggests that the continuous dynamic appearance of a JARID1B-positive subpopulation is essential to maintain tumor growth. There are thus a number of parallels between JARID1B and MITF expression both in terms of the dynamics of their expression and the properties they confer to tumour cells. Unfortunately, Roesch et al, did not specifically assess MITF expression in the slow cycling JARID1B-positive cells, that one would predict to have low MITF expression or at least low levels of 'active' MITF. Cheli et al, (Cheli et al., 2011) however, did not observe a consistent increase in JARID1B expression in the MITF low population. Previousy other markers such as CD133 (Monzani et al., 2007) or ABCB5 (Schatton et al., 2008; Zabierowski and Herlyn, 2008), have been used to characterise stem-like subpopulations in melanomas. Does this mean that there are multiple distinct slow cycling tumour cell populations characterised by different transcriptional programmes? Future studies should answer these questions.

5. Acknowledgements

We apologise to our many colleagues whose work we did not have space to discuss. This work was supported by grants from the CNRS, the INSERM, the Ligue Nationale contre le Cancer, the Institut national du Cancer (INCA) grant R08009AP and the Agence National de Recherche (ANR) Regulome project grant. ID is an 'équipe labellisée' of the Ligue Nationale contre le Cancer.

6. References

Alexaki, V.I., Javelaud, D., Van Kempen, L.C., Mohammad, K.S., Dennler, S., Luciani, F., Hoek, K.S., Juarez, P., Goydos, J.S., Fournier, P.J., Sibon, C., Bertolotto, C., Verrecchia, F., Saule, S., Delmas, V., Ballotti, R., Larue, L., Saiag, P., Guise, T.A. and Mauviel, A. (2010) GLI2-mediated melanoma invasion and metastasis. *J Natl Cancer Inst*, 102, 1148-1159.

Arozarena, I., Sanchez-Laorden, B., Packer, L., Hidalgo-Carcedo, C., Hayward, R., Viros, A., Sahai, E. and Marais, R. (2011) Oncogenic BRAF induces melanoma cell invasion by downregulating the cGMP-specific phosphodiesterase PDE5A. *Cancer Cell*, 19, 45-57.

Artandi, S.E. and DePinho, R.A. (2000) Mice without telomerase: what can they teach us about human cancer? *Nat Med*, 6, 852-855.

Artandi, S.E. and DePinho, R.A. (2010) Telomeres and telomerase in cancer. *Carcinogenesis*, 31, 9-18.

Bennett, D.C. (2008a) How to make a melanoma: what do we know of the primary clonal events? *Pigment Cell Melanoma Res*, 21, 27-38.

Bennett, D.C. (2008b) Ultraviolet wavebands and melanoma initiation. *Pigment Cell Melanoma Res*, 21, 520-524.

Bentley, D.J., Harrison, C., Ketchen, A.M., Redhead, N.J., Samuel, K., Waterfall, M., Ansell, J.D. and Melton, D.W. (2002) DNA ligase I null mouse cells show normal DNA repair activity but altered DNA replication and reduced genome stability. *J Cell Sci*, 115, 1551-1561.

Bhoumik, A. and Ronai, Z. (2008) ATF2: a transcription factor that elicits oncogenic or tumor suppressor activities. *Cell Cycle*, 7, 2341-2345.

Boyle, G.M., Woods, S.L., Bonazzi, V.F., Stark, M.S., Hacker, E., Aoude, L.G., Dutton-Regester, K., Cook, A.L., Sturm, R.A. and Hayward, N.K. (2011) Melanoma cell invasiveness is regulated by miR-211 suppression of the BRN2 transcription factor. *Pigment Cell Melanoma Res.*

Carreira, S., Goodall, J., Denat, L., Rodriguez, M., Nuciforo, P., Hoek, K.S., Testori, A., Larue, L. and Goding, C.R. (2006) Mitf regulation of Dia1 controls melanoma proliferation and invasiveness. *Genes Dev*, 20, 3426-3439.

Cheli, Y., Guiliano, S., Botton, T., Rocchi, S., Hofman, V., Hofman, P., Bahadoran, P., Bertolotto, C. and Ballotti, R. (2011) Mitf is the key molecular switch between mouse or human melanoma initiating cells and their differentiated progeny. *Oncogene*.

Chin, L., Garraway, L.A. and Fisher, D.E. (2006) Malignant melanoma: genetics and therapeutics in the genomic era. *Genes Dev*, 20, 2149-2182.

Cook, A.L., Donatien, P.D., Smith, A.G., Murphy, M., Jones, M.K., Herlyn, M., Bennett, D.C., Leonard, J.H. and Sturm, R.A. (2003) Human melanoblasts in culture: expression of BRN2 and synergistic regulation by fibroblast growth factor-2, stem cell factor, and endothelin-3. *J Invest Dermatol*, 121, 1150-1159.

Cook, A.L. and Sturm, R.A. (2008) POU domain transcription factors: BRN2 as a regulator of melanocytic growth and tumourigenesis. *Pigment Cell Melanoma Res*, 21, 611-626.

Delmas, V., Beermann, F., Martinozzi, S., Carreira, S., Ackermann, J., Kumasaka, M., Denat, L., Goodall, J., Luciani, F., Viros, A., Demirkan, N., Bastian, B.C., Goding, C.R. and Larue, L. (2007) Beta-catenin induces immortalization of melanocytes by suppressing p16INK4a expression and cooperates with N-Ras in melanoma development. *Genes Dev*, 21, 2923-2935.

Dennler, S., Andre, J., Verrecchia, F. and Mauviel, A. (2009) Cloning of the human GLI2 Promoter: transcriptional activation by transforming growth factor-beta via SMAD3/beta-catenin cooperation. *J Biol Chem*, 284, 31523-31531.

Dupin, E., Calloni, G., Real, C., Goncalves-Trentin, A. and Le Douarin, N.M. (2007) Neural crest progenitors and stem cells. *C R Biol*, 330, 521-529.

Dupin, E., Creuzet, S. and Le Douarin, N.M. (2006) The contribution of the neural crest to the vertebrate body. *Adv Exp Med Biol*, 589, 96-119.

Eisen, T., Easty, D.J., Bennett, D.C. and Goding, C.R. (1995) The POU domain transcription factor Brn-2: elevated expression in malignant melanoma and regulation of melanocyte-specific gene expression. *Oncogene*, 11, 2157-2164.

Fagiani, E., Giardina, G., Luzi, L., Cesaroni, M., Quarto, M., Capra, M., Germano, G., Bono, M., Capillo, M., Pelicci, P. and Lanfrancone, L. (2007) RaLP, a new member of the Src homology and collagen family, regulates cell migration and tumor growth of metastatic melanomas. *Cancer Res*, 67, 3064-3073.

Garrido, M.C. and Bastian, B.C. (2009) KIT as a therapeutic target in melanoma. *J Invest Dermatol*, 130, 20-27.

Giuliano, S., Cheli, Y., Ohanna, M., Bonet, C., Beuret, L., Bille, K., Loubat, A., Hofman, V., Hofman, P., Ponzio, G., Bahadoran, P., Ballotti, R. and Bertolotto, C. (2010) Microphthalmia-Associated Transcription Factor Controls the DNA Damage Response and a Lineage-Specific Senescence Program in Melanomas. *Cancer Res*, 70, 3813-3822.

Goding, C.R. (2000a) Melanocyte development and malignant melanoma. *Forum (Genova)*, 10, 176-187.

Goding, C.R. (2000b) Mitf from neural crest to melanoma: signal transduction and transcription in the melanocyte lineage. *Genes Dev*, 14, 1712-1728.

Goodall, J., Carreira, S., Denat, L., Kobi, D., Davidson, I., Nuciforo, P., Sturm, R.A., Larue, L. and Goding, C.R. (2008) Brn-2 represses microphthalmia-associated transcription factor expression and marks a distinct subpopulation of microphthalmia-associated transcription factor-negative melanoma cells. *Cancer Res*, 68, 7788-7794.

Goodall, J., Martinozzi, S., Dexter, T.J., Champeval, D., Carreira, S., Larue, L. and Goding, C.R. (2004a) Brn-2 expression controls melanoma proliferation and is directly regulated by beta-catenin. *Mol Cell Biol*, 24, 2915-2922.

Goodall, J., Wellbrock, C., Dexter, T.J., Roberts, K., Marais, R. and Goding, C.R. (2004b) The Brn-2 transcription factor links activated BRAF to melanoma proliferation. *Mol Cell Biol*, 24, 2923-2931.

Hawley, S.P., Wills, M.K., Rabalski, A.J., Bendall, A.J. and Jones, N. (2011) Expression patterns of ShcD and Shc family adaptor proteins during mouse embryonic development. *Dev Dyn*, 240, 221-231.

Hemesath, T.J., Steingrimsson, E., McGill, G., Hansen, M.J., Vaught, J., Hodgkinson, C.A., Arnheiter, H., Copeland, N.G., Jenkins, N.A. and Fisher, D.E. (1994) microphthalmia, a critical factor in melanocyte development, defines a discrete transcription factor family. *Genes Dev*, 8, 2770-2780.

Hodgkinson, C.A., Moore, K.J., Nakayama, A., Steingrimsson, E., Copeland, N.G., Jenkins, N.A. and Arnheiter, H. (1993) Mutations at the mouse microphthalmia locus are associated with defects in a gene encoding a novel basic-helix-loop-helix-zipper protein. *Cell*, 74, 395-404.

Hoek, K.S., Eichhoff, O.M., Schlegel, N.C., Dobbeling, U., Kobert, N., Schaerer, L., Hemmi, S. and Dummer, R. (2008) In vivo switching of human melanoma cells between proliferative and invasive states. *Cancer Res*, 68, 650-656.

Hoek, K.S. and Goding, C.R. (2010) Cancer stem cells versus phenotype-switching in melanoma. *Pigment Cell Melanoma Res*, 23, 746-759.

Hoek, K.S., Schlegel, N.C., Brafford, P., Sucker, A., Ugurel, S., Kumar, R., Weber, B.L., Nathanson, K.L., Phillips, D.J., Herlyn, M., Schadendorf, D. and Dummer, R. (2006) Metastatic potential of melanomas defined by specific gene expression profiles with no BRAF signature. *Pigment Cell Res*, 19, 290-302.

Hou, L. and Pavan, W.J. (2008) Transcriptional and signaling regulation in neural crest stem cell-derived melanocyte development: do all roads lead to Mitf? *Cell Res*, 18, 1163-1176.

Hughes, M.J., Lingrel, J.B., Krakowsky, J.M. and Anderson, K.P. (1993) A helix-loop-helix transcription factor-like gene is located at the mi locus. *J Biol Chem*, 268, 20687-20690.

Kashyap, V., Rezende, N.C., Scotland, K.B., Shaffer, S.M., Persson, J.L., Gudas, L.J. and Mongan, N.P. (2009) Regulation of stem cell pluripotency and differentiation involves a mutual regulatory circuit of the NANOG, OCT4, and SOX2 pluripotency transcription factors with polycomb repressive complexes and stem cell microRNAs. *Stem Cells Dev*, 18, 1093-1108.

Kim, N.W., Piatyszek, M.A., Prowse, K.R., Harley, C.B., West, M.D., Ho, P.L., Coviello, G.M., Wright, W.E., Weinrich, S.L. and Shay, J.W. (1994) Specific association of human telomerase activity with immortal cells and cancer. *Science*, 266, 2011-2015.

Klemm, J.D., Rould, M.A., Aurora, R., Herr, W. and Pabo, C.O. (1994) Crystal structure of the Oct-1 POU domain bound to an octamer site: DNA recognition with tethered DNA-binding modules. *Cell*, 77, 21-32.

Kobi, D., Steunou, A.L., Dembele, D., Legras, S., Larue, L., Nieto, L. and Davidson, I. (2010) Genome-wide analysis of POU3F2/BRN2 promoter occupancy in human melanoma cells reveals Kitl as a novel regulated target gene. *Pigment Cell Melanoma Res*, 23, 404-418.

Larue, L. and Beermann, F. (2007) Cutaneous melanoma in genetically modified animals. *Pigment Cell Res*, 20, 485-497.

Leisner, M., Stingl, K., Frey, E. and Maier, B. (2008) Stochastic switching to competence. *Curr Opin Microbiol*, 11, 553-559.

Levy, C., Khaled, M., Iliopoulos, D., Janas, M.M., Schubert, S., Pinner, S., Chen, P.H., Li, S., Fletcher, A.L., Yokoyama, S., Scott, K.L., Garraway, L.A., Song, J.S., Granter, S.R., Turley, S.J., Fisher, D.E. and Novina, C.D. (2010) Intronic miR-211 assumes the tumor suppressive function of its host gene in melanoma. *Mol Cell*, 40, 841-849.

Mazar, J., DeYoung, K., Khaitan, D., Meister, E., Almodovar, A., Goydos, J., Ray, A. and Perera, R.J. (2010) The regulation of miRNA-211 expression and its role in melanoma cell invasiveness. *PLoS One*, 5, e13779.

McGill, G.G., Horstmann, M., Widlund, H.R., Du, J., Motyckova, G., Nishimura, E.K., Lin, Y.L., Ramaswamy, S., Avery, W., Ding, H.F., Jordan, S.A., Jackson, I.J., Korsmeyer, S.J., Golub, T.R. and Fisher, D.E. (2002) Bcl2 regulation by the melanocyte master regulator Mitf modulates lineage survival and melanoma cell viability. *Cell*, 109, 707-718.

Monzani, E., Facchetti, F., Galmozzi, E., Corsini, E., Benetti, A., Cavazzin, C., Gritti, A., Piccinini, A., Porro, D., Santinami, M., Invernici, G., Parati, E., Alessandri, G. and La Porta, C.A. (2007) Melanoma contains CD133 and ABCG2 positive cells with enhanced tumourigenic potential. *Eur J Cancer*, 43, 935-946.

Moore, K.J. (1995) Insight into the microphthalmia gene. *Trends Genet*, 11, 442-448.

Nakai, S., Kawano, H., Yudate, T., Nishi, M., Kuno, J., Nagata, A., Jishage, K., Hamada, H., Fujii, H., Kawamura, K. and et al. (1995) The POU domain transcription factor Brn-

2 is required for the determination of specific neuronal lineages in the hypothalamus of the mouse. *Genes Dev*, 9, 3109-3121.

Ouhtit, A., Gaur, R.L., Abd Elmageed, Z.Y., Fernando, A., Thouta, R., Trappey, A.K., Abdraboh, M.E., El-Sayyad, H.I., Rao, P. and Raj, M.G. (2009) Towards understanding the mode of action of the multifaceted cell adhesion receptor CD146. *Biochim Biophys Acta*, 1795, 130-136.

Pasini, L., Turco, M.Y., Luzi, L., Aladowicz, E., Fagiani, E. and Lanfrancone, L. (2009) Melanoma: targeting signaling pathways and RaLP. *Expert Opin Ther Targets*, 13, 93-104.

Phillips, K. and Luisi, B. (2000) The virtuoso of versatility: POU proteins that flex to fit. *J Mol Biol*, 302, 1023-1039.

Pinner, S., Jordan, P., Sharrock, K., Bazley, L., Collinson, L., Marais, R., Bonvin, E., Goding, C. and Sahai, E. (2009) Intravital imaging reveals transient changes in pigment production and Brn2 expression during metastatic melanoma dissemination. *Cancer Res*, 69, 7969-7977.

Richards, H.W. and Medrano, E.E. (2009) Epigenetic marks in melanoma. *Pigment Cell Melanoma Res*, 22, 14-29.

Roesch, A., Fukunaga-Kalabis, M., Schmidt, E.C., Zabierowski, S.E., Brafford, P.A., Vultur, A., Basu, D., Gimotty, P., Vogt, T. and Herlyn, M. (2010) A temporarily distinct subpopulation of slow-cycling melanoma cells is required for continuous tumor growth. *Cell*, 141, 583-594.

Rothhammer, T. and Bosserhoff, A.K. (2007) Epigenetic events in malignant melanoma. *Pigment Cell Res*, 20, 92-111.

Rudolph, K.L., Chang, S., Lee, H.W., Blasco, M., Gottlieb, G.J., Greider, C. and DePinho, R.A. (1999) Longevity, stress response, and cancer in aging telomerase-deficient mice. *Cell*, 96, 701-712.

Ruthenburg, A.J., Allis, C.D. and Wysocka, J. (2007) Methylation of lysine 4 on histone H3: intricacy of writing and reading a single epigenetic mark. *Mol Cell*, 25, 15-30.

Ryan, A.K. and Rosenfeld, M.G. (1997) POU domain family values: flexibility, partnerships, and developmental codes. *Genes Dev*, 11, 1207-1225.

Santiago-Walker, A. and Herlyn, M. (2010) The ups and downs of transcription factors in melanoma. *J Natl Cancer Inst*, 102, 1103-1104.

Schatton, T., Murphy, G.F., Frank, N.Y., Yamaura, K., Waaga-Gasser, A.M., Gasser, M., Zhan, Q., Jordan, S., Duncan, L.M., Weishaupt, C., Fuhlbrigge, R.C., Kupper, T.S., Sayegh, M.H. and Frank, M.H. (2008) Identification of cells initiating human melanomas. *Nature*, 451, 345-349.

Schmit, T.L., Zhong, W., Setaluri, V., Spiegelman, V.S. and Ahmad, N. (2009) Targeted depletion of Polo-like kinase (Plk) 1 through lentiviral shRNA or a small-molecule inhibitor causes mitotic catastrophe and induction of apoptosis in human melanoma cells. *J Invest Dermatol*, 129, 2843-2853.

Schonemann, M.D., Ryan, A.K., Erkman, L., McEvilly, R.J., Bermingham, J. and Rosenfeld, M.G. (1998) POU domain factors in neural development. *Adv Exp Med Biol*, 449, 39-53.

Schonemann, M.D., Ryan, A.K., McEvilly, R.J., O'Connell, S.M., Arias, C.A., Kalla, K.A., Li, P., Sawchenko, P.E. and Rosenfeld, M.G. (1995) Development and survival of the endocrine hypothalamus and posterior pituitary gland requires the neuronal POU domain factor Brn-2. *Genes.Dev.*, 9, 3122-3135.

Shah, M., Bhoumik, A., Goel, V., Dewing, A., Breitwieser, W., Kluger, H., Krajewski, S., Krajewska, M., Dehart, J., Lau, E., Kallenberg, D.M., Jeong, H., Eroshkin, A., Bennett, D.C., Chin, L., Bosenberg, M., Jones, N. and Ronai, Z.A. (2011) A role for ATF2 in regulating MITF and melanoma development. *PLoS Genet*, 6, e1001258.

Steingrimsson, E. (2008) All for one, one for all: alternative promoters and Mitf. *Pigment Cell Melanoma Res*, 21, 412-414.

Steingrimsson, E., Moore, K.J., Lamoreux, M.L., Ferre-D'Amare, A.R., Burley, S.K., Zimring, D.C., Skow, L.C., Hodgkinson, C.A., Arnheiter, H., Copeland, N.G. and et al. (1994) Molecular basis of mouse microphthalmia (mi) mutations helps explain their developmental and phenotypic consequences. *Nat Genet*, 8, 256-263.

Strub, T., Giuliano, S., Ye, T., Bonet, C., Keime, C., Kobi, D., Le Gras, S., Cormont, M., Ballotti, R., Bertolotto, C. and Davidson, I. (2011) Essential role of microphthalmia transcription factor for DNA replication, mitosis and genomic stability in melanoma. *Oncogene*.

Sugitani, Y., Nakai, S., Minowa, O., Nishi, M., Jishage, K., Kawano, H., Mori, K., Ogawa, M. and Noda, T. (2002) Brn-1 and Brn-2 share crucial roles in the production and positioning of mouse neocortical neurons. *Genes Dev*, 16, 1760-1765.

Tassabehji, M., Newton, V.E. and Read, A.P. (1994) Waardenburg syndrome type 2 caused by mutations in the human microphthalmia (MITF) gene. *Nat Genet*, 8, 251-255.

Thomas, A.J. and Erickson, C.A. (2008) The making of a melanocyte: the specification of melanoblasts from the neural crest. *Pigment Cell Melanoma Res*, 21, 598-610.

Thomson, J.A., Murphy, K., Baker, E., Sutherland, G.R., Parsons, P.G., Sturm, R.A. and Thomson, F. (1995) The brn-2 gene regulates the melanocytic phenotype and tumorigenic potential of human melanoma cells. *Oncogene*, 11, 691-700.

Thurber, A.E., Douglas, G., Sturm, E.C., Zabierowski, S.E., Smit, D.J., Ramakrishnan, S.N., Hacker, E., Leonard, J.H., Herlyn, M. and Sturm, R.A. (2011) Inverse expression states of the BRN2 and MITF transcription factors in melanoma spheres and tumour xenografts regulate the NOTCH pathway. *Oncogene*.

Tomkinson, A.E. and Mackey, Z.B. (1998) Structure and function of mammalian DNA ligases. *Mutat Res*, 407, 1-9.

Wehrle-Haller, B. (2003) The role of Kit-ligand in melanocyte development and epidermal homeostasis. *Pigment Cell Res*, 16, 287-296.

Wellbrock, C., Rana, S., Paterson, H., Pickersgill, H., Brummelkamp, T. and Marais, R. (2008) Oncogenic BRAF regulates melanoma proliferation through the lineage specific factor MITF. *PLoS One*, 3, e2734.

2.1.3 Insight from gene expression profiling studies

An emerging body of evidence is re-defining the conventional genetic model of melanoma progression. Gene expression profiling studies using multi-center cohorts of patient tumors have previously revealed the existence of two major expression signatures (Hoek, 2007; Hoek et al., 2006). These signatures correlate to two distinct populations of melanoma cells, one with a predominantly proliferative phenotype and the other with a predominantly invasive phenotype. Subsequent transcriptional profiling studies in melanoma cells have revealed two discrete states of differentiation (Hoek, 2007; Tap et al., 2010). The first state results in a phenotype closely resembling primary human melanocytes, while the second results in a phenotype resembling neuronal stem cells (Hoek, 2007; Tap et al., 2010). Further, melanoma cells with a proliferative phenotype tend to be in a melanocytic differentiation state, while cells which acquire an invasive phenotype tend to dedifferentiate into a neuronal state. Several studies have demonstrated that melanoma has the ability to switch back-and-forth between these two phenotypes and/or differentiation states, triggered by factors such as microenvironmental conditions and therapeutic intervention (Hoek et al., 2008; Hoek and Goding, 2010). The ability of melanoma cells to constantly switch phenotypes undoubtedly contributes to the resistance of melanoma to treatment.

2.1.4 Cancer stem cells and melanoma

Traditional chemotherapy operates largely under the premise that all cancer cells have equal malignant potential, with drug therapy focused on decreasing the population of cells within the tumor. Recently, studies looking at melanoma and other cancers have introduced the concept that certain populations within the tumor, often referred to as cancer stem cells (CSCs), have increased tumor initiating capabilities along with increased resistance to traditional chemotherapeutic approaches (Dou et al., 2007; Grichnik et al., 2006; Schatton et al., 2008). Consequently, the ability to identify, study and manipulate cells with the highest tumor-initiating capacity will be critical for developing effective therapeutic strategies.

In the case of melanoma, the exact nature of CSCs remains controversial, with several putative CSC markers having been proposed in the literature (Zabierowski and Herlyn, 2008). These markers include ABCB5 (Schatton et al., 2008), CD271/NGFR (Boiko et al., 2010), and CD34 (Held et al., 2010). However, additional reports have demonstrated that tumor initiating capacity may actually be quite common among melanoma cells, and does not depend on the expression of any of the published putative melanoma CSC markers (Quintana et al., 2010; Quintana et al., 2008). In the context of cellular differentiation, studies have also found that like other cancers, melanoma exhibits similarities to embryonic stem cells (Klein et al., 2007; Postovit et al., 2007). The ability to correlate features of melanoma cells such as gene expression profiles with functional phenotypes such as tumor-initiating capacity (a hallmark of CSCs) will further delineate the role of cell fate in regulating melanoma progression.

2.1.5 Tumor heterogeneity and plasticity

While the cellular heterogeneity of tumors is a long-recognized phenomenon (Fidler, 1978), these recent studies highlight the variability within populations highlight regarding both gene signature and phenotypic plasticity. The concepts of phenotype switching and cancer stem cells in melanoma may both represent what happens within the tumor environment. Cancer stem cells may not be a fixed population, but rather a dynamically changing one resulting from the phenotype switching of more "differentiated" cells in a tumor. This type of model could reconcile both sets of observations, and implies an inherent plasticity of melanoma cells that would undoubtedly complicate therapeutic efforts and potentially contribute to the variability seen with the use of cell surface markers to isolate CSC populations. While the use of the term differentiated in this model may again conjure up pre-conceptions that this population may be either more terminal/benign or less lethal in the long term, this assumption requires further experimental confirmation.

2.2 The proliferative phenotype of melanoma cells

Since cell fate and differentiation in the setting of cancer most closely parallels phenotype, this review will focus in particular on phenotypic characteristics that have been the center of efforts to understand melanoma at the molecular level. The first of the two major phenotypes expressed by malignant melanoma cells is the proliferative phenotype. As the name suggests, this phenotype is associated with a high rate of proliferation, as well as minimal invasive potential (Hoek et al., 2008; Hoek et al., 2006). Two key features of this group of cells help to account for their proliferative nature, including the activity of microphthalmia-associated transcription factor (MITF) (Levy et al., 2006) as well as the activity of the canonical Wnt/β-catenin pathway (Chien et al., 2009a).

2.2.1 Microphthalmia transcription factor (MITF)

MITF is a transcription factor that plays a critical role in the differentiation of melanoblasts from other cells derived from the neural crest (Levy et al., 2006), and severe mutations of MITF impede the embryonic development of melanocytes (Goding, 2000). It also plays a critical role in the normal functioning of differentiated primary melanocytes, regulating genes involved in the manufacture of melanosomes and melanin (Hornyak, 2006). This multi-tasking potential has been summarized using a proposed "rheostat model" of MITF function (Carreira et al., 2006; Hoek and Goding, 2010), which describes three different scenarios: MITF function in normal, differentiated melanocytes; MITF function in proliferative melanoma cells; and decreased MITF expression as seen in invasive melanoma cells.

As previously mentioned, the primary role of MITF in a normally functioning melanocyte cell, where MITF expression is highest, is the regulation of genes involved in melanosome and melanin production (Lekmine et al., 2007; Levy et al., 2006). Some examples of the broad range of genes that affect pigmentation, whose expression is regulated by MITF, include melanocortin 1 receptor (*MC1R*), melanocortin 4 receptor (*MC4R*), tyrosinase (*TYR*) and melan-A (Lekmine et al., 2007; Levy et al., 2006). Other genes essential for normal melanocyte development, such as endothelin receptor type B (*EDNRB*) (Sato-Jin et al., 2008), $p21^{cip1}$ (Carreira et al., 2005; Sestakova et al., 2010) and $p16^{INK4}$ (Loercher et al., 2005), have also been shown to depend on MITF expression. Significantly, $p21^{cip1}$ and $p16^{INK4}$ are both regulators of the cell cycle, and are expressed when MITF levels are at their highest.

As melanocytes acquire activating mutations in critical signalling pathways such as the MAPK pathway, the cellular effects of MITF change. Although the exact mechanism of this change is still not clear, it is primarily thought to be the result of altered post-translational modification of MITF, causing MITF to be targeted towards a different set of genes (Hoek and Goding, 2010). According to the rheostat model, overall MITF activity is also thought to be lower in malignant melanoma cells as compared to melanocytes (Hoek and Goding, 2010). Consequently, MITF expression in this cell population results in suppression of senescence and increased proliferation, as well as decreased invasiveness, both hallmarks of melanoma cells in the proliferative gene expression cluster.

There have been many mechanisms proposed to help explain how MITF expression leads to increased proliferation of melanoma cells. For example, suppression of $p27^{kip1}$, or cyclin-dependent kinase inhibitor 1B (CDKN1B), is thought to be of primary importance in this process . The main function of $p27^{kip1}$ is to impede cell cycle progression at G1. In melanoma cells with a proliferative phenotype, there is decreased $p27^{kip1}$ expression (Carreira et al., 2006). This is thought to be the result of increased expression of diaphanous-related formin DIA1, a protein which is upregulated by MITF and has a role in the regulation of a wide variety of cellular functions, including actin polymerization and E-cadherin organization. DIA1 in turn increases degradation of $p27^{kip1}$ by S-phase kinase-associated protein 2 (*SKP2*), a gene which is regulated by DIA1 (Carreira et al., 2006). In addition, other genes upregulated by MITF in proliferative melanoma cells include *BCL2* and *CDK2* (Cheli et al., 2010). While BCL2 upregulation imparts apoptotic resistance on melanoma cells, increased expression of cyclin-dependent kinase 2 results in cell cycle dysregulation and thus increased proliferation (Cheli et al., 2010).

Besides increasing proliferation, MITF also contributes to the low invasive potential characteristic of melanoma cells in the "proliferative state". Based on the results of Carreira et al., the ability of MITF to inhibit invasion is likely dependent on its DIA1-mediated regulation of the RHO/ROCK pathway, a known promoter of invasiveness (Carreira et al., 2006). MITF also appears to be a negative regulator of the Notch signalling cascade, which is itself a driver of invasive potential (Thurber et al., 2011). The frequent dysregulation of MITF by gene amplification in melanoma cells (Garraway et al., 2005) further highlights the critical nature of MITF in melanoma progression, and in the regulation of melanoma cell fate.

2.2.2 Wnt/β-catenin signaling

The Wnt/β-catenin signaling pathway represents a morphogenic pathway that is critical for development and almost always dysregulated in the context of cancers (Chien et al., 2009a) . Constitutive activation of the Wnt/β-catenin pathway is a common feature of many cancers, and increased activity of this pathway in general is a feature which distinguishes proliferative melanoma cells from invasive ones (Hoek et al., 2006). In the context of cellular differentiation and melanoma, which is neural crest-derived, Wnt/β-catenin signaling is particularly relevant since this pathway plays a pivotal role in regulating the differentiation of precursor cells into either neurons or melanocytes (Dorsky et al., 1998) .

The key mediator of canonical Wnt/β-catenin pathway signalling is β-catenin, a protein whose degradation is inhibited upon Wnt ligand bidning, allowing its translocation to the nucleus where it regulates target gene expression (Chien et al., 2009a) . Wnt/β-catenin and MITF are intimately related in that β-catenin increases MITF expression (Dorsky et al., 2000b), while MITF can interact with β-catenin in cultured malignant melanoma cells to alter its downstream gene-targeting (Widlund et al., 2002). Like MITF, Wnt/β-catenin signalling is critical to the normal embryonic development of melanocytes, so much so that the Wnt3a ligand is one of only three factors needed to stimulate the development of a pluripotent human embryonic stem cell into a mature melanocyte (Fang et al., 2006).

The exact role of Wnt/β-catenin signaling in melanoma remains controversial, in part due to some differences in observed patient data and data obtained from murine models. Overall, increased activation of this pathway in approximately one-third of all melanomas is suggested by the presence of increased nuclear localization of β-catenin (Chien et al., 2009b), a surrogate marker for Wnt/β-catenin activation. More importantly, the activation of Wnt/β-catenin signaling has been unexpectedly associated with improved patient survival (Bachmann et al., 2005; Chien et al., 2009b). In addition, the presence of nuclear β-catenin in the majority of benign nevi (Bachmann et al., 2005; Kageshita et al., 2001; Maelandsmo et al., 2003) implicates a role for Wnt/β-catenin signaling in maintaining normal cellular homeostasis, and suggests that the dysregulaton of this pathway may contribute to the process of melanoma progression.

The interpretation of these observations in patients is complicated by studies using a mouse model expressing a constitutively-active β-catenin mutant under the transcriptional control of a melanocyte-specific promoter. This transgenic mouse model suggests that increased Wnt/β-catenin signalling contributes to the initial immortalizaton of melanoma cells by inhbiting the expression of $p16^{INK4a}$, a tumor suppressing protein which plays a key role in the induction of G1 cell cycle arrest in response to DNA damage (Delmas et al., 2007). Interestingly, although immortalization is often associated with proliferation, Delmas et al. show that in fact these two processes are effectively uncoupled during the process of malignant transformation in melanocytes (Delmas et al., 2007). However, despite facilitating the immortalization of melanocytes, the presence of a constitively-active β-catenin mutant was by itself not sufficient to generate spontaneous melanomas, which required concommitant activation of MAPK signaling through *Nras* mutation (Delmas et al., 2007).

With regards to the issue of differentiation and questions surrounding the cell of origin for melanoma, the comparison of Wnt/β-catenin signaling in both human patients and mice raise two interesting points. First, melanomas from the mouse model appear to originate from the bulge region of the hair follicle, which is the proposed niche for melanocytic stem cells (Delmas et al., 2007); by contrast, most patient melanomas arise from interfollicular epidermis rather than from the hair follicle. Second, while these studies utilize a constitutively active mutant of β-catenin (Delmas et al., 2007), these types of activating mutations are quite rare in patient melanomas (Lucero et al., 2010), where Wnt/β-catenin activation is thought to result primarily from secreted Wnt ligand. Intuitively, the activation of signaling by secreted Wnt ligand is subject to modulation by extrinsic factors including endogenous inhibitors (i.e. DKK1, SFRPs) (Chien et al., 2009a), which would permit a model more akin the the MITF rheostat. Interestingly, the activation of Wnt/β-catenin signaling through the forced expression of WNT3A rather than a mutant β-catenin results in decreased proliferation in vitro and in vivo, correlating with the increased expression of genes associated with melanocyte differentiation (Chien et al., 2009b).

2.3 The invasive phenotype of melanoma cells

The second major gene expression signature of melanoma cells results in a phenotype characterized by a high degree of invasiveness and relatively lower rates of proliferation. Both MITF as well as canonical Wnt/β-catenin signalling are markedly downregulated in this population of cells, with a concomitant upregulation of a variety of pro-invasive mediators (Hoek et al., 2006). Notably, invasive melanoma cells are defined by genes suggestive of increased noncanonical WNT5A signalling, increased Notch1 signaling, upregulation of TGF-β and Brn-2 transcription factor as well as loss of the AP-2 transcription factor, all of which are reviewed below.

2.3.1 WNT5A and non-canonical Wnt signaling

Whereas the canonical Wnt pathway is reliant on β-catenin signaling, the noncanonical Wnt pathway uses calcium-dependent mediators such as protein kinase C (PKC) to propagate the signal of its primary extracellular ligand, WNT5A (Chien et al., 2009a). Normally, WNT5A signalling plays an important role in the regulation of cell fate, embryogenic patterning and cell motility (Chien et al., 2009a). In many forms of cancer, including colon, breast and liver cancer, WNT5A acts as a tumor suppressor (Chien and Moon, 2007). In the context of melanoma cell differentiation, which is assessed largely through gene signatures, the continued appearance of WNT5A as a major determinant of melanoma clusters in transcriptional profiling studies speaks to its likely importance as a genetic marker (Bittner et al., 2000; Hoek, 2007; Hoek et al., 2006; Weeraratna et al., 2004).

Functionally, WNT5A is thought to contribute significantly to the invasive phenotype by regulating cellular migration, both through PKC and the re-distribution of cellular adhesion molecules (Dissanayake et al., 2007; Weeraratna et al., 2002; Witze et al., 2008). In addition, WNT5A signalling has been shown to inhibit the canonical Wnt/β-catenin pathway and consequently cause the downregulation of the downstream target genes of β-catenin (Chien et al., 2009b; Dissanayake et al., 2008), which may further contribute to its role in melanoma progression. The observation that WNT5A can be involved in the specification of dopaminergic neuronal cells (Castelo-Branco et al., 2003) and specification of axonal or synaptic function (Agalliu et al., 2009; Bodmer et al., 2009; Varela-Nallar et al., 2010) may also indicate a previously under-appreciated role of this pathway in the control of cellular differentiation. Conceivably, the role of WNT5A in neuronal cells may overlap with the phenotypic effects seen with WNT5A activation in melanoma cells, thereby contributing to whether these cells may display a phenotype that is neuronal as opposed to melanocyte-like. Alternatively, the expression of WNT5A in melanoma may simply be a reflection of cellular differentiation state, which would be consistent with transcriptional profiling studies where WNT5A is enriched in melanoma cells with a gene signature suggestive of neuroprogenitor cells (Tap et al., 2010).

2.3.2 Notch signaling

Another pathway implicated in melanoma is the Notch signaling cascade, which is one of the prototypical regulators of cell fate determination during embryonic development (Kopan and Ilagan, 2009). Like other primary transforming mutations in melanoma such as BRAF and NRAS, constitutive activation of the Notch1 receptor was in itself sufficient for the malignant transformation of human melanocytes (Pinnix et al., 2009). In fact, Notch1 signaling is also required for β-catenin-induced proliferation in melanoma cells with a proliferative phenotype (Balint et al., 2005). However, the expression of Notch is negatively regulated by MITF, and thus its contribution to cellular phenotype is most pronounced in invasive melanoma cells where MITF is down-regulated (Thurber et al., 2011). Reports that these Notch effects in melanoma are mediated through regulation of the MAPK and PI3K-Akt pathways (Liu et al., 2006a; Liu et al., 2006b) further highlight the convergence of critical pathways during melanoma progression.

Like Wnt signaling, the Notch pathway plays a critical role in the specification of cell fate during neural crest development, making it particularly relevant to melanoma biology (Cornell and Eisen, 2005). During embryonic development, Notch signaling is thought to regulate both the specification of neural crest, as well as the subsequent determination of secondary cell fate through differentiation into glial-based lineages (Cornell and Eisen, 2005). Engagement of Notch signaling can inhibit neurogenesis and neural differentiation, which may play some part in the role of this pathway in melanoma. Likewise in the context of stem- and progenitor cells, Notch signaling can have varied roles in regulating either the maintenance of stem cell phenotype or the differentiation of stem cells into mature lineages (Liu et al., 2010). Understanding the interplay between Notch and other signaling pathways will be vital to effectively leveraging this important regulator of cellular differentiation for therapeutic benefit.

2.3.3 Transforming growth factor-beta (TGFB)

The morphogen-based Nodal signaling pathway, representing a subset of transforming growth factor β (TGFB) signaling pathways, was perhaps the initial pathway of interest in melanoma with regards to the concept of 'differentiation therapy' (Hardy et al., 2010; Postovit et al., 2008a; Postovit et al., 2008b; Strizzi et al., 2009). Like many of the other pathways that participate in melanoma biology, Nodal is a morphogen ligand involved the determination of cell fate during development. Melanoma is characterized by the presence of increased levels of Nodal ligand coinciding with decreased expression of the secreted Nodal antagonist Lefty (Postovit et al., 2008a). Typical benign nevi appear to express low levels of Nodal, although a subset of congenital nevi express levels of Nodal by immunohistochemistry that are comparable to what is observed in melanoma (Yu et al., 2010). Analogous to its role in maintaining human embryonic stem cells in the undifferentiated state, Nodal signaling in melanoma is thought to regulate or facilitate the plasticity of tumor cells (Postovit et al., 2008a), thus eliciting considerable interest in the targeting of this pathway for therapeutic purposes.

Overall, the role of TGFB in melanoma pathogenesis is complex, given the variability of its effects based on a cell's stage of progression (Javelaud et al., 2008; Lasfar and Cohen-Solal, 2010). Whereas normal human melanocytes are exquisitely sensitive to the anti-proliferative effects of TGF-β, resistance to this effect begins to develop as malignant transformation occurs. However, proliferative melanoma cells do retain sensitivity to TGF-β, and thus in this population of melanoma cells TGF-β actually acts as a tumor suppressor (Hoek et al., 2006). Hoek et al. demonstrated that melanoma cells which clustered into the invasive, low MITF gene expression group also showed upregulation of many downstream targets of TGF-β (Hoek et al., 2006). Further, specific inhibition of the TGF-β signaling cascade via exogenous Smad7 significantly reduces the capacity of melanoma cells for anchorage-independent growth, a characteristic intrinsic to metastatic potential (Javelaud et al., 2005). An important mechanism by which TGF-β signaling is able to increase invasive potential is likely its ability to decrease MITF expression, which results in upregulation of the pro-invasive RHO/ROCK and Notch signaling cascades (Carreira et al., 2006; Thurber et al., 2011). It also induces the expression of factors which inhibit canonical Wnt signaling (Hoek et al., 2006), promotes angiogenesis through factors such as VEGF, and has broad immunosuppressive effects which may contribute to the therapeutic resistance of TGF-β expressing tumor cells (Javelaud et al., 2008).

A small but accumulating body of literature has also characterized the involvement in melanoma of bone morphogenic proteins (BMPs), which represent another subset of the TGFB superfamily (Hsu et al., 2005). Like TGFB, BMP7 can act in an autocrine fashion to inhibit melanoma cell growth (Hsu et al., 2008). Interestingly, the upregulation of BMP7 with melanoma progression coincides with upregulation of Noggin, an antagonist of BMP (Hsu et al., 2008). This finding parallels the observed acquisition of resistance to autocrine TGFB seen in melanoma cells compared to melanocytes (Krasagakis et al., 1999). In contrast, others have reported that BMPs including BMP7 promote melanoma cell migration and invasion (Rothhammer et al., 2005), suggesting that the current model for how BMPs affect melanoma is still incomplete. The observation that nevi display relatively low levels of BMP4 and BMP7 may reflect that these cells retain sensitivity to these ligands (Rothhammer et al., 2005), and would be consistent with a potential oncogenic role for BMPs during melanoma progression.

2.3.4 Brn-2

Brn-2 is a POU domain transcription factor which regulates melanocytic growth (Cook and Sturm, 2008; Thomson et al., 1995), and in the setting of melanoma, is upregulated by both the MAPK and β-catenin signaling pathways (Goodall et al., 2004a; Goodall et al., 2004b). Increased expression of Brn-2 is a hallmark of invasive melanoma cells, and its activity contributes to this phenotype through a variety of different mechanisms. For one, Brn-2 is a potent repressor of MITF expression, and downregulation of Brn-2 during melanoblast differentiation to a mature melanocyte is necessary to ensure adequate expression of MITF (Goodall et al., 2004a). In invasive melanoma cells however, Brn-2 is upregulated, leading to MITF depletion and increased metastatic potential. Pinner et al. demonstrated that Brn-2 upregulation is a key feature of invasive and metastatic melanoma cells through intravital imaging of GFP-tagged Brn-2 levels in melanoma (Pinner et al., 2009). The invasive and metastatic tumor cells also showed decreased pigmentation, a surrogate marker for de-differentiation as a result of a Brn-2-induced decrease in MITF expression. Besides acting as a repressor of MITF expression, Brn-2 increases invasive potential through its role as an activator of the Notch pathway. With siRNA knockdown of Brn-2 in the A2058 melanoma cell line, there is a resultant decrease in the expression of several Notch1-related target genes (Thurber et al., 2011). Interestingly, Brn-2 is one of only three factors necessary to facilitate the conversion of mouse fibroblasts into functional neurons (Vierbuchen et al., 2010), demonstrating the importance of this pathway not only in melanocyte biology, but also in neuronal biology. This observation is not entirely surprising given close links developmentally between melanocytes and other neural crest-derived cell types.

2.3.5 AP-2

The activity of AP-2, a 52kDa transcription factor, is vital to the normal embryonic development of neural crest cells, and also appears to play an important role in the differentiation of adult cells (Bar-Eli, 2001; Tellez et al., 2003). In normal human melanocytes, AP-2 is responsible for the regulation of a host of normal cellular functions, including DNA repair, cell cycle arrest and cell adhesion (Zhuang et al., 2007). However, in melanoma cells, the loss of AP-2 is a prominent feature associated with a switch to an invasive phenotype (Braeuer et al., 2011). It appears that this downregulation is the result of the increased activity of cAMP-responsive element binding (CREB) protein, a common feature in melanoma progression due to dysregulation of the MAPK pathway (Melnikova et al., 2010). Melnikova et al. showed that activation of PKA-dependent CREB signaling down-regulates AP-2 in invasive melanoma cells, while re-introduction of AP-2 into these cells restores a non-metastatic phenotype (Melnikova et al., 2010). By our definition, this effect of AP-2 would constitute forced differentiation, resulting in an altered cell fate. Further studies will be needed to address whether AP-2 and its regulation by PKA/CREB can utilized as a viable therapeutic strategy.

2.4 Classification of melanoma by states of differentiation

2.4.1 Relating gene signatures to the differentiation of cell lineages

Melanocytes develop from embryonic stem cells along two distinct lineages (Dorsky et al., 2000a; Thomas and Erickson, 2008). The classical lineage involves migration of neural crest cells (NCC) from the dorsal aspect of the neural tube. These pluripotent NCC initially have the ability to differentiate into a wide variety of cell types, including smooth muscle cells, peripheral neurons and glia, as well as melanocytes (Dorsky et al., 2000a; Thomas and Erickson, 2008). Certain extrinsic factors are necessary in order to induce melanocytic differentiation of these stem cells, and several have been identified, including mast cell growth factor (*MGF/KITLG*), endothelin 3 (*EDN3*) and SOX10.

Intriguingly, in the search for key intrinsic modulators of melanocytic differentiation, it appears as though one transcription factor acts as the universal regulator of this process: MITF (Goding, 2000). Mutations of the MITF gene cause neural crest cell dysfunction and marked impairment of normal pigmentation, as reflected in patients with a variant of Waardenburg Syndrome (Goding, 2000). Some typical markers of melanocytic differentiation include tyrosinase (TYR), melanoma antigen recognized by T-cells 1 (MART-1) and transmembrane glycoprotein NMB (GPNMB).

Not all melanocytes follow the same path of differentiation from the neural crest. If the transcription factor HMX1 is expressed in the dorsal root ganglia, NCCs instead migrate along the ventral aspect of the dorsal root, and are induced to differentiate towards a neuronal phenotype (Adameyko et al., 2009; Krispin et al., 2010). These neuronal and glial cells are then directed to expanding branches of peripheral neurons throughout the body. Among this population of ventrally-derived neuronal cells is a group of pluripotent stem cells known as Schwann Cell Precursors (SCPs). Adameyko et al. demonstrated that although these cells are fully capable of differentiating into Schwann cells, SCPs are also capable of differentiating along a melanocytic lineage, under the influence of growth factors such as IGF-1 and PDGF (Adameyko et al., 2009). Melanocytes spawned from this neuronal lineage have a gene expression profile defined by a lack of MITF or Wnt/β-catenin influence, and thus lack expression of many melanocyte-specific genes (Tap et al., 2010). Thus, the transcriptional profile closely parallels (and in fact may represent) invasive or stem cell-like melanoma cells (Hoek et al., 2006).

2.4.2 Melanoma gene signatures resembling melanocytes or neuronal precursors

Analogous to the two distinct clusters of gene expression profiles representing proliferative and invasive subpopulations of melanoma cells discussed in this chapter until now, there is also a large body of research which has used transcriptional profiling studies to identify two major differentiation states of melanoma cells. These differentiation states have previously been classified by Tap et al. as either the differentiated melanocyte group (DMG), or the neuronal precursor group (NPG) (Tap et al., 2010). Based on our description of the two distinct lineages of melanocytes, the differentiation state of melanoma cells in the DMG resembles melanocytes of the classical lineage, while the differentiation state of melanoma in the NPG resembles melanocytes of a neuronal lineage. The existence of these two distinct melanoma differentiation states is in keeping with the cancer stem cell theory, which is quickly gaining acceptance within the cancer research community as the missing link in our understanding of phenomena such as metastasis and therapeutic resistance (Zabierowski and Herlyn, 2008). This theory proposes that every tumor is made up of cells in various states of differentiation, with one subgroup made up of quickly dividing tumor cells which remain highly differentiated and another subgroup made up of tumor cells which take on a stem-like phenotype.

In relation to melanoma, the melanocytic subgroup of cells, or DMG, represents a population of tumor cells which express many of the markers of a differentiated melanocyte. These markers include TYR, MART-1, GPNMB, endothelin receptor type B (EDNRB) and neurturin (Tap et al., 2010). Melanoma cells belonging to the DMG are increasingly being referred to as the fast-growing, differentiated counterparts to stem cell-like tumor initiating melanoma cells. As with melanocytes which develop from NCC via the classical lineage under strong SOX10 influence, the well-differentiated population of melanoma tumor cells express a transcriptional profile which reflects the influence of MITF and Wnt/β-catenin signalling. Tap et al. postulate that melanoma cells belonging to the DMG develop as per the typical pattern of melanocyte development from the dorsal aspect of the neural tube (Tap et al., 2010). It would appear that melanoma cells in the DMG may in fact represent the same subgroup of highly proliferative, minimally invasive melanoma cells described by Hoek & Goding, and refered to as proliferative melanoma cells (Hoek and Goding, 2010; Tap et al., 2010).

The existence of a distinct subpopulation of cells within malignant tumors which retain key stem cell-like properties such as the capacity for self-renewal and differentiation is a hallmark of the cancer stem cell theory, and indeed melanoma tumors do contain populations of de-differentiated cells which resemble neuronal stem cells (Barnhill et al., 2004). Much like the neuronal melanocyte lineage which develops from NCC under the strong influence of the HMX1 transcription factor and a lack of SOX10 signalling, the stem-like NPG melanoma population expresses a relative lack of MITF and Wnt/β-catenin influence in its transrciptional profile (Tap et al., 2010). Instead, several cellular markers asociated with neuronal and not melanocytic cells are expressed, including neural crest nerve growth factor receptor CD271, glial fibrillary acidic protein (GFAP), neurofilament protein (NFP) and synaptophysin (Syn) (Boiko et al., 2010). Further, melanoma cells which express stem-like properties are highly invasive and minimally proliferative. Add to all of this the fact the transcriptional profile of the NPG reflects the strong influence of noncanonical WNT5A signalling, and we come to the reasonable conclusion that the de-differentiated population of neuronal melanoma cells identified by Tap et al. May in fact be equivalent to the invasive melanoma population described by Hoek & Goding (Hoek and Goding, 2010; Tap et al., 2010).

2.5 Phenotype switching and tumor heterogeneity

In contrast to the unidirectional genetic theory of melanoma progression is the fact that the proliferative transcriptional grouping is comprised of cell lines originating from primary tumors as well as from distant secondary metastases, while the invasive grouping predominantly contains pre-metastatic cells taken from the outer margins of a melanoma lesion, or metastatic melanoma cells collected during the actual process of intravascular migration (Eichhoff et al., 2010; Hoek et al., 2008). A Clark-like model of melanoma progression would instead predict that the proliferative grouping would be made up entirely of pre-metastatic cells, while the invasive grouping would contain mainly metastatic and post-metastatic cells (Miller and Mihm, 2006). However, evidence derived from several in vivo studies instead suggests that melanoma cells have the ability to cycle from a predominantly proliferative to a predominantly invasive phenotype, based on such influences as the tumor microenvironment and pharmaceutical therapies (Hoek and Goding, 2010).

One compelling study in support of phenotype switching as a source of melanoma heterogeneity was conducted by Pinner et al., in which it was shown through the use intravital imaging of melanoma cells that highly motile, intravasated metastatic melanoma cells reverted back to their pre-metastatic, proliferative phenotype once seeding at the site of secondary tumor metastasis occurred (Pinner et al., 2009). Specifically, whereas melanoma cells in the primary tumor as well as the secondary metastatic tumor were shown to have a phenotype defined by low levels of the transcription factor Brn-2 and a high level of pigmentation, highly motile, actively metastasizing melanoma cells were shown to express a predominantly Brn-2-high/pigment-low phenotype (Pinner et al., 2009).

In a patient-matched analysis of both a primary metastatic lesion and distant metastases, Eichhoff et al. demonstrated that, consistent with our description of proliferative and invasive melanoma phenotypes, cells in the primary and distant tumors expressed high levels of *MITF* and Melan-A, while cells in the "unstructured" regions of these tumors (areas from which metastatic cells are most likely to be derived) stained heavily for WNT5A and far less for Mitf and Melan-A (Eichhoff et al., 2010). Strikingly, this study also revealed late-stage metastatic melanoma cells adopted phenotypes and morphologies nearly identical to early-phase cells, indicating that melanoma cells have significant plasticity with regards to their gene expression profile (Eichhoff et al., 2010).

Lending further support to the existence of phenotype switching are the findings of Hoek et al., in which seed melanoma cells of either an exclusively proliferative or exclusively invasive phenotype were injected subcutaneously into immunocompromised mice (Hoek et al., 2008). Regardless of seed cell phenotype, the resultant tumors expressed both major gene signatures, and furthermore the signatures appeared to adhere to a strict geographic localization pattern within the tumor. Specifically, melanoma cells expressing a proliferative phenotype were predominantly found on the periphery of melanoma tumors, while the invasive melanoma cells were found within the core of the tumor. As the tumor invades to deeper levels of tissue, the cells within the tumor core are brought into contact with microenvironmental factors such as Nodal signaling proteins, which in turn drive melanoma invasion (Hoek et al., 2008).

2.6 Cell fate as a determinant of therapeutic response

2.6.1 The advent of targeted BRAF inhibitors for metastatic melanoma

One of the most promising targeted molecular therapies currently under development are small-molecule targeted kinase inhibitors such as PLX4720 (Tsai et al., 2008) and PLX4032 (Flaherty et al., 2010a; Halaban et al., 2010; Yang et al., 2010). This drug works by inhibiting the mutated form of BRAF, a key serine/threonine protein kinase in the mitogen-activated protein kinase (MAPK) pathway (Singh et al., 2008). Up to 40-60% of melanomas harbor activating BRAF mutations (Goel et al., 2006; Gorden et al., 2003; Greene et al., 2009), and of these mutations, most are the result of a single amino acid substitution in the activation loop of exon 15. The most common mutation is $BRAF^{V600E}$ mutation, which results in a 500-fold increase in kinase activity, and is the target of PLX4032 inhibition (Flaherty et al., 2010b). Indeed, the results of Phase I/II trials have been promising, with a demonstrated response rate of up to 80% (Roukos, 2011).

Exposure to drugs such as PLX4720 or PLX4032 results in a variety of anti-melanoma effects through the inhibition of the MAPK pathway and more specifically by mitigating aberrant activation of extracellular signal-regulated kinase (ERK), a downstream target of BRAF. As a result, the use of PLX4720 or PLX4032 in cells harbouring activating mutations of BRAF such as $BRAF^{V600E}$ demonstrate decreased levels of proliferation, impaired colony-forming capability and the induction of apoptosis (Tsai et al., 2008). Despite obvious excitement over the demonstrated response rate of PLX4032 thus far, talk of accelerated FDA approval and current Phase III clinical trials, questions still remain regarding the potential benefit of this drug on overall patient survival (Roukos, 2011).

2.6.2 The impact of cell fate on response to targeted BRAF inhibition

Despite producing startling initial results in some patients and achieving an overall response rate of around 80%, all melanomas sensitive to treatment with the V600 BRAF inhibitor PLX4032 eventually develop resistance, and some melanomas with the V600 BRAF mutation are resistant from the outset of treatment (Flaherty et al., 2010a). Thus, melanoma cells treated with PLX4032 make for an ideal model of mechanisms underlying the process of therapeutic resistance.

Transcriptional profiling provides some insight into the role of cell fate and PLX4032 resistance (Tap et al., 2010). In general, BRAF-mutant melanomas with a DMG (differentiated melanocyte group) gene expression signature had the least amount of resistance to growth inhibition by PLX4032, while melanoma cells with the NPG (neuronal precursor group) gene expression signature displayed the highest level of resistance to growth inhibition by PLX4032. However, the most interesting findings of this study stem from the characterization of initially sensitive cells which later acquired resistance. Contrary to the obvious conclusion that BRAF must have undergone further mutations thereby rendering PLX4032 unable to maintain its inhibitory effect, what investigators found instead was that the activity of several parallel signaling pathways was upregulated to compensate for the BRAF inhibition. Of note, levels of acquired drug resistance were highest in melanoma cells with mutated NRAS, a GTPase signaling molecule which allows for cross-talk between the PI3K-AKT and MAPK pathways.

In more general terms, it appears as though BRAF-mutated melanoma cells sensitive to PLX4032 uniformly revert to a less differentiated transcriptional profile resembling neuronal stem cells (Tap et al., 2010). Future studies will likely illuminate the exact role of cell fate in regulating the response to targeted BRAF inhibition. Understanding how the exact differentiation state of a cell (reflected by gene signature) affects phenotypes such as dependence on MAPK signaling, drug metabolism, and susceptibility to apoptosis will provide the foundation for developing therapies aimed at manipulating cell fate to therapeutic advantage.

3. Conclusion

Recent developments in our understanding of melanoma are particularly interesting with regards to thinking about forced differentiation as a potential therapeutic approach. Can we employ strong morphogen pathways to forcibly alter or refine melanoma cell fate in a manner that renders them more susceptible to therapies like targeted BRAF inhibition? Are morphogen pathways able to act as a 'master override' within a large tumor cell population to effectively decrease the heterogeneity that arises from dynamic phenotype switching? Is there a "differentiated" cancer cell state that is truly more benign and manageable compared to a parallel "undifferentiated" state?

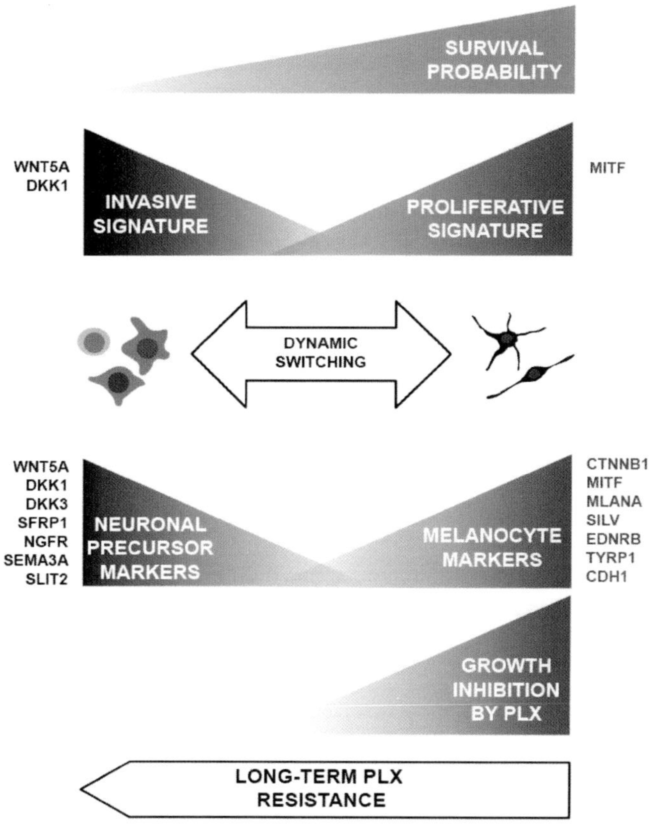

Fig. 1. **A summary of cell fate and differentiation in melanoma.** This model attempts to reconcile findings in the literature regarding cell fate and differentiation. In the middle, melanoma cells are shown transitioning dynamically between two states: 1) a neuroprogenitor-like state (left) highlighted by gene signatures enriched for inhibitors of Wnt/β-catenin signaling such as WNT5A and DKK1; and 2) a more melanocyte-like state (right) exhibiting a gene signature consistent with active Wnt/β-catenin signaling, and reflecting increased expression of melanocytic markers. Note that the continued exposure of cells to PLX4032 can promote the development of cells with largely a neuronal or invasive signature (left). The increased survival denoted on the right side (upper part of panel) reflects the clinical observation that increased Wnt/β-catenin signaling correlates with increased patient survival (Bachmann et al., 2005; Chien et al., 2009b).

Our traditional understanding of melanoma progression was based on the presumption that once a melanocyte acquired malignant potential, the constant accumulation of novel mutations conferred a progressively more aggressive phenotype as well as an increasing survival advantage to newly generated cancer cells. While it is true that key mutations such as the BRAF mutation targeted by PLX4032 are critical to melanoma pathogenesis, the sequence of intracellular events underlying the processes of tumor proliferation and metastasis in melanoma is far more dynamic than previously thought.

The recent characterization of distinct gene expression signatures in melanoma challenges our traditional model of melanoma progression. For one, two discreet transcriptional profiles would not be predicted by this model. Instead, we would expect a continuous spectrum of signatures representing the accumulation of new genetic mutations as melanoma became more aggressive. Secondly, we would expect that the transcriptional profiles of melanoma cells from secondary metastatic sites would bear less resemblance to cells in the primary tumor. Instead, proliferative melanoma cells from both primary and secondary sites are virtually identical, while the majority of invading and metastasizing melanoma cells express an invasive gene signature. Consequently, cell fate and the process of cellular differentiation are important for understanding the plasticity of melanoma cells and developing effective treatment strategies with durable long-term results.

4. Acknowledgment

A.J.C. is funded by a K08 Mentored Career Development Award from the NIH/NCI. This review was an attempt to summarize a broad and rapidly evolving field of research, and as is often the case with such ambitious undertakings, we were unable to include a comprehensive list of studies for this work. We apologize in advance for any unintended oversights that may have occurred. The authors would also like to thank Mr. Patrick O'Lin for editorial assistance during the preparation of this manuscript, and Mr. Ian A. Marsman for his assistance with mediating our international collaboration.

5. References

Adameyko, I., Lallemend, F., Aquino, J.B., Pereira, J.A., Topilko, P., Muller, T., Fritz, N., Beljajeva, A., Mochii, M., Liste, I., *et al.* (2009). Schwann cell precursors from nerve innervation are a cellular origin of melanocytes in skin. Cell *139*, 366-379.

Agalliu, D., Takada, S., Agalliu, I., McMahon, A.P., and Jessell, T.M. (2009). Motor neurons with axial muscle projections specified by Wnt4/5 signaling. Neuron *61*, 708-720.

Bachmann, I.M., Straume, O., Puntervoll, H.E., Kalvenes, M.B., and Akslen, L.A. (2005). Importance of P-cadherin, beta-catenin, and Wnt5a/frizzled for progression of melanocytic tumors and prognosis in cutaneous melanoma. Clin Cancer Res *11*, 8606-8614.

Balint, K., Xiao, M., Pinnix, C.C., Soma, A., Veres, I., Juhasz, I., Brown, E.J., Capobianco, A.J., Herlyn, M., and Liu, Z.J. (2005). Activation of Notch1 signaling is required for beta-catenin-mediated human primary melanoma progression. J Clin Invest *115*, 3166-3176.

Bar-Eli, M. (2001). Gene regulation in melanoma progression by the AP-2 transcription factor. Pigment Cell Res *14*, 78-85.

Barnhill, R., Piepkorn, M., and Busam, K.J. (2004). Pathology of melanocytic nevi and malignant melanoma (New York, Springer-Verlag).

Bittner, M., Meltzer, P., Chen, Y., Jiang, Y., Seftor, E., Hendrix, M., Radmacher, M., Simon, R., Yakhini, Z., Ben-Dor, A., *et al.* (2000). Molecular classification of cutaneous malignant melanoma by gene expression profiling. Nature *406*, 536-540.

Bodmer, D., Levine-Wilkinson, S., Richmond, A., Hirsh, S., and Kuruvilla, R. (2009). Wnt5a mediates nerve growth factor-dependent axonal branching and growth in developing sympathetic neurons. J Neurosci *29*, 7569-7581.

Boiko, A.D., Razorenova, O.V., van de Rijn, M., Swetter, S.M., Johnson, D.L., Ly, D.P., Butler, P.D., Yang, G.P., Joshua, B., Kaplan, M.J., *et al.* (2010). Human melanoma-initiating cells express neural crest nerve growth factor receptor CD271. Nature *466*, 133-137.

Braeuer, R.R., Zigler, M., Villares, G.J., Dobroff, A.S., and Bar-Eli, M. (2011). Transcriptional control of melanoma metastasis: The importance of the tumor microenvironment. Semin Cancer Biol *21*, 83-88.

Carreira, S., Goodall, J., Aksan, I., La Rocca, S.A., Galibert, M.D., Denat, L., Larue, L., and Goding, C.R. (2005). Mitf cooperates with Rb1 and activates p21Cip1 expression to regulate cell cycle progression. Nature *433*, 764-769.

Carreira, S., Goodall, J., Denat, L., Rodriguez, M., Nuciforo, P., Hoek, K.S., Testori, A., Larue, L., and Goding, C.R. (2006). Mitf regulation of Dia1 controls melanoma proliferation and invasiveness. Genes Dev *20*, 3426-3439.

Castelo-Branco, G., Wagner, J., Rodriguez, F.J., Kele, J., Sousa, K., Rawal, N., Pasolli, H.A., Fuchs, E., Kitajewski, J., and Arenas, E. (2003). Differential regulation of midbrain dopaminergic neuron development by Wnt-1, Wnt-3a, and Wnt-5a. Proc Natl Acad Sci U S A *100*, 12747-12752.

Cheli, Y., Ohanna, M., Ballotti, R., and Bertolotto, C. (2010). Fifteen-year quest for microphthalmia-associated transcription factor target genes. Pigment Cell Melanoma Res *23*, 27-40.

Chien, A.J., Conrad, W.H., and Moon, R.T. (2009a). A Wnt survival guide: from flies to human disease. J Invest Dermatol *129*, 1614-1627.

Chien, A.J., and Moon, R.T. (2007). WNTS and WNT receptors as therapeutic tools and targets in human disease processes. Front Biosci *12*, 448-457.

Chien, A.J., Moore, E.C., Lonsdorf, A.S., Kulikauskas, R.M., Rothberg, B.G., Berger, A.J., Major, M.B., Hwang, S.T., Rimm, D.L., and Moon, R.T. (2009b). Activated Wnt/beta-catenin signaling in melanoma is associated with decreased proliferation in patient tumors and a murine melanoma model. Proc Natl Acad Sci U S A *106*, 1193-1198.

Cook, A.L., and Sturm, R.A. (2008). POU domain transcription factors: BRN2 as a regulator of melanocytic growth and tumourigenesis. Pigment Cell Melanoma Res *21*, 611-626.

Cornell, R.A., and Eisen, J.S. (2005). Notch in the pathway: the roles of Notch signaling in neural crest development. Semin Cell Dev Biol *16*, 663-672.

Delmas, V., Beermann, F., Martinozzi, S., Carreira, S., Ackermann, J., Kumasaka, M., Denat, L., Goodall, J., Luciani, F., Viros, A., *et al.* (2007). Beta-catenin induces immortalization of melanocytes by suppressing p16INK4a expression and cooperates with N-Ras in melanoma development. Genes Dev *21*, 2923-2935.

Dissanayake, S.K., Olkhanud, P.B., O'Connell, M.P., Carter, A., French, A.D., Camilli, T.C., Emeche, C.D., Hewitt, K.J., Rosenthal, D.T., Leotlela, P.D., *et al.* (2008). Wnt5A regulates expression of tumor-associated antigens in melanoma via changes in signal transducers and activators of transcription 3 phosphorylation. Cancer Res *68*, 10205-10214.

Dissanayake, S.K., Wade, M., Johnson, C.E., O'Connell, M.P., Leotlela, P.D., French, A.D., Shah, K.V., Hewitt, K.J., Rosenthal, D.T., Indig, F.E., *et al.* (2007). The Wnt5A/protein kinase C pathway mediates motility in melanoma cells via the inhibition of metastasis suppressors and initiation of an epithelial to mesenchymal transition. J Biol Chem *282*, 17259-17271.

Dorsky, R.I., Moon, R.T., and Raible, D.W. (1998). Control of neural crest cell fate by the Wnt signalling pathway. Nature *396*, 370-373.

Dorsky, R.I., Moon, R.T., and Raible, D.W. (2000a). Environmental signals and cell fate specification in premigratory neural crest. Bioessays *22*, 708-716.

Dorsky, R.I., Raible, D.W., and Moon, R.T. (2000b). Direct regulation of nacre, a zebrafish MITF homolog required for pigment cell formation, by the Wnt pathway. Genes Dev *14*, 158-162.

Dou, J., Pan, M., Wen, P., Li, Y., Tang, Q., Chu, L., Zhao, F., Jiang, C., Hu, W., Hu, K., *et al.* (2007). Isolation and identification of cancer stem-like cells from murine melanoma cell lines. Cell Mol Immunol *4*, 467-472.

Dupin, E., Glavieux, C., Vaigot, P., and Le Douarin, N.M. (2000). Endothelin 3 induces the reversion of melanocytes to glia through a neural crest-derived glial-melanocytic progenitor. Proc Natl Acad Sci U S A *97*, 7882-7887.

Dupin, E., Real, C., Glavieux-Pardanaud, C., Vaigot, P., and Le Douarin, N.M. (2003). Reversal of developmental restrictions in neural crest lineages: transition from Schwann cells to glial-melanocytic precursors in vitro. Proc Natl Acad Sci U S A *100*, 5229-5233.

Eichhoff, O.M., Zipser, M.C., Xu, M., Weeraratna, A.T., Mihic, D., Dummer, R., and Hoek, K.S. (2010). The immunohistochemistry of invasive and proliferative phenotype switching in melanoma: a case report. Melanoma Res *20*, 349-355.

Fang, D., Leishear, K., Nguyen, T.K., Finko, R., Cai, K., Fukunaga, M., Li, L., Brafford, P.A., Kulp, A.N., Xu, X., *et al.* (2006). Defining the conditions for the generation of melanocytes from human embryonic stem cells. Stem Cells *24*, 1668-1677.

Fidler, I.J. (1978). Tumor heterogeneity and the biology of cancer invasion and metastasis. Cancer Res *38*, 2651-2660.

Flaherty, K., Puzanov, I., Kim, K., Ribas, A., McArthur, G.A., Sosman, J.A., O'Dwyer, P., Lee, R., Grippo, J.F., Nolop, K., *et al.* (2010a). Inhibition of mutated, activated BRAF in metastatic melanoma. N Engl J Med *363*, 809-819.

Flaherty, K.T., Hodi, F.S., and Bastian, B.C. (2010b). Mutation-driven drug development in melanoma. Curr Opin Oncol *22*, 178-183.

Garraway, L.A., Widlund, H.R., Rubin, M.A., Getz, G., Berger, A.J., Ramaswamy, S., Beroukhim, R., Milner, D.A., Granter, S.R., Du, J., *et al.* (2005). Integrative genomic analyses identify MITF as a lineage survival oncogene amplified in malignant melanoma. Nature *436*, 117-122.

Goding, C.R. (2000). Mitf from neural crest to melanoma: signal transduction and transcription in the melanocyte lineage. Genes Dev *14*, 1712-1728.

Goel, V.K., Lazar, A.J., Warneke, C.L., Redston, M.S., and Haluska, F.G. (2006). Examination of mutations in BRAF, NRAS, and PTEN in primary cutaneous melanoma. J Invest Dermatol *126*, 154-160.

Goodall, J., Martinozzi, S., Dexter, T.J., Champeval, D., Carreira, S., Larue, L., and Goding, C.R. (2004a). Brn-2 expression controls melanoma proliferation and is directly regulated by beta-catenin. Mol Cell Biol *24*, 2915-2922.

Goodall, J., Wellbrock, C., Dexter, T.J., Roberts, K., Marais, R., and Goding, C.R. (2004b). The Brn-2 transcription factor links activated BRAF to melanoma proliferation. Mol Cell Biol *24*, 2923-2931.

Gorden, A., Osman, I., Gai, W., He, D., Huang, W., Davidson, A., Houghton, A.N., Busam, K., and Polsky, D. (2003). Analysis of BRAF and N-RAS mutations in metastatic melanoma tissues. Cancer Res *63*, 3955-3957.

Greene, V.R., Johnson, M.M., Grimm, E.A., and Ellerhorst, J.A. (2009). Frequencies of NRAS and BRAF mutations increase from the radial to the vertical growth phase in cutaneous melanoma. J Invest Dermatol *129*, 1483-1488.

Grichnik, J.M., Burch, J.A., Schulteis, R.D., Shan, S., Liu, J., Darrow, T.L., Vervaert, C.E., and Seigler, H.F. (2006). Melanoma, a tumor based on a mutant stem cell? J Invest Dermatol *126*, 142-153.

Halaban, R., Zhang, W., Bacchiocchi, A., Cheng, E., Parisi, F., Ariyan, S., Krauthammer, M., McCusker, J.P., Kluger, Y., and Sznol, M. (2010). PLX4032, a selective BRAF(V600E) kinase inhibitor, activates the ERK pathway and enhances cell migration and proliferation of BRAF melanoma cells. Pigment Cell Melanoma Res *23*, 190-200.

Hardy, K.M., Kirschmann, D.A., Seftor, E.A., Margaryan, N.V., Postovit, L.M., Strizzi, L., and Hendrix, M.J. (2010). Regulation of the embryonic morphogen Nodal by Notch4 facilitates manifestation of the aggressive melanoma phenotype. Cancer Res *70*, 10340-10350.

Held, M.A., Curley, D.P., Dankort, D., McMahon, M., Muthusamy, V., and Bosenberg, M.W. (2010). Characterization of melanoma cells capable of propagating tumors from a single cell. Cancer Res *70*, 388-397.

Hoek, K.S. (2007). DNA microarray analyses of melanoma gene expression: a decade in the mines. Pigment Cell Res *20*, 466-484.

Hoek, K.S., Eichhoff, O.M., Schlegel, N.C., Dobbeling, U., Kobert, N., Schaerer, L., Hemmi, S., and Dummer, R. (2008). In vivo switching of human melanoma cells between proliferative and invasive states. Cancer Res *68*, 650-656.

Hoek, K.S., and Goding, C.R. (2010). Cancer stem cells versus phenotype-switching in melanoma. Pigment Cell Melanoma Res *23*, 746-759.

Hoek, K.S., Schlegel, N.C., Brafford, P., Sucker, A., Ugurel, S., Kumar, R., Weber, B.L., Nathanson, K.L., Phillips, D.J., Herlyn, M., *et al.* (2006). Metastatic potential of melanomas defined by specific gene expression profiles with no BRAF signature. Pigment Cell Res *19*, 290-302.

Hsu, M.Y., Rovinsky, S., Penmatcha, S., Herlyn, M., and Muirhead, D. (2005). Bone morphogenetic proteins in melanoma: angel or devil? Cancer Metastasis Rev *24*, 251-263.

Hsu, M.Y., Rovinsky, S.A., Lai, C.Y., Qasem, S., Liu, X., How, J., Engelhardt, J.F., and Murphy, G.F. (2008). Aggressive melanoma cells escape from BMP7-mediated autocrine growth inhibition through coordinated Noggin upregulation. Lab Invest *88*, 842-855.

Javelaud, D., Alexaki, V.I., and Mauviel, A. (2008). Transforming growth factor-beta in cutaneous melanoma. Pigment Cell Melanoma Res *21*, 123-132.

Javelaud, D., Delmas, V., Moller, M., Sextius, P., Andre, J., Menashi, S., Larue, L., and Mauviel, A. (2005). Stable overexpression of Smad7 in human melanoma cells inhibits their tumorigenicity in vitro and in vivo. Oncogene *24*, 7624-7629.

Kageshita, T., Hamby, C.V., Ishihara, T., Matsumoto, K., Saida, T., and Ono, T. (2001). Loss of beta-catenin expression associated with disease progression in malignant melanoma. Br J Dermatol *145*, 210-216.

Klein, W.M., Wu, B.P., Zhao, S., Wu, H., Klein-Szanto, A.J., and Tahan, S.R. (2007). Increased expression of stem cell markers in malignant melanoma. Mod Pathol *20*, 102-107.

Kopan, R., and Ilagan, M.X. (2009). The canonical Notch signaling pathway: unfolding the activation mechanism. Cell *137*, 216-233.

Krasagakis, K., Kruger-Krasagakes, S., Fimmel, S., Eberle, J., Tholke, D., von der Ohe, M., Mansmann, U., and Orfanos, C.E. (1999). Desensitization of melanoma cells to autocrine TGF-beta isoforms. J Cell Physiol *178*, 179-187.

Krispin, S., Nitzan, E., and Kalcheim, C. (2010). The dorsal neural tube: a dynamic setting for cell fate decisions. Dev Neurobiol *70*, 796-812.

Lasfar, A., and Cohen-Solal, K.A. (2010). Resistance to transforming growth factor beta-mediated tumor suppression in melanoma: are multiple mechanisms in place? Carcinogenesis *31*, 1710-1717.

Lekmine, F., Chang, C.K., Sethakorn, N., Das Gupta, T.K., and Salti, G.I. (2007). Role of microphthalmia transcription factor (Mitf) in melanoma differentiation. Biochem Biophys Res Commun *354*, 830-835.

Lens, M.B., and Dawes, M. (2004). Global perspectives of contemporary epidemiological trends of cutaneous malignant melanoma. Br J Dermatol *150*, 179-185.

Levy, C., Khaled, M., and Fisher, D.E. (2006). MITF: master regulator of melanocyte development and melanoma oncogene. Trends Mol Med *12*, 406-414.

Liu, J., Sato, C., Cerletti, M., and Wagers, A. (2010). Notch signaling in the regulation of stem cell self-renewal and differentiation. Curr Top Dev Biol *92*, 367-409.

Liu, Z.J., Xiao, M., Balint, K., Smalley, K.S., Brafford, P., Qiu, R., Pinnix, C.C., Li, X., and Herlyn, M. (2006a). Notch1 signaling promotes primary melanoma progression by activating mitogen-activated protein kinase/phosphatidylinositol 3-kinase-Akt pathways and up-regulating N-cadherin expression. Cancer Res *66*, 4182-4190.

Liu, Z.J., Xiao, M., Balint, K., Soma, A., Pinnix, C.C., Capobianco, A.J., Velazquez, O.C., and Herlyn, M. (2006b). Inhibition of endothelial cell proliferation by Notch1 signaling is mediated by repressing MAPK and PI3K/Akt pathways and requires MAML1. Faseb J *20*, 1009-1011.

Loercher, A.E., Tank, E.M., Delston, R.B., and Harbour, J.W. (2005). MITF links differentiation with cell cycle arrest in melanocytes by transcriptional activation of INK4A. J Cell Biol *168*, 35-40.

Lucero, O.M., Dawson, D.W., Moon, R.T., and Chien, A.J. (2010). A re-evaluation of the "oncogenic" nature of Wnt/beta-catenin signaling in melanoma and other cancers. Curr Oncol Rep *12*, 314-318.

Maelandsmo, G.M., Holm, R., Nesland, J.M., Fodstad, O., and Florenes, V.A. (2003). Reduced beta-catenin expression in the cytoplasm of advanced-stage superficial spreading malignant melanoma. Clin Cancer Res *9*, 3383-3388.

Melnikova, V.O., Dobroff, A.S., Zigler, M., Villares, G.J., Braeuer, R.R., Wang, H., Huang, L., and Bar-Eli, M. (2010). CREB inhibits AP-2alpha expression to regulate the malignant phenotype of melanoma. PLoS One *5*, e12452.

Miller, A.J., and Mihm, M.C., Jr. (2006). Melanoma. N Engl J Med *355*, 51-65.

Pinner, S., Jordan, P., Sharrock, K., Bazley, L., Collinson, L., Marais, R., Bonvin, E., Goding, C., and Sahai, E. (2009). Intravital imaging reveals transient changes in pigment production and Brn2 expression during metastatic melanoma dissemination. Cancer Res *69*, 7969-7977.

Pinnix, C.C., Lee, J.T., Liu, Z.J., McDaid, R., Balint, K., Beverly, L.J., Brafford, P.A., Xiao, M., Himes, B., Zabierowski, S.E., *et al.* (2009). Active Notch1 confers a transformed phenotype to primary human melanocytes. Cancer Res *69*, 5312-5320.

Postovit, L.M., Costa, F.F., Bischof, J.M., Seftor, E.A., Wen, B., Seftor, R.E., Feinberg, A.P., Soares, M.B., and Hendrix, M.J. (2007). The commonality of plasticity underlying multipotent tumor cells and embryonic stem cells. J Cell Biochem *101*, 908-917.

Postovit, L.M., Margaryan, N.V., Seftor, E.A., and Hendrix, M.J. (2008a). Role of nodal signaling and the microenvironment underlying melanoma plasticity. Pigment Cell Melanoma Res *21*, 348-357.

Postovit, L.M., Margaryan, N.V., Seftor, E.A., Kirschmann, D.A., Lipavsky, A., Wheaton, W.W., Abbott, D.E., Seftor, R.E., and Hendrix, M.J. (2008b). Human embryonic stem cell microenvironment suppresses the tumorigenic phenotype of aggressive cancer cells. Proc Natl Acad Sci U S A *105*, 4329-4334.

Quintana, E., Shackleton, M., Foster, H.R., Fullen, D.R., Sabel, M.S., Johnson, T.M., and Morrison, S.J. (2010). Phenotypic heterogeneity among tumorigenic melanoma cells from patients that is reversible and not hierarchically organized. Cancer Cell *18*, 510-523.

Quintana, E., Shackleton, M., Sabel, M.S., Fullen, D.R., Johnson, T.M., and Morrison, S.J. (2008). Efficient tumour formation by single human melanoma cells. Nature *456*, 593-598.

Rothhammer, T., Poser, I., Soncin, F., Bataille, F., Moser, M., and Bosserhoff, A.K. (2005). Bone morphogenic proteins are overexpressed in malignant melanoma and promote cell invasion and migration. Cancer Res *65*, 448-456.

Roukos, D.H. (2011). PLX4032 and melanoma: resistance, expectations and uncertainty. Expert Rev Anticancer Ther *11*, 325-328.

Sato-Jin, K., Nishimura, E.K., Akasaka, E., Huber, W., Nakano, H., Miller, A., Du, J., Wu, M., Hanada, K., Sawamura, D., *et al.* (2008). Epistatic connections between microphthalmia-associated transcription factor and endothelin signaling in Waardenburg syndrome and other pigmentary disorders. Faseb J *22*, 1155-1168.

Schatton, T., Murphy, G.F., Frank, N.Y., Yamaura, K., Waaga-Gasser, A.M., Gasser, M., Zhan, Q., Jordan, S., Duncan, L.M., Weishaupt, C., *et al.* (2008). Identification of cells initiating human melanomas. Nature *451*, 345-349.

Schmoeckel, C., Castro, C.E., and Braun-Falco, O. (1985). Nevoid malignant melanoma. Arch Dermatol Res *277*, 362-369.

Sestakova, B., Ondrusova, L., and Vachtenheim, J. (2010). Cell cycle inhibitor p21/ WAF1/ CIP1 as a cofactor of MITF expression in melanoma cells. Pigment Cell Melanoma Res *23*, 238-251.

Singh, M., Lin, J., Hocker, T.L., and Tsao, H. (2008). Genetics of melanoma tumorigenesis. Br J Dermatol *158*, 15-21.

Strizzi, L., Hardy, K.M., Seftor, E.A., Costa, F.F., Kirschmann, D.A., Seftor, R.E., Postovit, L.M., and Hendrix, M.J. (2009). Development and cancer: at the crossroads of Nodal and Notch signaling. Cancer Res *69*, 7131-7134.

Tap, W.D., Gong, K.W., Dering, J., Tseng, Y., Ginther, C., Pauletti, G., Glaspy, J.A., Essner, R., Bollag, G., Hirth, P., *et al.* (2010). Pharmacodynamic characterization of the efficacy signals due to selective BRAF inhibition with PLX4032 in malignant melanoma. Neoplasia *12*, 637-649.

Tellez, C., McCarty, M., Ruiz, M., and Bar-Eli, M. (2003). Loss of activator protein-2alpha results in overexpression of protease-activated receptor-1 and correlates with the malignant phenotype of human melanoma. J Biol Chem *278*, 46632-46642.

Thomas, A.J., and Erickson, C.A. (2008). The making of a melanocyte: the specification of melanoblasts from the neural crest. Pigment Cell Melanoma Res *21*, 598-610.

Thomson, J.A., Murphy, K., Baker, E., Sutherland, G.R., Parsons, P.G., Sturm, R.A., and Thomson, F. (1995). The brn-2 gene regulates the melanocytic phenotype and tumorigenic potential of human melanoma cells. Oncogene *11*, 691-700.

Thurber, A.E., Douglas, G., Sturm, E.C., Zabierowski, S.E., Smit, D.J., Ramakrishnan, S.N., Hacker, E., Leonard, J.H., Herlyn, M., and Sturm, R.A. (2011). Inverse expression states of the BRN2 and MITF transcription factors in melanoma spheres and tumour xenografts regulate the NOTCH pathway. Oncogene.

Tsai, J., Lee, J.T., Wang, W., Zhang, J., Cho, H., Mamo, S., Bremer, R., Gillette, S., Kong, J., Haass, N.K., *et al.* (2008). Discovery of a selective inhibitor of oncogenic B-Raf kinase with potent antimelanoma activity. Proc Natl Acad Sci U S A *105*, 3041-3046.

Tsao, H., Atkins, M.B., and Sober, A.J. (2004). Management of cutaneous melanoma. N Engl J Med *351*, 998-1012.

Varela-Nallar, L., Alfaro, I.E., Serrano, F.G., Parodi, J., and Inestrosa, N.C. (2010). Wingless-type family member 5A (Wnt-5a) stimulates synaptic differentiation and function of glutamatergic synapses. Proc Natl Acad Sci U S A *107*, 21164-21169.

Vierbuchen, T., Ostermeier, A., Pang, Z.P., Kokubu, Y., Sudhof, T.C., and Wernig, M. (2010). Direct conversion of fibroblasts to functional neurons by defined factors. Nature *463*, 1035-1041.

Weeraratna, A.T., Becker, D., Carr, K.M., Duray, P.H., Rosenblatt, K.P., Yang, S., Chen, Y., Bittner, M., Strausberg, R.L., Riggins, G.J., *et al.* (2004). Generation and analysis of melanoma SAGE libraries: SAGE advice on the melanoma transcriptome. Oncogene *23*, 2264-2274.

Weeraratna, A.T., Jiang, Y., Hostetter, G., Rosenblatt, K., Duray, P., Bittner, M., and Trent, J.M. (2002). Wnt5a signaling directly affects cell motility and invasion of metastatic melanoma. Cancer Cell *1*, 279-288.

Widlund, H.R., Horstmann, M.A., Price, E.R., Cui, J., Lessnick, S.L., Wu, M., He, X., and Fisher, D.E. (2002). Beta-catenin-induced melanoma growth requires the downstream target Microphthalmia-associated transcription factor. J Cell Biol *158*, 1079-1087.

Winkelmann, R.K., and Rocha, G. (1962). The dermal nevus and statistics. An evaluation of 1,200 pigmented lesions. Arch Dermatol *86*, 310-315.

Witze, E.S., Litman, E.S., Argast, G.M., Moon, R.T., and Ahn, N.G. (2008). Wnt5a control of cell polarity and directional movement by polarized redistribution of adhesion receptors. Science *320*, 365-369.

Yang, H., Higgins, B., Kolinsky, K., Packman, K., Go, Z., Iyer, R., Kolis, S., Zhao, S., Lee, R., Grippo, J.F., *et al.* (2010). RG7204 (PLX4032), a selective BRAFV600E inhibitor, displays potent antitumor activity in preclinical melanoma models. Cancer Res *70*, 5518-5527.

Yu, L., Harms, P.W., Pouryazdanparast, P., Kim, D.S., Ma, L., and Fullen, D.R. (2010). Expression of the embryonic morphogen Nodal in cutaneous melanocytic lesions. Mod Pathol *23*, 1209-1214.

Zabierowski, S.E., and Herlyn, M. (2008). Melanoma stem cells: the dark seed of melanoma. J Clin Oncol *26*, 2890-2894.

Zhuang, L., Lee, C.S., Scolyer, R.A., McCarthy, S.W., Zhang, X.D., Thompson, J.F., and Hersey, P. (2007). Mcl-1, Bcl-XL and Stat3 expression are associated with progression of melanoma whereas Bcl-2, AP-2 and MITF levels decrease during progression of melanoma. Mod Pathol *20*, 416-426.

Part 4

Tumor Progression and the Microenvironment

15

Role of Angiogenesis and Microenvironment in Melanoma Progression

Roberto Ria, Antonia Reale and Angelo Vacca
University of Bari
Italy

1. Introduction

The growth, survival and proliferation of cancer cells are guaranteed by a crosstalk between cancer cells themselves and surrounding host cells and extracellular matrix. An intense area of research has contributed to a better understanding of the pathophysiological modification of tumour progression, e.g., the role of microenvironment.

Human malignant melanoma is a highly metastatic tumour with poor prognosis and extreme resistance to treatment. It progresses through different steps: nevocellular nevi, dysplastic nevi (when these two entity can be identified as primary events in melanocytic neoplasia progression), in situ melanoma, radial growth phase melanoma (Breslow index ≤0.75 mm), vertical growth phase melanoma (index >0.75 mm), and metastatic melanoma (Breslow, 1970). Primary tumour grows horizontally through the epidermis; over time, a vertical growth phase component intervenes and melanoma increases its thickness and invades the dermis. Once a vertical growth phase has developed, there is a direct correlation between the tumour thickness and the number of metastases (Heasley et al., 1996).

Parallel with progression, melanoma acquires a rich vascular network. Melanoma neovascularization has been correlated with poor prognosis, shorter overall survival, ulceration and increased rate of relapse (Srivastava et al., 1988, 1989). This neovascularization is initiated and maintained by mean the secretion of various angiogenic cytokines, i.e. *Vascular Endothelial Growth Factor-A* (VEGF-A), *Fibroblast Growth Factor-2* (FGF-2), *Placental Growth Factor* (PGF) *-1* and *-2*, *Interleukin* (IL) *-8*, *Transforming Growth Factor-1* (TGF-1), by melanoma cells. Moreover cytokines production has been correlated to the transition from the radial to the vertical growth phase, and to the metastatic phase (Erhard et al., 1997; Marcoval et al., 1997; Salven et al., 1997).

2. Human melanoma

Human malignant melanoma originates from the melanocytes and manifests mainly on the skin. Rarely, melanomas can occur on the eye, the meninges, and the mucosa in different locations. The incidence of melanoma in white populations worldwide is increasing, especially in light skinned people with sun exposure. Melanomas are rare in populations with pigmented skin and almost always located on the mucosa or the palms of the hands or soles of the feet (Garbe et al., 2008).

The most important etiological factor for the development of a melanoma is UV radiation. Even in childhood, the influence of UV radiation results in the development of benign melanocytic neoplasms, in the form of melanocytic nevi. These are indicators of acquired mutations in the melanocytic system. The more melanocytic nevi someone has, the higher their risk of developing melanoma. Melanomas develop primarily in sites with the highest numbers of melanocytic nevi (Garbe et al., 2008).
Clinically and histologically, four different subtypes of melanoma can be distinguished, which have different patterns of mutation: superficially spreading melanoma; nodular melanoma; lentigo maligna melanoma; acral lentiginous melanoma. The criteria of the ABCDE rule are the main diagnostic criteria (Asymmetry; Border irregularity; Color; Diameter; Evolving). Staging (American Joint Committee on Cancer Staging System) is important for selecting the best therapeutic approach (Balch et al., 2001, 2009).

3. Tumour angiogenesis

Angiogenesis is the sprouting of new blood vessels from a pre-existing vasculature and it is a tightly regulated process (Stasi & Amadori, 2002). During embryogenesis two major processes of blood vessel formation are implicated in the development of the vascular system: vasculogenesis and angiogenesis (Risau, 1988).
Vasculogenesis starts from mesodermal-derived cells, the hemangioblasts, which differentiate both into angioblasts-endothelial cells and into hematopoietic stem cells. Vasculogenesis prevails in the embryo but it may have physiological roles in health and disease in adults (Iruela-Arispe & Dvorak, 1997). Both mechanisms, angiogenesis and vasculogenesis, occur in ischemic and tumour tissues in response to growth factors, such as VEGF and FGF-2, produced by tumour and stromal cells (Folkman et al., 2001). In some aggressive tumours the vessel wall is lined with only cancer cells as a mosaic of cancer cells and endothelial cells. This phenomenon is called *"vasculogenesis mimicry"* (Dome et al., 2007).
Angiogenesis is uncontrolled and unlimited in time, and essential for tumour growth, invasion and metastasis during the transition from the avascular to the vascular phase, the so-called angiogenic switch, in which the balance between angiogenesis inducers and inhibitors leans towards the former. The vascular phase is characterized by the new formation of vascular channels that enhance tumour cell proliferation, local invasion, and hematogenous metastasis.

3.1 Angiogenesis and human melanoma

New blood vessel formation is a prominent feature of human melanomas, indicating that these tumours have angiogenic activity (Mihm et al., 1975). The observation that cutaneous melanoma cells acquire the capacity to actively induce the growth of new blood vessels dates back to the earliest days of tumour angiogenesis research, when Warren and Shubik observed it after transplantation of human melanoma fragments into a hamster cheek pouch (Warren & Shubik, 1966). These studies were confirmed in later studies (Hubler & Wolf, 1976). Rapid angiogenesis of cutaneous melanomas dramatically enhances the risk of lethality and contributes to the progression of the most common type of young adults (Streit & Detmar, 2003).

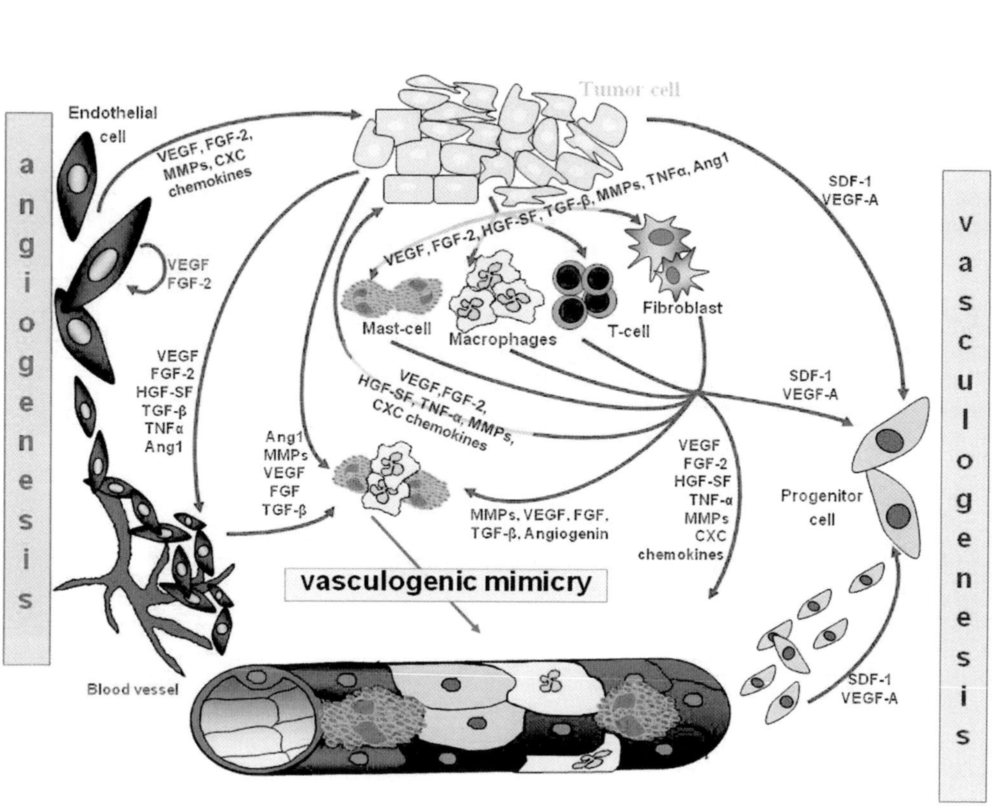

Fig. 1. Processes implied in neovessel formation tumor-induced

3.1.1 The role of angiogenic cytokines

Tumour angiogenesis depends mainly on the release by neoplastic cells of growth factors specific for endothelial cells, able to stimulate the growth of the host's blood vessels.

VEGF is expressed in most solid tumours and the VEGF receptors (VEGF-Rs) are predominant in endothelial cells surrounding or penetrating malignant tissue, but are absent from vascular cells in the surrounding normal tissue. This finding suggests that VEGF-Rs expression is induced in endothelial cells during tumour angiogenesis by VEGF secreted by tumour cells.

Secretion of VEGF-A isoform by melanoma cells has been correlated to the transition from the radial to the vertical growth phase, and to the metastatic phase (Erhard et al., 1997; Marcoval et al., 1997; Salven et al., 1997). Our previous studies indicated that increased microvascular density, strong VEGF-A tumour immunoreactivity, increased vascular diameter, and high number of vascular pillars—expression of the intussusceptive microvascular growth—are correlated to a high Breslow index (>3.6 mm).

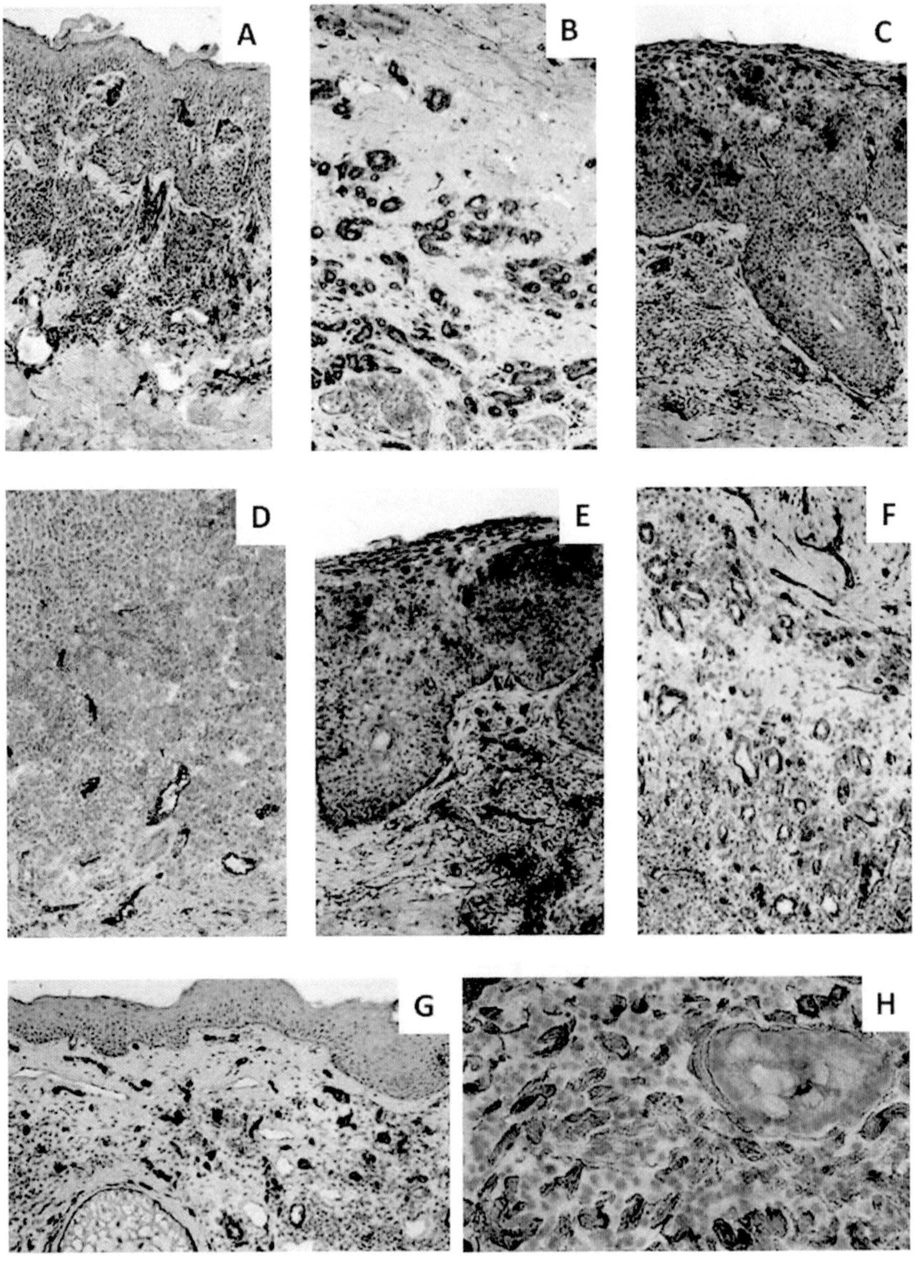

Fig. 2. Angiogenesis extent parallel with melanoma progression: A) common nevi, B) displastic nevi, C) microvessels under the base of melanoma, D) melanoma breslow 0.45 mm, E) melanoma breslow 1 mm, F) melanoma breslow >3 mm, G) advanced melanoma with inflammatory infiltrate, H) bowel metastasis of advanced melanoma

Salven et al. (1997) have demonstrated that up-regulation of VEGF-A expression in metastatic melanoma is associated with an increase in the number of tumour-infiltrating inflammatory cells expressing VEGF-A.

FGF-2 regulates endothelial cell proliferation and angiogenesis by both autocrine and paracrine mechanisms. Since FGF-2 is devoid of the classic signal peptide for secretion, tumour cells release this factor by exocytosis from endoplasmic reticulum. Significant amounts of FGF-2 were found to be associated with extracellular matrix as well as with basement membrane of the newly formed blood vessels in human melanomas. Digestion of extracellular matrix by matrix metalloproteinases of melanoma or endothelial origin promotes release of matrix bound FGF-2, which, in turn, stimulates endothelial cell proliferation and vascular tube formation in melanomas. We and other authors (Salven et al., 1997) have demonstrated a significant correlation between melanoma progression, percentage of FGF-2-expressing tumour cells, and the number of mast cells which, in turn, secrete other angiogenic molecules, such as VEGF-A.

Another important stimulator of melanoma angiogenesis is PGF. PGF-1 and -2 are expressed by melanoma cells and are known to bind neuropilin-1 and -2 receptors expressed on endothelial cells (Odorisio et al., 2006). In addition, PGF acts through binding VEGF-R1 inducing the mobilization and recruitment of VEGF-R1+ hematopoietic precursors from bone marrow and enhancing blood vessel maturation by acting on VEGF-R1-expressing smooth muscle cells/pericytes (Donnini et al., 1999). Moreover, PGF forms heterodimers with VEGF-A and enhances melanoma angiogenesis by activating VEGF-R2 on endothelial cells (Donnini et al., 1999; Luttun et al., 2004).

IL-8 expression was found to be very little in normal epidermis and benign melanocytic lesions. However, it is dramatically increased in the majority of cutaneous melanomas. Its serum levels in patients are significantly elevated compared to healthy individuals and correlate with advanced disease stage as well as with overall survival (Bar-Eli et al., 1999). Melanoma-derived IL-8 is able to induce endothelial cell migration, modulate vascular permeability, and enhance actin stress fiber formation. These activities resulted in enhanced angiogenesis, rapid tumour growth, and increased metastatic potential (Mahler et al., 2004; Melnikova & Bar-Eli, 2006). Liu et al. (2005) have demonstrated that TGF-1 is able to enhance expression of IL-8 in human melanoma cells and promote angiogenesis in several mouse xenograft models.

Melanotransferrin, a member of the transferrin family, which is comprised of serum transferrin, lactoferrin and ovotransferrin, is highly expressed on melanoma cells compared to normal melanocytes. It exerts an angiogenic response quantitatively similar to that elicidated by FGF-2, and its angiogenic activity may depend on activation of endogenous VEGF. We have demonstrated that melanotransferrin contributes to angiogenesis during melanoma progression, and is likely associated with VEGF overexpression.

4. Tumour microenvironment

Neoplastic cells are influenced by their microenvironment and viceversa. The specific organ microenvironment determines the extent of cancer cell proliferation, angiogenesis, invasion and survival (Park et al., 2000; Liotta & Kohn, 2001). These data indicate that a permissive stromal environment is important in supporting tumour progression in combination with genetic alterations.

Tumour cells are surrounded by an infiltrate of inflammatory cells, namely lymphocytes, neutrophils, macrophages and mast cells, which communicate via a complex network of intercellular signalling pathways, mediated by surface adhesion molecules, cytokines and their receptors.

The inflammatory cell infiltrate, particularly macrophages, may contribute to tumour angiogenesis, and there are many reports of associations between macrophage infiltration, vascularity and prognosis. Tumour-associated macrophages accumulate in poorly vascularized hypoxic or necrotic areas (Leek et al., 1999) and respond to experimental hypoxia by increasing the release of VEGF and FGF-2 and a broad range of other factors, such as *Tumour Necrosis Factor-alpha* (TNF-α), urokinase and matrix metalloproteinases (Bingle et al., 2002). Moreover, activated macrophages synthesize and release inducible nitric oxide synthase, which increases blood flow and promotes angiogenesis (Jenkins et al., 1995). Lastly, the angiogenic factors secreted by macrophages stimulate mast cell migration (Gruber et al., 1995).

Chemokines also have a role: some CXC chemokines, such as IL-8 are pro-angiogenic (Bernardini et al., 2003). Chemokines may exert their regulatory activity on angiogenesis directly or as a consequence of leucocyte infiltration and/or the induction of growth factor expression. Malignant melanoma is also associated with a dramatic host response composed of mast cells at the tumour periphery.

Mast cells infiltrate hyperplasias, dysplasias and invasive fronts of carcinomas (but not the core of solid tumours), where they degranulate in close apposition to capillaries and epithelial basement membranes. Mast cells contain many angiogenic factors and a variety of cytokines, such as TGF-β, TNF-α, IL-8, FGF-2, VEGF, implicated in normal, as well as tumour-associated neoangiogenesis.

Angiogenesis in human malignant melanoma, measured as microvessel counts, is highly correlated with both the percentage of tumour cells reactive to FGF-2 and mast cells counts (as total cell and tryptase-positive cell counts), and these parameters increase with tumour progression.

Two distinct types of human mast cells have been described based on the protease composition of their secretory granules: mast cells containing chymase, carboxypeptidase, cathepsin and tryptase and mast cells containing tryptase only. Tryptase, a protease unique to the mast cells secretory granules, acts as a mitogen for fibroblasts, smooth muscle cells, and epithelial cells (Brown et al., 1995; Cairns & Walls, 1996).

Blair and colleagues (Blair et al., 1997) have shown that mast cell-released tryptase plays an important role in neovascularization. Tryptase induces the formation of capillary structures by either directly acting on endothelial cells or by facilitating the early stages of angiogenesis. In fact, tryptase activates latent matrix metalloproteinases and plasminogen activator (Stack & Johnson, 1994), which degrade the extracellular matrix, a critical step in these stages (Mignatti & Rifkin, 1993).

Mast cells are strikingly associated with angiogenesis in tumours, namely haemangioma, carcinomas, lymphoma and multiple myeloma where they are preferentially accumulated in the peripheral areas of the tumour, within the surrounding connective tissue, and rest near or around blood or lymphatic vessels. Mast cells are recruited and activated via several factors secreted by tumour cells: the c-kit receptor (Norrby & Woolley, 1993), FGF-2, VEGF-A and *Platelet-Derived Endothelial Cell Growth Factor* (PD-ECGF), which are operative at picomolar concentrations (Gruber et al., 1995).

The fact that mast cells contribute to the induction of tumour angiogenesis stems from studies on mast cell-deficient mice, which display slow angiogenesis, and its restoration after local reconstitution of mast cells (Starkley et al., 1988; Toth et al., 2000). Moreover, in malignant breast lesions the number of mast cells with tryptase activity was significantly higher than in benign lesions (Kankunnen et al., 1997) and mast cells derived from human renal tumour tissues contained tryptase (Beil et al., 1998).

Tryptase-positive mast cells may contribute, at least partly, to the melanoma-associated angiogenesis. Furthermore, tumour-derived FGF-2 may have pleiotropic influences, first on tumour invasion, by elevating proteolytic enzymes , second on angiogenesis, by paracrine stimulation of endothelial cell growth, and third on recruitment and activation of mast cells, which express the FGF-2 receptor. Mast cells, in their turn, secrete FGF-2 stored in their secretory granules, which further stimulates endothelial cell growth and amplifies the FGF-2 paracrine stimulatory loop on angiogenesis.

4.1 Integrin signalling and extracellular matrix enzymes

Parallel with the angiogenic switch, an increasing number of tumour cells express the laminin receptor, which enables their adhesion to the vascular wall, favouring tumour cell extravasation and metastases. Our data indicate that melanoma cells express the 67-kDa laminin receptor in step with the progression from the nevocellular to the dysplastic nevi, and from the primary to the metastatic tumour. This expression enables melanoma cell adhesion to the vascular wall and together with the increased vascular network favours tumour cell extravasation and metastasis.

Overexpression of $\alpha v\beta 3$, $\alpha v\beta 5$, $\alpha 2\beta 1$, and $\alpha 5\beta 1$ integrins has been correlated with the transition from primary to metastatic melanoma (Bosserhoff, 2006). In turn, integrins overexpression stimulates matrix metalloproteinases -2 and -7 in melanoma cells, increasing their invasive potential (Kuphal et al., 2005).

Melanoma and tumour stromal cells express several matrix metalloproteinases, including matrix metalloproteinases -1, -2, -3, -7, -9, -14, -15, -16, as well as *Tissue Inhibitors of Matrix Metalloproteinases* such as TIMP-1, -2, and -3 (Hofmann et al., 2000a). Matrix metalloproteinases overexpression has been correlated with increased microvascular density, Bcl-2 overexpression, and low survival rate. The most extensively studied matrix metalloproteinases in melanomas are the isoforms -2 and -9.

The expression and activation of both enzymes have been correlated to the invasive and metastatic phenotypes of the tumours (Hofmann et al., 2000b; Kerkela & Saarialho-Kere, 2003; Nikkola et al., 2005; Cotignola et al., 2007; Schnaeker et al., 2004) in which they are constitutively expressed and highly associated with atypia and dedifferentiation into melanocytic lesions. Matrix metalloproteinase -2 expression was highly correlated with the metastatic spread and low survival rates (Hofmann et al., 2000a). Moreover, functional activity of matrix metalloproteinases is required for tumour progression. Overexpression of Membrane-Type- Matrix Metalloproteinase in melanoma cells induced activation of matrix metalloproteinase -2 which is crucial for extracellular matrix degradation. Matrix metalloproteinase -2 and Membrane-Type- Matrix Metalloproteinase + tumour cells were often restricted to the interface between the tumour invasive part and stroma (Durko et al., 1997; Hofmann et al., 2000b).

Expression of matrix metalloproteinases is not restricted to tumour cells but is also found abundantly in stromal cells indicating a major contribution of host-derived proteases to tumour progression (Wojtowicz-Praga et al., 1998). Also matrix metalloproteinase -1 expression is highly associated with melanoma progression (Nikkola et al., 2005). Matrix metalloproteinase -9 expression in melanoma cells was found exclusively during the horizontal growth phase but not during the vertical phase. This clearly suggests that expression of matrix metalloproteinase -9 is an early event in melanoma progression (Kerkela & Saarialho-Kere, 2003).

Several studies using either cell lines or animal models have demonstrated that the balance between matrix metalloproteinases and their inhibitors finally determines melanoma progression (Hofmann et al., 2000b; Wojtowicz-Praga et al., 1998; Rudek et al., 2001; Jin et al., 2006; Wojtowicz-Praga et al., 1996; Bodey et al., 2001; Airola et al., 1999). Overexpression of TIMP-1, -2, and -3 significantly reduces melanoma tumour cell invasion, migration, growth and metastasis, and significantly reduces tumour neovascularization in several tumour models (Anand-Apte et al., 1996). *Urokinase Plasminogen Activator and Its Receptor* (uPA/uPAR) have been demonstrated to play a crucial role in several stages of melanoma progression including tumour cell migration, invasion, and metastasis. uPA secreted from melanoma cells is able to regulate endothelial cell functions including migration and the organization of endothelial cells into tube-like structures (Mueller, 1996; Delbaldo et al., 1994; Hearing et al., 1988).

The extracellular matrix enzymes and their inhibitors play also an important role in cancer dysregulated angiogenesis (Roy et al., 2009; Huang et al., 2009). These enzymes are the major degrading enzymes produced by angiogenic endothelial cells for migration through extracellular matrix during neovessel formation. Moreover, matrix metalloproteinases and TIMPs may act as regulators of signalling pathways through the cleavage of nonmatrix substrates, including cytokines, chemokines, and growth factors. In the last fifteen years, different extracellular matrix proteins and cleavage products have been identified. These molecules possess the ability to regulate vascular development, repair and function. Therefore, possible regulatory mechanisms in vascular biology controlled by different cleavage products of basement membrane proteins (e.g., endostatin and tumstatin, endorepellin), their activation by proteases and inhibitors, such as matrix metalloproteases, cathepsins, tissue inhibitors of matrix metalloproteinases and cystatin, have been reviewed in Suhr et al. (2009).

Integrin-Linked Kinase (ILK) is a highly conserved serine-threonine protein kinase involved in cell-extracellular matrix interactions, cytoskeletal organization and cell signalling. Overexpression of ILK in epithelial cells leads to anchorage-independent growth with increased cell cycle progression. ILK upregulation strongly correlates with melanoma progression, invasion and inversely correlates with 5-year survival of melanoma patients (Wani et al., 2011). However, the molecular mechanism by which ILK enhances melanoma progression is currently unknown. The proangiogenic molecule IL-6 is the downstream target of ILK in melanoma cells. Wani et al. (2011) have demonstrated that ILK overexpression increases IL-6, whereas silencing of ILK suppressed IL-6 expression at both messenger RNA and protein levels. ILK also alteres the activity and subcellular localization of Nuclear Factor-KappaB (NF-κB) subunit p65. ILK enhances the IL-6 gene transcription by promoting the binding of NF-κB p65 to IL-6 promoter. Moreover, ILK overexpression in melanoma cells enhances the tube-forming ability of endothelial cells in vitro and microvessel formation in vivo (Wani et al., 2011).

5. Hypoxia in melanoma progression

Solid tumours, including melanomas, are characterized by areas of hypoxia/anoxia that result from an imbalance between oxygen supply and consumption in proliferating tumour cells. This imbalance is further exacerbated by a compromised tumour vasculature (Vaupel & Mayer, 2007).

The presence of hypoxia within a tumour is an independent marker of a poor prognosis for patients with various cancer types including cutaneous melanomas. Because stringent hypoxia/anoxia (<0.5% O_2) is toxic for normal and tumour cells, it can promote tumour progression by selecting cells with mutations that allow them to survive in these extreme conditions. Furthermore, hypoxia activates signalling pathways that trigger neovascularization and that facilitate tumour cell invasion, migration, adhesion, and metastasis (Bedogni & Broome Powell, 2009).

Metastasis is a complex multi-step process in which tumour cells have to acquire an invasive/migratory phenotype, enter the blood and lymphatic flow, survive anoikis and the immune response, and once localized to a distant site, survive in a likely hostile environment and proliferate. This process is relatively inefficient and only few cells within a tumour mass will have all the requirements that will allow them to successfully metastasize. Tumour hypoxia can influence most of the stages of metastasis (Bedogni & Broome Powell, 2009).

Hypoxia has been involved in a Epithelial-Mesenchymal Transition-like process where tumour cells change from an epithelial non-motile phenotype to a mesenchymal migratory phenotype and gain the ability to invade other tissues. Epithelial-Mesenchymal Transition is accompanied by specific changes in gene expression, such as down-regulation of E-cadherin. Tumour hypoxia or loss of *von Hippel-Lindau* (VHL) which leads to *Hypoxia-Inducible Factor* (HIF) stabilization, down-regulates E-cadherin (Yang & Wu, 2008). Furthermore, hypoxia through HIF-1, increases invasion by regulating genes, such as matrix metalloproteinase-2, that are involved in the degradation and remodelling of the extracellular matrix (Krishnamachary et al., 2003).

Via induction of pro-angiogenic factors such as VEGF, IL-8 and angiopoietin- 2, tumour hypoxia contributes to tumour angiogenesis providing cancer cells with access to blood vessels which is made easier by the leakiness of the tumour vasculature. HIF-1 can also increase resistance to anoikis by down-regulating the expression of $\alpha5$ integrin which mediates survival signals in the presence of extracellular matrix and apoptotic signals when cells lack adhesion to a substrate. Finally, by increasing the expression of lysyl oxidase, hypoxia/HIF-1 contributes to cancer metastasis in part by facilitating the recruitment of bone marrow derived cells to the metastatic niche, which prepares a receptive environment for cancer cells (Erler et al., 2009, 2006).

A direct role of hypoxia in advanced melanoma is slowly starting to emerge. HIF-1 has been shown to play a critical role in uveal melanoma progression by increasing the expression of a number of target genes involved in invasion. HIF-1 is regarded as one of the critical biomarkers that most accurately can predict uveal melanoma metastasis. Furthermore, a recent study by Qi et al. (2008), supports a role in melanomagenesis and metastasis of Siah2. Siah2, recently found to be regulated by the Serine/Threonine Protein Kinase Akt, is an inhibitor of Prolyl Hydroxylase Domain Protein function and therefore enhances hypoxia dependent HIF-1α stabilization by further inhibiting Prolyl Hydroxylase Domain Protein -1 and -3 in hypoxia. The authors found that blocking the axis Siah2-Spry2 leads to decreased

HIF-1*α* stabilization, and results in a significant reduction of metastasis in a metastatic melanoma mouse model. This observation correlated with findings in human samples where reduced expression of the Siah2 substrates Prolyl Hydroxylase Domain Protein-3 and Spry2 and increased HIF-1*α* are characteristic of more advanced melanoma (Bedogni & Broome Powell, 2009).
A role of HIF signalling in melanomagenesis is further supported by the work of Giatromanolaki et al. (2003). In this study, HIF-1*α* and HIF-2*α* were found to be expressed in 28 and 65% of melanoma samples respectively, and HIF-2*α*, together with VEGF and vascular density, was associated with poor overall disease survival.
In summary, these observations strongly support a role of hypoxia and HIF signalling in melanomagenesis and melanoma metastasis (Bedogni & Broome Powell, 2009).

6. Antiangiogenic therapies

Different molecular targets of antiangiogenic molecules can be recognized, so various antiangiogenic agents are currently in clinical trials for melanoma.
Thalidomide was withdrawn from the market due to its teratogenecity, but in recent years its use has been focused on its anti-angiogenic properties (Frankset al., 2004; Kirchmair et al., 2007; Son et al., 2006). In fact, Thalidomide has been found to have antiangiogenic and anti-inflammatory properties, and accordingly it has been used as a therapeutic agent in some malignant tumours including liver, renal cell, and breast carcinomas (Singhal & Mehta, 2002).
We ourselves demonstrated that Thalidomide inhibits many genes which codify for angiogenic cytokines and their relative receptors in endothelial cells. Moreover, we have demonstrated that Thalidomide reduce the fundamental activity of activated endothelial cells (i.e. proliferation, migration, chemotaxis) as well as vessel formation in the Matrigel assay. It has been also proposed that the teratogenic property of Thalidomide involves in production of *Reactive Oxygen Species* (ROS), leading to subsequent DNA damage (Maniotis et al., 1999). When Thalidomide-induced ROS formation is inhibited, the anti-angiogenesis properties of Thalidomide will be reduced.
Thalidomide inhibits vasculogenic mimicry channel and mosaic vessels formation in melanoma through the regulation of vasculogenic factors, and it can induce necrosis of tumour cells, which may be related with the NF-kB signalling pathway (Zhang et al., 2008).
In advanced melanoma Thalidomide has obtained some promising results when used as single agent. Pawlak and Legha (Pawlak & Legha, 2004), published a study evaluating single-agent Thalidomide in metastatic malignant melanoma, showing no objective responses, but seven cases of stable disease.
Other single agent phase II studies (Reiriz et al., 2004; Eisen et al., 2000) demonstrated stable disease in a few patients, with 30% of the patients included in these trials having ocular melanoma. In another phase II study Thalidomide has shown limited activity in patients with metastatic melanoma against melanoma metastases in the *Central Nervous System* (CNS) (Lene et al., 2008). However, the minor effects founded on peripheral tumour manifestations, has led to the conclusion that Thalidomide might be part of the treatment strategy for these patients.
On the basis of these promising but non optimal results and since Thalidomide exhibits low oral bioavailability due to limitations in solubility, some experimental modification of oral preparation have been tested to improve the delivery of Thalidomide and its therapeutical

activity (Kale et al., 2008). Its complexation with sulfobutyl ether-7 beta-cyclodextrin has demonstrated to increase stability, oral bioavailability, drug absorption, and distribution through solubilization of Thalidomide in experimental animals.

The safety and tolerability of adjuvant treatment with subcutaneous *Granulocyte Macrophage Colony-Stimulating Factor* (GM-CSF) administered in combination with escalating doses of Thalidomide in patients with surgically resected stage II (T4), III, or IV melanoma at high risk for recurrence has been also evaluated (Lutzky et al., 2009). This therapy has obtained promising results with a 42% overall survival at 2.6 years. However, the high incidence of life-threatening events, particularly thrombosis, that are unacceptable in the adjuvant setting, render the up-front antithrombotic prophylaxis necessary for further evaluation of this combination.

Many studies are also focused on the effects of Thalidomide on advanced melanoma in combination with Interferon alpha 2 b (Hutchins et al., 2007; Vaishampayan et al., 2007), Temozolomide (Quirt et al., 2007; Atkins et al., 2008), and Dacarbazine (Ott et al., 2009) with encouraging results. The combination of Pegylated Interferon and Thalidomide was evaluated in a phase II trial (Vaishampayan et al., 2007). Pegylated Interferon was administered at a dose of 0.5 microg/kg subcutaneously weekly and Thalidomide 200 mg orally daily. Dose escalation of Thalidomide to 300 mg daily was feasible in some patients. This combination was well tolerated but failed to demonstrate clinical efficacy in pretreated metastatic melanoma. In fact, no objective responses were obtained, and only three patients achieved disease stabilization.

The addition of Thalidomide to Temozolomide with or without whole brain irradiation does not appear to provide a substantial advantage in the treatment of patients with CNS metastasis from melanoma but seems to add only toxicity. An initial study (Hwu et al., 2003) reported considerable activity (32%response rate) for the Temozolomide and Thalidomide combination in the treatment of patients with systemic metastases from melanoma. This study combining Temozolomide in the prolonged administration schedule and Thalidomide at 200 mg/day with dose escalation to 400 mg/day produced 1 complete response and 11 partial responses in 38 patients with advanced melanoma and a median survival of 9.5 months. Evidence of response in CNS metastases was also reported in this setting. Subsequent results in a combined 53 evaluable patients in the *Cytokine Working Group* (CWG) and *Cancer and Leukemia Group B* (CALGB) studies are clearly disappointing (Quirt et al., 2007). Fatigue and an increased risk of thromboembolic events, without meaningfully increasing the modest CNS antitumour activity previously noted with the Temozolomide and whole brain irradiation combination (Margolin et al., 2002) or either Temozolomide (Agarwala et al., 2004) or whole brain irradiation alone (Fife et al., 2004). The conclusions of this study are consistent with the results of a CALGB trial using a similar regimen (Krown et al., 2006). This trial was stopped after 16 patients were enrolled because of excessive toxicity that included severe fatigue and sudden death in 1 patient and thromboembolic events (pulmonary embolism and deep vein thrombosis) in 4 patients. No tumour responses were observed in 14 evaluable patients.

Given the virtual lack of efficacy observed for the Temozolomide and Thalidomide combination against systemic disease in these 2 studies, the lack of significant CNS tumour response or major impact on overall survival is not surprising.

Similar results have been obtained when Thalidomide has been combined with Temozolomide alone in patients with stage IV malignant melanoma without active brain metastases (Joseph et al., 2010). In this phase II study patients received Thalidomide (200mg/d escalated to 400mg/d for patients <70, or 100mg/d escalated to 250mg/d for patients ≥70) plus Temozolomide (75mg/m2/d × 6 weeks then 2 weeks rest). The progression free survival was 15% at 6 month and the overall survival was 35% at 1 year. Enrolled patients obtained only partial response with a response rate of 13%. Authors conclude that this combination of Thalidomide and Temozolomide does not appear to have a clinical benefit that exceeds Dacarbazine alone and they not recommend it further for phase III trials or for standard community use.

Similar results have been obtained when Thalidomide has been associated to Dacarbazine in the treatment of patients with advanced melanoma (Ott et al., 2009). Of the 13 patients evaluable for response of that enrolled in this phase II trial, 1 patient had a partial response, 3 patients had stable disease and 9 patients had progressive disease. No complete responses were achieved. 1 patient withdrew due to toxicity. Grade III/IV constipation, peripheral neuropathy, fatigue, edema and rash were attributed to Thalidomide addition. The authors conclude that Thalidomide dose escalation beyond 200 mg/day was limited by unacceptable toxicity and this combination yielded activity insufficient to proceed with additional trials.

In the last years Lenalidomide, a less toxic analogue of Thalidomide, has been tested in vitro and in vivo. Lenalidomide has been showed good efficacy in hematologic and non hematologic cancer with a good toxicity profile (Zeldis et al., 2011). Promising preliminary results have been obtained in a study recruit 13 patients with stage IV malignant melanoma (Bartlett et al., 2004). Despite the fact that clinical response was not the primary end-point of the study and that the patients had not responded to prior therapy, clear evidence of drug activity in rapidly progressing malignant melanoma with one partial response and two minor responses of visceral disease have been obtained.

Subsequent studies (Glaspy et al., 2009; Eisen et al., 2010) have demonstrated that treatment with Lenalidomide (25 mg/d) has a manageable safety profile in patients with previously treated metastatic malignant melanoma. Although no benefit in tumour response, time to progression, or overall survival has been achieved in these patients, future trials for treatment of metastatic malignant melanoma with Lenalidomide should be conduct which focus its use in combination therapies (Lu et al., 2009).

On the basis of preclinical findings indicating that continuous low dose (metronomic) chemotherapy is thought to inhibit tumour angiogenesis, the evaluation of antiangiogenic potency of various chemotherapeutic drugs for metronomic chemotherapy, particularly Taxol, is ongoing for its efficacy (Drevs et al., 2004). In a pivotal study, 20 patients received paclitaxel 10 mg/m^2 for 96 hours weekly as a continuous intravenous infusion and oral celecoxib 400 mg twice daily. One patient achieved a partial response, and 3 of 20 patients (15%) had stable disease for >6 months. The median time to progression was 57 days, and the median overall survival was 212 days. These findings support a role for metronomic therapy in patients with advanced melanoma. (Bhatt et al., 2010).

A newest approach to cancer therapy is to target the multicellular biological entity of the tumour microenvironment. This type of combination causes an inhospitable microenvironment for tumour cells and represent a great promise for clinical use. (Blansfield et al., 2008).

Semaxanib, a small molecule inhibitor of the VEGFR-2 tyrosine kinase, has shown encouraging results in patients with metastatic melanoma (Kuenen et al., 2003; Peterson, et al., 2004) in whom it has also been evaluated in combination with Thalidomide to assess the efficacy, tolerability, pharmacokinetic, and pharmacodynamic characteristics (Mita et al.,

2007). This last study has demonstrated that the combination Semaxanib-Thalidomide is feasible and has also demonstrated antitumour activity in patients with metastatic melanoma who had failed prior therapy. Twelve patients were enrolled in this study and received 44 courses of Semaxanib at the fixed dose of 145 mg/m2 intravenously twice-weekly in combination with Thalidomide, commencing at 200 mg daily with intrapatient dose escalation as tolerated. The principal toxicities included deep venous thrombosis, headache, and lower extremity edema. Out of ten patients evaluable for response, one complete response lasting 20 months and one partial response lasting 12 months were observed. Additionally, four patients had stable disease lasting from 2 to 10 months. These results indicate that the combination of Semaxanib and Thalidomide is feasible and demonstrated anti-tumour activity in patients with metastatic melanoma who had failed prior therapy.

Another way to inhibit angiogenesis is the inhibition of matrix metalloproteinase activity. In the early 1990, matrix metalloproteinase inhibitors generated great enthusiasm among several research groups wishing to take them to clinical trials. Preclinical trials of matrix metalloproteinase inhibitors were very promising, showing minimum side effects compared to other drugs available at the time. Several current inhibitors, which have been tested in preclinical and clinical trials, are broad category matrix metalloproteinase inhibitors. Pharmacological inhibitors such as Prinomastat, Batimastat, and its analog Marimastat, which interfere with the catalytic site of the matrix metalloproteinases, were the first inhibitors studied in detail. Most of the inhibitors tested in clinical trials were not very promising due to the lack of positive outcomes and the appearance of substantial drug side effects, which were not observed in preclinical studies. Therefore, most of the inhibitor clinical trials were terminated following phase 3 clinical trials (Quirt et al., 2002; Pavlaki & Zucker, 2003; Coussens et al., 2002).

Good therapeutic effects have been obtained in little studies with the combination of Bevacizumab (the anti-VEGF monoclonal antibody) and chemotherapy in advanced melanoma. Moreover, preclinical data strongly support the use of a combination of Bevacizumab and Erlotinib, a tyrosine kinase receptors inhibitor (Varker et al., 2007; Perez et al., 2009; Vásquez et al., 2009; Schicher et al., 2009).

PI-88, a potent inhibitor of heparanase, demonstrates an overall survival and time to progression similar to standard chemotherapy (Basche et al., 2006). In a phase II trial (Lewis et al., 2008) a total of 44 patients were enrolled with about 60% of them previously treated. The median time to progression and overall survival was 1.7 months and 9 months, respectively. One (2.4%) patient achieved a partial response and six (14.6%) had stable disease as best response. At the end of six cycles of treatment, three of the 41 evaluable patients had non-progressive disease. Treatment was generally well tolerated with serious bleeding occured in two patients and positive anti-platelet antibody test in three patients. One of these four patients experienced an associated thrombosis. These results indicate that in patients with advanced melanoma, PI-88 demonstrates an overall survival and time to progression similar to standard chemotherapy with evidence of activity that warrantee further investigation.

Preclinical data suggest that the ectopic expression of alphaIIb beta3 in melanoma cells can be exploited as a novel target of antibody therapy (Mitjans et al., 2000).

Although most of these study have obtained encouraging results, further evaluations of therapeutic strategies that target multiple angiogenesis pathways may be warranted in patients with advanced melanoma and other malignancies.

Finally, antiangiogenic therapy might have the unintended effect of promoting tumour metastasis by increasing vasculogenic mimicry as an alternative circulatory system (Qu et al., 2010). When the endothelium-dependent vessels are inhibited by the effective angiogenesis inhibitors, the hypoxia of tumour cells caused by antiangiogenesis may increase vasculogenic mimicry compensatively which can replace the job of endothelium-dependent vessels to maintain the tumour blood supply and provide a convenient route of tumour metastasis.

7. Conclusion

Tumour microenvironment plays a crucial role in the pathophysiology of human melanoma. It is involved in the crosstalk between melanoma cells and the microenvironment cells, which increases the survival, proliferation and migration of tumour cells themselves, and represents the substrate for angiogenesis which favours disease progression. Due to interaction with active microenvironment, neoplastic cells also acquire drug resistance giving less opportunity to therapy response.

Many research studies have tried to better understand the biological mechanisms and the genetic basis of all the interactions between tumour cells and the microenvironment cells. VEGF, FGF-2, IL-6, IL-8, macrophages, mast cells, and many others cells and molecules, play important roles in this process.

State the important role of angiogenesis in melanoma progression and diffusion, it represents a good target for biological therapies. Several molecules targeting the tumour microenvironment are actually evaluated in clinical trials and other compounds are in preclinical developing. However the initial results obtained with these compounds are promising, these approaches should be further developed.

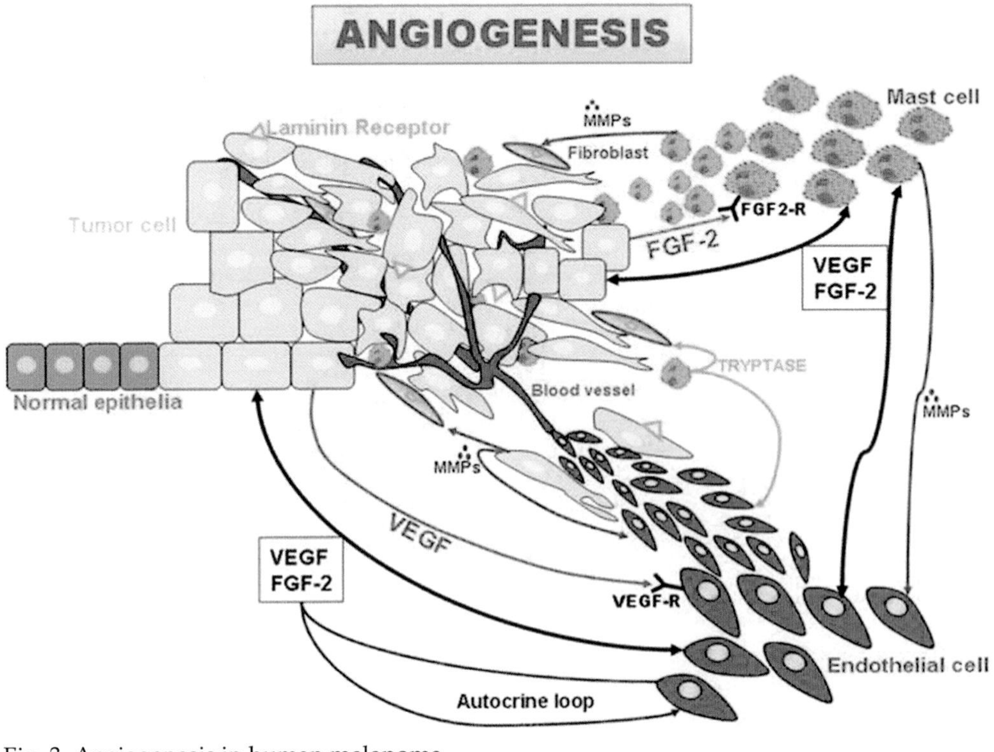

Fig. 3. Angiogenesis in human melanoma

8. Acknowledgments

The Authors would like to thank Prof. Franco Dammacco, Prof. Domenico Ribatti, and Prof. Beatrice Nico for their technical support.

We would also like to thank to Prof. Cecilia Perillo for the English revision of the manuscript.

This work was supported by Associazione Italiana per la Ricerca sul Cancro (AIRC), Investigator Grant and Special Program Molecular Clinical Oncology 5 per mille n. 9965, Milan, Italy.

9. References

Agarwala, S.S., Kirkwood, J.M., Gore, M., Dreno, B., Thatcher, N., Czarnetski, B., Atkins, M., Buzaid, A., Skarlos, D., & Rankin, E.M. (2004). Temozolomide for the treatment of brain metastases associated with metastatic melanoma: a phase II study. *J ClinOncol.*, Vol. 22, No., pp. 2101-2107

Airola, K., Karonen, T., Vaalamo, M., Lehti, K., Lohi, J., Kariniemi, A.L., Keski-Oja, J., & Saarialho-Kere, U.K. (1999). Expression of collagenases-1 and -3 and their inhibitors TIMP-1 and -3 correlates with the level of invasion in malignant melanomas. *British Journal of Cancer,* Vol.80, No.5-6, pp. 733–743

Anand-Apte, B., Bao, L., Smith, R., Iwata, K., Olsen, B.R., Zetter, B., & Apte, S.S. (1996). A review of tissue inhibitor of metalloproteinases-3 (TIMP-3) and experimental analysis of its effect on primary tumour growth. *Biochemistry and Cell Biology*, Vol. 74, No.6, pp. 853–862

Atkins, M.B., Sosman, J.A., Agarwala, S., Logan, T., Clark, J.I., Ernstoff, M.S., Lawson, D., Dutcher, J.P., Weiss, G., Curti, B., & Margolin, K.A. (2008). Temozolomide, Thalidomide, and whole brain radiation therapy for patients with brain metastasis from metastatic melanoma: a phase II cytokine working group study. *Cancer*, Vol. 113, No. 8, pp. 2139–2145

Balch, C.M., Soong, S.J., Gershenwald, J.E., Thompson, J.F., Reintgen, D.S., Cascinelli, N., Urist, M., McMasters, K.M., Ross, M.I., Kirkwood, J.M., Atkins, M.B., Thompson, J.A., Coit, D.G., Byrd, D., Desmond, R., Zhang, Y., Liu, P.Y., Lyman, G.H., & Morabito, A. (2001). Prognostic factors analysis of 17,600 melanoma patients: validation of the American Joint Committee on Cancer melanoma staging system. *J Clin Oncol.*, (Aug 15 2001), Vol.19, No.16, pp. 3622-34

Balch, C.M., Gershenwald, J.E., Soong, S.J., Thompson, J.F., Atkins, M.B., Byrd, D.R., Buzaid, A.C., Cochran, A.J., Coit, D.G., Ding, S., Eggermont, A.M., Flaherty, K.T., Gimotty, P.A., Kirkwood, J.M., McMasters, K.M., Mihm, M.C. Jr, Morton, D.L., Ross, M.I., Sober, A.J., & Sondak, V.K. (2009). Final version of 2009 AJCC melanoma staging and classification. *J Clin Oncol.*, (Dec 20 2009), Vol.27, No.36, pp. 6199-206

Bar-Eli, M. (1999). Role of interleukin-8 in tumour growth and metastasis of human melanoma. *Pathobiology*, Vol. 67, No. 1, pp. 12–18

Bartlett, J.B., Michael, A., Clarke, I.A., Dredge, K., Nicholson, S., Kristeleit, H., Polychronis, A., Pandha, H., Muller, G.W., Stirling, D.I., Zeldis, J., & Dalgleish, A.G. (2004). Phase I study to determine the safety, tolerability and immunostimulatory activity of Thalidomide analogue CC-5013 in patients with metastatic malignant melanoma and other advanced cancers. *British Journal of Cancer*, No. 90, pp. 955–961

Basche, M., Gustafson, D.L., Holden, S.N., O'Bryant, C.L., Gore, L., Witta, S., Schultz, M.K., Morrow, M., Levin, A., Creese, B.R., Kangas, M., Roberts, K., Nguyen, T., Davis, K., Addison, R.S., Moore, J.C., & Eckhardt, S.G. (2006). A phase I biological and pharmacologic study of the heparanase inhibitor PI-88 in patients with advanced solid tumours, *Clinical Cancer Research*, Vol. 12, No. 18, pp. 5471–5480

Bedogni, B., & Broome Powell M. (2009). Hypoxia, melanocytes and melanoma - survival and tumour development in the permissive microenvironment of the skin. *Pigment Cell Melanoma Res*, 22(2):166-74

Beil, W.J., Fureder, W., Wiener, H., Grosschmidt, K., Maier, U., Schedle, A., Bankl, H.C., Lechner, K., & Valent, P. (1998). Phenotypic and functional characterization of mast cells derived from renal tumour tissues. *Exp. Hematol.*, No. 26, pp. 158–169

Bernardini, G., Ribatti, D., Spinetti, G., Morbidelli, L., Ziche, M., Santoni, A., Capogrossi, M.C., & Napolitano, M. (2003). Analysis of the role chemokines in angiogenesis. *J Immunol Methods*, No. 273, pp. 83–101

Bhatt, R.S., Merchan, J., Parker, R., HK, Wu., Zhang, L., Seery, V., Heymach, J.V., Atkins, M.B., McDermott, D., & Sukhatme, V.P. (2010). A phase 2 pilot trial of low-dose, continuous infusion, or "metronomic" paclitaxel and oral celecoxib in patients with metastatic melanoma. *Cancer*, Vol. 116, No. 7, pp. 1751-6

Bingle, L., Brown, N.J., & Lewis, C.E. The role of tumour associated macrophages in tumour progression: implications for new anticancer therapies. (2002). *J Pathol.*, No. 196, pp. 254–65

Blair, R.J., Meng, H., Marchese, M.J., Ren, S., Schwartz, L.B., Tonnesen, M.G., & Gruber, B.L. (1997). Human mast cells stimulate vascular tube formation. Tryptase is a novel, potent angiogenic factor. *J. Clin. Invest.*, No. 99, pp. 2691–2700

Blansfield, J.A., Caragacianu, D., Alexander, H.R. 3rd, Tangrea, M.A., Morita, S.Y., Lorang, D., Schafer, P., Muller, G., Stirling, D., Royal, R.E., & Libutti, S.K. (2008). Combining agents that target the tumour microenvironment improves the efficacy of anticancer therapy. *Clin Cancer Res*, Vol. 14, No. 1, pp. 270-80

Bodey, B., Gr¨oger, A.M., Siegel, S.E., & Kaiser, H.E. (2001). Invasion and metastasis: the expression and significance of matrix metalloproteinases in carcinomas of the lung. *In Vivo*, Vol. 15, No. 2, pp. 175–180

Bosserhoff, A. K. (2006). Novel biomarkers inmalignant melanoma. *Clinica Chimica Acta*, Vol. 367, No. 1-2, pp. 28–35

Breslow, A. (1970) Thickness, cross-sectional areas and depth of invasion in the prognosis of cutaneous melanoma. *Annals of Surgery*, Vol. 172, No. 5, pp. 902–908

Brown, J.K., Jones, C.A., Tyler, C.L., Ruoss, S.J., Hartmann, T., & Caughey, G.H. (1995). Tryptase-induced mitogenesis in airway smooth muscle cells. *Chest*, No. 107, pp. 95S–96S

Cairns, J.A. & Walls, A.F. (1996). Mast cell tryptase is a mitogen for epithelial cells: stimulation of IL-8 production and intercellular adhesion molecule-1 expression. *J. Immunol.*, No. 157, pp. 275–283

Clark, J.C., Moon, J., Hutchins, L.F., Sosman, J.A., Kast, W.M., Da Silva, D.M., Liu, P.Y., Thompson, J.A., Flaherty, L.E., & Sondak, V.K. (2010). Phase II Trial of Combination Thalidomide plus Temozolomide in Patients with Metastatic Malignant Melanoma: Southwest Oncology Group S0508. *Cancer*, Vol. 116, No. 2, pp. 424–431

Cotignola, J., Reva, B., Mitra, N., Ishill, N., Chuai, S., Patel, A., Shah, S., Vanderbeek, G., Coit, D., Busam, K., Halpern, A., Houghton, A., Sander, C., Berwick, M., & Orlow, I. (2007). Matrix metalloproteinase-9 (MMP-9) polymorphisms in patients with cutaneous malignant melanoma. *BMC Medical Genetics*, Vol. 8, Article 10

Coussens, L.M., Fingleton, B., & Matrisian, L. M. (2002). Matrix metalloproteinase inhibitors and cancer: trials and tribulations. *Science*, Vol. 295, No. 5564, pp. 2387–2392

Delbaldo, C., Masouye, I., Saurat, J.-H., Vassalli, J.-D., & Sappino, A.-P. (1994). Plasminogen activation in melanocytic neoplasia. *Cancer Research*, Vol. 54, No. 16, pp. 4547–4552

Dome, B., Hendrix, M.J., Paku, S., Tóvári, J., & Tímár, J. (2007). Alternative vascularisation mechanisms in cancer: pathology and therapeutic implications. *Am J Pathol.*, No. 170, pp. 1-15

Donnini, S., Machein, M. R., Plate, K. H., & Weich, H. A. (1999). Expression and localization of placenta growth factor and P1GF receptors in human meningiomas. *Journal of Pathology*, Vol. 189, No. 1, pp. 66–71

Drevs, J., Fakler, J., Eisele, S., Medinger, M., Bing, G., Esser, N., Marmé, D., & Unger, C. (2004). Antiangiogenic potency of various chemotherapeutic drugs for metronomic chemotherapy. *Anticancer Research*, Vol. 24, No. 3A, pp. 1759–1763

Durko, M., Navab, R., Shibata, H. R., & Brodt, P. (1997). Suppression of basement membrane type IV collagen degradation and cell invasion in human melanoma cells expressing an antisense RNA for MMP-1. *Biochimica et Biophysica Acta*, Vol. 1356, No. 3, pp. 271–280

Eisen, T., Boshoff, C., Mak, I., Sapunar, F., Vaughan, M.M., Pyle, L., Johnston, S.R., Ahern, R., Smith, I.E., & Gore, M.E. (2000). Continuous low dose Thalidomide: A phase II study in advanced melanoma, renal cell, ovarian and breast cancer. *Br J Cancer.*, Vol. 82, pp. 812-7

Eisen, T., Trefzer, U., Hamilton, A., Hersey, P., Millward, M., Knight, R.D., Jungnelius, J.U., & Glaspy. (2010). J. Results of a Multicenter, Randomized, Double-Blind Phase 2/3 Study of Lenalidomide in the Treatment of Pretreated Relapsed or Refractory Metastatic Malignant Melanoma. *Cancer*, No. 116, pp. 146–54

Erhard, H., Rietveld, F. J. R., van Altena, M. C., Bröcker, E.B., Ruiter, D.J., & de Waal , R.M. (1997). Transition of horizontal to vertical growth phase melanoma is accompanied by induction of vascular endothelial growth factor expression and angiogenesis, *Melanoma Research*, Vol. 7, No. 2, pp. S19–S26

Erler, J.T., Bennewith, K.L., Nicolau, M., Dornhofer, N., Kong, C., Le, Q.T., Chi, J.T., Jeffrey, S.S., & Giaccia, A.J. (2006). Lysyl oxidase is essential for hypoxia-induced metastasis. *Nature*, No. 440, pp. 1222–1226

Erler, J.T., Bennewith, K.L., Cox, T.R., Lang, G., Bird, D., Koong, A., Le, Q.T., & Giaccia AJ. (2009). Hypoxia induced lysyl oxidase is a critical mediator of bone marrow cell recruitment to form the premetastatic niche. *Cancer Cell.*, No. 15, pp. 35–44

Fife, K.M., Colman, M.H., Stevens, G.N., Firth, I.C., Moon, D., Shannon, K.F., Harman, R., Petersen-Schaefer, K., Zacest, A.C., Besser, M., Milton, G.W., McCarthy, W.H., & Thompson, J.F. (2004). Determinants of outcome in melanoma patients with cerebral metastases. *J Clin Oncol.*, Vol. 22, pp. 1293-1300

Folkman, J., Browder, T., & Palmblad, J. (2001). Angiogenesis research: guidelines for translation to clinical application. *Thromb Haemost.*, No. 86, pp. 23-33

Franks, M.E., Macpherson, G.R., & Figg, W.D. (2004). Thalidomide. *Lancet*, No. 363, pp. 1802-1811;

Garbe, C., Terheyden, P., Keilholz, U., Kölbl, O., & Hauschild, A. (2008). Treatment of Melanoma. *Dtsch Arztebl Int.*, Vol. 105, No. 49, pp. 845-51

Giatromanolaki, A., Sivridis, E., Kouskoukis, C., Gatter, K.C., Harris, A.L., & Koukourakis, M.I. (2003). Hypoxia-inducible factors 1alpha and 2alpha are related to vascular endothelial growth factor expression and a poorer prognosis in nodular malignant melanomas of the skin. *Melanoma Res.*, No. 13, pp. 493–501

Glaspy, J., Atkins, M.B., Richards, J.M., Agarwala, S.S., O'Day, S., Knight, R.D., Jungnelius, J.U., & Bedikian, A.Y. (2009). Results of a Multicenter, Randomized, Double-Blind, Dose-Evaluating Phase 2/3 Study of Lenalidomide in the Treatment of Metastatic Malignant Melanoma. *Cancer*, No. 115, pp. 5228–36

Gruber, B.L., Marchase, M.J., & Kaw, R. (1995). Angiogenic factors stimulate mast cell migration. *Blood*, No. 86, pp. 2488–93

Hearing, V. J., Law, L. W., Corti, A., Appella, E., & Blasi, F. (1988). Modulation of metastatic potential by cell surface urokinase of murine melanoma cells. *Cancer Research*, Vol. 48, No. 5, pp.1270–1278

Heasley, D.D., Toda, S., & Mihm Jr., M.C. (1996). Pathology of malignant melanoma. *Surgical Clinics of North America*, Vol. 76, No. 6, pp. 1223–1255

Hofmann, U.B., Westphal, J.R., Van Muijen, G.N.P., & Ruiter, D.J. (2000a). Matrix metalloproteinases in human melanoma. *Journal of Investigative Dermatology*, Vol. 115, No. 3, pp. 337–344

Hofmann, U.B., Westphal, J.R., Zendman, A.J.W., Becker, J.C., Ruiter, D.J., & Van Muijen, G.N.P. (2000b). Expression and activation of matrix metalloproteinase-2 (MMP-2) and its colocalization with membrane-type I matrix metalloproteinase (MTI-MMP) correlate with melanoma progression. *Journal of Pathology*, Vol. 191, No. 3, pp. 245–256

Huang, S.C., Sheu, B.C., Chang, W.C., Cheng, C.Y., Wang, P.H., & Lin, S. (2009). Extracellular matrix proteases—cytokine regulation role in cancer and pregnancy. *Frontiers in Bioscience*, Vol. 14, pp. 1571–1588

Hubler, Jr W., & Wolf, Jr J. (1976). Melanoma. Tumour angiogenesis and human neoplasia. *Cancer*, No. 38, pp. 187-192

Hutchins, L.F., Moon, J., Clark, J.I., Thompson, J.A., Lange, M.K., Flaherty, L.E., & Sondak, V.K. (2007). Evaluation of interferon alpha-2B and Thalidomide in patients with disseminated malignant melanoma, phase 2, SWOG 0026. *Cancer*, Vol. 110, No. 10, pp. 2269–2275

Hwu, W.J., Krown, S.E., Menell, J.H., Panageas, K.S., Merrell, J., Lamb, L.A., Williams, L.J., Quinn, C.J., Foster, T., Chapman, P.B., Livingston, P.O., Wolchok, J.D., &

Houghton, A.N. (2003). Phase II study of Temozolomide plus Thalidomide for the treatment of metastatic melanoma. *J Clin Oncol.*, Vol. 21, pp. 3351-3356

Iruela-Arispe, M.L., & Dvorak, H.F. (1997). Angiogenesis: a dynamic balance of stimulators and inhibitors. *Thromb Haemost.*, No. 78, pp. 672-677

Jenkins, D.C., Charles, I.G., Thompson, L.L., Moss, D.W., Holmes, L.S., Baylis, S.A., Rhodes, P., Westmore, K., Emson, P.C., & Moncada, S. (1995). Role of nitric oxide in tumour growth. *Proc Natl Acad Sci USA*, No. 92, pp. 4392–6

Jin, X., Yagi, M., Akiyama, N., Hirosaki, T., Higashi, S., Lin, C.Y., Dickson, R.B., Kitamura, H., & Miyazaki, K. (2006). Matriptase activates stromelysin (MMP-3) and promotes tumour growth and angiogenesis. *Cancer Science*, Vol. 97, No. 12, pp. 1327–1334

Kale, R., Tayade, P., Saraf, M., & Juvekar, A. (2008). Molecular encapsulation of Thalidomide with sulfobutyl ether-7 beta-cyclodextrin for immediate release property: enhanced in vivo antitumour and antiangiogenesis efficacy in mice. *Drug Dev Ind Pharm*, Vol. 34, No. 2, pp. 149-56

Kankunnen, J.P., Harvima, I.T., & Naukkarinen, A. (1997). Quantitative analysis of tryptase and chimase containing mast cells in benign and malignant breast lesions. *Int. J. Cancer*, No. 72, pp. 385–388

Kerkela, E., & Saarialho-Kere, U. (2003). Matrix metalloproteinases in tumour progression: focus on basal and squamous cell skin cancer. *Experimental Dermatology*, Vol. 12, No. 2, pp. 109–125

Kirchmair, R., Tietz, A.B., Panagiotou, E., Walter, D.H., Silver, M., Yoon, Y.S., Schratzberger, P., Weber, A., Kusano, K., Weinberg, D.H., Ropper, A.H., Isner, J.M., & Losordo, D.W. (2007). Therapeutic angiogenesis inhibits or rescues chemotherapy-induced peripheral neuropathy: taxol- and Thalidomide-induced injury of vasa nervorum is ameliorated by VEGF. *Mol Ther*, Vol. 15, No. 1, pp. 69-75

Krishnamachary, B., Berg-Dixon, S., Kelly, B., Agani, F., Feldser, D., Ferreira, G., Iyer, N., LaRusch, J., Pak, B., Taghavi, P., & Semenza, G.L. (2003). Regulation of colon carcinoma cell invasion by hypoxia-inducible factor 1. *Cancer Res.*, 63:1138–1143

Krown, S.E., Niedzwiecki, D., Hwu, W.J., Hodgson, L., Houghton, A.N., & Haluska, F.G. (2006). Phase II study of Temozolomide and Thalidomide in patients with metastatic melanoma in the brain: high rate of thromboembolic events (CALGB 500102). *Cancer.*, Vol. 107, pp. 1883-1890

Kuenen, B.C., Tabernero, J., Baselga, J., Cavalli, F., Pfanner, E., Conte, P.F., Seeber, S., Madhusudan, S., Deplanque, G., Huisman, H., Scigalla, P., Hoekman, K., & Harris, A.L. (2003). Efficacy and toxicity of the angiogenesis inhibitor SU5416 as a single agent in patients with advanced renal cell carcinoma, melanoma, and soft tissue sarcoma. *Clinical Cancer Research*, Vol. 9, No. 5, pp. 1648–1655

Kuphal, S., Bauer, R., & Bosserhoff, A.K. (2005). Integrin signalling in malignant melanoma. *Cancer and Metastasis Reviews*, Vol.24, No. 2, pp. 195–222

Leek, R.D., Lander, R.J., Harris, A.L., & Lewis, C.E. (1999). Necrosis correlates with high vascular density and focal macrophages infiltration in invasive carcinoma of the breast. *Br J Cancer*, No. 79, pp. 991–5

Lene, W., Vestermark, Larsen, S., Lindeløv, B., & Bastholt, L. (2008). A phase II study of Thalidomide in patients with brain metastases from malignant melanoma. *Acta Oncologica*, Vol. 47, pp. 1526-1530

Lewis, K.D., Robinson, W.A., Millward, M.J., Powell, A., Price, T.J., Thomson, D.B., Walpole, E.T., Haydon, A.M., Creese, B.R., Roberts, K.L., Zalcberg, J.R., & Gonzalez, R. (2008). A phase II study of the heparanase inhibitor PI-88 in patients with advanced melanoma. *Invest New Drugs*, Vol. 26, No. 1, pp. 89-94

Liotta, L., & Kohn, E.C. (2001). The microenvironment of the tumour-host interface. *Nature*, No. 411, pp. 375–9

Liu, G., Zhang, F., Lee, J., & Dong, Z. (2005). Selective induction of interleukin-8 expression in metastatic melanoma cells by transforming growth factor-β1. *Cytokine*, Vol. 31, No. 3, pp. 241–249

Lu L., Payvandi, F., Wu, L., Zhang, L.H., Hariri, R.J., Man, H.W., Chen, R.S., Muller, G.W., Hughes, C.C., Stirling, D.I., Schafer, P.H., & Bartlett, J.B. (2009). The anti-cancer drug Lenalidomide inhibits angiogenesis and metastasis via multiple inhibitory effects on endothelial cell function in normoxic and hypoxic conditions. *Microvascular Research*, Vol. 77, No. 2, pp. 78–86

Luttun, A., Autiero, M., Tjwa, M., & Carmeliet, P. (2004). Genetic dissection of tumour angiogenesis: are PlGF and VEGFR-1 novel anti-cancer targets? *Biochimica et Biophysica Acta*, Vol. 1654, No. 1, pp. 79–94

Lutzky, J., Weber, R., Nunez, Y., Gillett, M., & Spitler, L. (2009). A phase 1 study of granulocyte macrophage colony-stimulating factor (sargramostim) and escalating doses of Thalidomide in patients with high-risk malignant melanoma. *Journal of Immunotherapy*, Vol. 32, No. 1, pp. 79–85

Mahler, D.A., Huang, S., Tabrizi, M., & Bell, G.M. (2004). Efficacy and safety of a monoclonal antibody recognizing interleukin-8 in COPD: a pilot study. *Chest*, Vol. 126, No. 3, pp. 926–934

Maniotis, A.J., Folberg, R., Hess, A., Seftor, E.A., Gardner, L.M., Pe'er, J., Trent, J.M., Meltzer, P.S., & Hendrix, M.J. (1999). Vascular channel formation by human melanoma cells in vivo and vitro: vasculogenic mimicry. *Am J Pathol.*, Vol. 155, pp. 739-752

Marcoval, J., Moreno, A., Graells, J., Vidal, A., Escribà, J.M., Garcia-Ramírez, M., & Fabra, A. (1997). Angiogenesis and malignant melanoma. Angiogenesis is related to the development of vertical (tumourigenic) growth phase. *Journal of Cutaneous Pathology*, Vol. 24, No. 4, pp. 212–218

Margolin, K., Atkins, B., Thompson, A., Ernstoff, S., Weber, J., Flaherty, L., Clark, I., Weiss, G., Sosman, J., II Smith, W., Dutcher, P., Gollob, J., Longmate, J., & Johnson, D. (2002). Temozolomide and whole brain irradiation in melanoma metastatic to the brain: a phase II trial of the Cytokine Working Group. *J Cancer Res Clin Oncol.*, Vol. 128, pp. 214-218

Melnikova, V.O., & Bar-Eli, M. (2006). Bioimmunotherapy for melanoma using fully human antibodies targeting MCAM/MUC18 and IL-8. *Pigment Cell Research*, Vol. 19, No. 5, pp. 395–405

Mignatti, P., & Rifkin, D.B. (1993). Biology and biochemistry of proteinases in tumour invasion. *Physiol. Rev.*, No. 73, pp. 161–195

Mihm, Jr M., Clark, Jr W., & Reed, R. (1975). The clinical diagnosis of malignant melanoma. Semin. *Oncol.*, No. 2, pp. 105-118

Mita M.M., Rowinsky, E.K., Forero, L., Eckhart, S.G., Izbicka, E., Weiss, G.R., Beeram, M., Mita, A.C., de Bono, J.S., Tolcher, A.W., Hammond, L.A., Simmons, P., Berg, K., Takimoto, C., & Patnaik, A. (2007). A phase II, pharmacokinetic, and biologic study of semaxanib and Thalidomide in patients with metastatic melanoma. *Cancer Chemotherapy and Pharmacology*, Vol. 59, no. 2, pp. 165–174

Mitjans, F., Meyer, T., Fittschen, C., Goodman, S., Jonczyk, A., Marshall, J.F., Reyes, G., & Piulats, J. (2000). In vivo therapy of malignant melanoma by means of antagonists of αv integrins. *International Journal of Cancer*, Vol. 87, No. 5, pp. 716–723

Mueller, M.B. (1996). Different roles for plasminogen activators and metalloproteinases inmelanomametastasis. *Current Topics in Microbiology and Immunology*, Vol. 213, pp. 65–80

Nikkola, J., Vihinen, P., Vuoristo, M.-S., Kellokumpu-Lehtinen, P., Kahari, V.M., & Pyrh¨onen, S. (2005). High serum levels of matrix metalloproteinase-9 and matrix metalloproteinase-1 are associated with rapid progression in patients with metastatic melanoma. *Clinical Cancer Research*, Vol. 11, No. 14, pp. 5158–5166

Norrby, K., & Woolley, D. (1993). Role of mast cells in mitogenesis and angiogenesis in normal tissue and tumour tissue. *Adv. Biosci.*, No. 89, pp. 71–115

Odorisio, T., Cianfarani, F., Failla, C.M., & Zambruno, G. (2006). The placenta growth factor in skin angiogenesis. *Journal of Dermatological Science*, Vol. 41, No. 1, pp. 11–19

Ott, P.A., Chang, J.L., Oratz, R., Jones, A., Farrell, K., Muggia, F., & Pavlick, A.C. (2009). Phase II trial of Dacarbazine and Thalidomide for the treatment of metastatic melanoma. *Chemotherapy*, Vol. 55, No. 4, pp. 221–227

Park, C.C., Bissell, M.J., & Barcellos-Hoff, M.H. (2000). The influence of the microenvironment on the malignant phenotype. *Mol Med Today*, No. 6, pp. 324–9

Pavlaki, M., & Zucker, S. (2003). Matrix metalloproteinase inhibitors (MMPIs): the beginning of phase I or the termination of phase III clinical trials. *Cancer and Metastasis Reviews*, Vol. 22, No. 2-3, pp. 177–203

Pawlak, W.Z., & Legha, S.S. (2004). Phase II study of Thalidomide in patients with metastatic melanoma. *Melanoma Res*, Vol. 14, pp. 57-62

Perez, D.G., Suman, V.J., Fitch, T.R., Amatruda, T. 3rd, Morton, R.F., Jilani, S.Z., Constantinou, C.L., Egner, J.R., Kottschade, L.A., & Markovic, S.N. (2009). Phase 2 trial of carboplatin, weekly paclitaxel, and biweekly bevacizumab in patients with unresectable stage IV melanoma: a North Central Cancer Treatment Group study, N047A. *Cancer*, Vol. 115, No. 1, pp. 119–127

Peterson, A.C., Swiger,S., Stadler, S.M., Medved, M., Karczmar, G., & Gajewski, T.F.(2004). Phase II study of the Flk-1 tyrosine kinase inhibitor SU5416 in advanced melanoma. *Clinical Cancer Research*, Vol. 10, No. 12, part 1, pp. 4048–4054

Qi, J., Nakayama, K., Gaitonde, S., Goydos, J.S., Krajewski, S., Eroshkin, A., Bar-Sagi, D., Bowtell, D., & Ronai, Z. (2008). The ubiquitin ligase Siah2 regulates tumourigenesis and metastasis by HIF-dependent and -independent pathways. *Proc Natl Acad Sci USA*, No. 105, pp. 16713–16718

Qu, B., Guo, L., Ma, J., & Lv, Y. (2010). Antiangiogenesis therapy might have the unintended effect of promoting tumour metastasis by increasing an alternative circulatory system. *Medical Hypotheses*, Vol. 74, No. 2, pp. 360–361

Quirt, I., Bodurth, A., Lohmann, R., Rusthoven, J., Belanger, K., Young, V., Wainman, N., Stewar, W., Eisenhauer, E.; National Cancer Institute of Canada Clinical Trials Group. (2002). Phase II study of marimastat (BB-2516) in malignant melanoma: a clinical and tumour biopsy study of the National Cancer Institute of Canada Clinical Trials Group. *Investigational New Drugs*, Vol. 20, No. 4, pp. 431–437

Quirt, I., Verma, S., Petrella, T., Bak, K., & Charette,M. (2007). Temozolomide for the treatment of metastatic melanoma: a systematic review. *Oncologist*, Vol. 12, No. 9, pp. 1114–1123

Reiriz, A.B., Richter, M.F., Fernandes, S., Cancela, A.I., Costa, T.D., DiLeone, L.P., & Schwartsmann, G. (2004). Phase II study of Thalidomide in patients with metastatic malignant melanoma. *Melanoma Res*, Vol. 14, pp. 527-31

Risau, W., Sariola, H., Zerwes, H.G., Sasse, J., Ekblom, P., Kemler, R., & Doetschman, T. (1988). Vasculogenesis and angiogenesis in embryonic stem-cell-derived embryoid bodies. *Development*, No. 102, pp. 471-478

Roy, R., Yang, J., & Moses, M.A. (2009). Matrix metalloproteinases as novel biomarkers and potential therapeutic targets in human cancer. *Journal of Clinical Oncology*, Vol. 27, No. 31, pp. 5287–5297

Rudek, M.A., Figg, W.D., Dyer, V., Dahut, W., Turner, M.L., Steinberg, S.M., Liewehr, D.J., Kohler, D.R., Pluda, J.M., & Reed, E. (2001). Phase I clinical trial of oral COL-3, a matrix metalloproteinase inhibitor, in patients with refractory metastatic cancer. *Journal of Clinical Oncology*, Vol. 19, No. 2, pp. 584–592

Salven, P., Heikkil¨a, P., & Joensuu, H. (1997). Enhanced expression of vascular endothelial growth factor in metastatic melanoma. *British Journal of Cancer*, Vol. 76, No. 7, pp. 930–934

Schicher, N., Paulitschke, V., Swoboda, A., Kunstfeld, R., Loewe, R., Pilarski, P., Pehamberger, H., Hoeller, C. (2009). Erlotinib and bevacizumab have synergistic activity against melanoma. *Clinical Cancer Research*, Vol. 15, No. 10, pp. 3495–3502

Schnaeker, E.-M., Ossig, R., Ludwig, T., Dreier, R., Oberleithner, H., Wilhelmi, M., & Schneider, S.W. (2004). Microtubule-dependent matrix metalloproteinase-2/matrix metalloproteinase-9 exocytosis: prerequisite in human melanoma cell invasion. *Cancer Research*, Vol. 64, No. 24, pp. 8924–8931

Singhal, S., & Mehta, J. (2002). Thalidomide in cancer. *Biomedicine and Pharmacotherapy*, Vol. 56, No. 1, pp. 4–12

Son, M.J., Kim, J.S., Kim, M.H., Song, H.S., Kim, J.T., Kim, H., Shin, T., Jeon, H.J., Lee, D.S., Park, S.Y., Kim, Y.J., Kim, J.H., & Nam, D.H. (2006). Combination treatment with Temozolomide and Thalidomide inhibits tumour growth and angiogenesis in an orthotopic glioma model. *Int J Oncol.*, Vol. 28, No. 1, pp. 53-59

Srivastava, A., Laidler, P., Davies, R.P., Horgan, K., & Hughes, L.E. (1988). The prognostic significance of tumour vascularity in Dermatology Research and Practice 5 intermediate-thickness (0.76–4.0mm thick) skin melanoma. A quantitative histologic study. *American Journal of Pathology*, Vol. 133, No. 2, pp. 419–423

Srivastava, A., Hughes, L.E., Woodcock, J.P., & Laidler, P. (1989). Vascularity in cutaneous melanoma detected by Doppler sonography and histology: correlation with tumour behaviour. *British Journal of Cancer*, Vol. 59, No. 1, pp. 89–91

Stack, M.S. & Johnson, D.A. (1994). Human mast cell tryptase activates single-chain urinary-type plasminogen activator (pro-urokinase). *J. Biol. Chem.*, No. 269, pp. 9416–9419

Starkey, J.R., Crowle, P.K., & Taubenberg, S. (1988). Mast cell-deficient W/Wv mice exhibit a decreased rate of tumour angiogenesis. *Int. J. Cancer*, No. 42, pp. 48–52

Stasi, R., & Amadori, S. (2002). The role of angiogenesis in hematologic Malignancies. *J of Hematotherapy & stem cell research*, No. 11, pp. 49-68

Streit, M., & Detmar, M. (2003). Angiogenesis, lymphangiogenesis, and melanoma metastasis. *Oncogene*, No. 22, pp. 3172-3179

Suhr, F., Brixius, K., & Bloch, W. (2009). Angiogenic and vascular modulation by extracellular matrix cleavage products. *Current Pharmaceutical Design*, Vol. 15, No. 4, pp. 389–410

Toth, T., Toth-Jakatics, R., Jimi, S., Takebayashi, S., & Kawamoto, N. (2000). Cutaneous malignant melanoma: correlation between neovascularization and peritumour accumulation of mast cells overexpressing vascular endothelial growth factor. *Hum. Pathol*, No. 31, pp. 955–960

Vaishampayan, U.N., Heilbrun, L.K., Marsack,C., Smith, D.W., & Flaherty, L.E. (2007). Phase II trial of pegylated interferon and Thalidomide in malignant metastatic melanoma. *Anti-Cancer Drugs*, Vol. 18, No. 10, pp. 1221–1226

Varker, K.A., Biber, J.E., Kefauver, C., Jensen, R., Lehman, A., Young, D., Wu, H., Lesinski, G.B., Kendra, K., Chen, H.X., Walker, M.J., & Carson, W.E. 3rd. (2007). A randomized phase 2 trial of bevacizumab with or without daily low-dose interferon alfa-2b in metastatic malignant melanoma. *Annals of Surgical Oncology*, Vol. 14, No. 8, pp. 2367–2376

Vásquez, L.M., Somani, S., Altomare, F., & Simpson, E.R., (2009). Intracameral bevacizumab in the treatment of neovascular glaucoma and exudative retinal detachment after brachytherapy in choroidal melanoma. *Canadian Journal of Ophthalmology*, Vol. 44, No. 1, pp. 106–107

Vaupel, P., & Mayer, A. (2007). Hypoxia in cancer: significance and impact on clinical outcome. *Cancer Metastasis Rev.*, No. 26, pp. 225–239.

Wani, A.A., Jafarnejad, S.M., Zhou, J., & Li, G. (2011). Integrin-linked kinase regulates melanoma angiogenesis by activating NF-κB/interleukin-6 signalling pathway. *Oncogene*, PMID 21278793

Warren, B.A., & Shubik, P. (1966). The growth of the blood supply to melanoma transplants in the hamster cheek pouch. *Lab. Invest.*, No. 15, pp. 464-478

Wojtowicz-Praga, S., Low, J., Marshall, J., Ness, E., Dickson, R., Barter, J., Sale, M., McCann, P., Moore, J., Cole, A., & Hawkins, M.J. (1996). Phase I trial of a novel matrix metalloproteinase inhibitor batimastat (BB-94) in patients with advanced cancer. *Investigational New Drugs*, Vol. 14, No. 2, pp. 193–202

Wojtowicz-Praga, S., Torri, J., Johnson, M., Steen, V., Marshall, J., Ness, E., Dickson, R., Sale, M., Rasmussen, H.S., Chiodo, T.A., & Hawkins, M.J. (1998). Phase I trial of Marimastat, a novel matrix metalloproteinase inhibitor, administered orally to patients with advanced lung cancer. *Journal of Clinical Oncology*, Vol. 16, No. 6, pp. 2150–2156

Yang, M.H., & Wu, K.J. (2008). TWIST activation by hypoxia inducible factor-1 (HIF-1): implications in metastasis and development. *Cell Cycle*, No. 7, pp. 2090–2096

Zeldis, J.B., Knight, R., Hussein, M., Chopra, R., Muller, G., & Ann, N.Y. (2011) A review of the history, properties, and use of the immunomodulatory compound Lenalidomide. *Acad Sci.*, Vol. 1222, No. 1, pp. 76-82

Zhang, S., Li, M., Gu, Y., Liu, Z., Xu, S., Cui, Y., & Sun, B. (2008). Thalidomide influences growth and vasculogenic mimicry channel formation in melanoma. *Journal of Experimental and Clinical Cancer Research*, Vol. 27, No. 1, article 60

16

Stromal Microenvironment Alterations in Malignant Melanoma

Svetlana Brychtova, Michala Bezdekova, Jaroslav Hirnak, Eva Sedlakova, Martin Tichy and Tomas Brychta
Palacky University Olomouc
Czech Republic

1. Introduction

The stromal microenvironment has become recognized as a major factor maintaining physiological functions of the cells and tissue integrity and it sensitively responds to pathological conditions including malignant transformation. The development of an altered stromal microenvironment in response to carcinoma is a common feature of many tumours. Induced stromal changes significantly contribute to malignant cell invasion and cancer progression. The chapter concerns about the most important stromal alterations involved in progression of malignant melanoma. It has been documented that one of the reasons, why melanoma cells escape apoptosis is a result of multicellular nature of the disease, in which melanoma cells are embedded in a tissue microenvironment of multiple cell types.

2. Malignant melanoma

Malignant melanoma is known as a highly aggressive tumour, the prognosis of which is difficult to predict. This tumour represents a paradox among all solid tumours because, despite the fact that many prognostic markers have been identified, there is very little understanding of their biological significance. In fact, the prognosis of malignant melanoma is still only based on histological criteria such as tumour size, depth of invasion, ulcerations and mitotic activity. However, these parameters do not allow precise prognosis. A small-sized tumour can metastasize very early, and, on the other hand, tumours of advanced stages may remain localized for many years (Heenen & Laporte, 2003). Many epidemiological, clinical, *in vitro* and *in vivo* studies have provided insight into the biology of the disease. In melanoma cells, numbers of mutations and/or deregulated expression of B-Raf, N-Ras, CDK2A, MDM2, PTEN, p53 have been recognised, but in addition to genetic abnormalities, it has been shown that interactions between tumour cells and surrounding stromal environment are significant. Melanoma cells are embedded in a tissue microenvironment of multiple cell types including keratinocytes, fibroblasts, endothelial cells and immunoregulatory cells.

2.1 Tumour stroma and malignant melanoma

The interactive signalling between tumour and stroma is very heterogeneous and contributes to the formation of the so-called “tumour organ”. Stroma is a compilation of cells including fibroblasts/myofibroblasts, epithelial, fat, immune, vascular and smooth muscle cells along with extracellular matrix and extracellular molecules (Fig.1). While none of these cells are malignant themselves, due to their interactions with each other and directly or indirectly with cancer cells, they acquire an abnormal phenotype and altered function to form a permissive and supportive environment for tumour, known as the reactive tumour stroma, which largely determines the phenotype of the tumour. This abnormal interplay consisting of cell-cell contact and active molecular crosstalk further drives the cancer stroma phenotype and may result in permanent alterations in cell function. The whole process is similar to wound healing; in fact, tumours are called never-healed wounds. The relative amount of stroma and its composition vary considerably from tumour to tumour and do not correlate with the degree of tumour malignancy.

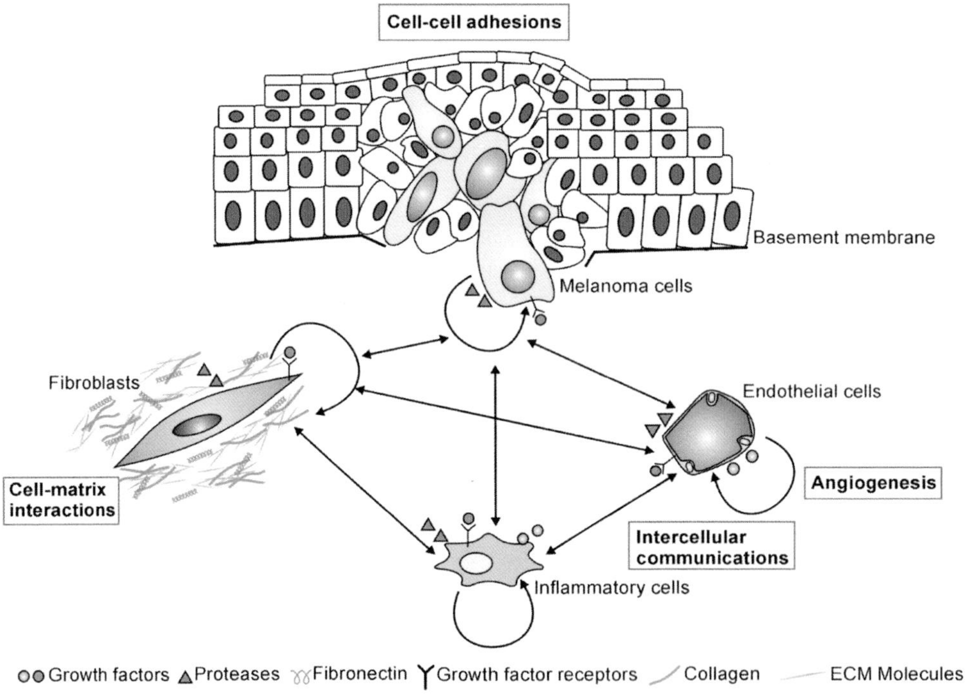

Fig. 1. Interactions between melanoma cells and activated stromal microenvironment are complicated and complex, and include changes in cell-cell adhesions, cell- matrix and cell-cell interactions and angiogenesis.

2.1.1 Stromal microenvironment

A large range of molecules including growth factors and their receptors, degradation and remodelling enzymes, extracellular matrix (ECM) molecules, cytokines, interleukins, formation of bioactive fragments are produced to disrupt normal tissue homeostasis and act in a paracrine manner to induce angiogenesis, the inflammatory response, changes in extracellular matrix composition and increased protease activity (Bhowmick et al., 2004), which affect differentiation, proliferation, migration and invasion of malignant cells, and support tumour spread and invasion. There is also increasing evidence that tumour stroma can have a more direct role in tumorigenesis by acting as a mutagen. As tumours progress, the cells display increased genetic instability. Conditions in the tumour microenvironment including oxidative stress, low pH environment and nutrient deprivation contribute to genetic instability through the induction of enhanced mutagenesis and an impaired DNA damage pathway (Bindra & Glazar, 2005). Alterations of the microenvironment are not the same within the whole tumour mass, conditions in the central region, where hypoxia and necrosis occur, differ from more viable areas found toward the periphery.

2.1.2 Carcinoma-associated fibroblasts

One of the most important components of stromal microenvironment are stromal fibroblasts. The main function of normal fibroblasts is synthesis of fibrillar extracellular matrix including collagens I, III, V and fibronectin. They also contribute to basal membrane formation by secretion of collagen IV and laminin. Carcinoma-associated fibroblasts (CAFs) can form a foetal-like environment. Through production of a variety of growth factors including basic fibroblast growth factor (bFGF), platelet-derived growth factor (PDGF), epidermal growth factor (EGF), transforming growth factor alpha (TGF-alpha) and the family of vascular endothelial growth factors (VEGFs) A, B and C. Fibroblasts are capable of modulating complicated interactions between epithelial and mesenchymal cells. Fibroblasts can also act as antigen-presenting cells and so importantly regulate the immune response. Besides maintaining homeostasis and integrity of healthy tissues, fibroblasts fundamentally contribute to tissue healing by formation of granulation tissue and scarring. In cancers, CAFs or myofibroblasts are believed to be a major part of a tumorous stroma. Such fibroblasts are phenotypically and genotypically different from normal fibroblasts (Bhowmick et al., 2004). They become highly proliferating cells with decreased apoptotic potential and increased migratory capacity.

CAFs promote tumour progression by secreting growth factors and pro-migratory ECM components, as well as up-regulating the expression of serine proteases and matrix metalloproteinases that degrade and remodel the ECM. They also contribute to tumorous neoangiogenesis. Moreover, CAFs can promote progression of pre-malignant lesions or even act as a direct mutagen stimulating the progression of a non-tumorigenic cell population to a tumorigenic one (Bhowmick et al., 2004). On the other hand, fibroblasts may also inhibit tumour growth. However, only normal fibroblasts possess these abilities. The mechanisms are still not clear, though the reduction of TGF or modulation of the immune response via interleukin-1 (IL-1), interleukin-6 (IL-6) or inhibition of T-lymphocyte apoptosis have been described (Silzle et al., 2004). In *in vivo* models of melanoma genesis, both the early vertical phase and the late radial phase were repressed (Proia & Kuperwasser, 2005). Thus normalization of the stromal microenvironment should be able to slow or even reverse tumour progression.

2.2 Tumour changes in malignant melanoma

In skin, under normal condition, tissue homeostasis determines whether a cell remains quiescent, proliferates, differentiates, or undergoes apoptosis. Melanocytes, after cell division, separate and migrate along the basement membrane; finally, they extend their dendrites and establish multiple contacts with keratinocytes and Langerhans cells. In the state of homeostasis, keratinocytes control growth and behaviour of melanocytes through a complicated and complex system of paracrine growth factors and cell-cell adhesion molecules. Once this delicate homeostatic balance is altered, melanocyte proliferation and migration is stimulated, which can lead to nevi or even malignant melanoma development. Melanoma cells escape from the control of keratinocytes through several mechanisms including a decrease or loss of intercellular adhesions by down-regulation of receptors and proteins important for their communication with keratinocytes (E-cadherin, P-cadherin), loss of their anchorage to the basement membrane, because of altered expression of the extracellular matrix-binding integrin family, and up-regulation of receptors and signalling molecules important for melanoma-melanoma and melanoma-fibroblast interaction such as N-cadherin.

The growth of melanoma is associated with cumulating stromal alterations. The molecular changes associated with the transformation of melanoma cells from the radial growth phase (RGP) to the vertical growth phase (VGP) and the metastatic phenotype are not very well defined. However, some of the genes that are critical for melanoma progression have been demonstrated. For example, the switch from RGP to VGP and the metastatic phenotype are associated with loss of the AP-2 alpha transcription factor. This loss resulted in overexpression of MCAM/UC18, MMP, and lack of c-KIT expression (Leslie & Bar-Eli, 2005). AP-2 alpha also regulates two G protein-coupled receptors (GPCRs), the thrombin receptor protease-activated receptor (PAR-1) and platelet-activating factor receptor (PAFR). In turn, PAR-1 regulates the expression of gap junction protein connexin 43 and the tumour suppressor maspin. Activation of PAR-1 also leads to overexpression and secretion of proangiogenic factors such as IL-8, VEGFs, PDGF, as well as certain integrins. The ligands for these GPCRs, thrombin and PAF, are secreted by stromal cells, emphasizing the importance of the melanoma microenvironment for the progression of the disease (Braeuer et al., 2010). Other studies have shown that AP-2 alpha regulates additional genes involved in melanoma growth including E-cadherin, p21/WAF-1, Her2, Bcl-2, FAS/APO-1, plasminogen activator inhibitor-1 (PAI-1), hepatocyte growth factor (HGF) and insulin-like growth factor receptor 1 (IGFR-1). The factor is a p53 binding partner, and has been shown to stimulate p53-dependent transcription (Melnikova & Bar-Eli, 2008). Additionally, the transition of melanoma cells from RGP to VGP is associated with overexpression of transcription factors CREB/ATF-1 (cAMP-responsive element binding protein/activating transcription factor-1). Two mechanisms how overexpression of CREB and ATP-1 contributes to the aggressive phenotype have been identified. The first one is overexpression of the metalloproteinase MMP-2 and the adhesion molecule MCAM/UC18; in the second mechanism both proteins act as survival factors for melanoma cells.

In malignant melanoma, tumour stroma interactions involve five main mechanisms influencing the growth and invasion of malignant cells, activation of which determine each other reciprocally: (1) changes in intercellular adhesion such as the cadherin, catenin, Snail and claudin families, (2) up-regulation of growth factors and their receptors, (3) activation of transcription factors (the family of signal transducers and activators of transcription, STATs), (4) stimulation of angiogenesis, and (5) immune cell response.

2.2.1 Cell-cell adhesions

In normal epithelial structures, cell-cell junctions play an important role in the maintenance, integrity and morphology of the epithelium (Alami et al., 2003). It has been reported that the E-cadherin/beta-catenin system of adhesion molecules plays a crucial role in these processes

(Weis & Nelson, 2006). E-cadherin is a cell adhesion transmembrane molecule, a member of a family of functionally related transmembrane glycoproteins that mediate Ca2+-dependent intercellular adhesion. The adhesion is mediated via interaction with adjacent cells through their N-terminal ectodomains and the cytoplasmic terminal tail of E-cadherin links specifically to beta-catenin that binds directly to the cytoskeletal actin. A deficiency in E-cadherin causes loss of adherent junctions (AJs), which leads to impaired intercellular signalling, but not to direct tumour transformation. It has been reported that dysfunction or disruption of cell adhesion molecules accompanies the invasiveness and metastatic behaviour of malignant cells. Protein beta-catenin is a molecular sensor that integrates cell-cell junctions and cytoskeletal dynamics with signalling pathways affecting morphogenesis, tissue homeostasis, and intercellular communication within tissues (Perez-Moreno & Fuchs, 2006). Generally, beta-catenin has a dual function. It plays a key role in cell-cell adhesion by linking cadherins to alpha-catenin and cytoskeletal actin (Weis & Nelson, 2006). In the absence of Wnt signal, beta-catenin is constitutively down-regulated by a multicomponent destruction complex containing GSK3 beta (glycogen synthase kinase 3 beta), axin and the tumour suppressor APC (adenomatous polyposis coli). These proteins promote the phosphorylation of serine and threonine residues in the NH2-terminal region of beta-catenin. Beta-catenin is then degraded by casein kinase CK1 and protein phosphatases PP2A and PP2C through the ubiquitin-proteasome pathway. Wnt signalling inhibits this process, leading to an accumulation of beta-catenin in the nucleus, which promotes the formation of transcriptionally active complexes with members of the Tcf/lef family (T-cell factor/lymphoid enhancer factor). The Tcf/beta-catenin heterodimers act as bipartite transcription factors and activate expression of the specific Wnt responsive genes that encode proteins regulating cell cycle, e.g. c-Myc, cyclin D1 and Pitx2 (Tetsu & McCormick, 1999). Alterations in beta-catenin-mediated regulation have been demonstrated mainly during cancer development, where mutations of the beta-catenin gene *CTNNB1* result in disruption of a large number of cellular functions leading to loss of growth control and neoplastic change (Voeller et al., 1998; Garcia-Rostan et al., 1999).

The classical E-, N- and P- cadherins are expressed during various stages of melanoma progression. In the skin environment, E-cadherin expressed by keratinocytes and melanocytes prevents melanocytes from division without killing the cells, and P-cadherin is expressed only on the surfaces of basal layer, but not by keratinocytes or melanocytes (Satyamoorthy & Herlyn, 2002). During embryonic development, expression of cadherin subtypes correlates with the migration and segregation of different cell layers and the cell populations. An increase of E-cadherin expression is induced on the surfaces of melanoblasts prior to their entry into the epidermis, thereby forming an E-cadherin-high/P-cadherin-low population. The cadherin expression pattern then diversifies, giving rise to three populations: (1) an E-cadherin-/P-cadherin-negative dermal population, (2) an E-cadherin-high/P-cadherin-low epidermal population, and (3) an E-cadherin-/P-cadherin-mediate to -high follicular population. In all three populations, the patterns of expression are region specific. During melanoma development, expression of E-cadherin is progressively lost and becomes heterogeneous. In nevus cells, it is predominantly distributed diffusely in the cytoplasm, while in melanoma cells, it is completely absent. This may impair loss of terminal differentiation to melanocytes by disrupting the complex formation between cadherin, catenin and cytoskeleton required for strong intercellular adhesion. Despite the loss of E-cadherin by melanoma cells, these cells express high levels of N-cadherin and this switching of the profile is thought to promote their interaction with fibroblasts and endothelial cells. This may facilitate melanoma cells to migrate into the dermis and enter the vasculature (Perlis & Herlyn, 2004). In malignant melanoma, each of three cadherin molecules has been evaluated as a prognostic marker in multiple retrospective cohort studies of varying quality with different results. In multivariable analysis, decreased levels of P-cadherin have been shown to be associated with faster disease progression in thin (<2mm) lesions, but did not reach significance for all-cause mortality in another study (Pacifico et al., 2005). Gain of N-cadherin expression was significantly associated with increased all-cause mortality in one univariate long-rank analysis and did not retain its significance. Decreased levels of E-cadherin have been associated with a metastatic phenotype, where lower mean levels of the protein were shown in metastatic melanomas. Significant negative trends of E-cadherin were also shown with Breslow thickness (Kreizenbeck et al., 2008) On the other hand, improved survival was described in a group of patients with retained E-cadherin expression. Interesting data were published by Kreizenbeck et al. (2008) who evaluated simultaneous expression of cadherins. Worse outcomes were described in a subset of melanomas that successfully completed epithelial-mesenchymal transition (EMT) - down-regulation of E- and P-cadherins and up-regulation of N-cadherin. But unexpectedly, one group, despite having the highest levels of N-cadherin in the entire cohort, displayed the best survival. In this group, E-cadherin continued to be expressed. Thus, high levels of N-cadherin should not always be a feature of EMT, but high levels of the protein may recapitulate a very early but noninvasive, developmental phenotype.

In malignant melanoma, both the loss of E-cadherin and mutations of beta-catenin, leading to a more stable non-degradable protein, have been reported. Patients with N-cadherin and beta-catenin co-expression yielded a 3.29-fold increased risk of death (Kreizenbeck et al., 2008). The impact of beta-catenin expression depends on its subcellular distribution, where nuclear translocation of the protein represents an unfavourable prognosis, while cytoplasmic locations were associated with increased disease-free survival.

The mechanism of down-regulation of E-cadherin in malignant melanoma is still unknown. One possibility involves promoter inactivation attributable to hypermethylation. Furthermore, loss of activating protein-2 transcription factor expression as a potential activator of E-cadherin has been suggested. Also mutations in E-cadherin gene resulting in a functionally inactive protein have been detected. Ultraviolet irradiation leading to secretion of endothelin 1 can also down-regulate E-cadherin in melanocytes and melanoma cells (Jamal & Schneider, 2002), as well as tumour invasion. One of the strongest E-cadherin repressors is the protein Snail 1. Snail is a zinc-finger transcription factor involved in the process that facilitates cell movement during embryonic development. Snail 1 expression leads to the acquisition of fibroblastic properties by epithelial cells, facilitating their migration. In malignant melanoma, up-regulation of Snail 1 has been observed. Besides down-regulation of E-cadherin, Snail 1 is also known to promote the nuclear localization of beta-catenin. Furthermore, Snail suppresses the expression of claudins and occludins (De Craene et al., 2005). Snail has been described to affect transcriptional expression of CYLD (a tumour suppressor) in melanoma cells, which finally results in N-cadherin and cyclin D1 overexpression. The Snail family is activated by TGF-beta. Other known Snail inductors manifesting high metastatic potential and often exhibiting loss of functional tight junctions (TJs) include RAS or ILK (integrin-linked kinase) (Massoumi et al., 2009). Furthermore, mutation of BRAF can lead to up-regulation of Snail as well (Massoumi et al., 2009).

Besides AJs, cell-cell adhesions are maintained through tight junctions. In contrast to the role of AJs, the role of TJ proteins in cancer is less well understood. TJs are the most apical cell-

cell contacts and are important for a barrier function that regulates the passage of ions, water, macromolecules, and a fence function that maintains cell polarity. A number of integral membrane proteins associated with TJs have been identified including occludin, junctional adhesion molecules and the claudin family consisting of at least 24 members (Dhawan et al., 2005). Tumour cells, particularly in those cancers that manifest high metastatic potential, often exhibit loss of functional TJs. For example, levels of zonula occludens (ZO-1, ZO-2) and occludins are decreased during tumour formation and metastasis. There are differences in claudin family expression in various tumours. While a decrease of claudin-7 has been found, levels of claudin-1, -2 and -3 are frequently elevated. Claudins encode proteins with 4 transmembrane domains, and their N- and C-terminal ends are located in the cytoplasm. Members of the claudin family interact with each other. In addition, the C-terminal domain of claudins also serves as a binding site for interactions with other TJs that are potentially involved in signalling. Furthermore, claudins have been reported to recruit and promote the activation of MMP-2, suggesting potential involvement in invasion and metastasis. Claudin-1 was also recently identified as a probable target of beta-catenin/Tcf signalling. It has also been demonstrated that claudin-1 inhibition increases E-cadherin expression. Expression of various claudins is regulated by EGF and TGF-beta. As claudins regulate paracellular transport, they are usually found at the cell membrane. However, these proteins have been shown to alter their subcellular localization during malignant progression. Benign lesions and less aggressive melanomas express claudin-1 in the nucleus, whereas aggressive melanomas have an abundance of the protein in the cytoplasm. It has been reported that for the regulation and cytoplasmic localization of claudin expression, protein kinases such as protein kinase A (PKA) and protein kinase C (PKC) are important. In benign nevi and early stage melanomas, claudin is largely expressed in the nucleus, while highly metastatic melanoma cells tend to have increased claudin-1 in the cytoplasm and at the membrane (French et al., 2009). It is curious that in cases where claudin-1 is low, it is predominantly nuclear, despite abundant active PKA. This observation implies that the levels of claudin-1 may need to reach a certain threshold prior to being shuttled out of the nucleus. The significance of claudin-1 in the nucleus is unclear. It is known that the nuclear expression of other TJs can inhibit proliferation. But different results were obtained by others, claiming that nuclear translocation correlates with oncogenic transformation and proliferation. Cytoplasmic claudin-1 location can induce dramatic EMT, resulting in increased cell motility and metastatic potential.

2.2.2 Epithelial-mesenchymal transition

All the above-mentioned proteins (cadherins, catenin, Snail and claudins) are crucially involved in epithelial-mesenchymal transition. EMT refers to the process, in which an epithelial cell disengages from its parent tissue by losing mediators of homotypic and/or heterotypic cell-cell interactions in exchange for morphology and adhesions marker profiles consistent with a mesenchymal cell and is regarded as the first necessary step for invasion and metastasis (Kreizenbeck et al., 2008). This pathway is especially appropriate for melanoma, because EMT recapitulates a pivotal phase of melanocyte development. Normal melanocyte precursors are derived from the neural crest. During embryogenesis, these cells undergo the first EMT to disengage from the neural crest and then subsequently migrate through the embryonic mesenchyme until they reach their terminal locations distributed throughout the dermal/epidermal junction where they subsequently undergo reverse EMT to facilitate interactions with local keratinocytes.

EMT plays an important role not only in skin morphology but also in wound repair, tissue fibrosis and cancer progression (Nakamura & Tokura, 2011). In malignant melanoma, EMT contributes to the promotion of metastatic phenotype in primary tumour by supporting specific adhesive, invasive, and migratory properties, and it is important for promoting transition to the VGP. EMT is the result of the expression of mesenchymal gene products such as fibronectin, vimentin and metalloproteinases, and the invasion and inhibition of E-cadherin. For EMT induction in melanomas, all genetic abnormalities including common mutations and/or deregulated expression of B-Raf, N-Ras and PTEN seem to synergize with microenvironmental factors including cell-cell interaction and angiogenic efficiency. In addition, it has been shown that hypoxia promotes melanocyte transdifferentiation and melanoma migratory and invasive abilities through up-regulating of genes normally associated with the extracellular matrix remodelling and invasion. These genes include laminin, urokinase and genes encoding matrix metalloproteinases. Furthermore, different microenvironments may be selective for higher levels of B-Raf-dependent and B-Raf-independent ERK1/2 activation. These microenvironments are critical for tumour cell proliferation and spread. It has been shown that expression levels of phosphorylated ERK1/2 are not always correlated with the station status of B-Raf or N-Ras, suggesting that other factors promote ERK1/2 activation. Among these factors are growth factor autocrine loops such as the CDF-dependent activation of c-Kit, and extracellular signals. The above findings exemplify how the microenvironment can complement aberrant genetic changes to promote melanomagenesis and to support an invasive cell phenotype (Lin et al., 2010). In contrast to a general conception that invasion and dissemination occur during the later vertical phase, recent findings show that early dissemination of tumour cells that have not fully progressed contributes to subsequent development of metastasis. Moreover, B-RAF mutation is associated with constitutive hyperactivation of survival/antiapoptotic pathways such as the MAPK, NF-kappaB, and PI3K/AKT, which may also initiate EMT. All pathways cross-talk and regulate each other's activities and functions. For instance, the NF-kappaB pathway directly regulates EMT through the transcription of gene products involved in EMT such as COX-2. Metalloproteinases and VEGFs in metastatic lesions directly and indirectly induce Snail through the transcriptional up-regulation. Snail in turn suppresses the expression of the metastasis suppressor gene product Raf kinase inhibitor protein RKIP (inhibits the MAPK and NF-kappaB pathways) as well as PTEN (inhibits the PI3K/AKT pathway). Hyperactivation of NF-kappaB greatly increases the metastatic potential, while knockdown of NF-kappaB reverses the mesenchymal-like phenotype and suppresses the motility and invasion capacity of melanoma cells (Lin et al., 2010).

EMT accelerates cancer metastasis through not only enhanced invasion but also via induction of immunosuppression. Human melanocytes with typical EMT features after Snail transduction induce regulatory T cells and impair dendritic cells *in vitro* and *in vivo*. Intratumoral injection with a Snail-specific monoclonal antibody inhibits tumour growth and metastasis followed by an increase of tumour-specific tumour-infiltrating lymphocytes and systemic immune response (Kudo-Saito et al., 2009).

Moreover, there are several new theories that EMT may also contribute to formation of malignant stroma when normal or cancer epithelial cells may be a source of carcinoma-associated fibroblasts largely involved in cancer progression.

2.2.3 Growth factors in melanoma progression

There is a large number of growth factors and their receptors and cytokines, which by means of autocrine and paracrine effects are associated with melanoma progression. Those considered to have the highest impact are dealt with in this review.

Fibroblast growth factors

Fibroblast growth factors (FGFs) are proteins with diverse functions in development, repair, and metabolism. The 22-member human FGF gene family includes FGF 1 - FGF 23; FGF 15 has not been identified in humans (Itoh, 2010). FGFs can be subdivided by their action mechanism into three groups: (1) the intracellular FGF 11/12/13/14 subfamily, (2) the hormone-like (endocrine) FGF 19/21 (23) subfamily, and (3) the canonical FGF subfamily comprising FGF 1/2/5, FGF 3/4/6, FGF 7/10/22, FGF 8/17/18 and FGF 9/16/20 (Itoh & Ornitz, 2008). Canonical FGFs mediate their biological responses as extracellular proteins by binding to and activating cell surface tyrosine kinase FGF receptors (FGFRs) including FGFR-1, -2 and -3 with heparin/heparan sulfate as a cofactor. They act as local signalling molecules in an autocrine/paracrine manner. Two members of the FGF family, acidic FGF (FGF1) and predominantly basic FGF (FGF-2), are related to melanoma progression. Basic FGF (bFGF) protein is known as a mitogen stimulating proliferation of mesenchymal, epithelial and neuroectodermal cells. The protein has been shown to stimulate proliferation of human melanocytes and also to support the growth and invasion of melanoma cells. The aberrant expression of bFGF occurs at an early stage of melanocyte lesions affecting growth and cell dedifferentiation. The protein is expressed not only by melanocytes or melanoblasts, but also by stromal cells, especially by activated fibroblasts. It is believed that aberrant expression of the protein even belongs to early changes stimulating proliferation and dedifferentiation of melanocytic lesions. Increased bFGF expression can be induced by exposure to UV radiation, with abnormal expression of the protein resulting in inactivation of some tumour suppressors. Halaban et al. (1988) found bFGF only in malignant melanoma cells and characterized it as a significant autocrine factor influencing melanoma growth. However, these findings have not been confirmed by other studies (Ugurel et al., 2001), where bFGF has also been described in cells of conventional benign nevi, although significantly less often. It seems to be more probable that bFGF cannot be considered a marker of melanocyte transformation and it can stimulate cell growth under benign as well malignant conditions. On the other hand, when bFGF was cleaved by thrombin, which imparted its biological activity, proliferation, chemotaxis and invasion of melanoma cells were observed (Totta et al., 2009). The function of bFGF may also be influenced by varying subcellular localization. Whilst in malignant melanomas, the protein is localized in the cytoplasm, its nuclear expression predominates in nevus cells. Cytoplasmic localization is associated with stimulation of VEGF and HIF expression in tumorous and stromal cells via activation of a variety of kinases such as PI-3K and MAPK. This location may reflect an aberrant form of the bFGF molecule, which is either incapable of nuclear transport or a possible defect in the bFGF-driven cascade may exist. It is possible that the different localization may be a key to another effect of bFGF, for example on the growth of malignant lesions and/or stimulation of fibrotization and maturation of benign nevi. In advanced stage III or IV melanomas, a significant increase in plasma bFGF levels has been found. These results even show that increased bFGF is a more sensitive parameter than detection of S-100 protein or VEGF. The protein bFGF is suggested to be one of the candidates of early detection of lymph node metastases (Kurschat et al., 2007).

Hepatocyte growth factor

Hepatocyte growth factor/scatter factor (HGF/SF) is a potent angiogenic factor and mediator of epithelial cell motility, morphogenesis and angiogenesis. HGF is a mediator of mesenchymal-epithelial interactions that stimulates cell proliferation, migration and morphogenesis through its receptor c-met. HGF/SF is an essential mesenchyme-derived factor in epithelial–mesenchymal (or stromal) interactions during organogenesis, maintaining homeostasis and regeneration of a variety of normal tissues. Moreover, HGF/SF is involved in tumorigenesis *in vivo* (Bellusci et al., 2004). The protein is considered to be expressed by CAFs and contributes to the microenvironment alteration (Dali et al., 2007). Delehedde et al. (2001) showed that HGF/SF is secreted by melanoma cells. HGF induces fibronectin expression and its extracellular assembly on the surface of melanoma cells through activation of the mitogen-activated protein (MAP) kinase pathway, and induction and transcriptional activation of early growth response 1. Altogether this autocrine HGF signalling seems to have important implications in regulation of melanoma progression.

Transforming growth factor beta

TGF-beta is a paracrine growth factor, which under normal physiological conditions maintains tissue homeostasis via proliferation and apoptosis. It also has strong immunosuppressive effects. On the contrary, in cancers, this factor stimulates cell proliferation and growth and can protect malignant cells from the attack by the immune system.

TGF-beta modulates the microenvironment to the benefit of tumour growth and invasion (Lázár-Molnár et al., 2000). TGF-beta stimulates angiogenesis, CAF proliferation, and extracellular matrix and cytokine production. It is also considered to be involved in EMT (Prud'homme, 2007). TGF-beta is generally secreted in an inactive form and requires prior activation. It has been documented that most mammalian cells including melanoma cells, express TGF-beta (Moretti et al., 1999), while melanocytes can produce latent TGF-beta only after stimulation by exogenous growth factors such as insulin-like growth factor 1. TGF-beta is a marker of advanced progression of malignant melanomas (Moretti et al., 1999). TGF-beta has an inhibitory effect on melanocytes and early lesions, but not on advanced stage melanomas. In some cases, it switches to an autocrine stimulator (Lázár-Molnár et al., 2000). However, the role of TGF-beta as a potential autocrine growth factor is more complex. Experimentally, factors such as TGF-beta can induce normal fibroblasts to become activated and express alpha SMA (smooth muscle actin), but it is not clear if these cells acquire other characteristics of CAFs, and if the phenotype is stable, or if they can recover again to a normal state.

Platelet-derived growth factor

PDGF drives cellular responses including proliferation, survival, migration and deposition of extracellular matrix and tissue remodelling factors (Hoch & Soriano, 2003). Besides its mitogenic activity, this factor has its own transforming ability. The important sources of the protein are not only malignant cells themselves, but also activated macrophages, fibroblasts, smooth muscle and endothelial cells and epidermal keratinocytes. PDGF acts through the platelet-derived growth factor receptor (PDGFR) family of receptors tyrosine kinases. These receptors are expressed by a range of cell types, in which they regulate cell growth and proliferation by activation of signalling pathways that include BRAF-MAPK and PI-3 pathways. PDGF is a known stimulator of tumorous stroma especially by its ability to modulate and activate stromal fibroblasts. Also important is its role in stimulation of angiogenesis. But PDGF contributes to morphological changes of new blood and lymph vessels, which are typical for tumorous microcirculation. It has been reported that molecules activated by PDGF via its receptors increase interstitial fluid pressure and in this way contribute to tumour chemoresistance. On the other hand, when PDGFRs and their ligands are blocked, there is increased therapeutic drug delivery to a tumour region (Ogawa et al., 2008).

Expression of PDGF in benign melanocytic lesions is low, a significant increase has been described in melanomas. Higher PDGF expression is documented not only in cells of primary skin melanomas but also in their metastases, emphasizing its importance as a growth factor in melanoma progression. Thus, PDGF has become a potential aim in anti-melanoma therapy that not only influences melanoma cells themselves but also importantly modulates a stromal response.

Epidermal growth factor receptor

EGFR belongs to the family of tyrosine kinase receptors governing cell proliferation, differentiation and transformation in a range of malignancies, mainly through activation of PI-3KAKT and MAPK pathways. EGFR also inhibits apoptosis and stimulates cell migration. EGFR has a direct effect on the stromal microenvironment including stimulation of angiogenesis and an increase of MMP-1 levels, which potentiate invasion of cancer cells. EGFR may also raise metastatic potential including inhibition of TGF-beta or MMP activation.

The main EGFR ligands include EGF and TGF-alpha. While increased expression of EGFR has been well described in many cancers such as colon, stomach, lung and breast carcinomas, where it correlates with a worse prognosis, its role in melanoma biology is less clear. EGFR is one of factors whose phosphorylation and activation are influenced by UV radiation. But in some cases, induction of apoptosis in cells exposed to UV radiation accompanied by inhibition of EGFR expression has been demonstrated. Transactivation of EGFR may also lead to increased stability of poly(ADP-ribose) polymerase (PARP) protein involved in DNA repair and associated with UV stress. *In vitro* studies have shown increased cell proliferation, when EGFR was transfected to melanoma cell lines. This is in contrast to *in vivo* studies using implantation of melanoma cells, where decreased EGFR together with growth inhibition have been documented. It seems that EGFR levels are modulated during melanoma growth, with one of important modulators being the immune system (Diaz et al., 2009). EGFR is increased not only in melanoma lesions including both early- and late-stage melanomas but also in benign nevi. It seems probable that different effector pathways are activated. Anti-apoptotic and proliferating effects predominate in melanoma cells while in nevi, DNA repairs are stimulated. What conditions and mechanisms determine the function is not clear. FGF 1 is related to the achievement of an angiogenic phenotype of melanoma cells.

Vascular endothelial growth factors

VEGFs possess the leading role among the factors regulating tumour angiogenesis. VEGFs and their receptors have been established as distinctive proteins playing a role in endothelial cell proliferation and/or elongation, migration and vascular morphogenesis. VEGFs are produced by a variety of cell types including keratinocytes, macrophages, mast cells, smooth muscle cells, endothelial cells and fibroblasts. VEGF-A is the most well-characterized member of the family of structurally related proteins that act as endothelial cell (EC) mitogens and angiogenic factors. VEGF-A is a dimeric glycoprotein with structural homology to PDGF (Ferrara et al., 1991). One of the most striking characteristics of the factor is its ability to induce vascular permeability. This enhanced permeability leads to subsequent fibrin deposition in the extracellular matrix that can then serve as a scaffold for migrating endothelial cells. VEGF-C, a structural homologue with VEGFs and PDGF, has been shown to stimulate the growth of the lymphatic endothelium and thus induce lymphangiogenesis.

The known responses of VEGFs are mediated through their receptors (VEGFRs) including VEGFR-1 (Flt-1), VEGFR-2 (KDR/Flk-1) and VEGFR-3. The activation of VEGFRs by its ligands results in enhanced permeability of the vasculature and increased migration and proliferation of endothelial cells, making them also major targets for therapy (Rosen, 2002). VEGFs bind and activate two receptors, VEGFR-1 and VEGFR-2. The binding-affinity of VEGFR-1 for VEGF-A is one order of magnitude higher than that of VEGFR-2, whereas the kinase activity of VEGFR-1 is about 10-fold weaker than that of VEGFR-2 (Shibuya, 2006). VEGFR-1 plays a dual role: (1) a negative role in angiogenesis in the embryo most likely by tramping VEGF, and (2) a positive role in adulthood in a tyrosine kinase-dependent manner. VEGFR-2 has strong tyrosine kinase activity and it transduces the major signals for angiogenesis. VEGFR-2 is a direct signal transducer for pathological angiogenesis including cancer (Shibuya, 2006). VEGF-C binds and activates VEGFR-2 and VEGFR-3. VEGFR-3 is essential for the development of the lymphatic vasculature. Experimental tumours that overexpress VEGFR-3 ligands induce lymphatic vessel sprouting and enlargement and show enhanced metastasis to regional lymph nodes (Laakkonen et al., 2007). In melanocytic lesions, VEGF-A was shown to be expressed in benign as well malignant lesions, but malignant melanomas product the protein in significantly higher levels. However, there are different findings considering VEGF-A expression in moles, and some authors strictly deny their expression in nevus cells and they correlate increased production of the protein only with malignant transformation (Gorski et al., 2003; Goydos et al., 2003). Moreover, VEGF-A has been correlated to the transition from the radial to vertical growth phase. But it seems more likely that the factors can regulate angiogenesis under benign and malignant conditions and their detection can serve for differentiation of biological character of the lesion . The most important impact has deregulated and prolonged expression of VEGF-A in melanomas. Contrary to this, VEGF-C was shown to be mostly negative in nevi, and its expression seems to be directly associated with malignant transformation. Both factors are expressed already in early-stage melanomas, and it has been documented that the expression is regulated not only by hypoxia-inducible factor (HIF) caused by hypoxic conditions in larger tumours but also by numbers of cytokines and growth factors (Kyzas et al., 2005). VEGFs are significantly increased in stromal elements surrounding melanoma cells, especially in advanced melanomas. Local levels of VEGFs precede their serological levels described in stage IV melanoma (Pelletier et al., 2005).

VEGFRs are specific not only for endothelial cells but also for fibroblasts, tumour and immune cells. The role of VEGFRs is well recognised during embryonic development, but their impact in tumours is less clear (Shibuya, 2006). While some melanomas express increased levels of the receptors, others are completely negative. VEGFs are likely to be at least partly independent on their receptors. On the other hand, there are results exhibiting better prognosis of tumours, which express VEGFR-1. One explanation may be that VEGFs may bound-out free VEGFs and thus block their effector pathway (Yamaguchi et al., 2007). From this point of view, it may be possible that VEGFR-negative melanomas would have a worse prognosis.

2.2.4 Activation of transcriptional factors

In melanoma progression, a variety of transcriptional factors have been described. The leading role is believed to belong to the c-Myc oncoprotein and STAT family.

c-Myc

It is known that the c-Myc proto-oncogene stimulates cell proliferation and inhibits differentiation. The protein has also its own transforming potential. Increased expression of c-Myc was described already in early stages of melanoma development, but significant deregulation was mostly bound to advanced stages. Autocrine production of c-Myc by melanoma cells stimulates their growth and dedifferentiation, but simultaneously c-Myc may stimulate proliferation of fibroblasts in a paracrine way and thus form tumorous stroma (Gu et al., 2001). Moreover, c-Myc has been found to be expressed in increased levels by stromal fibroblasts. Such production markedly contributes to stromal autoregulation.

In tissues, the c-Myc oncoprotein is stabilized and its effector function is therefore potentiated by FGF (Lepigue et al., 2004). It has been demonstrated that oncogenic signals outgoing from CAFs may stimulate transformation of a non-tumorous cell population to a tumorous one. c-Myc is one of molecules that through the stromal compartment may transform cells and/or contribute to accumulation of mutations and to selection of more aggressive cell clones.

Signal transducers and transcriptional activators

STATs form a family of 7 proteins (STAT 1, 2, 3, 4, 5A, 5B and 6), which are involved in activation of a variety of genes. Some of them are involved in malignant transformation (Yu & Jove, 2004). These proteins have dual roles as cytoplasmic signalling proteins and as nuclear transcriptional factors that activate a diverse set of genes including some that are implicated in malignant progression. In normal cells, STAT proteins transmit cytoplasmic signals from polypeptide cytokines, specifically interferon (IFN) and IL-6, and growth factors that have receptors with intrinsic or associated tyrosine kinase activity, especially EGFR and PDGF.

STATs are activated by phosphorylation at TYR 701, which results in their dimerization and translocation to the nucleus, where they directly regulate gene expression. The phosphorylation may also be mediated by some non-receptor kinases such as SRC and BCR-ABL. Physiologically, ligand-dependent activation of STATs is a transient process lasting for several minutes to several hours. In tumours, their constitutive activation associated with their increased transcriptional initiation and stimulation of cell proliferation has been described. STATs have been shown to inhibit apoptosis by an increase of anti-apoptotic proteins such as BCL-XL and surviving, or a decrease by p53 protein. Moreover, STATs may stimulate expression of cyclins D1 and D2 and c-Myc oncoprotein.

STATs markedly regulate tumour angiogenesis by increased expression of VEGFs and HIF-1. They may also modulate the immune response, when both decrease of pro-inflammatory and stimulation of anti-inflammatory cytokines and chemokines have been demonstrated. STATs are also able to inhibit dendritic cell differentiation, which may result in an induction of cell tolerance. STATs may stimulate migration and invasion of malignant cells via induction of MMP-2 as well. Despite close structural homology of the STAT family, the responses of its individual members differ, depending on activating ligands.

STAT 1 and STAT 2 respond to interferons, STAT 3 to IL-6, STAT 4 and STAT 6 to IL-12/16, whereas STAT 5 is activated mainly by growth factors and prolactin. In malignant melanoma, increased levels of STAT 3 have been found, in comparison with moles, where their concentrations are generally low (Messina et al., 2008). STAT 3 is associated with an increased metastatic potential as its deregulated levels were observed in advanced and metastatic melanomas. In several STAT- negative cell lines, increased apoptosis or G1 arrest have been demonstrated. STAT 3 may affect the response to IFN-alpha adjuvant therapy in melanoma cells. On the one hand, a decreased antiproliferative effect of the cytokine may be observed. On the other hand, its activation may stimulate tumour progression. Similar effects on melanoma formation and progression are seen in STAT 5, which is associated with Bcl-2 overexpression. STAT 1 seems to have an opposite role with its pro-apoptotic and anti-angiogenic effects (Ho et al., 2006). Inducibility of STAT 1 activation significantly and favourably influences disease-free interval and overall survival. By contrast, low expression of STAT 1 after administration of IFN-alpha may mean that the tumour is resistant to the therapy. Wang et al. (2007) suggested to evaluate the STAT 1/STAT 3 ratio, with a high ratio referring to a favourable clinical response. The critical antitumour action seems to be the activation of STAT 1 in immune effector cells.

2.3 Angiogenesis

Angiogenesis is an example of how tumour stroma differs from normal connective tissue. The induction of new blood vessel growth into tumours from pre-existing vascular beds has been reported as a parameter of potential prognostic value in solid tumours, as it may facilitate tumour growth and metastasis (Miller, 2004). By contrast, normal adult vasculature is generally quiescent in nature, with endothelial cells dividing approximately every 10 years. Extensive angiogenesis occurs normally only during the female reproductive cycle and in body repair processes such as wound healing.

It has been shown that for their growth beyond 1-2 mm in size, solid tumours require constant vascular growth and remodelling (Folkman, 1990). In tumour growth, angiogenesis is uncontrolled and unlimited in the time and the transition from the avascular to the vascular phase is called the angiogenic switch, in which the balance between angiogenesis inducers and inhibitors lean towards the former (Ribatti et al., 2007). Studies on human breast carcinomas have even shown that vascular stroma formation occurs before invasion by tumour cells (Gallagher et al., 2005). Tumour vasculature differs from non-tumour not only by an increased number of newly formed vessels, but also by their different structure, organization and function, instead of regular arrangement. The vessels are distributed irregularly, being morphologically heterogeneous and typically thin-walled. The basal membranes are incomplete, partly degraded, with a reduced amount of laminin. They have activated endothelial cells and often lack pericytes in the periphery. The typical hallmark of tumour vasculature is its increased permeability. The origin of the vessels is mostly in activated and proliferating endothelial cells, but they may also be formed from circulation bone marrow progenitor cells.

In melanoma, parallel with progression, tumours acquire a rich vascular network, whereas an increasing number of tumour cells express the laminin receptor, which enables their adhesion to the vascular wall, favouring tumour cells extravasation and metastases (Mahabeleshwar & Byzova, 2007). Melanoma neovascularization has been correlated with poor overall survival, ulceration and increased rate of relapse (Ribatti et al., 2005).

Numerous cytokines, growth factors and extracellular matrix enzymes are associated with neoangiogenesis. They are produced by tumour cells themselves, but their important sources also include stromal elements such as fibroblasts, macrophages, mast cells and endothelial cells, as well as epidermal keratinocytes. The central role is played by the VEGF family via direct stimulation of endothelial cell migration and proliferation, permeability and adhesion among endothelial and tumour cells (Fig. 2).

Very important in tumour angiogenesis is bFGF, which can stimulate vascularization by activation of HIF-1 and the subsequent release of VEGFs or it may also act synergistically with VEGFs, but with distinctive effects on vessel function and with different consequences on tumour oxygenation and viability. Tumours with bFGF expression are characterized by

a striking heterology in blood vessel diameter with numerous large-calibre vessels. FGF down-regulation has a profound impact on microvessel morphology, causing a significant decrease in diameter heterogeneity and disappearance of large-calibre vessels. FGFs do not possess the ability to mediate a chemotactic response for pericytes and myofibroblasts, as is known for VEGFs (Giavazzi et al., 2003).
Other important stimulators of melanoma angiogenesis are PDGF and TGF-beta that directly stimulate VEGF-A secretion, or IGF 2, EGFR, HSP 90, STAT 3 acidosis and hypoxia that stimulate VEGF indirectly through activation of HIF gene transcription.
An important role is also played by placental growth factor (PGF), which binds neuropilin-1 and neuropilin-2 receptors expressed on endothelial cells. In addition, PGF acts through binding to VEGFR-1 inducing the mobilization and recruitment of hematopoietic precursors from bone marrow. Moreover, PGF forms heterodimers with VEGF-A and enhances melanoma angiogenesis by activating VEGFR-2 on endothelial cells (Ria et al., 2010). Endothelial cell migration and vascular permeability may also be induced by IL-6 derived from melanoma cells. It is known that levels of the cytokine dramatically increase in majority of melanomas and are correlated with rapid tumour growth and increased metastatic potential. Integrins overexpressed on melanoma cells may also contribute to melanoma progression and increased metastatic potential by stimulating MMP-2 and MMP-7 (Kuphal et al., 2005). MMP overexpression has been correlated with increased microvascular density, Bcl-2 overexpression and low survival rate. Several studies using either cell lines or animal models have demonstrated that the balance between MMPs and their inhibitors (TIMPs) finally determines melanoma progression. Overexpression of TIMPs reduces melanoma cell invasion, migration, tumour neovascularization and risk of metastases. MMPs and TIMPs may act as regulators of signalling pathways through the cleavage of non-matrix substrates including cytokines, chemokines and growth factors.

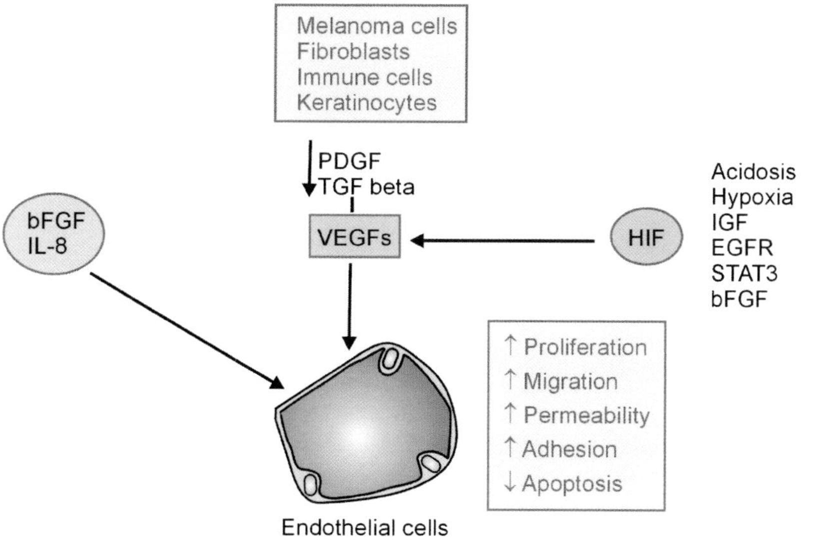

Fig. 2. Main factors involved in melanoma angiogenesis.

2.4 Therapy of malignant melanoma

Up to now, there has been no effective curative treatment of malignant melanoma beyond surgical excision of the primary lesion. Chemotherapy and immunotherapy have thus failed to make an impact on survival in the metastatic setting, while immunotherapy leads to modest improvement in survival in the adjuvant setting. Recent data have shed light on anti-melanoma targeted therapies, whereas successful management of malignant melanoma treatment will benefit from the identification of essential regulatory pathways and molecular switches underlying the plastic tumour cell phenotype and its unique interactions with the microenvironment.

This review presents data on the most promising agents in development. However, it is important to note that all these agents have been used singly or in combination with chemotherapy. It has become quite apparent that the inhibition of one pathway can lead to up-regulation of other related or redundant pathways. This may negatively affect its activity or likely lead to resistance. Therefore, combination of therapies utilizing these agents seems to be most promising approach in the future. Targeted molecular therapeutics are tailored to genetic abnormalities that are associated with tumour progression. These possible targets in melanoma include the RAS-MAPK and PI3K/AKT signal transduction pathways, resistance to apoptosis, the proteasome, melanoma-induced angiogenesis, and immunotherapy (Tab.1). Most agents are in early phase trials, although some have already reached phase III evaluation. As knowledge and experience with targeted therapy advance, new challenges appear to be arising particularly in terms of resistance and appropriate patient selection.

Inhibitors of RAS-MAPK signal transductor pathway	Sorafenib
Inhibitors of the PI3K/AKT signal transduction pathway	Rapamycin and its analogues RAD001, AP23573m and CCI-779 Imatinib mesylat R115777 (Lonafarnib)
Reversing resistance to apoptosis	Oblimerson sodium YM155
Inhibitors of the proteasome	Bortezomib
Anti-angiogenic therapy	Bevacizumab Thalidomide Anti-angiogenic isoforms of VEGF Vitaxin (MEDI-552)
Immunotherapy	Interleukin-2 Interluekin-2 with peptide vaccination Ipilimumab

Table 1. Targeted therapy in malignant melanoma

2.4.1 Inhibitors of the RAS-MAPK signal transduction pathway

The importance of the RAS-MAPK signal transduction pathway for the genesis of melanoma has been highlighted by the discovery of activating BRAF mutations in 60% of cutaneous melanoma. Constitutive activation of the RAS pathway occurs through mutational activation of the RAS oncogene and of downstream components. Numerous inhibitors have been developed including direct inhibitors of RAF such as sorafenib.

Sorafenib

Currently, only preliminary results of small- to medium sized phase II clinical trials are available for metastatic melanoma. In addition to blocking BRAF in tumour cells, it was also found that sorafenib blocks other receptors effectively, including VEGFR2, PDGFR, Flt3 (FMS-like tyrosine kinase), c-Kit and RET receptor kinases. As a single agent, however, Sorafenib seems to have little or no antitumour activity in advanced melanoma patients (Ott et al., 2010). The most promising results so far have been observed for combination of multikinase inhibitor sorafenib and chemotherapy, whereas sorafenib has been found to enhance the response of melanoma to regional chemotherapy. The main toxicities observed were grade 3/4 chemotherapy-related neutropenia and thrombocytopenia. No serious additional toxicity of sorafenib added to carboplatin and paclitaxel was obvious (Kirkwood et al., 2006). Discovery of markers for predicting response to sorafenib might be useful. In melanomas, it has been documented that high VEGFR2 expression is associated with response, whereas high ERK1/2 is associated with resistance (Jilaveanu et al., 2011).

2.4.2 Inhibitors of the PI3K/AKT signal transduction pathway

The phosphoinositide 3-kinase (PI3K) pathway is responsible for the production of 3-phosphoinositide lipid molecules that serve as second messengers in the cells. The pathway controls a cascade of signals that regulates basic cellular properties including survival, motility and apoptosis resistance. Multiple mechanisms for activation of the pathway have been identified such as amplification and overexpression of tyrosine kinase receptors and their ligands, c-kit or mutation of the PTEN tumour suppressor gene. Molecular cloning identified an additional family, whose catalytic domains bear resemblance to PI3K. Based on their sequence homology, the kinases were named PI3K-related kinases (PIKKs). They include several subfamilies such as the TOR family, ataxia telangiectasia gene product and the DNA-dependent protein kinase (Kirkwood et al., 2006). In melanoma therapy, the TOR subfamily is targeted by rapamycin and its analogues RAD001, AP23573m and CCI-779, from which especially the last molecule seems to have a promising therapeutic effect. Toxicity is mild, predominantly comprised of stomatitis, diarrhoea, a skin rash and hyperlipidemia.

R115777 (tipifarnib)

Farnesyl transferase inhibitors (FTIs) inhibit the farnesylation of proteins, which are involved in RAS downstream signalling pathway including the RAF-MEK-ERK (MAPK) and PI3K-AKT-mTOR (AKT). They have a major role in melanoma progression. Current findings suggest that R115777 inhibits mTOR signalling and may therefore represent an effective alternative for melanoma treatment. In particular, the combination of the FTI with the RAS inhibitor sorafenib synergistically inhibited melanoma cell growth, significantly enhanced sorafenib-induced apoptosis and completely suppressed invasive tumour growth.

Imatinib

The presence of c-kit and PDGF on the surface of at least some melanomas encouraged the exploration of these agents in melanoma patients. Imatinib is known as a c-kit and PDGF inhibitor. But an imatinib phase II study showed no objective clinical responses and no patient was progression-free at 6 months. Moreover, significant grade 3 and 4 toxicity was observed (Sosman & Puzanov, 2011). Based on the results, it was concluded that imatinib is inactive as single-agent therapy for metastatic melanoma.

Erlotinib

Erlotinib is a small-molecule inhibitor specific for the EGFR kinase, based on competing with ATP for binding to the intracellular catalytic domain of the receptor kinase, thereby inhibiting autophosphorylation of the receptor critical for binding to downstream signalling proteins. Whereas no influence on tumour cell proliferation was seen with erlotinib monotherapy, preclinical studies demonstrated decreased invasive potential of its combination with bevacizumab (anti-VEGF therapy), providing promising rationale for clinical studies.

2.4.3 Reversing resistance to apoptosis

One of the major consequences of the constitutive activation of the MAPK and PI3K/AKT pathways is the induction of tumour cell resistance to apoptosis. This resistance is believed to be an element of the resistance of melanoma to the classical therapy. Members of the anti-apoptotic Bcl-2 family have been successfully targeted to render tumour cells more susceptible to apoptosis.

Oblimersen sodium is an anti-Bcl-2 oligonucleotide that selectively targets Bcl-2 RNA for degradation by RNase H, thereby decreasing Bcl-2 protein production. Although the drug did not increase overall survival, the application was associated with a significant increase of durable response (exceeding 6 months). The use of oblimersen can improve multiple outcomes in patients with advanced melanoma in combination with dacarbazine. The adverse effects of the therapy include fever, neutropenia and thrombocytopenia (Tawbi & Nimmagadda, 2009).

Another targeted molecule of this class is survivin, which has been found to be highly expressed in most cancers. YM155 is a small molecule that has been demonstrated in preclinical models to suppress the function of survivin.

2.4.4 Inhibitors of the proteasome

The proteasome is a multienzyme complex that serves as a major protein in degradation pathway. The proteasome controls the levels of proteins that are important for cell cycle progression and apoptosis including cyclins, caspases, Bcl-2, and NF-kappaB. In cancers, deregulation of the ubiquitin-proteasome pathway may contribute to tumour progression, drug resistance and altered immune surveillance. Bortezomib was identified as a leading candidate of proteasome inhibitors correlated with growth-inhibitory effect. But a phase II study of bortezomib was terminated due to a lack of responses, and it was concluded that single-agent bortezomib administration was not efficacious in metastatic melanoma. Patients demonstrated grade 3 toxicity including sensory neuropathy, thrombocytopenia, constipation, fatigue, ileus and infections without neutropenia.

2.4.5 Anti-angiogenic therapy

Targeting tumour angiogenesis has several advantages over standard chemotherapy including independence on tumour cell resistance, broad applicability to tumour of different histogenesis and the potential to develop very specific therapies with minimal toxicities, because neoangiogenesis is not required for normal adult tissues. Because VEGF has a key role in tumour angiogenesis, numerous compounds have been developed to counteract its angiogenic effect.

Bevacizumab

Bevacizumab is an anti-VEGF monoclonal antibody, received FDA approval for colorectal cancer therapy in US in 2005 (Kirkwood et al., 2006). Bevacizumab is currently being tested in metastatic melanoma. The effect of bevacizumab on tumour cells is indirect and not necessarily lethal with no direct anti-proliferative effect. This is probably why as a single agent it is not very active, but bevacizumab therapy seems to be promising when combined with anti-proliferative agents. It is combined with low- and high-dose IFN-alpha. This chemotherapy is comprised of carboplatin and paclitaxel, imatinib mesylate, and lastly with erlotinib. The addition of bevacizumab to conventional chemotherapy has been shown to control tumour growth and progression more effectively than chemotherapy alone. This is probably explained by bevacizumab´s ability to dampen the effect of VEGF up-regulation induced by chemotherapy. Adverse response include infrequently increased risk of grade 3/4 hypertension, but also bleeding relating death was documented (Yang et al., 2010).

Anti-angiogenic isoforms of VEGF

These isoforms are generated by differential splicing of exon 8 being widely expressed in normal human tissue but down-regulated in cancer. Endogenous anti-angiogenic VEGF isoforms are cytoprotective for endothelial, epithelial and neuronal cells suggesting both an improved safety profile and an explanation for unpredictable anti-VEGF side effects. It has been demonstrated that administration of recombinant VEGF(165)b inhibits angiogenesis in colorectal carcinoma and malignant melanoma. Splicing factors and their regulatory molecules alter splice site selection and cells can switch from the anti-angiogenic VEGF isoforms to the pro-angiogenic ones. Splice site selection in cancer opens up the possibility of using splicing factor inhibitors as novel anti-angiogenic therapeutics.

Thalidomide

The precise mechanism of thalidomide anti-angiogenic activity remains unknown, however some of its effect may result from blocking angiogenic factors such as VEGF. Thalidomide has also been suggested to have immunomodulating effect by decreasing cyclooxygenase-2 activity. Thalidomide is a potent inhibitor TNF-alpha and decreases the density of TNF-alpha induced adhesion molecules such as ICAM-1 and VCAM. Thalidomide also causes induction of NK (natural killer) cells and increases the levels of IL-1, IL-2 receptors and INF-gamma leading to tumour cell lysis and modulates immune system to induce anticancer activity. Thalidomide has also antiproliferative and proapototic properties through induction of cell growth arrest at the G1 phase, downregulation of NF-kappaB and activation of caspase 8 (Tawbi & Nimmagada, 2009). Because thalidomide alone showed poor activity, various combination have been used in metastatic melanoma. The combinations, however, failed to demonstrate clinical efficacy.

The main toxicities are dose-dependent neuropathy, constipation, anorexia, skin rash, fatigue, but to the most serious belong deep venous thrombosis and pulmonary embolism.

Vitaxin (MEDI-552)

Vitaxin is a monoclonal antibody targeted against the $\alpha v\beta 3$ integrin expressed by endothelial and melanoma cells but not by normal melanocytes. Tumours from patients with stage IV melanoma seem to express the integrin more intensely. MEDI-552 potentially blocks tumour growth causing cell apoptosis and impairment of angiogenesis. The drug alone showed no objective response, whereas the combination with chemotherapy demonstated mild response rate. Grade 3 and 4 adverse events were chiefly neutropenia and thrombocytopenia (Sosman & Puzanov, 2011).

2.4.6 Immunotherapy

IL-2 is a potent immune modulator that stimulates activation and proliferation of T lymphocytes. Treatment with high-dose IL-2 leads to objective tumour responses. Treatment is typically reserved for younger, fitter patients and requires intensive monitoring. The therapy is associated with substantial toxicity including oliguria, renal failure, hepatotoxicity, edema, sepsis, and death (Algazi et al., 2010).

IL-2 with peptide vaccination

Recent data suggest that vaccination against the melanoma peptide antigen gp-100 may improve the efficacy of high-dose IL-2 (Algazi et al., 2010).

Anti-CTLA4 antibodies

The T cell surface protein, CTLA4, competes with CD28 for B7. It is a second surface protein of antigen presenting cells that acts as a costimulatory molecule for T lymphocytes. Binding of CTLA4 to B7 inhibits T-cell proliferation, thus anti-CTLA4 antibodies have been developed to abrogate these inhibitory interactions and break immune tolerance to melanoma. Ipilimumab is an anti-CTLA4 antibody that have led to modest rates of objective tumour response. Common observed toxicities included grade 3 and 4 immune-related events such as colitis, dermatitis, hepatitis, acute pancreatitis and hypophysitis (Di Giacomo et al., 2011).

Combined approaches are already being tested. Some of the most promising combination development are listed in Table 2. All trials are planned with an emphasis on tumour biology. Molecular characterization of the tumour before the therapy followed by treatment examining inhibitory effects on the targets will be critical to understand the clinical results.

Sorafenib + bevacizumab
Sorafenib + CCI-779
Sorafenib + R115777
Bevacizumab + CCI-779
Bevacizumab + R115777

Table 2. The most promising combinations for melanoma therapy

3. Conclusions

Stroma alterations in malignant melanoma are observed already in early stage tumours and are further cumulated as tumours progress. A deeper understanding the factors modulating melanoma microenvironment is necessary and would potentially lead to a new therapeutic approach.

4. Acknowledgement

This work was supported by grants GACR P304/10/1070 and MSM 6198959216 from the Czech Ministry of Education.

5. References

Alami, J.; Williams, BR. & Yeger, H. (2003). Differential expression of E-cadherin and beta catenin in primary and metastatic Wilms's tumours. *Molecular pathology : MP*, Vol. 56, No. 4, (August 2003), pp. 218-225, ISSN 1366-8714

Algazi, AP.; Soon, CW. & Daud, AI. (2010). Treatment of cutaneous melanoma: current approaches and future prospects. *Cancer management and research [electronic resource]*, Vol. 2, (August 2010), pp. 197-211, ISSN 1179-1322

Bellusci, S.; Moens, G.; Gaudino, G.; Comoglio, P.; Nakanuta, T.; Thiery, JP. & Jouanneau, J. (1994). Creation of an hepatocyte growth factor/scatter factor autocrine loop in carcinoma cells induces invasive properties associated with increased tumorigenicity. *Oncogene*, Vol. 9, No. 4, (April 1994), pp.1091-1099, ISSN 0950-9232

Bhowmick, NA.; Neilson, EG.& Moses, HL. (2004). Stromal fibroblasts in cancer initiation and progression. *Nature*, Vol. 432, No.7015, (November 2004), pp.332-337, ISSN 0028-0836.

Bindra, RS. & Glazer, PM. (2005).Genetic instability and the tumor microenvironment: towards the concept of microenvironment-induced mutagenesis. *Mutation research*, Vol. 569, No.1-2, (January 2005), pp. 75-85, ISSN 0027-5107

Braeuer, RR.; Zigler, M.; Villares, GJ.; Dobroff, AS. & Bar-Eli, M. (2011). Transcriptional control of melanoma metastasis: The importance of the tumor microenvironment. *Seminars in cancer biology*, Vo. 21, No. 2, (April 2011), pp. 83-88, ISSN 1044-579X

De Craene, B.; Gilbert, B.; Stove, C.; Bruyneel, E.; van Roy, F. & Berx, G. (2005). The transcription factor snail induces tumor cell invasion through modulation of the epithelial cell differentiation program. *Cancer research*, Vol. 65, No. 14, (July 2005), pp. 6237-6244, ISSN 0008-5472

Delehedde, M.; Sergeant, N.; Lyon, M.; Rudland, PS. & Fernig, DG. (2001). Hepatocyte growth factor/scatter factor stimulates migration of rat mammary fibroblasts through both mitogen-activated protein kinase and phosphatidylinositol 3-kinase/Akt pathways. *European journal of biochemistry/ FEBS*, Vol. 268, No.16, (August 2001), pp. 4423-4429, ISSN 0014-2956

Di Giacomo, AM.; Danielli, R.; Calabrò, L.; Bertocci, E.; Nannicini, C.; Giannarelli, D.; Balestrazzi, A.; Vigni, F.; Riversi, V.; Miracco, C.; Biagioli, M.; Altomonte, M. & Maio M. (2011). Ipilimumab experience in heavily pretreated patients with melanoma in an expanded access program at the University Hospital of Siena (Italy). *Cancer immunology, immunotherapy*, Vol. 60, No. 4, (April 2011), pp. 467-477, ISSN 0340-7004

Diaz, A.; Suarez, E.; Blanco, R.; Lopez, A. & Montero, E. (2009). Epidermal growth factor receptor modulates the tumorigenic potential of melanoma. *Frontiers in bioscience*, (January 2009), Vol. 14, pp. 159-166, ISSN 1945-0494

Dhawan, P.; Singh, AB.; Deane, NG.; No, Y.; Shuku, SR.; Schmidt, C.; Neff, J.; Washington, MK. & Beauchamp, RD. (2005). Claudin-1 regulates cellular transformation and metastatic behavior in colon cancer. *The Journal of clinical investigation*, Vol. 115, No. 7, (July 2005), pp. 1765-1776, ISSN 0021-9738

Ferrara, N.; Houck, KA.; Jakeman, LB.; Winer, J. & Leung,DW. (1991). The vascular endothelial growth factor family of polypeptides. *Journal of cellular biochemistry*, Vol. 47, No. 3, (November 1991), pp. 211-218, ISSN 0730-2312

Folkman J. (1990). What is the evidence that tumors are angiogenesis dependent? *Journal of the National Cancer Institute*, Vol. 82, No. 1, (January 1990), pp. 4-6, ISSN 0027-8874

French, AD.; Fiori, JL.; Camilli, TC.; Leotlela, PD.; O'Connell, MP.; Frank, BP.; Subaran, S.; Indig, FE.; Taub, DD. & Weeraratna, AT. (2009). PKC and PKA phosphorylation affect the subcellular localization of claudin-1 in melanoma cells. *I International journal of medical sciences [electronic ressource*, Vol. 6, No. 2, (2009); pp. 93-101, ISSN 1449-1907

Gallagher, PG.; Bao, Y.; Prorock, A.; Zigrino, P.; Nischt, R.; Politi, V.; Mauch, C.; Dragulev, B. & Fox, JW. (2005). Gene expression profiling reveals cross-talk between melanoma and fibroblasts: implications for host-tumor interactions in metastasis. *Cancer research*, Vol. 65, No. 10, (May 2005), pp. 4134-4146, ISSN 0008-5472

Garcia-Rostan, G.; Tallini, G.; Herrero, A.; D'Aquila, TG.; Carcangiu, ML. & SIMM, DL. (1999). Frequent mutation and nuclear localization of beta-catenin in anaplastic thyroid carcinoma. *Cancer research*. 1999 Apr 15;59(8):1811-1815, ISSN 0008-5472

Giavazzi, R.; Sennino, B.; Coltrini, D.; Varovalo, A.; Dossi, R.; Ronca, R.; Tosatti, MP. & Presta, M. (2003). Distinct role of fibroblast growth factor-2 and vascular endothelial growth factor on tumor growth and angiogenesis. *Journal of pathology informatics*, Vol. 162, No. 6, (June 2003), pp. 1913-1926, ISSN 2153-3539

Gorski, DH.; Leal, AD. & Goydos, JS. (2003). Differential expression of vascular endothelial growth factor-A isoforms at different stages of melanoma progression. *Journal of the American College of Surgeons*, Vol. 197, No. 3, (September 2003), pp. 408-18, ISSN 1072-7515

Goydos, JS. & Gorski, DH. (2003). Vascular endothelial growth factor C mRNA expression correlates with stage of progression in patients with melanoma. *Clinical cancer research : an official journal of the American Association for Cancer Research*, Vol. 9, No. 16 Pt.1, (December 2003), pp.5962-5967, ISSN 1078-0432

Gu, X.; Fu, X.; Yang, Y.; Sun, T. & Juany, L. (2001). Expression characteristics of c-fos, c-myc and bFGF in early burn tissue. *Chinese medical journal*, Vol. 114, No.9, (September 2001), pp. 925-928, ISSN 0366-6999

Halaban, R.; Kwon, BS.; Ghosh, S.; Delli Bovi, P. & Baird, A. (1988). bFGF as an autocrine growth factor for human melanomas. *Oncogene research*, Vol. 3, No.2, (September 1988), pp. 177-186, ISSN 0890-6467

Heenen, M. & Laporte, M. (2003). Molecular markers associated to prognosis of melanoma. *Annales de dermatologie et de vénéréologie*, Vol.130, No. 11, pp. 1025-1031, ISSN 0151-9638

Ho, HH. & Ivashkiv, LB. (2006). Role of STAT3 in type I interferon responses. Negative regulation of STAT1-dependent inflammatory gene activation. *The Journal of biological chemistry*. Vol. 281, No. 20, (May 2006), pp. 14111-14118, ISSN 0021-9258

Hoch, RV. & Soriano, P. (2003). Roles of PDGF in animal development. *Development*, (October 2003), Vol. 130, No. 20, pp. 4769-4784, ISSN 0950-1991

Itoh, N. & Ornitz, DM. (2008). Functional evolutionary history of the mouse Fgf gene family. *Developmental dynamics : an official publication of the American Association of Anatomists* , Vol. 237, No. 1, (January 2008), pp. 18-27, ISSN 1058-8388

Itoh, N. (2010). Hormone-like (endocrine) Fgfs: their evolutionary history and roles in development, metabolism, and disease. *Cell and tissue research*, Vol. 342, No. 1, (October 2010), pp. 1-11, ISSN 0302-766X

Jamal, S. & Schneider, RJ.; UV-induction of keratinocyte endothelin-1 downregulates E-cadherin in melanocytes and melanoma cells. *The Journal of clinical investigation* , Vol. 110, No. 4, (August 2002), pp. 443-452, ISSN 0021-9738

Kirkwood, JM.; Moschos, S. & Wang, W. (2006). Strategies for the development of more effective adjuvant therapy of melanoma: current and future explorations of antibodies, cytokines, vaccines, and combinations. *Clinical cancer research : an official journal of the American Association for Cancer Research.*, Vol. 12, No. 7 Pt 2, (Apríl 2006), pp. 2331s-2336s, ISSN 1078-0432

Kreizenbeck, GM.; Berger. AJ.; Subtil, A.; Rimm, DL. & Gould Rothberg, BE. (2008). Prognostic significance of cadherin-based adhesion molecules in cutaneous malignant melanoma. *Cancer epidemiology, biomarkers and prevention*, Vol. 17, No. 4, (April 2008), pp. 949-958, ISSN 1055-9965

Kudo-Saito, C.; Shirako, H.; Takeuchi, T. & Kawakami, Y. (2009). Cancer metastasis is accelerated through immunosuppression during Snail-induced EMT of cancer cells. *Cancer cell*, Vol. 15, No. 3, (March 2009), pp. 195-206, ISSN 1535-6108

Kuphal, S.; Bauer, R. & Bosserhoff, AK. (2005). Integrin signaling in malignant melanoma. *Cancer metastasis reviews*, Vol. 24, No. 2, (June 2005), pp. 195-222, ISSN 0167-7659

Kurschat, P.; Eming, S.; Nashan, D.; Krieg, T. & Mauch, C. (2007). Early increase in serum levels of the angiogenesis-inhibitor endostatin and of basic fibroblast growth factor in melanoma patients during disease progression. *The British journal of dermatology*, Vol. 156, No. 4, (April 2007), pp. 653-658, ISSN 0007-0963

Kyzas, PA.; Stefanou, D.; Batistatou ,A. & Agnantis, NJ. (2005). Hypoxia-induced tumor angiogenic pathway in head and neck cancer: an in vivo study. *Cancer letters*, Vol. 225, No. 2, (July 2005), pp. 297-304, ISSN

Laakkonen, P.; Waltari, M.; Holopainen, T.; Takahashi, T. Pytowski, B.; Steiner, P.; Hicklin, D.; Persaud, K.; Tonra, JR.; Witte, L. & Alitalo, K. (2007). Vascular endothelial growth factor receptor 3 is involved in tumor angiogenesis and growth. *Cancer research*, Vol. 67, No. 2, (January 2007), pp. 593-599, ISSN 0008-5472

Lázár-Molnár, E.; Hegyesi, H.; Tóth, S. & Falus, A. (2000). Autocrine and paracrine regulation by cytokines and growth factors in melanoma. *Cytokine*, Vol. 12, No. 6, (June 2000), pp. 547-554, ISSN 1043-4666

Lepique, AP.; Mores, MS.; Rocha, KM.; Eichler, CB.; Hajj, GN.; Schwindt, TT. & Armelin, HA. (2004). Sněžana c-Myc protein is stabilized by fibroblast growth factor 2 and destabilized by ACTH to control cell cycle in mouse Y1 adrenocortical cells. *Journal of molecular endokrinology*, Vol. 33, No. 3, (December 2004), pp. 623-638, 0952-5041

Leslie, MC. & Bar-Eli, M. (2005). Regulation of gene expression in melanoma: new approaches for treatment. *Journal of cellular biochemistry*, Vol. 94, No.1, (January 2005), pp. 25-38, ISSN 0730-2312

Lin, K.; Baritaki, S.; Militello, L.; Malaponte, G.; Bevelacqua, Y. & Bonavida, B. (2010). The Role of B-RAF Mutations in Melanoma and the Induction of EMT via Dysregulation of the NF-κB/Snail/RKIP/PTEN. *Genes & cancer*, Vol. 1, No. 5, (May 2010), pp. 409-420, ISSN 1947-6019

Mahabeleshwar, GH. & Bytová, TV. (2007). Angiogenesis in melanoma. *Seminars in oncology*, Vol. 34, No. 6, (December 2007), pp. 555-565, ISSN 0093-7754

Massoumi, R.; Kuphal, S.; Hellerbrand, C.; Haas, B.; Wild, P.; Spruss,T.; Pfeifer, A.; Fässler, R. & Bosserhoff, AK. (2009). Down-regulation of CYLD expression by Snail promotes tumor progression in malignant melanoma. *Journal of experimental medical science*, Vol. 206, No. 1, (January 2009), pp. 221-232, ISSN 0022-099X

Melnikova, VO. & Bar-Eli, M. (2008). Transcriptional control of the melanoma malignant phenotype. *Cancer biology & therapy*, Vol. 7, No. 7 (July 2008), pp. 997-1003, ISSN 1538-4047

Mesina, JL.; Yu, H.; Riker, AI, Monster, PN.; Jove, RL. & Daud, AI. (2008). Activated stat-3 in melanoma. *Cancer control : journal of the Moffitt Cancer Center*, Vol. 15, No. 3, (July 2008), pp. 196-201, ISSN 1073-2748

Miller, KD. (2004). Recent translational research: antiangiogenic therapy for breast cancer - where do we stand? *Breast cancer research : BCR, Vol. 6, No. 3,* (2004), pp. 128-132, ISSN 1465-5411

Moretti, S.; Pinzi, C.; Spallanzani, A.; Berti, E.; Chiarugi. A.; Mazzoli, S.; Fabiani, M. Vallecchi, C. & Herlyn, M. (1999). Immunohistochemical evidence of cytokine networks during progression of human melanocytic lesions. *International journal of cancer. Journal international du cancor*, Vol.84, No. 2, (April 1999), pp. 160-168, ISSN 0020-7136

Mueller, MM. & Fusenig, NE. (2002) Tumor-stroma interactions directing phenotype and progression of epithelial skin tumor cells. *Differentiation; research in biological diversity*, Vol. 70, No. 9-10, (December 2002), pp. 486-497, ISSN 0301-4681

Nakamura, M. & Tokura, Y. (2011). Epithelial-mesenchymal transition in the skin. *Journal of dermatological science*, Vol. 61, No. 1, (January 2011), pp. 7-13, ISSN 0923-1811

Ogawa, Y.; Kawamura, T.; Furuhashi, M.; Tsukamoto, K. & Shimada, S. (2008) Improving chemotherapeutic drug penetration in melanoma by imatinib mesylate. *Journal of dermatological science*,Vol. 51, No. 3, (September 2008), pp. 190-199. ISSN 0923-1811

Ott, PA.; Hamilton, A.; Min, C.; Safarzadeh-Amiri, S.; Goldberg, L.; Yoon, J.; Yee, H.; Buckley, M.; Christos, PJ.; Wright, JJ.; Polsky, D.; Osman, I.; Liebes, L. & Pavlick, AC. (2010). A phase II trial of sorafenib in metastatic melanoma with tissue correlates. *PloS one [electronic resource]*, Vol. 5, No. 12, (December 2010), pp. e15588, ISSN 1932-6203

Pacifico, MD.; Grover, R.; Richman, PI.;, Buffa, F.; Daley, FM. & Wilson, GD. (2005). Identification of P-cadherin in primary melanoma using a tissue microarrayer: prognostic implications in a patient cohort with long-term follow up. *Annals of plastic Surgery*, Vol. 55, No. 3, (September 2005), pp. 316-320, ISSN 0148-7043

Pelletier, F.; Bermont, L.; Puzenat, E.; Blanc, D.; Cairey-Remonnay, S.; Mougin, C.; Laurent, R.; Humbert, P. & Aubin, F.(2005). Circulating vascular endothelial growth factor in cutaneous malignant melanoma. *The British journal of dermatology*, Vol. 152, No. 4, (April 2005), pp. 685-689, ISSN 0007-0963

Perez-Moreno, M. & Fuchs, E. (2006). Catenins: keeping cells from getting their signals crossed. *Developmental cell*, Vol. 11, No. 5, (November 2006), pp. 601-612, ISSN 1534-5807

Perlis, C. & Herlyn, M. (2004) Recent advances in melanoma biology. *The oncologist*, Vol. 9, No. 2, (April 2004), pp. 182-187, ISSN 1083-7159

Proia, DA. & Kuperwasser, C. (2005). Stroma: tumor agonist or antagonist. *Cell cycle*, Vol. 4, No. 8, (August 2005), pp. 1022-1025, ISSN 1538-4101

Prud'homme, GJ. (2007). Pathobiology of transforming growth factor beta in cancer, fibrosis and immunologic disease, and therapeutic considerations. Laboratory investigation; a journal of technical methods and patology, Vol. 87, No. 11, (November 2007), pp. 1077-1091, ISSN 0023-6837

Ria, R.; Reale, A.; Castrovilli, A.; Mangialardi, G.; Dammacco, F.; Ribatti, D. & Vacca, A. (2010). Angiogenesis and progression in human melanoma.*Dermatol Dermatology research and practice [electronic resource]*, Vol. 2010, (2010), pp. 185687, ISSN 1687-6105

Ribatti, D.; Nico, B.; Crivellato, E. & Vacca, A. (2007). The structure of the vascular network of tumors. *Cancer letters*, Vol. 248, No. 1, (Apríl 2007), pp. 18-23, ISSN 0304-3835

Ribatti, D.; Nico, B.; Floris, C.; Mangieri, D.; Piras, F.; Ennas, MG.; Vacca, A. & Sirigu, P. (2005).Microvascular density, vascular endothelial growth factor immunoreactivity in tumor cells, vessel diameter and intussusceptive microvascular growth in primary melanoma.*Oncol Rep*, Vol. 14, No. 1, (June 2005), pp. 81-84, ISSN 1021-335X

Rosen, LS. (2002). Clinical experience with angiogenesis signaling inhibitors: focus on vascular endothelial growth factor (VEGF) blockers. *Cancer control : journal of the Moffitt Cancer Center*,Vol. 9, No.2 Suppl), (Mar-Apr 2002), pp. 36-44, ISSN 1073-2748

Satyamoorthy, K. & Herlyn, M. Cellular and molecular biology of human melanoma. Cancer biology & therapy, Vol.1, No. 1, (Jan-Feb 2002), pp.14-17, ISSN 1538-4047

Shibuya, M.(2006). Differential roles of vascular endothelial growth factor receptor-1 and receptor-2 in angiogenesis. *Journal of biochemistry and molecular biology*, Vol. 39, No. 5, (September 2006), pp. 469-478, ISSN 1225-8687

Silzle, T.; Randolph, G.; Kreutz, M. & Kunz-Schughart, LA. (2004) The fibroblast: sentinel cell and local immune modulator in tumor tissue. *International journal of cancer. Journal international du cancer*, Vol. 108, No. 2, (January 2004), pp. 173-180, ISSN 0020-7136

Sosman, JA. & Puzanov, I. (2006). Molecular targets in melanoma from angiogenesis to apoptosis. *Clinical cancer research : an official journal of the American Association for Cancer Research.*, Vo. 12, No. 7 Pt 2, (Apríl 2006), pp. 2376s-2383s, ISSN 1078-0432

Tawbi, H. & Nimmagadda, N. (2009). Targeted therapy in melanoma. Biologics : targets & therapy, Vol. 3, (2009), pp. 475-484, ISSN 1177-5475

Tetsu, O. & McCormick, F. (1999). Beta-catenin regulates expression of cyclin D1 in colon carcinoma cells. *Nature*, Vol. 398, No. 6726, (April 1999), pp. 422-426, ISSN 0028-0836

Totta, P.; De Cristofaro, R.; Giampietri, C.; Aguzzi, MS.; Faraone, D.; Capogrossi, MC. & Facchiano, A. (2009). Thrombin-mediated impairment of fibroblast growth factor-2 activity. *The FEBS journal*, Vol. 276, No. 12, (June 2009), pp. 3277-3289, ISSN 1742-464X

Ugurel, S.; Rappl, G.; Tilgen, W. & Reinhold , U. (2001). Increased serum concentration of angiogenic factors in malignant melanoma patients correlates with tumor progression and survival. *Journal of clinical oncology : official journal of the American Society of Clinical Oncology*, Vol. 19, No. 2, (January 2001), pp. 577-583, ISSN 0732-183X

Voeller, HJ.; Truica, CI. & Gelmann, EP. (1998). Beta-catenin mutations in human prostate cancer. *Cancer research*, Vol. 58, No. 12, (June 1998), pp. 2520-2523, ISSN 0008-5472

Wang, W.; Edington, HD.; Rao, UN. & Kulic, DM. (2007). Land SR, Ferrone S, Kirkwood JM. Modulation of signal transducers and activators of transcription 1 and 3 signaling in melanoma by high-dose IFNalpha2b. *Clinical cancer research : an official journal of the American Association for Cancer Research*, Vol. 13, No. 5, (March 2007), pp. 1523-1531, ISSN 1078-0432

Weis, WI. & Nelson, WJ. (2006). Re-solving the cadherin-catenin-actin conundrum. *The Journal of biological chemismy*, Vol. 281. No. 47, (November 2006), pp. 35593-35597, ISSN 0021-9258

Yamaguchi, T.; Bando, H.; Mori, T.; Takahashi, K.; Matsumoto, H.; Yasutome, M. Weich, H. & Toi, M. (2007). Overexpression of soluble vascular endothelial growth factor receptor 1 in colorectal cancer: Association with progression and prognosis. *Cancer science*, Vol. 98, No. 3, (March 2007), pp.405-410, ISSN 1347-9032

Yang, H.; Jager, MJ. & Grossniklaus, HE. (2010). Bevacizumab suppression of establishment of micrometastases in experimental ocular melanoma. *Investigative ophthalmology & visual science*, Vol. 51, No. 6, (June 2010), pp. 2835-2842, ISSN 0146-0404

Yu, H. & Jove, R. (2004). The STATs of cancer--new molecular targets come of age. *Nature reviews. Cancor*, Vol. 4, No. 2, (February 20

17

Current Insight Into the Metastatic Process and Melanoma Cell Dissemination

Isabelle Bourgault-Villada[1], Michelle Hong[2], Karen Khoo[2], Muly Tham[2], Benjamin Toh[2], Lu-En Wai[2] and Jean-Pierre Abastado[2]

[1]*AP-HP, Hôpital Ambroise Paré, Boulogne Billancourt and Université de Versailles Saint-Quentin, Versailles,*
[2]*Singapore Immunology Network, BMSI, A-STAR*
[1]*France*
[2]*Singapore*

1. Introduction

Tumour metastasis is the primary cause of death in cancer patients, and cutaneous melanoma is one of the most highly metastatic cancers. While early stage melanomas are almost always curable, despite new and promising treatments (Flaherty et al., 2010; Hodi et al., 2010), advanced unresectable melanomas (Stage III and IV) have a much worse prognosis (Shivers et al., 1998). Similarly, once uveal melanomas have metastasized, they are irremediably lethal (Kivela et al., 2006).

Until recently, tumour cell dissemination was thought to be a late event in cancer progression (Fearon and Vogelstein, 1990). But the advent of sensitive and reliable techniques for detecting circulating tumour cells has revealed that tumour cells can disseminate long before the primary tumour reaches a clinically detectable size. A growing body of convergent studies, including those from our laboratory, confirms this finding in both mice and humans.

If some cancer cells disseminate before diagnosis and if metastases develop from these disseminated cancer cells, how can the treatment of the primary tumour impact disease progression? Or might it be more efficient to focus therapeutic intervention on the control of the disseminated cancer cells?

This new paradigm of early dissemination implies that disseminated cancer cells remain dormant or under control for prolonged periods of time, often for decades, before developing into overt metastases. It is not yet clear why only some disseminated cancer cells develop into metastases and why not all patients with disseminated cancer cells develop metastatic disease. Tumour-initiating cells may only represent a small fraction of disseminated cancer cells, as proposed by the cancer stem cell hypothesis. Alternatively, disseminated cancer cells may require additional adaptation to their new environment or specific signals delivered by their new environment to exit from dormancy (the metastatic niche model). It is certain that the immune system plays a crucial role in controlling the dormancy of disseminated cancer cells, since both acquired and iatrogenic immune

suppression accelerates the development of metastases. A better understanding of the immune mechanisms keeping disseminated melanoma cells in a state of dormancy could lead to the development of interventions to help to slow down cancer progression, improve the treatment of advanced melanomas and increase patient survival. In this regard, immunotherapies such as cancer vaccines or anti-CTLA4 monoclonal antibodies (which prevent T lymphocyte anergy) are likely to be most successful if used to delay the onset of metastasis in patients with dormant disseminated cancer cells and minimal disease.
In this chapter, we will review our current understanding of the metastatic process and discuss possible therapeutic implications. We will address some of the key questions arising from recent data, and their relevance to the treatment of patients. For example, if metastases derive from cancer cells that have already disseminated at the time of diagnosis, how do the size of the primary tumour and the extent of lymph node invasion still predict survival? Are there any features of the primary tumour that correlate with early dissemination, or does the primary tumour itself contribute to the growth of disseminated cancer cells? And how do the answers to these questions impact on our ability to understand which individuals will develop metastatic disease and how to best manage patients for maximum survival benefit?

2. The process of metastasis

Metastasis is a multistep process in which cancer cells derived from the primary tumour migrate to regional or distant sites where they reinitiate their development (Chiang and Massague, 2008). Cancer cells can disseminate directly through the blood or may enter the circulatory system via the lymphatics (Wong and Hynes, 2006). While tumour cells are reliant on the blood for their dissemination, the circulatory system is essentially a hostile environment; intravenously injected cancer cells are cleared after just a few days. To successfully use the blood circulation to colonize a new site, cancer cells must enter the vessel, brave the substantial shear forces of the blood flow and then arrest their movement in order to extravasate and invade the tissue. Lymph may be gentler to disseminated cancer cells, in part because shearing forces there are lower, but lymph nodes may serve as filters. Each type of cancer exhibits a preferred metastatic profile. For example ocular melanomas typically metastasize to the liver; cutaneous melanomas prefer the skin, lungs, liver, bones and brain; while prostate cancers often spread to the bones, liver, brain and lung (Weinberg, 2007). The reasons underlying such preferences for different metastatic sites are important to understand. In some cases the sites where circulating cancer cells stop may be determined by physical restrictions imposed by the vasculature. For example, large cancer cells might be more likely to be arrested in small lung capillaries. Alternatively, chemokines may be exploited by tumour cells in order to actively target specific organs; breast cancer cells expressing CXCR4 are preferentially attracted to organs expressing the CXCR4 ligand CXCL12 (Helbig et al., 2003; Muller et al., 2001). Similarly, expression of CCR7 by B16 melanoma cells increases their homing to lymph nodes and the outgrowth of lymph node metastases (Wiley et al., 2001). However, homing is only a small part of determining the eventual pattern of metastasis, as the ability of the cancer cells to survive and proliferate in their ectopic location is a key factor. This is evidenced by the fact that less than 0.01% of circulating cancer cells will successfully develop into metastases (Chambers et al., 2002; Luzzi et al., 1998). As originally hypothesized in 1889 by Paget, circulating cancer cells will only develop into overt metastasis if they encounter a favourable environment (Paget, 1989).

This has been clearly demonstrated in the RETAAD model of melanoma. RETAAD mice are transgenic for the human RET oncogene, which is specifically expressed in melanocytes. These fully immune-competent mice develop spontaneous uveal melanoma. While cancer cells derived from the primary eye tumor disseminate to all tested organs and tissues, metastases develop almost exclusively in the skin, muscles, lungs and reproductive tract (Eyles et al., 2010).

3. Initial routes of dissemination

Cancer cells disseminate through the blood and the lymph, although it can be challenging to discern which route is preferred by different tumours. Cutaneous melanomas were thought to disseminate mainly through the lymph, but some visceral metastases occur without lymph node invasion. In addition, it had been claimed that ocular melanoma disseminates exclusively through the blood (Clarijs et al., 2001), however, data from both humans and mice now indicate dissemination via the lymph as well (Boonman et al., 2004; Harris et al., 2007). Tumour growth itself is associated with profound alterations of the blood and lymph vessels that may be advantageous to disseminating cells. The growth of a tumour requires the development of new blood vessels in and around the lesion. These newly-generated vessels convey nutrients and oxygen to the growing tumour, but are also used by cancer cells to escape the primary tumour and disseminate. The relatively high leakiness of tumour-associated blood vessels may also facilitate cancer cell intravasation. Similarly, tumour growth is associated with lymphangiogenesis (the growth of lymphatic vessels) both within and around the tumour and in the tumour-draining lymph node. Using the RETAAD model of spontaneous melanoma, we found that the growth of lymphatic vessels precedes melanoma cell migration to the draining lymph node and correlates with the size of the primary tumour. This suggests that the primary tumour secretes factors which favour lymphangiogenesis in the draining lymph node. Tumour tissues are also chronically inflamed, and inflammation encourages both angiogenesis and lymphangiogenesis. This may, at least in part, contribute to the well-established link between tumour inflammation and cancer progression. It is therefore reasonable to consider that melanomas can disseminate through the lymph or through the blood and that the actual route of dissemination may vary according to local conditions.

4. Early cancer cell dissemination

Until recently, cancer cell dissemination was thought to be a late event in disease progression (Fearon and Vogelstein, 1990; Fidler and Hart, 1982; Fidler and Kripke, 1977). Metastasis was believed to occur once the primary tumour had reached a certain size. Indeed the risk of metastatic disease increases with the size of the primary tumour. The recent advent of sensitive and reliable techniques to detect circulating tumour cells has revealed that tumour cells can in fact disseminate long before the primary tumour reaches a clinically detectable size (Pantel and Brakenhoff, 2004; Wharton et al., 1999). In the RETAAD model, melanoma cells can be detected in all tissues and organs by the time mice are two weeks of age, while the primary tumour is only visible after 5 to 8 weeks. In human uveal melanoma, calculation of tumour doubling times also suggests that metastases derive from tumour cells that disseminate on average three years before the primary tumour is diagnosed (Eskelin et al., 2000). Moreover, at the time of dissemination, the size of the primary tumour represents less than 1% of its final size at the time of diagnosis. Even though 98% of patients are free of metastasis at the time of surgery, about 50% of them will eventually succumb to metastatic disease (Eskelin et al., 2000). Similar conclusions have been reached in other types of cancer. For example, whole exome sequencing of pancreatic tumours has confirmed that metastases derive from cells that disseminate roughly three years before diagnosis (Luebeck, 2010). Strikingly, Vinokurava et al. reported five cases of patients with non-invasive cervical intraepithelial neoplasia (CIN) who relapsed 4 to 12 years after radical hysterectomy. Cervical tumours are caused by random integration of the human papilloma virus (HPV) genome, and mapping the site of HPV integration confirmed a common clonal origin of the primary lesions (CIN) and metachronous metastases (Vinokurova et al., 2005). Remarkably this implies that transformed cells can even spread from pre-invasive cervical lesions, and go on to cause clinical disease. In summary, a growing body of convergent findings in both mice and humans shows that tumour cell dissemination can be an early event in cancer progression and sometimes occurs even before the primary tumour is diagnosed.

5. What drives cancer cell dissemination?

Cancer cells within the primary tumour compete with each other for space and nutrients. The evolution of cancer cells is therefore likely to be affected by this competition, and selection should favour cancer cells with advantageous characteristics (Gatenby and Gillies, 2008). What could be the selective pressure responsible for the early acquisition of a motile phenotype by the cancer cells in the primary tumour? If disseminated cancer cells remain dormant for prolonged periods of time, metastasis is unlikely to be positively selected: selection is blind to the future. Perhaps unexpectedly, hints may come from the analysis of tumour shapes. Primary tumours often display a multinodular, papilloma-like structure. The shape of the primary tumour correlates with the risk of disease progression (Goutzanis et al., 2008; Tambasco and Magliocco, 2008) and is therefore linked to metastatic propensity. In silico modelling suggests that tumour multinodularity results from the competition among cancer cells for nutrients (Ferreira et al., 2002; Mallet and De Pillis, 2006). This competition is particularly keen in non-vascularised tumours. We showed that such multinodular growth is determined by intercellular adhesion, adhesion between cells and the extra-cellular matrix and cancer cell motility (Narang, 2011). Importantly, these in silico models show that under nutrient-limited conditions, tumour growth is faster if it is multinodular. Therefore, acquisition of a metastatic phenotype could be selected because it favours the growth of the primary tumour (Norton, 2005); dissemination would be more of an accidental by-product resulting from the acquisition of cellular behaviours aimed at benefitting the primary tumour. This would explain why the risk of metastasis correlates with primary tumour size.

6. Cancer cell dissemination and mesenchymal transition

In order to disseminate, cancer cells need to detach from the primary tumour and become motile. Cancer cells must therefore decrease expression of various adhesion molecules such as cadherins and catenins, increase expression of proteases (e.g. matrix metalloproteinases

or MMP) able to degrade the extracellular matrix, and enhance their motility. So how do cancer cells simultaneously acquire this panel of phenotypic changes? Epithelial to Mesenchymal transition (EMT) is often considered the first step of cancer cell progression toward metastasis. The term EMT traditionally refers to the formation of mesenchymal cells (loosely adherent, often motile cells embedded in the extracellular matrix) from a primitive epithelium during embryonic development (Thiery, 2002). The process of EMT is associated with down-regulation of cell surface molecules involved in intercellular contacts and up-regulation of mesenchymal markers (vimentin, N-cadherin). Similar changes are indeed observed during carcinoma progression. It is therefore likely that the mechanism by which sessile carcinoma cells become motile resembles EMT. Even though melanocytes are not of epithelial origin, expression of mesenchymal markers correlates with tumour aggressiveness and propensity to metastasize.
Melanocytes and melanocyte stem cells derive from melanoblasts, a non-pigmented cell population which migrates from the neural crest during embryonic development (Thomas and Erickson, 2008). Therefore, acquisition of a motile phenotype by melanoma cells only requires re-expression of a previously silenced pathway. Weinberg and coll. have shown that ectopic expression of just a few genes in human melanocytes was sufficient to make them tumourigenic and highly metastatic (Gupta et al., 2005). The same set of genes transferred into fibroblasts or epithelial cells resulted in only localized tumour formation. Therefore, cells of melanocytic origin are more prone to undergo mesenchymal transition, and lineage-specific factors contribute to the tendency of melanoma to metastasize.

7. Clinical relevance

If cancer cell dissemination can occur early on during disease development, it is likely that many patients already have cancer cells disseminated throughout their body at diagnosis. A recent meta-analysis including 38,918 patients with cutaneous melanoma showed that patients whose primary tumour had a Breslow's thickness above 1 mm, was ulcerated and/or had a mitotic index above 1 mitose / mm^2 were at higher risk of melanoma-related death, even in the absence of invaded nodes and metastasis (Balch et al., 2009). Because metastases have a long latency period, it has been hypothesized that these early disseminating cancer cells were unable to develop into metastases, supporting the traditional notion that the spread of cells causing metastases occurred late during disease. Accordingly, accumulation of additional genetic changes would be required for the development of full-blown metastatic potential. However, recent studies in mouse models of breast cancer and melanoma have shown that early disseminating cancer cells are fully competent to develop into metastases (Eyles et al., 2010; Husemann et al., 2008). Moreover, genetic comparison of primary human tumours, disseminated cancer cells and metastases confirmed that metastases do derive from early disseminating cancer cells (Klein, 2009). The interesting question of the factors controlling this long-term latency of early disseminated tumour cells is then raised. The immune system is likely to play a major role, but if so, does the treatment of the primary tumour impact disease progression and is there really any benefit from removing the tumour-draining lymph node? More than 30 years ago, B. Fisher predicted that if cancer (in this case, breast cancer) were a systemic disease from its inception, the extent of local treatment should not affect patient survival (Fisher, 1980). Several of his predictions also hold true for melanoma, in particular for primary tumours presenting with pejorative prognostic factors.

8. Tumour excision

It has been known for more than 50 years that melanoma cells often disseminate locally (up to 5 cm away) around the primary tumour. Initially it seemed logical to excise these distant cells by using a large enough surgical margin. A first randomised prospective trial was conducted in the 1970's to determine whether there was any significant clinical benefit associated with a 5 cm margin excision compared to a 2 cm margin (Wargo and Tanabe, 2009). No statistically significant difference was observed in distant metastases or overall survival. This conclusion was counter-intuitive and difficult to accept, and so at least four other prospective randomized studies were conducted between 1980 and 2000 to determine the optimal margin of excision for cutaneous melanomas (Balch et al., 2001; Balch et al., 1993; Cohn-Cedermark et al., 2000; Ringborg et al., 1996; Thomas et al., 2004; Veronesi and Cascinelli, 1991; Veronesi et al., 1988). These trials compared various margins from 1 to 5 cm, in melanomas of different thickness and in a total of 2,861 patients. None of these trials found any survival benefit associated with the larger excision. Similarly, the survival of patients with anal melanoma is not different whether they are treated by local tumour excision or rectal resection (Kiran et al., 2010). Regardless, the consensus in clinical practice is to use large margins to excise thick primary tumours.

Besides their obvious implications for melanoma management, these observations lead to important theoretical conclusions. There is no doubt that some cancer cells are left behind after a narrow excision of the primary tumour, but the patient is able to control these cancer cells to the extent that they do not affect patient survival. Alternatively, these cells may not play a major role in the development of the distant metastases that cause patient death because metastases develop from cancer cells that have already disseminated at the time of surgery, and not from residual cancer cells left in the vicinity of the primary tumour. But since surgery cures most early stage patients, one has to conclude that only some primary tumours have the properties that favour metastases, and that most patients are able to control the disseminated cancer cells. A systemic biological process, for example the immune system, is therefore able to prevent the proliferation of cancer cells, provided they are not too numerous.

9. Sentinel lymph node biopsy

Infiltration of melanoma cells in the tumour-draining lymph node has also been extensively studied. The results of sentinel lymph node biopsy followed by examination using H&E stains and immunohistochemistry is one of the most reliable predictors of patient survival. However, it is now recognized that not all tumour-draining lymph nodes containing disseminated cancer cells will progress into palpable metastases. The number and localisation of the disseminated cancer cells within the lymph node seem to be important. In one study, 50% of patients with thin primary tumours had tumour-draining lymph nodes containing melanoma cells, as judged by RT-PCR, but 85% of them survived more than 5 years (Shivers et al., 1998). In addition, the melanoma-specific survival of patients with subcapsular deposits less than 1 mm in diameter is the same as that of patients with negative lymph nodes (Starz et al., 2004). However it is not clear whether these few cells are fully-fledged melanoma cells or whether they represent sub-capsular nevi. In any case, the patient's own immune system is probably able to cope with a limited number of cancer cells disseminated in the draining lymph node. One could even argue that the presence of cancer cells in the draining lymph node might facilitate the induction of an anti-melanoma immune response (Ochsenbein et al., 2001). Using various mouse tumour models, including the B16 melanoma model, these authors suggested that tumour-specific induction of protective cytotoxic T cells (CTLs) could depend on sufficient tumour cells reaching secondary lymphatic organs. However, whether this finding holds for human tumours is unclear.

For almost 20 years, patients with intermediate or thick primary melanomas (Breslow's depth above 1 mm) have been advised to undergo sentinel lymph node biopsy (SLNBx) and this procedure has become a standard approach (Wargo and Tanabe, 2009). When metastatic cells are identified in the sentinel lymph node, a complete regional lymph node dissection (CRLND) is performed. Indeed, the result of SLNBx and CRLND accurately predicts patient survival. The 5-year survival of patients with positive SLNBx (72.3%) is significantly shorter than that of patients with negative SLNBx (90.2%; $p<0.001$) (Baldwin et al., 2010). In addition, the efficacy of adoptive immune therapy depends on the number of metastatic lymph nodes (Khammari et al., 2007). Patients presenting with a single metastatic lymph node benefit from adoptive treatment with tumour-infiltrating lymphocytes (prolonged overall survival $p=0.0125$; decreased relapse rate $p=0.022$), but not those with more than one invaded node. However, four controlled studies have shown that there is no survival benefit associated with early removal of non-palpable lymph nodes (Balch et al., 2000; Cascinelli et al., 1998; Sim et al., 1986; Veronesi et al., 1982; Zitelli, 2008). The prospective randomized Multi-centre Selective Lymphadenectomy Trial (MSLT-1), conducted between 1994 and 2002 with 1269 patients, clearly confirmed that there is no survival benefit for patients undergoing wide excision and SLNBx with immediate CRLND if nodal micrometastases were detected compared to those undergoing wide excision and postoperative observation of regional lymph nodes with therapeutic lymph node dissection (lymphadenectomy) if nodal relapse occurred (Baldwin et al., 2010; Morton et al., 2006). The Sunbelt Melanoma trial analysed the survival of patients with minimal infiltration of the sentinel lymph node by melanoma cells. Patients whose SLNBx was negative by standard immunopathology/immunochemistry methods, but positive by RT-PCR, were randomized to observation or CRLND treatment; but interestingly, no difference in overall survival was found between the two groups (McMasters et al., 2001). In conclusion, while lymph node invasion correlates with shorter survival, early removal of non-palpable lymph nodes containing micrometastases does not improve survival. It is still unknown whether removal of palpable metastatic lymph nodes improves survival, but this question is being addressed by the MSLT-II trial.

Similar conclusions have been reached in studies on other types of cancer. For example, Sleeman et al. analysed 7 randomized clinical studies, totalling 3,351 patients with breast cancer (Sleeman et al., 2011). None of these studies showed any overall survival or disease-free survival benefit from removing tumour-draining lymph nodes. A recent report also compared 891 breast cancer patients with metastasis-containing sentinel lymph nodes undergoing either sentinel lymph node dissection alone or complete axillary lymph node dissection (Giuliano et al., 2011). Five years after surgery, no significant difference in the rates of overall survival (91.8% vs 92.5%) or disease-free survival (82.2% vs 83.9%) was observed. In the same indication, Bidart et al. found that 82% of patients with tumour cells in the bone marrow do not relapse at least for the 6 years of the study (Bidard et al., 2008). Veronesi et al. performed a meta-analysis with an average follow up of 30 years. While the presence of tumour cells in the internal lymph nodes was a strong predictor of patient survival, extensive lymphadenectomy did not change survival (Veronesi et al., 1999). Collectively, these observations confirm that patients are able to control disseminated cancer cells for prolonged period of times, provided they are not too numerous.

10. Reasons to remove the tumour-draining lymph nodes

Despite the lack of clinical evidence supporting a benefit of extensive lymph node dissection, there are theoretical reasons to believe that removal of invaded draining lymph nodes may be beneficial. Firstly, cancer cells secrete factors that facilitate metastasis. Cytokines such as TGF-β, which is abundantly secreted by tumours can suppress the anti-tumour immune response. Tumours also secrete GM-CSF which plays a crucial role in the accumulation of myeloid-derived suppressor cells (MDSC). We found that tumours in RETAAD mice also secrete chemokines that attract MDSC. MDSC favour tumour cell proliferation, metastasis, and dampen the immune response. In melanoma patients, regulatory T cells, which suppress the immune response, are twice as frequent in metastatic lymph nodes as in tumour-free nodes (Viguier et al., 2004). Primary tumours also secrete growth factors that directly stimulate the proliferation of disseminated cancer cells or micrometastases. Tumour supernatants have also been involved in the development of the cellular clusters of non-tumoural cells that facilitate organ colonization by the cancer cells. These clusters have been referred to as pre-metastatic niches (Kaplan et al., 2005). In summary, large tumour masses participate in immunosuppression to favour tumour growth, and some studies show that surgery to remove such masses could improve the functionality of the anti-tumour response (Tatsumi et al., 2002). It is therefore difficult to argue against the removal of any detectable tumour cell.

11. Reasons not to remove tumour-draining lymph nodes

There are also theoretical reasons explaining why lymph node removal does not improve survival, or could even be deleterious. Surgery may sometimes result in the spread of cancer cells into the circulation, as has been shown in colorectal and prostate cancers (Yamaguchi et al., 2000). This has also been reported for cutaneous and uveal melanoma (De Giorgi et al., 2010). Surgery also induces inflammation, and the link between inflammation and cancer progression is well established. Wound healing is known to induce local production of TGFβ and bFGF, which promotes the growth of B16 tumours in experimental models (Hofer et al., 1998). Similarly, trauma facilitates the implantation of mammary carcinoma cells (Murthy et al., 1989). Alteration of the lymphatic drainage may further worsen these effects. Lymph node removal reduces fluid drainage and favours oedema development which may also cause increased inflammation. While inflammation stimulates lymphangiogenesis (Angeli and Randolph, 2006), inhibitors of lymphangiogenesis have been shown to increase local inflammation. Conversely, stimulation of lymphangiogenesis reduces chronic skin inflammation (Huggenberger et al., 2010). All these studies are consistent with the idea that inefficient drainage increases inflammation. Inflammation induced by extensive surgery could then favour angiogenesis and suppress the anti-tumour immune response. Since suppression of angiogenesis (Holmgren et al., 1995; Naumov et al., 2006) and the immune response (Eyles et al., 2010) are considered the main mechanisms controlling dormancy of disseminated cancer cells, this would explain how surgery can influence the outgrowth of distant micrometastases.

In fact, there is substantial evidence, especially in colorectal cancer, that surgery contributes to metastasis (van der Bij et al., 2009). In melanoma patients, similar observations have been reported. Tseng et al noted the cases of two patients with giant upper extremity melanomas and no sign of progression for years. However, six months after surgery, both patients developed extensive metastatic disease (Tseng et al., 2009). Using the RETAAD model of uveal melanoma, we found that early removal of the primary eye tumour does not always reduce metastasis. In a few instances, incomplete enucleation was followed by rapid local recurrence, accelerated tumour growth and increased dissemination. Similarly, removal of the mandibular lymph node which drains the primary eye tumour resulted in increased angiogenesis and accelerated melanoma cell dissemination in this model. Taken together, these observations indicate that surgery aimed at removing the primary tumour and cancer cells disseminated locally could stimulate the growth of distant metastases. To address this issue and the considerable morbidity associated with CRLND, Murali et al. recently established a set of clinical and histo-pathological features predicting the negativity of non-sentinel lymph nodes (Murali et al., 2010). Murali et al. recommend low risk patients to be spared unnecessary surgery.

12. Immune surveillance and immune control of disseminated cancer cells

The immune surveillance theory originally proposed by L. Thomas (Thomas, 1959) and F. Burnet (Burnet, 1970) in the 50's proposes that the immune system plays a critical role in preventing cancer development and progression. This idea was initially broadly accepted, and then almost universally rejected, until the last decade when R. Schreiber, M. Smyth and their colleagues conclusively showed that the immune system controls not only the incidence of specific cancers in mice, but also interacts in a complex way with the tumour to shape its immune profile (Dunn et al., 2004). It is now recognized that both immunodeficient animals (Swann and Smyth, 2007) and patients under immunosuppression (Peto, 2001) have a higher incidence of cancer. The immune system is not only important to eliminate subclinical primary tumours. It plays a crucial role in controlling the dormancy of disseminated cancer cells, since immune suppression also accelerates the development of metastases. While pregnancy does not increase the risk of melanoma (Lens and Bataille, 2008), it may accelerate the development of metastatic disease (Sato et al., 2008; Youn et al., 2010). We also showed that RETAAD mice depleted of $CD8^+$ T cells develop visceral metastases much earlier than control mice (Eyles et al., 2010; Lengagne et al., 2008). Pathological examination of the lungs of CD8-depleted animals revealed a higher density of proliferating cancer cells. This suggests that $CD8^+$ T cells control metastatic dormancy through their anti-proliferative activity (for example by secreting cytostatic cytokines) rather than by direct cytotoxicity. Striking evidence for a role of the immune system in controlling disseminated cancer cells in humans comes from iatrogenic cases of allogeneic melanoma after organ transplantation (Penn, 1996). MacKie et al. reported two cases of such melanoma developing in patients grafted with the kidneys of a donor who had been treated for superficial melanoma without any detectable metastases 16 years before the transplantation (MacKie et al., 2003). Some disseminated melanoma cells apparently survived in the donor for this long period of time and escaped from dormancy only after transplantation into the immune-suppressed recipients. Tumour cells can escape immune control through a variety of mechanisms (Mapara and Sykes, 2004; Zou, 2005). In fact, the development of metastases in cancer patients with active anti-tumour immune responses is one of the most disturbing paradoxes of cancer immunology. Indeed, in most cancer patients, anti-tumour T cell responses can be detected. For the first time in 2010, the US Food and Drug Administration approved a therapeutic cancer vaccine, Provenge, to treat asymptomatic or minimally symptomatic metastatic hormone-refractory prostate cancer (Kantoff et al., 2010). While significant progress has been made in increasing the strength and quality of the immune response induced by candidate cancer vaccines, clinical benefits are still limited (Rosenberg et al., 2004). Cancer vaccines have most frequently been tested in advanced cancer patients with bulky tumours. Work in preclinical models however, suggests that such vaccines may be more efficient at controlling the dormancy of disseminated cancer cells.

13. Conclusion

Most patients with early stage melanoma are cured by local surgery. However, extensive surgical treatment of more advanced patients may not always be beneficial because some primary tumour cells have the capacity to disseminate early during disease progression. Distant metastases may not develop from nodal metastases detected at diagnosis but rather from cancer cells already disseminated throughout the body. Once the main tumoural mass has been removed, the immune system of the patient should be able to cope with the residual cancer cells. In these patients, extensive surgery may even accelerate the outgrowth of distant metastases by adversely affecting the immune response and favouring the escape of disseminated cancer cells from dormancy. Collectively, the data presented in this review plead for a limited surgery of the primary tumour combined with systemic adjuvant therapy.

14. References

Angeli, V., and Randolph, G.J. (2006). Inflammation, lymphatic function, and dendritic cell migration. Lymphat Res Biol *4*, 217-228.

Balch, C.M., Gershenwald, J.E., Soong, S.J., Thompson, J.F., Atkins, M.B., Byrd, D.R., Buzaid, A.C., Cochran, A.J., Coit, D.G., Ding, S., *et al.* (2009). Final version of 2009 AJCC melanoma staging and classification. J Clin Oncol *27*, 6199-6206.

Balch, C.M., Soong, S., Ross, M.I., Urist, M.M., Karakousis, C.P., Temple, W.J., Mihm, M.C., Barnhill, R.L., Jewell, W.R., Wanebo, H.J., and Harrison, R. (2000). Long-term results of a multi-institutional randomized trial comparing prognostic factors and surgical results for intermediate thickness melanomas (1.0 to 4.0 mm). Intergroup Melanoma Surgical Trial. Ann Surg Oncol *7*, 87-97.

Balch, C.M., Soong, S.J., Smith, T., Ross, M.I., Urist, M.M., Karakousis, C.P., Temple, W.J., Mihm, M.C., Barnhill, R.L., Jewell, W.R., *et al.* (2001). Long-term results of a prospective surgical trial comparing 2 cm vs. 4 cm excision margins for 740 patients with 1-4 mm melanomas. Ann Surg Oncol *8*, 101-108.

Balch, C.M., Urist, M.M., Karakousis, C.P., Smith, T.J., Temple, W.J., Drzewiecki, K., Jewell, W.R., Bartolucci, A.A., Mihm, M.C., Jr., Barnhill, R., and et al. (1993). Efficacy of 2-cm surgical margins for intermediate-thickness melanomas (1 to 4 mm). Results of a multi-institutional randomized surgical trial. Ann Surg *218*, 262-267; discussion 267-269.

Baldwin, B.T., Cherpelis, B.S., Sondak, V., and Fenske, N.A. (2010). Sentinel lymph node biopsy in melanoma: Facts and controversies. Clin Dermatol *28*, 319-323.

Bidard, F.C., Vincent-Salomon, A., Gomme, S., Nos, C., de Rycke, Y., Thiery, J.P., Sigal-Zafrani, B., Mignot, L., Sastre-Garau, X., and Pierga, J.Y. (2008). Disseminated tumor cells of breast cancer patients: a strong prognostic factor for distant and local relapse. Clin Cancer Res *14*, 3306-3311.

Boonman, Z.F., van Mierlo, G.J., Fransen, M.F., Franken, K.L., Offringa, R., Melief, C.J., Jager, M.J., and Toes, R.E. (2004). Intraocular tumor antigen drains specifically to submandibular lymph nodes, resulting in an abortive cytotoxic T cell reaction. J Immunol *172*, 1567-1574.

Burnet, F.M. (1970). The concept of immunological surveillance. Prog Exp Tumor Res *13*, 1-27.

Cascinelli, N., Morabito, A., Santinami, M., MacKie, R.M., and Belli, F. (1998). Immediate or delayed dissection of regional nodes in patients with melanoma of the trunk: a randomised trial. WHO Melanoma Programme. Lancet *351*, 793-796.

Chambers, A.F., Groom, A.C., and MacDonald, I.C. (2002). Dissemination and growth of cancer cells in metastatic sites. Nat Rev Cancer *2*, 563-572.

Chiang, A.C., and Massague, J. (2008). Molecular basis of metastasis. N Engl J Med *359*, 2814-2823.

Clarijs, R., Schalkwijk, L., Ruiter, D.J., and de Waal, R.M. (2001). Lack of lymphangiogenesis despite coexpression of VEGF-C and its receptor Flt-4 in uveal melanoma. Invest Ophthalmol Vis Sci *42*, 1422-1428.

Cohn-Cedermark, G., Rutqvist, L.E., Andersson, R., Breivald, M., Ingvar, C., Johansson, H., Jonsson, P.E., Krysander, L., Lindholm, C., and Ringborg, U. (2000). Long term results of a randomized study by the Swedish Melanoma Study Group on 2-cm versus 5-cm resection margins for patients with cutaneous melanoma with a tumor thickness of 0.8-2.0 mm. Cancer *89*, 1495-1501.

De Giorgi, V., Pinzani, P., Salvianti, F., Panelos, J., Paglierani, M., Janowska, A., Grazzini, M., Wechsler, J., Orlando, C., Santucci, M., *et al.* (2010). Application of a filtration- and isolation-by-size technique for the detection of circulating tumor cells in cutaneous melanoma. J Invest Dermatol *130*, 2440-2447.

Dunn, G.P., Old, L.J., and Schreiber, R.D. (2004). The three Es of cancer immunoediting. Annu Rev Immunol *22*, 329-360.

Eskelin, S., Pyrhonen, S., Summanen, P., Hahka-Kemppinen, M., and Kivela, T. (2000). Tumor doubling times in metastatic malignant melanoma of the uvea: tumor progression before and after treatment. Ophthalmology *107*, 1443-1449.

Eyles, J., Puaux, A.L., Wang, X., Toh, B., Prakash, C., Hong, M., Tan, T.G., Zheng, L., Ong, L.C., Jin, Y., *et al.* (2010). Tumor cells disseminate early, but immunosurveillance limits metastatic outgrowth, in a mouse model of melanoma. J Clin Invest *120*, 2030-2039.

Fearon, E.R., and Vogelstein, B. (1990). A genetic model for colorectal tumorigenesis. Cell *61*, 759-767.

Ferreira, S.C., Jr., Martins, M.L., and Vilela, M.J. (2002). Reaction-diffusion model for the growth of avascular tumor. Phys Rev E Stat Nonlin Soft Matter Phys *65*, 021907.

Fidler, I.J., and Hart, I.R. (1982). Biological diversity in metastatic neoplasms: origins and implications. Science *217*, 998-1003.

Fidler, I.J., and Kripke, M.L. (1977). Metastasis results from preexisting variant cells within a malignant tumor. Science *197*, 893-895.

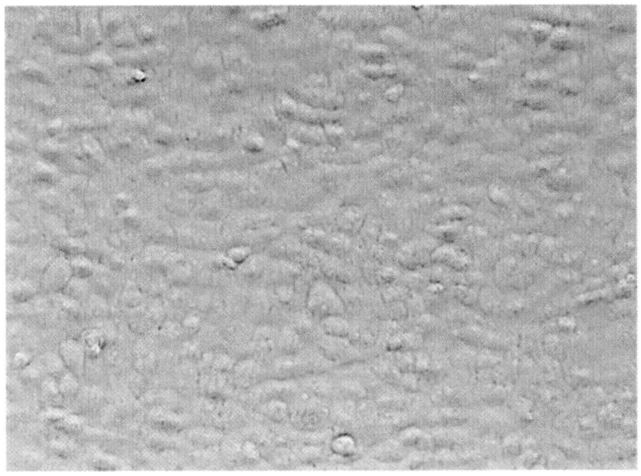

Fig. 1. Morphology of 2D C918 uveal melanoma cultures. In traditional 2D cultures, C918 uveal melanoma cells formed a monolayer of cells on the bottom surface of the tissue culture wells (200x magnification).

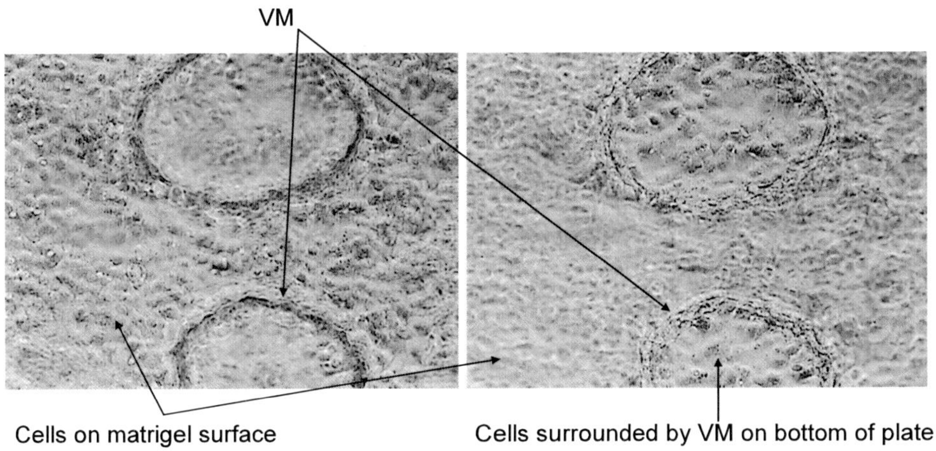

Fig. 2. Morphology of 3D C918 uveal melanoma cultures. Pictures of a 3D C918 uveal melanoma culture with focus either on cells growing on the Matrigel surface (left panel) or on cells growing on the bottom of the tissue culture well (right panel). Vasculogenic mimicry (VM) patterns are also marked by arrows (200x magnification).

3.2 VM-forming melanoma cells have increased resistance against cisplatin

Starting 4 to 5 days after the initiation of cultures, when 2D cultures formed monolayers and cells in 3D cultures formed morphologically distinct tumor cell subpopulations including VM patterns, cultures were exposed to various concentrations of cisplatin (Del Bello et al., 2003; Feldman et al., 2004; Bowden et al., 2010) and observed daily for toxicity. Cisplatin concentrations tested in the experiments ranged from 30 to 300 μM and fresh culture media containing cisplatin were added to the cultures daily. Control cultures not exposed to cisplatin remained viable and demonstrated growth. However, cultures exposed to cisplatin demonstrated dose dependant toxicity (Table 1). Interestingly, we found that VM-forming tumor cells demonstrated prolonged survival following cisplatin treatment relative to other tumor cell subpopulations in 3D cultures and relative to cells grown in 2D (Table 1, Figs 3 to 8). For instance, it took 6 days until 300 μM cisplatin destroyed more than 99% of cells forming VM in 3D cultures while other cell subpopulations in 3D cultures and cells grown in 2D cultures were destroyed by 4 and 3 days, respectively (Table 1). Even more pronounced differences were detected at 100 μM cisplatin concentrations as destruction of VM-forming tumor cells never reached 99% in 3D cultures during a 7-day observation period while other cell subpopulations in 3D cultures and cells grown in 2D cultures were destroyed by 4 and 3 days, respectively (Table 1). These findings indicate that VM-forming tumor cells have increased resistance against the cytotoxic effects of cisplatin in 3D uveal melanoma cultures.

	2D	**3D**		
	Cells on surface of plate	Cells on surface of Matrigel	VM	Cells on surface of plate
No CPL Control	NA (>7 days)	NA (>7 days)	NA (>7 days)	NA (>7 days)
CPL 30 μM	NA (>7 days)	NA (>7 days)	NA (>7 days)	NA (>7 days)
CPL 100 μM	3 days	4 days	NA (>7 days)	4 days
CPL 300 μM	3 days	4 days	6 days	4 days

Table 1. Time (days) elapsed from the initiation of cisplatin treatment to destruction of more than 99% of C918 uveal melanoma cells in 2D cultures and destruction of more than 99% of various C918 cell subpopulations in 3D cultures during a 7-day observation period. Abbreviations: 2D = two-dimensional cultures; 3D = three-dimensional cultures; VM = cells forming vasculogenic mimicry patterns; CPL = cisplatin; NA (>7 days) = not applicable, cell death did not reach 99% during the 7-day observation period.

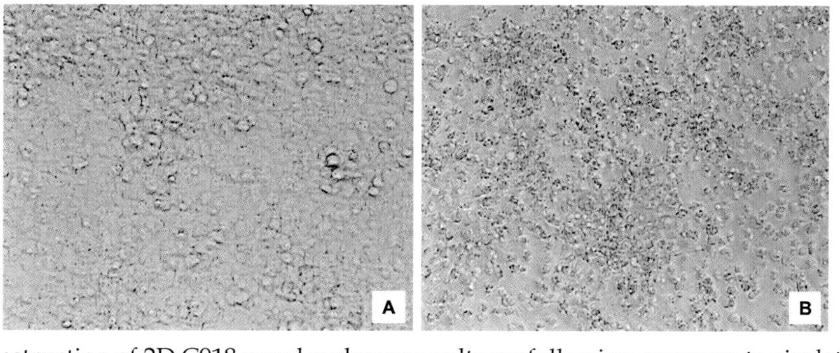

Fig. 3. Destruction of 2D C918 uveal melanoma cultures following exposure to cisplatin for four days. Panel A shows cultures grown in regular culture medium. Panel B shows destruction of cells that were cultured in medium containing 100 μM cisplatin. Magnification: 100x.

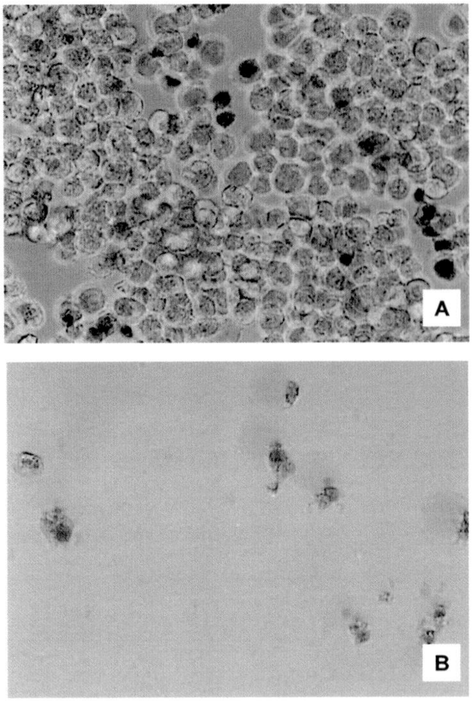

Fig. 4. Trypan blue staining in 2D C918 uveal melanoma cultures following 100 μM cisplatin treatment for seven days. While the majority of cells are viable (negative for trypan blue) in untreated control cultures (panel A), no viable (trypan blue-negative) C918 uveal melanoma cells are detected after 100 μM cisplatin treatment (panel B) (200x magnification).

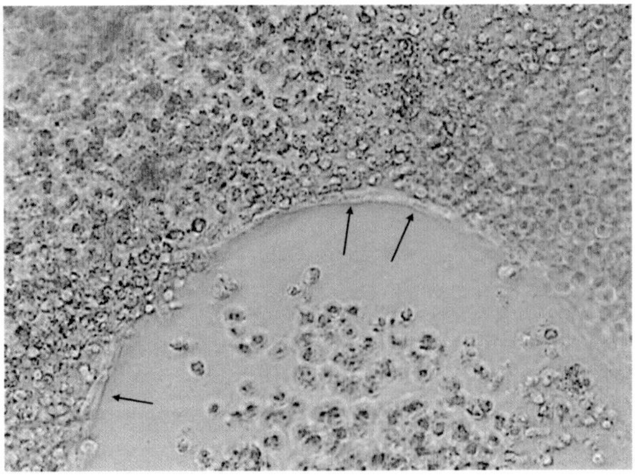

Fig. 5. Effect of 100 μM cisplatin on 3D C918 uveal melanoma cultures. All cells but those forming VM patterns demonstrate extensive destruction by 100 μM cisplatin in 3D cultures of C918 uveal melanoma cells three days after initiation of cisplatin treatment. Arrows point to VM (100x magnification).

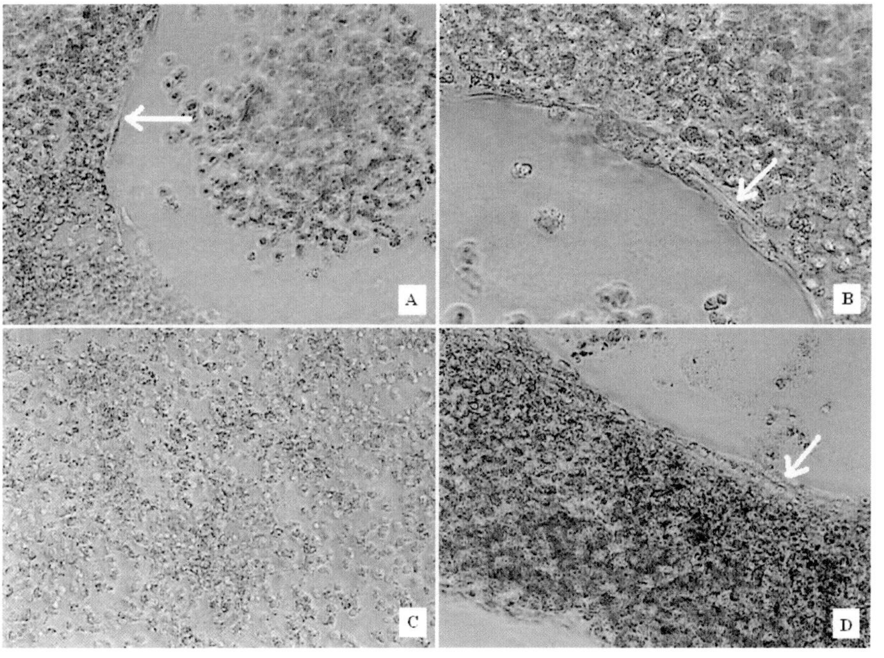

Fig. 6. Effect of 100 μM cisplatin on the morphology of 2D and 3D C918 uveal melanoma cultures. All cells but those forming VM patterns (arrows) are destroyed by 100 μM cisplatin in 3D cultures exposed for four days to cisplatin (panels A, B, and D). Destruction of 2D cultures exposed for four days to cisplatin (panel C). Magnification: 100x.

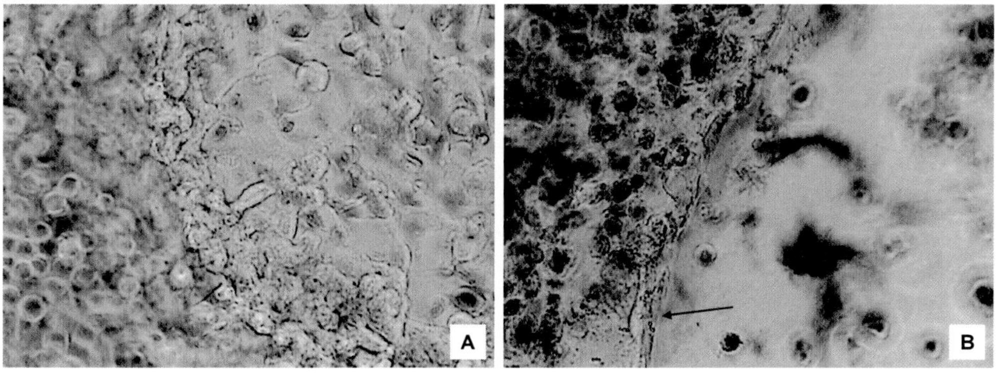

Fig. 7. Trypan blue staining in 3D C918 uveal melanoma cultures exposed for four days to regular medium (panel A) or to medium containing 100 μM cisplatin (panel B). Note that the majority of cells are viable (negative for trypan blue) in the control cultures in panel A. In contrast, only some of the cells associated with VM formation are viable (negative for trypan blue) in 3D cultures four days after 100 μM cisplatin treatment. Arrow in panel B points to VM (200x magnification).

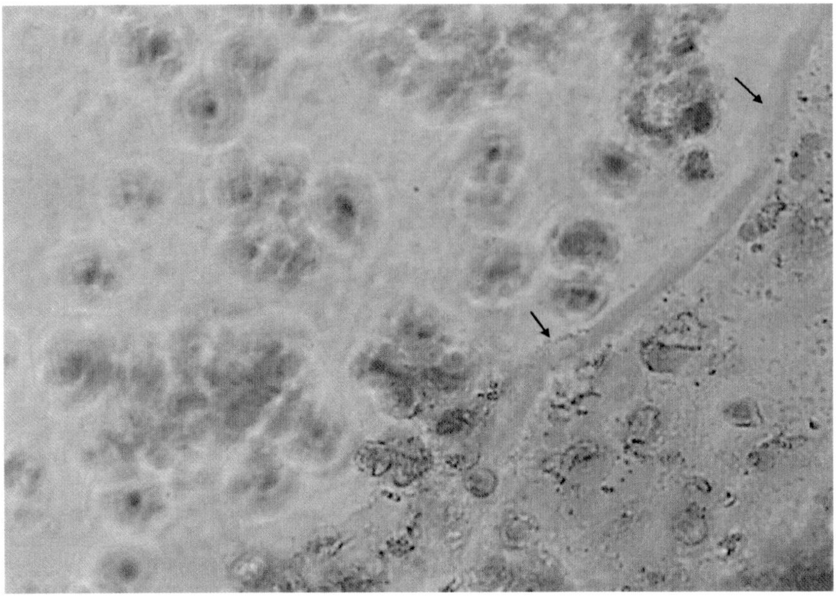

Fig. 8. Trypan blue staining in a 3D C918 uveal melanoma culture following 100 μM cisplatin treatment for seven days. Only some of the cells associated with VM formation (arrows) are viable (negative for trypan blue). Magnification: 200x.

3.3 VM-forming melanoma cells have increased resistance against cadmium

Starting 4 to 5 days after the initiation of cultures, when 2D cultures formed monolayers and cells in 3D cultures formed morphologically distinct tumor cell subpopulations including VM patterns, cultures were exposed to various concentrations of cadmium chloride (Yokouchi et al., 2007) and observed daily for toxicity. Cadmium chloride concentrations tested in the experiments ranged from 20 to 1000 μM. Fresh culture media containing cadmium chloride were added to the cultures daily for up to 4 weeks. Control cultures not exposed to cadmium chloride remained viable and demonstrated growth for several weeks. However, cultures exposed to cadmium chloride in the culture medium demonstrated dose dependant toxicity (Table 2). Similarly to the observations made with cisplatin, VM-forming tumor cells demonstrated prolonged survival following cadmium treatment relative to other tumor cell subpopulations in 3D cultures and cells grown in 2D (Table 2, Figs 9 through 14). Specifically, at 200 μM cadmium chloride concentration, destruction of VM-forming tumor cells never reached 99% in 3D cultures during a 16-day observation period while other cell subpopulations in 3D cultures and cells grown in 2D cultures were completely destroyed by 4 and 3 days, respectively (Table 2). Interestingly, as presented in the next section in detail, if cadmium chloride treatment was stopped sixteen days after initiation of drug treatment, residual still viable cells in VM patterns served as foci of new tumor growth (Fig. 16 through 18). These findings indicate that VM-forming tumor cells have increased resistance against the cytotoxic effects of cadmium chloride in 3D uveal melanoma cultures.

	2D	3D		
	Cells on surface of plate	Cells on surface of Matrigel	VM	Cells on surface of plate
No Cd Control	NA (>16 days)	NA (>16 days)	NA (>16 days)	NA (>16 days)
Cd 20 μM	NA (>16 days)	NA (>16 days)	NA (>16 days)	NA (>16 days)
Cd 200 μM	4 days	4 days	NA (>16 days)	4 days
Cd 400 μM	2 days	2 days	2 days	2 days
Cd 1000 μM	2 days	2 days	2 days	2 days

Table 2. Time (days) elapsed from the initiation of cadmium chloride ($CdCl_2$) treatment to destruction of more than 99% of C918 uveal melanoma cells in 2D cultures and destruction of more than 99% of various C918 cell subpopulations in 3D cultures during a 16-day observation period. Abbreviations: 2D = two-dimensional cultures; 3D = three-dimensional cultures; VM = cells forming vasculogenic mimicry patterns; Cd = cadmium chloride ($CdCl_2$); NA (>16 days) = not applicable, cell death did not reach 99% during the 16-day observation period.

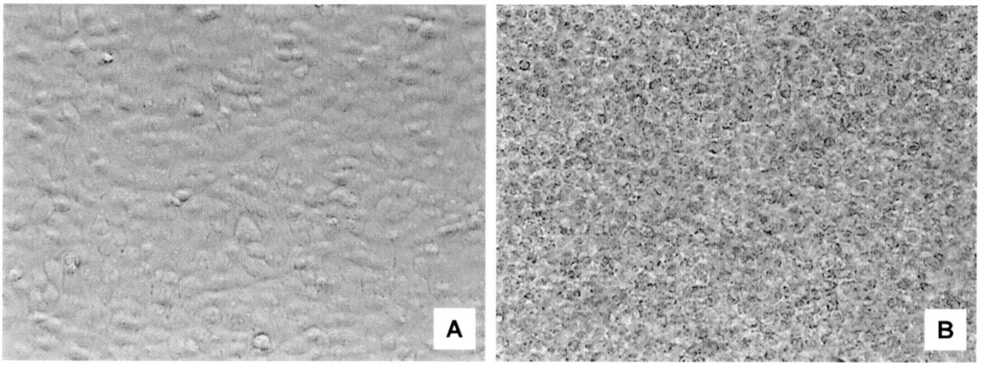

Fig. 9. Effect of 200 μM cadmium chloride on 2D C918 uveal melanoma cultures. Panel A shows cultures grown in regular culture medium. Panel B shows destruction of cells that were cultured in medium containing 200 μM cadmium chloride for four days. Magnification: 100x.

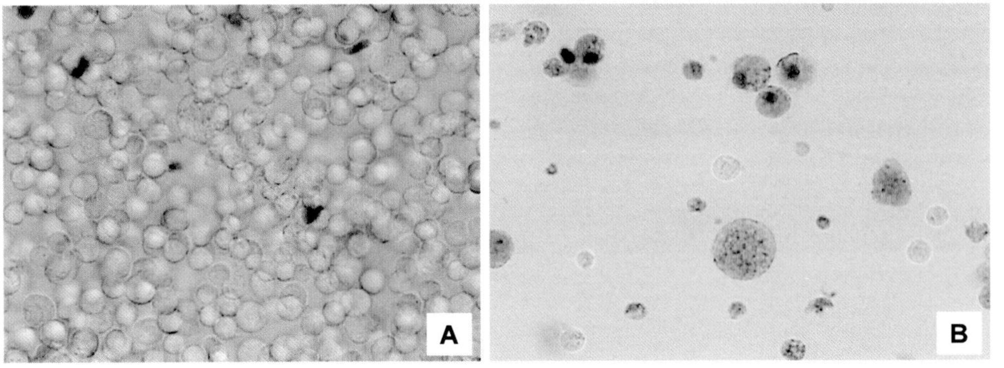

Fig. 10. Trypan blue staining in 2D C918 uveal melanoma cultures following 200 μM cadmium treatment for four days. While the majority of cells are viable (negative for trypan blue) in untreated control cultures (panel A), no viable (trypan blue-negative) C918 uveal melanoma cells are detected after 200 μM cadmium treatment (panel B) (200x magnification).

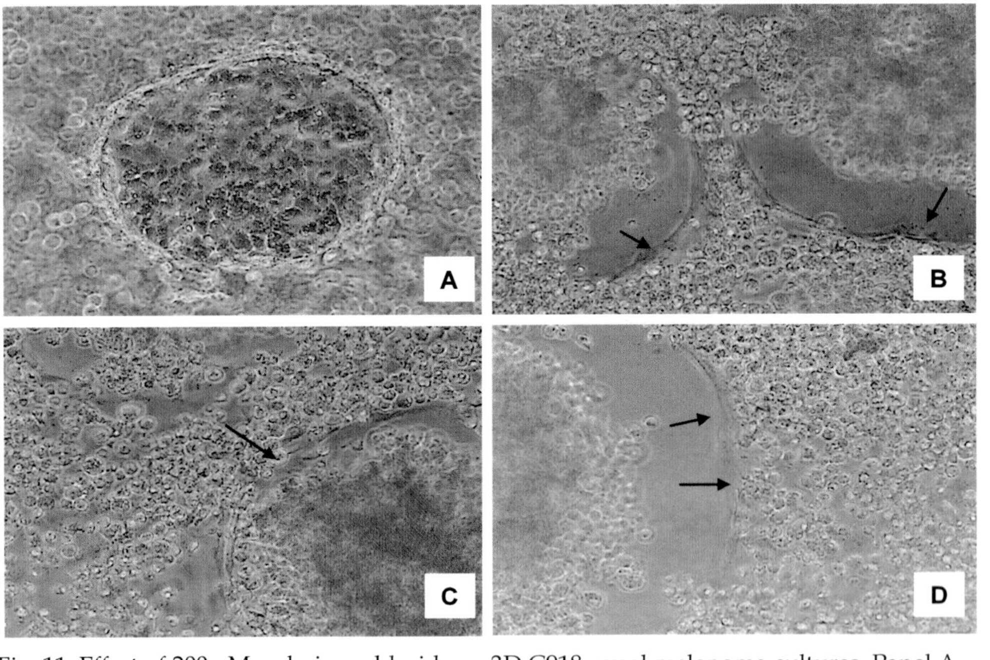

Fig. 11. Effect of 200 μM cadmium chloride on 3D C918 uveal melanoma cultures. Panel A shows a 3D culture grown in regular medium for nine days and is notable for an abundance of viable-appearing cells. Panels B through D show 3D cultures grown in medium containing 200 μM cadmium chloride for nine days. Note that all but some cells forming VM patterns are destroyed by the cadmium chloride treatment. Arrows point to VM in panels B, C, and D. Magnification: 200x.

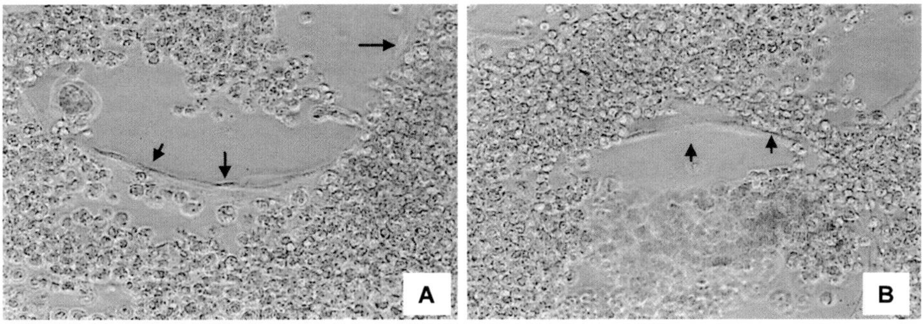

Fig. 12. Effect of exposure of 3D C918 uveal melanoma cultures to 200 μM cadmium chloride for nine days (A) or ten days (B). Note that all but some cells forming VM patterns (arrows) are destroyed by the cadmium chloride treatment. Magnification: 200x.

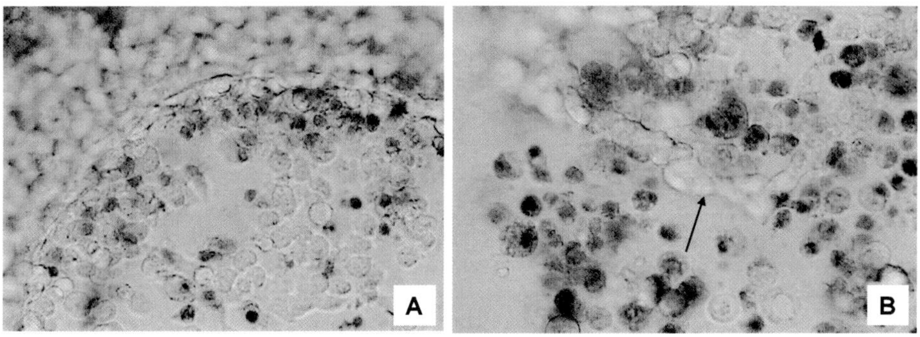

Fig. 13. Trypan blue staining in 3D C918 uveal melanoma cultures exposed for four days to regular medium (A) or to medium containing 200 μM cadmium chloride (B). The majority of cells are viable in the control cultures (A). Only some cells associated with VM formation are viable (negative for trypan blue) after cadmium treatment (arrow) (200x magnification).

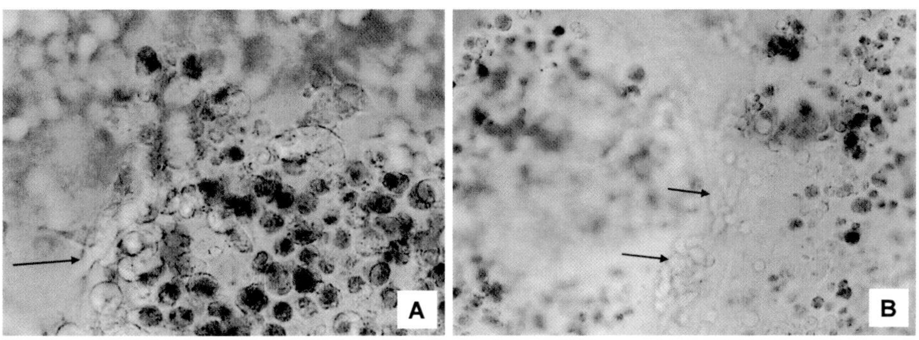

Fig. 14. Trypan blue staining in 3D C918 uveal melanoma cultures exposed for four days to 200 μM cadmium chloride. Only some tumor cells associated with VM formation (arrows) are viable (negative for trypan blue). 200x magnification.

3.4 VM-forming melanoma cells may serve as foci of renewed growth once drug treatment is stopped

Findings presented above indicate that VM-forming tumor cells have increased resistance against the cytotoxic effects of cadmium chloride in 3D uveal melanoma cultures. Interestingly, if cadmium chloride treatment was stopped sixteen days after initiation of drug treatment, residual still viable cells associated with VM patterns appeared to serve as foci of new tumor growth in the 3D cultures (Fig. 15 through 18).

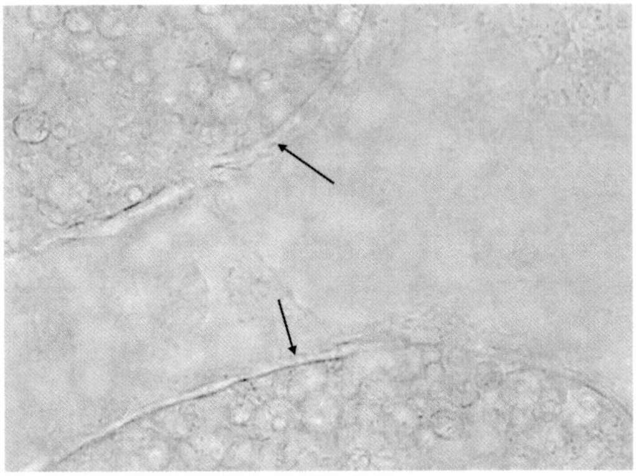

Fig. 15. Morphology of a 3D C918 melanoma culture one day after cadmium chloride treatment was stopped. Three-dimensional cultures of C918 uveal melanoma cells were exposed for sixteen days to medium containing 200 μM cadmium chloride resulting in the destruction of all cells but some cells forming VM (arrows). There is no evidence of cell growth from the VM yet. Magnification: 200x.

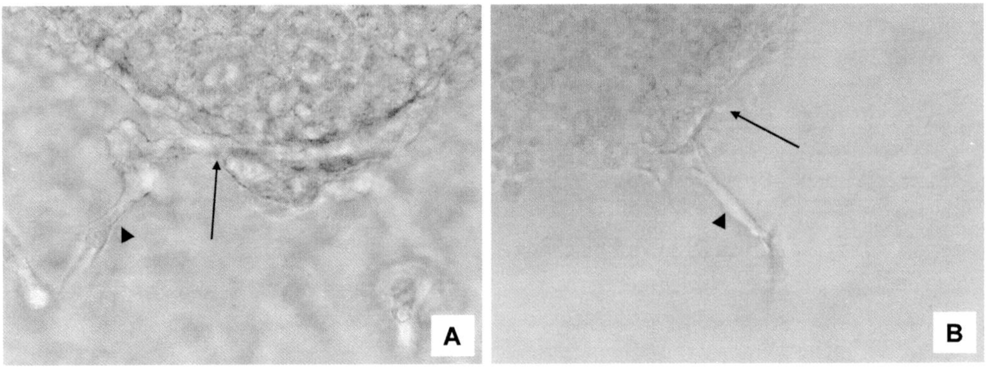

Fig. 16. Cells growing out from VM patterns four days following withdrawal of cadmium chloride treatment. Three-dimensional cultures of C918 uveal melanoma cells were exposed for sixteen days to medium containing 200 μM cadmium chloride resulting in the destruction of all cells but some forming VM (arrows). Note focus of resumed melanoma cell growth (arrowheads) from VM. Magnification: 200x.

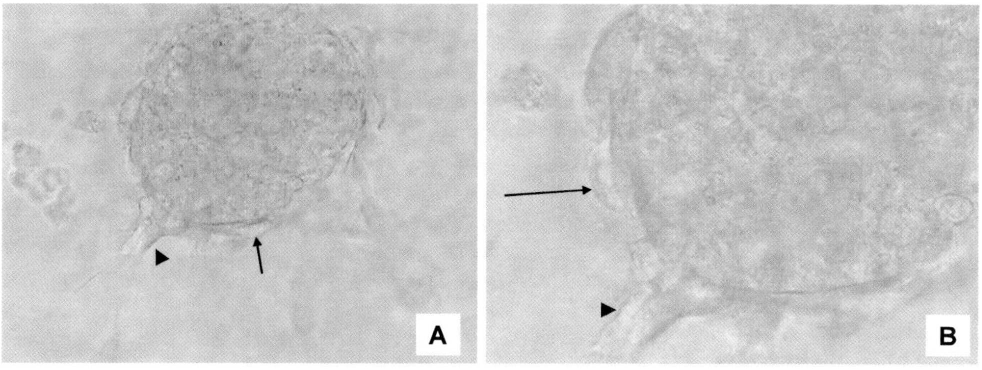

Fig. 17. Cells growing out from VM patterns four days following withdrawal of cadmium chloride treatment. Three-dimensional cultures of C918 uveal melanoma cells were exposed for sixteen days to medium containing 200 μM cadmium chloride resulting in the destruction of all cells but some forming VM (arrows). Note focus of resumed melanoma cell growth (arrowheads) from VM. Magnification: 100x (A), 200x (B).

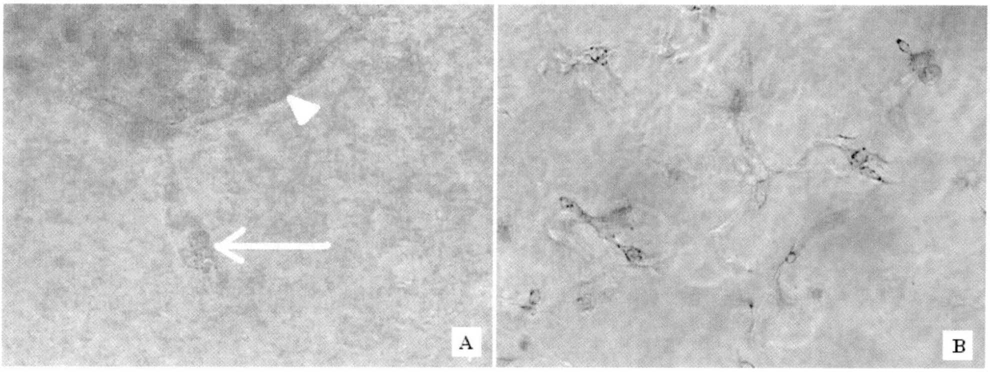

Fig. 18. Cells growing out from VM patterns following withdrawal of cadmium chloride treatment. Three-dimensional cultures of C918 uveal melanoma cells were exposed for sixteen days to medium containing 200 μM cadmium chloride resulting in the destruction of all cells but some of those associated with VM. Panel A shows cultures two days after drug withdrawal. Focus of resumed melanoma cell growth (arrow) is associated with VM (arrowhead). Panel B shows cultures nine days after drug withdrawal (200 x magnification).

4. Conclusions

While VM formation is clearly a marker of highly invasive tumor phenotype *in vivo*, mechanisms by which VM may contribute to adverse outcome are not well understood (Folberg et al., 1993; Maniotis et al., 1999; Folberg et al., 2000; Hendrix et al., 2003; Folberg and Maniotis, 2004; Lin et al., 2005; Döme et al, 2007). We have shown here that in 2D cultures, C918 uveal melanoma cells grow in monolayers and in 3D cultures, C918 cells form a number of morphologically distinct tumor cell subpopulations that include cells that form

VM patterns. Importantly, we found that following exposure to cytotoxic agents, VM-forming tumor cells demonstrate prolonged survival relative to other tumor cell subpopulations in 3D cultures and cells grown in 2D. Additional observations suggested that drug resistant VM-forming tumor cells may serve as foci of new tumor growth once cytotoxic drug levels drop. While confirmation of these observations in *in vivo* studies and other tumor types will be essential, our findings reported here suggest that increased drug resistance is a mechanism by which VM-forming tumor cells contribute to adverse outcome. As VM patterns have been described in a wide variety of malignant neoplasms, observations of this current report are of great potential significance.

5. Acknowledgments

This work was supported by fellowship grants to Andras Voros and Eva Gagyi by the Rosztoczy Foundation.

6. References

Abbott, A. (2003). Biology's new dimension. *Nature* 2003, 424:870–872.

Bowden, NA; Ashton, KA; Avery-Kiejda, KA; Zhang, XD; Hersey, P; Scott, RJ. (2010). Nucleotide excision repair gene expression after cisplatin treatment in melanoma.*Cancer Research*; 70:7918.

Del Bello, B; Valentini, MA; Comporti, M; Maellaro, E. (2003). Cisplatin-induced apoptosis in melanoma cells: role of caspase-3 and caspase-7 in Apaf-1 proteolytic cleavage and in execution of the degradative phases. *Ann N Y Acad Sci*; 1010:200-204.

Döme, B; Hendrix, MJ; Paku, S; Tóvári, J; Tímár, J. (2007). Alternative vascularization mechanisms in cancer. Pathology and therapeutic implications. *Am J Pathol* 170(1): 1-15.

Friedrich, MJ. (2003). Studying cancer in 3 dimensions. *JAMA* 2003; 290:1977–1979.

Feldman, ED; Pingpank, JF; Alexander Jr, RA.(2004) Regional treatment options for patients with ocular melanoma metastatic to the liver. *Ann Surg Oncol;* 11(3):290–297.

Folberg, R; Pe'er, J; Gruman, LM; Woolson, RF; Jeng, G; Montague, PR; Moninger, TO; Yi, H; Moore, KC. (1992). The morphologic characteristics of tumor blood vessels as a marker of tumor progression in primary human uveal melanoma: a matched case-control study. *Human Pathology* 23: 1298-1305.

Folberg, R; Rummelt, V; Parys-Van Ginderdeuren, R; Hwang, T; Woolson, RF; Pe'er, J; Gruman, LM. (1993). The prognostic value of tumor blood vessel morphology in primary uveal melanoma. *Ophthalmology* 100: 1389-1398.

Folberg, R; Hendrix, MJ; Maniotis, AJ. (2000). Vasculogenic mimicry and tumor angiogenesis. *Am J Pathol*; 156:361-381.

Folberg, R; Arbieva, Z; Moses, J; Hayee, A; Sandal, T; Kadkol, S; Lin, AY; Valyi-Nagy, K; Setty, S; Leach, L; Chévez-Barrios, P; Larsen, P; Majumdar, D; Pe'er, J; Maniotis, AJ. (2006). Tumor cell plasticity in uveal melanoma - Microenvironment directed dampening of the invasive and metastatic genotype and phenotype accompanies the generation of vasculogenic mimicry patterns. *Am J Pathol*; 169:1376-1389.

Folberg, R; Leach, L; Valyi-Nagy, K; Lin, AY; Apushkin, MA; Ai, Z; Barak, V; Majumdar, D; Pe'er, J; Maniotis, AJ. (2007). Modeling the behavior of uveal melanoma in the liver. *Invest Ophthalmol Vis Sci*; 48:2967-2974.

Folberg, R; Maniotis, AJ. (2004). Vasculogenic mimicry. *APMIS;* 112: 508-525.

Folberg, R; Kadkol, S; Frenkel, S; Valyi-Nagy, K; Jager, MJ; Pe'er, J; et al. (2008). Authenticating Cell Lines in Ophthalmic Research Laboratories. *Invest Ophthalmol Vis Sci;* 49 (11): 4697-4701.

Frank, NY; Schatton, T; Kim, S; Zhan, Q; Wilson, BJ; Ma, J; Saab, KR; Osherov, V; Widlund, HR; Gasser, M; Waaga-Gasser, AM; Kupper, TS; Murphy, GF; Frank, MH. (2011). VEGFR-1 expressed by malignant melanoma initiating cells is required for tumor growth. *Cancer Res;* 71(4):1474-1485.

Ghosh, S; Spagnoli, GC; Martin, I; Ploegert, S; Demougin, P; Heberer, M; Reschner, A. (2005). Three-dimensional culture of melanoma cells profoundly affects gene expression profile: A high density oligonucleotide array study. *J Cell Physiol;* 204:522-531.

Hendrix, MJC; Seftor, EA; Hess, AR; Seftor, RE. (2003). Vasculogenic mimicry and tumour-cell plasticity: lessons from melanoma. *Nature Reviews Cancer* 3: 411-421.

Jacks, T; Weinberg, RA. (2002). Taking the study of cancer cell survival to a new dimension. *Cell;* 111:923–925.

Lin, AY; Maniotis, AJ; Valyi-Nagy, K; Majumdar, D; Setty, S; Kadkol, S; Leach, L; Pe'er, J; Folberg, R. (2005). Distinguishing fibrovascular septa from vasculogenic mimicry patterns. *Arch Pathol Lab Med;* 129(7):884-889.

Maniotis, AJ; Folberg, R; Hess, A; Seftor, EA; Gardner, LMG; Pe'er, J; Trent, JM; Meltzer, PS; Hendrix, MJ. (1999). Vascular channel formation by human melanoma cells in vivo and in vitro: vasculogenic mimicry. *Am J Pathol;* 155:739-752.

Maniotis, AJ; Valyi-Nagy, K; Karavitis, J; Moses, J; Boddipali, JV; Wang, Y; Nuñez, R; Setty, S; Arbieva, Z; Bissell, MJ; Folberg, R. (2005). Chromatin organization measured by Alu I restriction enzyme changes with malignancy and is regulated by the extracellular matrix and the cytoskeleton. *Am J Pathol;* 166:1187-1203.

Nelson, CM; Bissell, MJ. (2005). Modeling dynamic reciprocity: engineering three-dimensional culture models of breast architecture, function, and neoplastic transformation. *Semin Cancer Biol;* 15:342–352.

Sandal, T; Valyi-Nagy, K; Spencer, VA; Folberg, R; Bissell, MJ; Maniotis, AJ. (2007). Epigenetic reversion of breast carcinoma phenotype is accompanied by changes in DNA sequestration as measured by AluI restriction enzyme-*Am J Pathol;*170(5):1739-1749.

Schmeichel, KL; Bissell, MJ. (2003). Modeling tissue-specific signaling and organ function in three dimensions. *J Cell Sci;* 116:2377–2388.

Schmidmaier, R; Baumann, P. (2008). Anti-adhesion evolves to a promising therapeutic concept in oncology. *Curr Med Chem;* 15:978-990.

Smalley, KS; Lioni, M; Herlyn, M. (2006). Life isn't flat: taking cancer biology to the next dimension. *In vitro Cell Dev Biol Anim ;* 42:242–247.

Vescio, RA; Redfern, CH; Nelso, TJ; Udoretz, S; Stern, PH; Hoffman, RM. (1987). In vivo-like drug responses of human tumors growing in three-dimensional gel-supported primary culture. *Proc Natl Acad Sci USA;* 84:5029-5033.

Valyi-Nagy, K; Folberg, R; Valyi-Nagy, T; Maniotis, AJ. (2007). Susceptibility of uveal melanoma to herpes simplex virus type 1: the role of tumor invasiveness, the extracellular matrix and chromatin sequestration. *Exp Eye Res;* 84:991-1000.

Valyi-Nagy, K; Dosa, S; Kovacs, SK; Bacsa, S; Voros, A; Shukla, D; Folberg, D; Valyi-Nagy, T. (2010). Identification of virus resistant tumor cell subpopulations in three dimensional uveal melanoma cultures. *Cancer Gene Therapy*; 17:223-234.

Xu, F; Burg, KJL. (2007). Three-dimensional polymeric systems for cancer cell studies. *Cytotechnology*; 54:135–143.

Yokouchi, M; Hiramatsu, N; Hayakawa, K; Kasai, A; Takano, Y; Yao, J; Kitamura, M. (2007). Atypical, bidirectional regulation of cadmium-induced apoptosis via distinct signaling of unfolded protein response. *Cell Death and Differentiation*;14:1467–1474.

Wang, F; Weaver, VM; Petersen, OW; Larabell, CA; Dedhar, S; Briand, P; Lupu, R; Bissell, MJ. (1998). Reciprocal interactions between beta1-integrin and epidermal growth factor receptor in three-dimensional basement membrane breast cultures: a different perspective in epithelial biology. *Proc Natl Acad Sci USA*; 95:14821–14826.

Weaver, VM; Petersen, OW; Wang, F; Larabell, CA; Briand, P; Damsky, C; Bissell, MJ. (1997). Reversion of the malignant phenotype of human breast cells in three-dimensional culture and in vivo by integrin blocking antibodies. *J Cell Biol*; 137:231–245.

19

The Role of Adhesion Receptors in Melanoma Metastasis and Therapeutic Intervention Thereof

Alexander, Michael[1,2,3] and Bendas, Gerd[3]
[1]*Department of Genomics, LIFE & BRAIN Center GmbH, University of Bonn, Bonn,*
[2]*Institute of Human Genetics, University of Bonn, Bonn,*
[3]*Pharmaceutical Institute, Department of Pharmaceutical Chemistry II, University of Bonn, Bonn,*
[1,2,3]*Germany*

1. Introduction

The metastatic spread of solid tumors is the most fatal complication in malignant diseases and the major cause of tumor-related mortality. This is of high relevance for malignant melanoma which are highly proliferating tumors with aggressive metastatic tendency. The majority of melanoma cells tend to metastasize primary via the lymph system and secondary into different organs, most likely distant skin regions, liver, lungs, brain, and heart via hematogenous distribution, which is associated with bad prognosis. The molecular mechanisms of the metastatic processes are complex and not fully elucidated. Although cytostatic agents or anti-angiogenetic drugs (e.g. Avastin/bevacizumab) affect, beside their effects on the primary tumors, also the growth and development of metastases, there is at present no antimetastatic pharmacological strategy in the clinics to interfere with tumor cell dissemination or spread.

Adhesion receptors are strongly involved in the process of tumor cell metastasis, either by deregulation of adhesive functions and subsequently the detachment of tumor cells from the primary tumor and the overcoming of tissue borders, or by mediating manifold cell contacts with blood components in the phase of hematogenous distribution. An intensive and ongoing preclinical research provided essential insight and several postulated factors and mechanisms for the hematogenous dissemination, i.e. the interaction of tumor cells with the different blood elements, soluble factors and cells. P- and L-selectin, members of a family of carbohydrate binding adhesion receptors are regarded as functional key players in the contact formation of tumor cells with platelets and leukocytes, thus facilitating microemboli formation and accelerating metastatic dissemination. The antimetastatic activities of heparin, confirmed by a number of prospective clinical trials, are to a large extent ascribed to the inhibition of these two selectins.

Besides the important role of selectins, integrins as ubiquitary cell adhesion receptors are also involved in the mediation of manifold adhesive interactions in the metastasis of tumor cells. Integrins bind ligands of the extracellular matrix (ECM), such as fibronectin, collagen, laminin and vitronectin to stabilize cell attachment with the surrounding tissues or to mediate migration in the metastatic cascade. Furthermore, integrins mediate cellular contacts of the tumor cells to platelets, leukocytes, and endothelium. However, in contrast to the selectins, the integrin function has hardly been considered as target for antimetastatic approaches.

Integrins possess important tasks in cell signalling that can be summarized as defining the cellular shape, mobility, invasion and cell cycle regulation. The regulation of these processes via contribution of the actin and microtubule cytoskeletons is well known to be controlled by Rho-GTPases (Ras homologue; guanosintriphosphatases), which belong to the superfamily of Ras-GTPases (Rat adeno sarcoma). GTPases of the Ras-superfamily are important for cell proliferation, metastasis, migration, apoptosis, gene expression and multiple other functions in the cell. Since the integrin signalling is also cross-linked to the function of GTPases, a therapeutic influence on the GTPase activity could be a novel and attractive approach to control integrin bindings. Recent data on the treatment of melanoma cells with lysophosphatidylcholine (LysoPC) referred to reduced integrin functions, which might be related to reduced GTPase signalling.

This book chapter will deal with the molecular function of adhesion receptors in the process of hematogenous metastasis of melanoma cells and the therapeutic potential and prospects to interfere with adhesion receptor activity as an antimetastatic approach. The focus was put on the integrins, which will be explained with their functions, abilities and connections to other indispensable proteins, such as cytoskeletal components in the context of cancer and metastasis. Finally the hypothesis to influence the integrin functions in metastatic cascade at a signalling level will be introduced and discussed as an interesting novel target for antimetastatic approaches.

2. The metastasis of melanoma cells

2.1 The course of the metastatic cascade

Tumor cell metastasis is a complex cascade which consists of various molecular events. Metastatic cells have to exit the primary tumor by a deregulation of the cellular contacts, have to migrate the basement membrane of the tumor, degrade the extracellular matrix and intravasate lymphatic vessels or local post capillary veins. Several factors are known which contribute to the malignant transformation of melanocytes and melanoma development and progression, including microenvironmental influences, or UV radiation for triggering a cascade of proinflammatory factors and mediators (Lee & Herlyn 2006; Schwarz & Luger 1989).

Once in the blood system, the tumor cells have to escape the immune surveillance and physical stress of the blood stream to finally seed at the vascular bed at distant organs. This is the rate-limiting step of the metastatic cascade before they can extravasate and form metastases (**Figure 1**).

An insight into the hematogenous phase of tumor cell distribution is given by numerous animal models of experimental metastasis, which dominantly used melanoma cell lines due to their rapid metastatic colonization tendency (Ludwig et al., 2004; Bereczky et al., 2005; Ludwig et al., 2006; Mousa et al., 2006; Niers et al. 2009). Although these models do not completely recapitulate the natural processes of metastatic spread, the timely defined presence of tumor cells in the blood systems allows for characterization and evaluation of cellular contacts within the phase of hematogenous distribution.

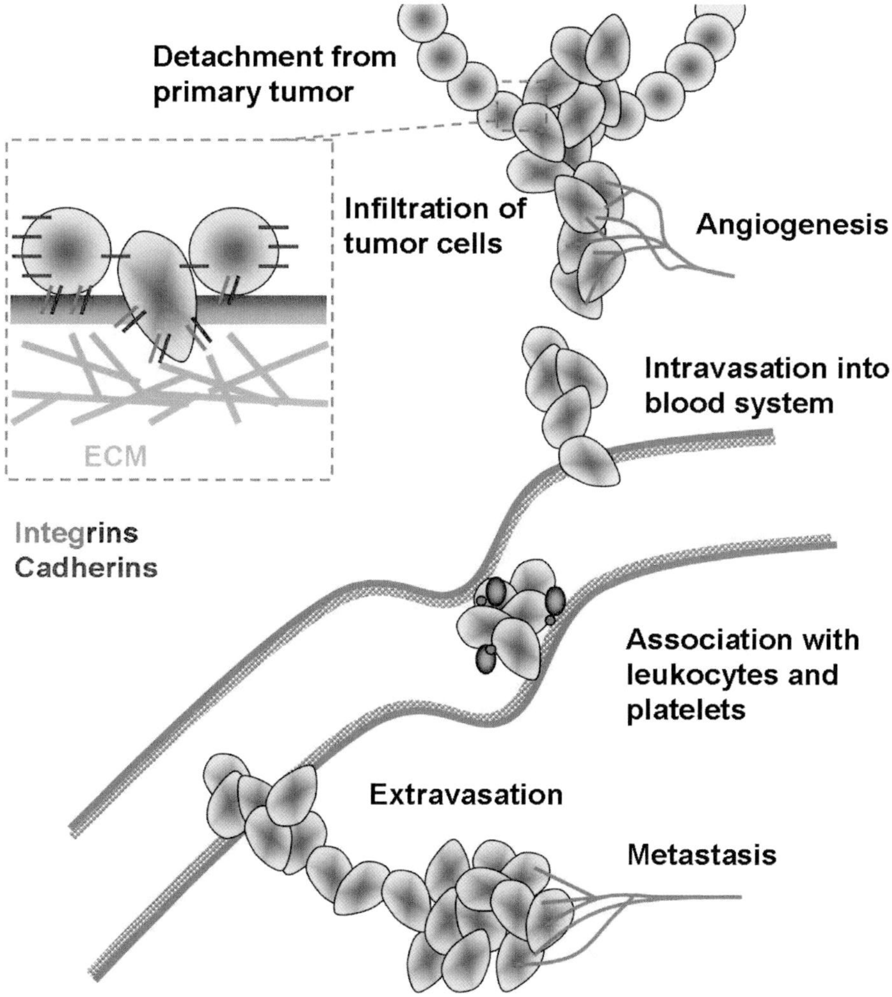

Fig. 1. Schematic representation of the hematogenous metastasis.
The illustration give insights into the step-by-step process of the hematogenous metastasis: Detachment of tumor cells from primary tumor; overcoming of ECM, intravasation into the blood system, association with platelets and leukocytes to prevent shear forces and immune defense, transport through the organism, physical arrest or arrest via interaction with the vascular endothel, extravasation, generation of micrometastases and angiogenesis to the blood supply.
Modified from (Guo W. & Giancotti F. G., 2004)

The massive interaction of tumor cells forming a platelet cloak is a vital strategy to evade the immune defense and was shown to correlate with metastatic progression. Furthermore, the recruitment of leukocytes to form microemboli is thought to support microvascular arrest at distant sites and contributes to activation of endothelial cells. In general, tumor cell and/or leukocyte interaction with the microenvironment at site of colonization induces an inflammatory-like activation of endothelial cells during the initial steps of metastasis progression, including the chemokine network and different procoagulative factors (Lazennec & Richmond, 2010). However, cellular adhesion receptors play a pivotal role for this complex cellular communication.

2.2 The impact of selectins on the hematogenous tumor cell dissemination

The selectins, a family of carbohydrate binding proteins, represent the crucial importance linked with hematogenous metastasis (Läubli & Borsig, 2010). P-selectin, expressed by platelets is dominant for the platelet contact of tumor cells. Its role for protecting the tumor cells and facilitating metastatic progression is confirmed by experiments using P-selectin knock-out mice, which displayed strongly attenuated experimental metastasis (Ludwig et al., 2004; Kim et al., 1998). It became evident that P-selectin, expressed by activated endothelial cells also contributes to the metastatic progression (Ludwig et al., 2004). L-selectin, which is constitutively expressed by all types of leukocytes, supports the comprehension of leukocyte into the microemboli and vascular contact formation and activation (Laubli et al., 2006). Endothelial activation is associated with the upregulation of other adhesion receptors, such as E-selectin or the integrin ligand vascular cell adhesion molecule-1 (VCAM-1), which again advises to the inflammatory-like reaction (Auguste et al., 2007).
Consequently, the competitive blocking of the selectin function appears as a promising therapeutic approach to interfere with the metastatic cascade.

2.3 The role of heparin for antimetastatic approaches

The evidence for those selectin-blocking approaches came indirectly from clinical efforts to treat cancer-associated thromboembolic events, which are frequent complications in malignant diseases. Heparin, or low molecular weight heparin (LMWH) are the anticoagulant drug of choice in the clinical treatment or prophylactic treatment of cancer-associated thrombosis. Based on the retrospective evaluation of clinical data, which referred to a survival benefit of heparin treated cancer patients, a number of prospective clinical trials have been lauchned (Zacharski & Lee, 2008). Animal experiments supported the assumption that heparin hardly affects the primary tumor but interferes with the process of metastasis. Several molecular mechanisms exist to explain the antimetastatic efficiency of heparin. The reader is referred to excellent reviews in this field (Borsig, 2010; Casu et al. 2008) from which the inhibitory capacity of heparin towards P- and L-selectin binding should be highlighted here.
Heparin as a highly sulfated, acidic polysaccharide has the ability to compete with the natural mucin-like selectin ligands. The capacity of heparin to interfere with P- and L-selectin binding has already been described in the early 90th (Skinner et al., 1991), but in the context of tumor cell metastasis the heparin effects as competitors of P- and L-selectins were accumulated during the last decade. Further insight was obtained into the structural requirements of heparin for selectin binding (Hostettler et al., 2007), and binding affinities of heparin to both selectins were shown to be in the low micromolar range (Simonis et al., 2007).

2.4 Integrins as targets for heparin

The platelet integrin IIb IIIa also contributes to the bond formation between platelets and melanoma cells via fibronectin or vWF to melanoma integrins. A recent study reported that heparin has also an inhibitory capacity to this binding (Zhang et al., 2009). Thrombin, interacting with its receptor PAR-1 on melanoma cells (protease-activated receptors-1) has a strong impact for regulating this interaction. PAR-1, which is predominantly overexpressed in malignant melanoma cells induces diverse procoagulant and metastatic events, such as matrix degradation, secretion of angiogenetic factors or integrin activation (Melnikova et al., 2008).

Melanoma integrins can also directly contribute to the firm adhesion to the vasculature. The integrin $\alpha 4\beta 1$ (very late activation antigen-4, VLA-4), which interacts with the VCAM-1 as counter receptor, is described as another pathway for endothelial arrest of malignant melanoma cells (beside osteosarcoma and rhabdomyosarcoma cells), thereby promoting the transmigration (Okahara et al., 1994; Liang & Dong, 2008) and metastasis (Garofalo et al., 1995; Schadendorf et al., 1995). Although these finding suggest that the inhibition of VLA-4 could be promising in the treatment of melanoma metastasis, and despite VLA-4 inhibition by antibodies or small molecules is a vital strategy to interfere with pathological inflammations, such approaches have not been described so far in the cancer field. We could recently show that the VLA-4/VCAM-1 interaction of murine or human melanoma cell lines can be efficiently blocked by heparin (Schlesinger et al., 2009). Nevertheless, beside those approaches for a competitive blockade of integrin receptor function, the manifold signalling functions of integrins open a new way for a therapeutic interference, which will be discussed below.

3. The biology of integrins in the context of cell adhesion processes and metastasis

In addition to the selectin-mediated cell adhesion processes in metastasis, the protein families of immunoglobulins (IGs), cadherins and integrins play important roles - in the case of malfunction - in the development and progression of melanoma metastasis.

Several members of the IG superfamily such as ICAM-1, L1CAM and MCAM/MUC18 are significantly associated with progression of melanoma metastasis (Meier et al., 2006; Yamada et al., 2006; Johnson et al., 1997). The MUC18/MCAM expression confers metastatic potential and increased tumorigenicity to human melanoma cells (Johnson et al., 1999). A switch of the cadherin molecules from E-cadherin to N-cadherin is responsible for the disassociation of melanoma cells from keratinocytes. The loss of E-cadherin function is connected with the upregulation/induction of MUC18/MCAM and $\alpha v\beta 3$ integrin in melanocytic cells in vitro and with changes in the levels and the cellular distribution of the transcriptional regulator β-catenin in melanomas in vivo (Johnson et al., 1999). Thus, melanoma cell invasion through the dermis is mediated by this change (Hsu et al., 1996; Hsu et al., 2000).

One of the most prominent examples that is frequently associated with the progression of melanoma is the integrin $\alpha 4\beta 1$ (VLA-4) (Braeuer et al, 2011). It was observed that VLA-4 overexpression and interaction with VCAM-1 is clearly correlated with experimental lung metastasis and the tumor stage (Schadendorf et al., 1995; Okahara et al., 1994). Due to the fact that the interaction of VLA-4 and VCAM-1 and other integrins are of great interest as possible targets for melanoma cancer therapy, the following chapter will handle with details on the integrin family and their structural and functional connections in the context of cancer metastasis.

3.1 The general structure of integrins

The integrins are large and complex transmembrane glycoproteins which act as adhesion receptor molecules that are responsible for the mediation of attachment and anchorage between cells or to the underlying extracellular matrix (ECM) (Morgan et al., 2007). In detail they span the plasma membrane and work alongside other proteins such as cadherins and selectins to mediate cell-cell and cell-matrix interaction and communication. One important task of integrins is the binding of the cell surface and ECM components such as fibronectin, vitronectin, collagen, and laminin.

Many cells have multiple types of integrins on their surface. That means the use of integrin-targeted reagents is not specific for all but for a few or one specific integrin. This provides additional mechanistic insights into the functions of integrin adhesion receptors.

The structure of integrins can be divided in two distinct chains, the α- and β-subunit (**Figure 2**) which form a non-covalent heterodimer (Morgan et al., 2007; Lau et al., 2009; Shattil et al., 2010). In mammals, 18 α- and 8 β-integrin genes have been characterized that encode polypeptides that combine to form 24 unique, canonical α/β receptors out of 144 possible combinations. The Drosophila genome encodes only five α- and two β-subunits, and the Caenorhabditis nematodes possess two α and one β genes (Shattil et al., 2010; Morgan et al., 2007; Humphries, 2000). In addition, variants of some integrin subunits are formed by differential splicing, for example four variants of the beta-1 subunit exist (Hynes, 2002).

Both the α- and β-subunits form separate tails, which penetrate the plasma membrane and possess small cytoplasmic domains (Nermut et al., 1988; Lau et al., 2009). The extracellular α/β-domains are relatively huge compared to the short cytoplasmic domain and the structure of each subunit is conserved between isoforms, excluding a subset of α-subunits, which include an inserted 'A-domain' in their ligand-binding pocket (Shattil et al., 2010; Morgan et al., 2007). The pathway of extracellular binding of integrins to intracellular transformation of the binding is most often mediated by the cytoplasmic tail of the β-subunit (Morgan et al., 2007).

3.2 The cellular functions of integrins

Concerning the function, integrins are involved in a wide range of biological activities, including immune patrolling, cell migration, defining cellular shape, cell cycle regulation, growth, invasion, proliferation, differentiation, survival/apoptosis and binding to cells by certain viruses (Desgrosellier & Cheresh, 2010; Assoian & Klein, 2008).

The integrin proteins act as receptors which are able to communicate between the ECM and the cell. They also transport information from the status inside the cell to the extracellular space. This allows rapid and flexible responses in both directions. Thus integrin tasks can be divided into two main functions: Attachment of the cell to the ECM and signal transduction from the ECM to the cell. Within the past decade it has become apparent that adhesion molecules such as integrins play an important role for the mediation of critical cytosolic signalling events in the cell (Stupack, 2007).

Integrins act to regulate complex processes in cancer disease such as angiogenesis, tumor growth and metastasis (Hynes, 2002), and the signalling has a dramatic impact on cell proliferation, survival and motility. For this reason they have become attractive therapeutic targets for the development of pharmaceutical compounds. Several effective integrin antagonists are now under clinical evaluation (Stupack, 2007).

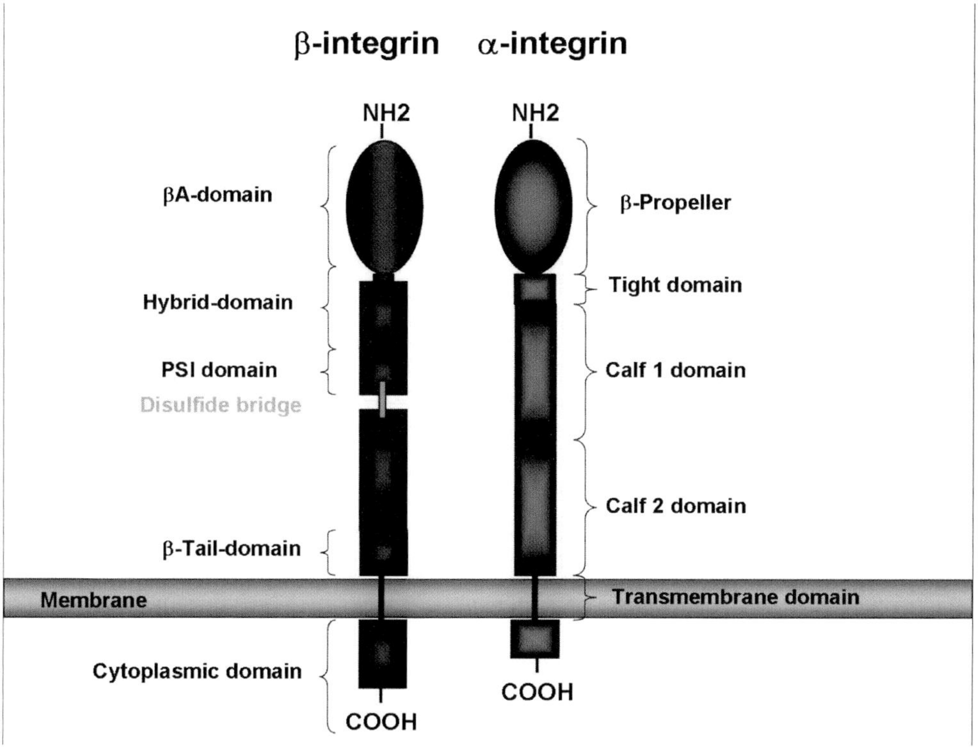

Fig. 2. Domain architecture of the heterodimeric transmembrane domains which show how integrins are designed to act as bidirectional signalling machines. Integrins are heterodimeric adhesive receptors consisting of an α- and a β-subunit. The ligand binding site is provided by the N-terminal domain of the α- and β-integrin subunits (the β-propeller and the βA domain, respectively) which are assembled in most integrins by non-covalent interactions to form a "head". It is known that in 8 α integrin subunits (α1, α2, α10, α11, αL, αM, αX and αD), the αA domain, which is homologous to the βA domain of the β-integrin subunit, is inserted into the β-propeller domain. This is the main ligand-binding site in these integrins. Integrins that lack an A domain (e.g. the depicted schematic architecture of αIIbβ3 integrin), the βA domain forms the main ligand-binding site. The PSI-domain (plexin, semaphorin and integrin) is at the N terminus of the β-integrin subunit, but is joined by disulfide bonds to more C-terminal residues. The remaining C-terminal extracellular domains of the α- and β-subunit comprise two long 'legs' which are anchored in the PM. The low affinity state of the integrin for its ligands is maintained by non-covalent interactions between the α- and β-integrin transmembrane and cytoplasmic domains. Figure is modified from (Shattil et al., 2010); α-subunit and β-subunit

In particular integrins operate as mechanistic biosensors in a context-dependent manner. On one hand, integrins that ligate substrate-immobilized ligands typically transduce positive signals into the cell. On the other hand, antagonized or unligated integrins promote negative signalling into the cell, which leads to cell cycle arrest or apoptosis. Thus, integrins constantly interrogate the local ECM and modulate cell behaviour accordingly. Typically, receptors inform a cell of the molecules in its environment and the cell evokes a response. Integrin receptors have two ways of signalling. They are able to perform outside-in signalling - response to molecules in its environment - and they also operate in an inside-out mode (Huveneers & Danen, 2009; Shattil et al., 2010; (**Figure 3**)). Therefore they are known as bidirectional, allosteric molecular signalling machines, although the relationship between specific conformations and activation remains controversial (Hynes, 2002; Shattil et al., 2010).

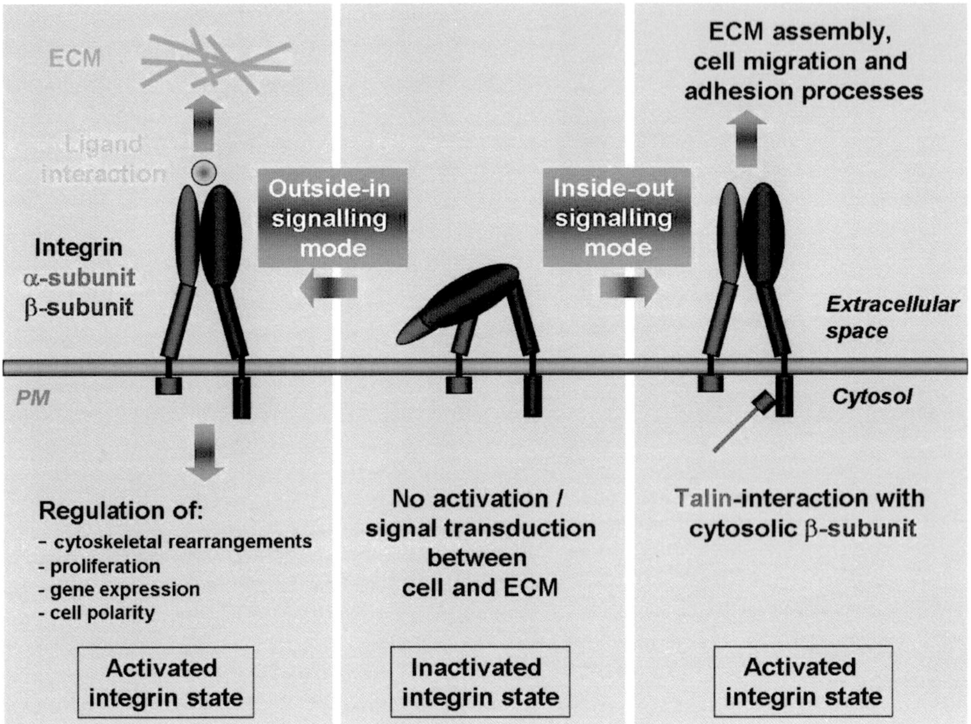

Fig. 3. Cellular signalling modes of integrins.
The two ways of integrin signalling can be divided in "outside-in" (left) and "inside-out" (right) modes. Both directions have different biological and biochemical consequences. In the case of "outside-in" signalling, binding of integrins to their extracellular ligands changes the conformation of the integrin and - because many of the ligands are multivalent - contributes to integrin clustering. The combination of these two events leads to intracellular signals that control cell polarity, cytoskeletal structure, gene expression, cell survival and proliferation. During 'inside-out' signalling, an intracellular activator, such as talin or kindlins, binds to the β-integrin tail, leading to conformational changes that result in increased affinity for extracellular ligands (integrin 'activation'). Inside-out signalling controls adhesion strength and enables sufficiently strong interactions between integrins and ECM proteins to allow integrins to transmit the forces required for cell migration and ECM remodelling and assembly. Both modes of signalling are often closely linked; for example, integrin activation can increase ligand binding, resulting in outside-in signalling. Conversely, ligand binding can generate signals that cause inside-out signalling. Modified from (Shattil et al., 2010)

As mentioned before, the cytoplasmic tail of the β-subunit is known to be the main region of mediating protein interaction (e.g. talin, a cytoskeletal protein), signal transduction and direct integrin activation (Shattil et al., 2010; Morgan et al., 2007).

4. The integrins in the context of signal transduction processes

The mechanisms of integrin interaction at the cytoplasmic side are strongly connected to the regulation of GTPases. For example, activated Rac1 and RhoA transduce signals to integrin activation via phospholipase **D** (**PLD**) and **p**hosphatidyl**i**nositol-4-**p**hosphate **5-k**inase **1γ** (**PIP5K1γ**) (Tybulewicz & Henderson, 2009). Furthermore it is known that integrin signalling is inhibited by RhoH through an unknown mechanism. In this case, integrin signalling leads to the activation of the GEF **αPIX** (**P**AK-**i**nteracting e**x**change factor-**α**) and the following activation of Rac1 and **PAK** (**p**21-**a**ctivated **k**inase) (Tybulewicz & Henderson, 2009). PAKs are well known to serve as targets for the small GTPases Cdc42 and Rac and they have been implicated in a wide range of biological activities, such as regulating the cell motility and morphology (PAK1), involvement in apoptotic processes (PAK2), or in the rapid cytoskeletal reorganization in dendritic spines (PAK3) or mediation of filopodia formation (PAK4).
Integrin signalling works predominantly through the recruitment and activation of **S**rc-**f**amily **k**inases (**SFKs**). Most integrins recruit **f**ocal **a**dhesion **k**inase (**FAK**) through their cytoplasmic domain of the β-subunit (Guo & Giancotti, 2004). FAK works as a phosphorylation-regulated scaffold to recruit Src to focal adhesions. From this important point of origin, several signal pathways influence the cell proliferation, survival and migration (**Figure 4**). Activating signalling via FAK, **p**hosphatidyl**i**nositol **3-k**inase (**PI3K**) over **p**hospha**t**i**d**yl**in**ositol-**3,4,5-trisphosphate** (**PtdIns(3,4,5)P$_3$**) to AKT and **p**rotein **k**inase **B** (**PKB**) can induce the mentioned effects (e.g. adhesion, cell proliferation, etc.). In addition, there is a direct crosstalk via GEF to activate Rac (another possibility for activation is from SFK via CAS, Crk and DOCK180 to Rac) which in turn can activate PAK, **Jun** amino-terminal **k**inase (**JNK**) and **n**uclear **f**actor **kappa-B** (**NFκB**) (Parsons & Parsons, 1997; Schlaepfer & Hunter, 1998; Cary *et al*, 1999). Furthermore FAK can activate **e**xtracellular signal-**r**egulated **k**inase/**m**itogen-**a**ctivated **p**rotein **k**inase (**ERK/MAPK**) by recruiting the Rap1 GEF C3G through Crk. Rap1 is then able to activate ERK/MAPK through B-Raf. An alternative way for ERK/MAPK activation is via the direct recruitment of **g**rowth-factor-**r**eceptor-**b**ound-**2** (**GRB2**) and **s**on-**o**f-**s**evenless (**SOS**) complex. Here, certain integrins, including α5β1, α1β1 and αvβ3, are coupled to palmitoylated SFKs through their α-subunits. The palmitoylated SFKs recruit and phosphorylate the adaptor Shc, which combines with GRB2–SOS to activate ERK/MAPK signalling from Ras (Wary *et al.*, 1996; 1998).
Beside the interaction of integrins with SFKs mentioned before, some integrins are able to interact directly with SFKs via the cytoplasmic tail of their β-subunits (Arias-Salgado et al., 2003). As an example, the α6β4 integrin is palmitoylated at its β-subunit. This palmitoylation is required for the incorporation of the complete α6β4 integrin in lipid rafts where the receptor is able to interact with SFKs that are similarly palmitoylated (Gagnoux-Palacios et al., 2003). Here, the SFKs phosphorylate several tyrosine residues in the cytoplasmic domain of β4, which causes the recruitment of SHC and activation of Ras-ERK/MAPK and PI3K signalling (Mainiero et al., 1995; 1997; Shaw et al., 1997; 2001). The known pathways that integrins can activate through SFKs are sufficient for the induction of cell migration, invasion and proliferation or to confer some protection from apoptosis on cells.

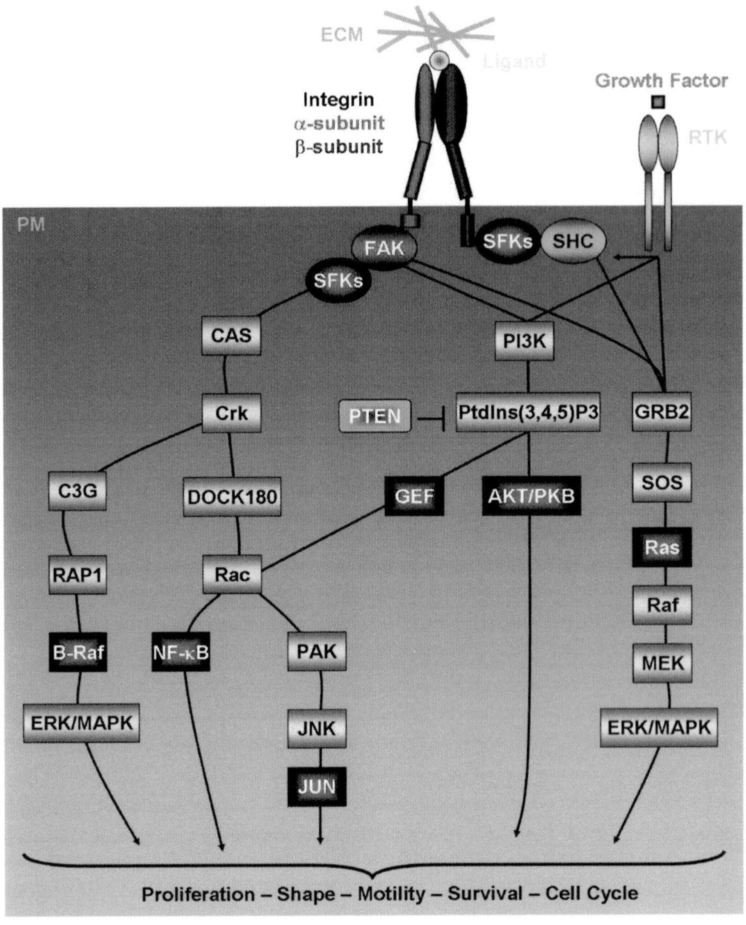

Fig. 4. General overview of alternative integrin signalling pathways.
The figure shows a section of the possible signalling cascades which lead to the activation of cellular survival proliferation and migration. Further details to the interactions are explained in the main text.
Modified from (Guo & Giancotti, 2004).

In addition to the α6β4 integrin, α4β1 (VLA-4) and αLβ2 have been identified to colocalize with the lipid raft marker GM-1 in T-cells. Disruption of raft integrity through depletion of membrane cholesterol with methyl-β-cyclodextrin (MbCD) completely disrupted α4β1 cluster formation, implying that the lipid rafts are required for α4 integrin clusters (Leitinger & Hogg, 2002). The integrins αvβ3, αIIbβ3 and α2β1 are associated with specific integrin interacting proteins in cholesterol-dependent microdomains distinct from classical rafts (Green et al., 1999). These results hypothesize that the mechanism of membrane compartmentalization - as identified for the mentioned integrins - also operates in other integrin-signalling systems, which might be an explanation for several specific aspects of diverse integrins.

5. Possible ways for pharmacological antimetastatic approaches by intervention with integrins on the plasma membrane and signalling level

The integrins, especially the integrin VLA-4 has been for longer time in the interest as target for the design of small molecule competive inhibitors as potential antiinflammatory drugs (Singh et al, 2004).

Concerning the "non-competitive" influence on integrins, there basically exist two different ways for integrin modulation: An interference with the signal transduction at the cytoplasmatic site or an influence on the integrin compartmentalization at the plasma membrane. As mentioned before the influence on integrins is mainly mediated via the cytoplasmatic tail of their β-subunits which allows the inside-out signalling (Arias-Salgado et al., 2003).

In general, integrins essentially need the specific membrane positioning and membrane anchorage of signalling proteins like GTPases of the Ras-superfamily for their signalling processes. The distribution of Ras proteins is determined by different C-terminal lipid modifications. Extensive experimental studies on Ras-GTPases have revealed that the proteins only operate at the plasma membrane (Meder & Simons, 2005; Pechlivanis & Kuhlmann, 2006). Several publications have pointed out the importance of Ras compartmentalization for signal transduction (Roy et al. 2002; Chiu et al., 2002). In particular, the palmitoylation allows the anchorage for H-Ras / N-Ras and the spatial and temporal organization plus segregation of the GTPases signal transfer duration. The time of PM-Golgi apparatus cycling, for N-Ras the transfer time from the PM to the Golgi apparatus during cycling, was remarkably shortened compared to H-Ras (Rocks et al., 2010; Rocks et al., 2005). This is in line with their palmitoylation status - two palmitoyl anchors for H-Ras and one palmitoyl anchor for N-Ras. Therefore, impact on the GTPase localization by affecting the membrane characteristics might have strong consequences for the integrin activity too.

In addition to the α6β4 integrin mentioned before, which possesses as laminin-5 receptor unique functions in epithelial growth and carcinoma invasion (Mainiero et al., 1997; Shaw et al., 1997) a palmitoylation of the β4-subunit as a prerequisite for the incorporation of α6β4 in rafts and the compartmentalization with SFKs (Gagnoux-Palacios et al., 2003), other integrins were also reported to depend critically on their membrane localization. The α4β1 integrin (VLA-4) was also identified to be localized in lipid rafts, which revealed that lipid rafts also play a key role in regulating integrin activity, function and its further downstream signalling (Leitinger & Hogg, 2002; Schadendorf et al., 1995; Okahara et al., 1994). Non-raft integrins are excluded from the rafts by cytoskeletal constraints and are no more able to perform signalling from raft microdomains (Leitinger & Hogg, 2002). Thus, the positioning of integrins inside or outside of rafts for their physical interaction with important signalling switches, such as GTPases or FAKs depends critically on the surrounding lipid composition. Consequently, an influence on the membrane characteristics and lipid composition of tumor cells appears as attractive way to influence integrin activities.

In a recent study, such an aspect of attenuated melanoma metastasis has been reported (Jantscheff et al., 2011), which refers to reduced receptor mediated binding by non-competively interfering with integrin function. This study is based on earlier findings that empty liposomes consisting of saturated phosphatidylcholine (PC) displayed strong antimetastatic effects in a murine pancreatic mice model (Graeser et al., 2009). Jantscheff et al. (2011) postulated that liposomes, passively accumulated in the tumor, release LysoPC as a degradation product of the saturated PC which affects the capability of tumor cells for metastases. In order to follow this hypothesis, the authors incubated murine melanoma B16.F10 cells with physiological and increased concentrations of saturated LysoPC. The melanoma cells fastly removed the LysoPC from the medium which was accompanied by a radical shift in tumor cell membrane fatty acid composition towards saturated fatty acids. This had strong morphological and functional consequences for the tumor cells. Electron microscopic images suggested that the changed membrane composition leads to a strong increase in number and size of filopodial-like membrane protrusions. It became evident that these morphological changes are based on cytoskeletal contractions. However, these concentrations of LysoPC used did not possess direct cytotoxicity. An induction of apoptosis could also be excluded.

The functional basis for antimetastatic effects of LysoPC became exposed by investigating the adhesion receptor binding. As mentioned before, melanoma cells make use of their integrin VLA-4 binding the endothelial ligand VCAM-1 for vascular arrest in the metastatic cascade. LysoPC incubation affected crucially the VLA-4 activity in a concentration dependent manner, although the expression levels of this integrin were not changed. Exceeding the physiological LysoPC concentration, the melanoma cells lost their ability for VCAM-1 binding. Furthermore, even though the treated cells exhibited a remarkably augmented number of protrusions, the cell motility on fibronectin as essential requirement for distinct steps of metastasis, e.g. tissue transmigration was significantly attenuated. In addition, the interaction with platelets via P-selectin was also strongly diminished, which is a further factor for reduced metastasis. These in vitro findings were totally reflected in a syngenic intravenous lung-invasion model. Using ex vivo-treated B16.F10 cells, LysoPC concentrations above the threshold (450 µM) resulted in significantly reduced metastasis-like lesions in lung tissue.

The search for the molecular basis of these promising data is ongoing yet, but might lead to some preliminary postulations. On the one hand, biophysical aspects of membrane properties and their change by the saturated lipids can be discussed to affect integrin function. On the other hand, an interference of LysoPC with the integrin signalling at the level of GTPases can be assumed.

Referring to the first assumption, a balance between saturated and unsaturated fatty acids is a fundamental biophysical determinant of membrane fluidity (Mansilla et al., 2008). The so-called homeoviscous adaptation is highly regulated and influences important membrane properties as flexibility, and lipid raft composition (Mansilla et al., 2008; Stulnig et al., 2001; Callaghan et al., 1993; Hac-Wydro et al., 2007). This strongly indicates that the addition of exogenous fully hydrogenated LysoPC and the subsequent change of membrane composition might have a clear impact on the deregulation of these factors. Since the integrin function is dependent on several aspects of membrane compartmentation (as described before), a reduced VLA-4 function could result from changes in e.g. raft domains.

Concerning the expression of important signalling proteins, we observed slightly reduced gene expression of the GTPases RhoA, RhoB and others after LysoPC exposition (300 µM and 450 µM) indicating an altered signal transduction in the context of membrane shape and adhesion (Alexander M. et al., 2010; 2011). RhoA and RhoB are known to participate in the regulaton of cytoskeleton, proliferation, formation of filopodia, lamellipodia, stress fibers and adhesion complexes (Hall A., 1998; Bishop & Hall, 2000; Etienne-Manneville & Hall, 2002; Etienne-Manneville & Hall, 2001; Hall A., 2009). Thus, activation of Rho GTPases is necessary for signalling between cells and ECM and for maintenance of cell shape and associated focal adhesion complexes (Burridge & Wennerberg, 2004).

Furthermore, one main part of cellular crosstalk and adhesion is the signal transduction via the integrins and SFKs (Mainiero et al., 1995; 1997; Shaw et al., 1997; 2001). In addition, to the reduced gene expression of GTPases, we also identified that several integrin subunits (ITGA4, ITGA2 and ITGB1) are reduced in transcription by LysoPC exposition in a concentration-dependent manner (Alexander M. et al., 2010). Thus, one can assume interplay between the LysoPC incubation and the altered adhesion, membrane morphology and gene expression of the examined melanoma cells.

The exact signal pathway that is affected by LysoPC exposition has to be investigated in future analyses due to the fact that not only one or a few defined signal pathways are triggering the adhesion process via integrins **(Figure 4)**. Nevertheless it is suggested that - due to the kind of deregulated genes - the ERK/MAPK pathway may be one key part of the promising antimetastatic effects initiated by LysoPC.

Genes which are regulated in expression levels by the ERK/MAPK pathway could influence the processes of invasion and adhesion. It is not completely understood if ERK/MAPK is activated or inhibited by LysoPC but specific kinases such as the dual-specificity phosphatase 1 (DUSP1) - a member of the threonine-tyrosine dual-specificity phosphatases - are deregulated by LPC treatment. Several members of the dual-specificity phosphatase (DUSPs) family are able to dephosphorylate MAPK isoforms with different specificity, cellular and tissue localization (Bermundez et al., 2010; Calvisi et al., 2008; Liu et al., 2007). The MAP kinases phosphatase (MKP) DUSP1/MKP-1 was shown to dephosphorylate ERKs (extracellular-regulated kinases), JNK and p38MAPKs (Liu et al., 2007). DUSP1 displays a rather broad specificity for inactivation of the ERK, p38 and JNK MAP kinases (Keyse, 2008). In addition, DUSP1 has detectable binding to ERK in vivo and is suggested to act as a positive activator of ERK in EGFR-mutant lung cancer cell lines independent of the ability to bind to ERK (Britson et al., 2009). Recent findings support the involvement of DUSPs in cancer progression and resistance (Bermundez et al., 2010) due to the fact that abnormalities in MAPK signalling have important consequences for processes critical to the development and progression of human cancer.

LysoPC exhibit a comparable chemical structure to the experimental anticancer drugs miltefosine and edelfosine **(Figure 5)**. The treatment of cancer cells with those alkylphosphocholines (APCs), which are able to incorporate into specific membrane compartments can disturb the well balanced and organized lipid network and thus influence the signalling of associated proteins. Such effects were reported for edelfosine and miltefosine, which are known to induce changes in receptor interaction and consequently signalling processes (Ausili et al., 2008; Gajate et al., 2009; Mollinedo & Gajate, 2010).

Since LysoPC possess a remarkably rapid uptake in the membranes of cancer cells, a comparable cellular mechanism by the critical alteration of the integrity and functionality of specific membrane microdomains could be hypothesized for LysoPC with regard to the global gene expression data. Although LysoPC possesses an evident similarity in chemical structure compared to the APCs, LysoPC seems to activate different signalling pathways. One difference is that exposition with edelfosine leads to selective promotion of apoptosis in leukemic cells (Mollinedo et al., 1997; Gajate et al., 2000; 2004).

Edelfosine was tested as a pharmaceutical compound against prostate cancer (Berdel et al., 1981), human brain tumors, lung tumors and other cancer types (Berdel et al. 1984; Denizot et al., 2001; Haugland et al., 1999; Houlihan et al., 1987; Kosano & Takatani, 1988; Ausili et al., 2008). In detail, edelfosine exposition leads to accumulation in lipid rafts (van der Luit et al., 2002; Gajate et al., 2004) and to a reorganization of the lipid and protein composition of

1

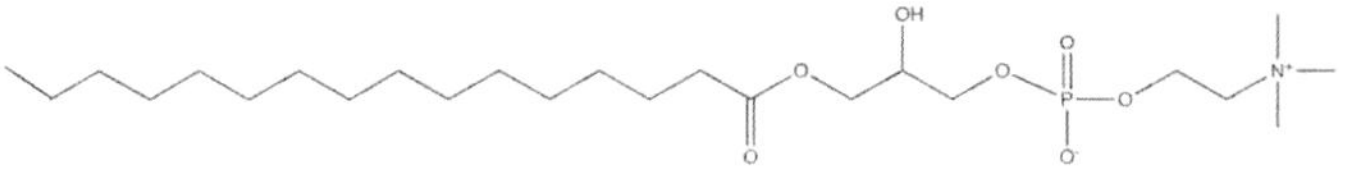

2

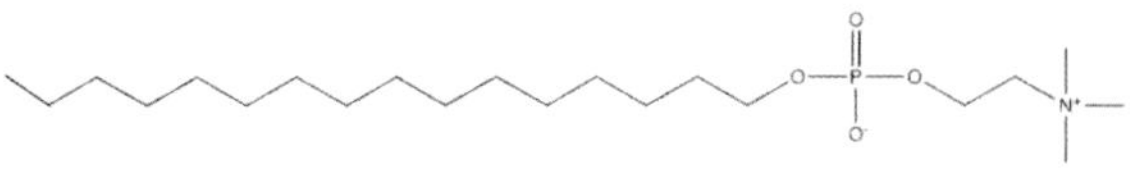

3

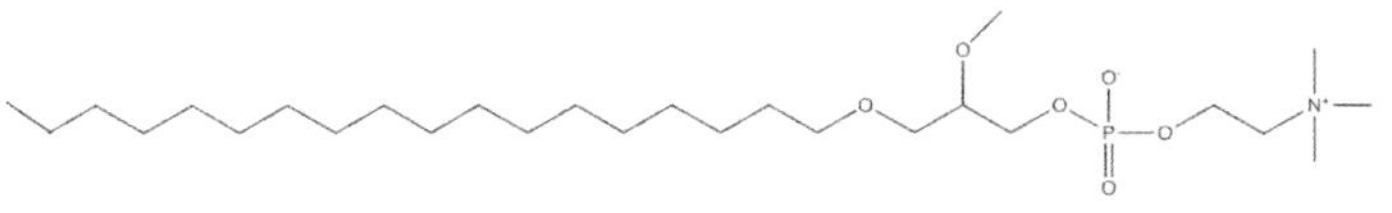

4

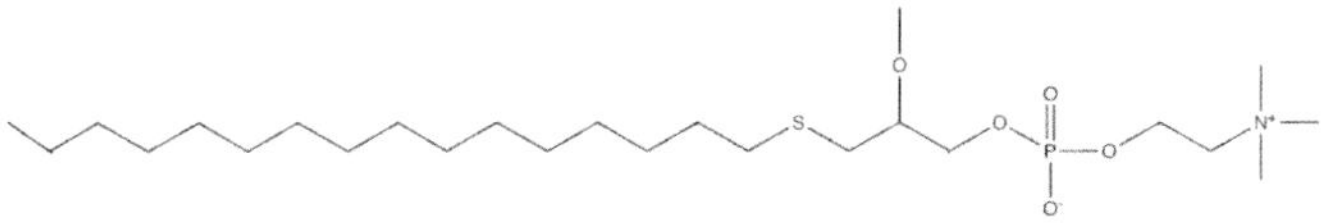

Fig. 5. Chemical structures of: Lysophosphatidylcholine (1), Miltefosine (2), Edelfosine (3) and Ilmofosine (4).

membrane caveolae (Gajate et al., 2004; Zaremberg et al., 2005; Gajate & Mollinedo, 2007). In a multiple myeloma animal model, oral administration of edelfosine showed a potent in vivo anti-myeloma activity and the drug accumulated preferentially in the tumor (Mollinedo et al., 2010). These data suggest that edelfosine incorporation in lipid rafts leads to a redistribution of sterols from the plasma membrane (Zaremberg et al., 2005). The redistribution of a major lipid raft component - they consist of cholesterol, glycolipids und sphingolipids - is likely to alter the biophysical properties of the lipid raft microdomain with putative important consequences for cell fate, due to the fact that the association of raft-targeted proteins is strongly assumed to be altered. However, there are no data available how edelfosine affects the integrin status of tumor cells.

In addition, the APC analog miltefosine (hexadecylphosphocholine) acts as another membrane-directed anti-tumoral and also anti-leishmanial drug (Santa-Rita et al., 2004). It activates anti-tumor effects against a broad spectrum of established tumor cell lines and solid tumors (Boggs et al., 1998; Wieder et al., 1998; Rybczynska et al., 2001; Jendrossek et al., 2002). Initial clinical studies have shown promising results: for example, miltefosine may be used for the treatment of cutaneous metastases of mammary carcinomas (Clive et al., 1999; Jimenez-Lopez et al., 2010).

Presently it remains open whether the antimetastatic effects and the serious affect on integrin activity by LysoPC are in line or on a comparable mechanistic level with the APC membrane effects. Future studies will provide insight into the hypotheses on membrane effects and the consequences for integrin localization and signalling. However, the non-competitive influence on the integrin activity by changing the lipid microenvironment appears as an interesting approach to interfere with integrin function in tumor cell metastasis.

6. Conclusion

The mortality rate of melanoma diseases is to a great extent related to the high tendency to form metastases via the lymph and blood system. An increasing insight into the molecular mechanisms of hematogenous metastasis offers new therapeutic options to interfere with the metastatic spread. Cellular adhesion receptors appear as attractive targets in that context, since adhesion molecules mediate several key events to allow the tumor cells the survival in the blood system and the settlement in the vascular bed of distant organs.

For a competitive blockade of the adhesion receptor function, heparin or non-anticoagulative heparin products possess most promises, since heparin is clinically accepted as anticoagulant and numerous preclinical data confirm the capacity of heparin to interfere with the selectins and selected integrins.

A novel strategy refers to a non-competitive influence on the adhesion receptors. A recent example is given by studies using LysoPC to melanoma cells, which drastically reduced the binding capacity of the integrin VLA-4 and thus, metastatic rate in mice. Although the exact molecular mechanisms are not fully elucidated, this might open new potential therapeutic options to reduce metastasis by interfering with adhesion molecules at the signalling level.

7. Acknowledgment

We thank Ulrich Massing for proof reading of the manuscript.

8. References

Lee, J.T. & Herlyn, M. (2006). Microenvironmental influences in melanoma progression. J. Cell Biochem. Vol. 110; No.4, pp. 862-872

Schwarz, T. & Luger, T.A. (1989). Effect of UV irradiation on epidermal cell cytokine production. J. Photochem. Photobiol. B Vol4, No.1, pp. 35448-35457

Ludwig, R.J.; Boehme, B.; Podda, M.; et al. (2004). Endothelial P-selectin as a target of heparin action in experimental melanoma lung metastasis. Cancer Res Vol. 64, pp. 2743–2750

IBereczky, B.; Gilly, R.; Raso, E.; et al. (2005). Selective antimetastatic effect of heparins in preclinical human melanoma models is based on inhibition of migration and microvascular arrest. Clin. Exp. Metastasis Vol. 22, pp. 69–76

Ludwig, R.J.; Alban, S.; Bistrian,R.; et al. (2006). The ability of different forms of heparins to suppress P-selectin function in vitro correlates to their inhibitory capacity on bloodborne metastasis in vivo. Thromb Haemost Vol. 95, pp. 535–40

Mousa, S.A.; Linhardt, R.; Francis, J.L. & Amirkhosravi, A. (2006). Anti-metastatic effect of a non-anticoagulant low-molecular-weight heparin versus the standard low molecular-weight heparin, enoxaparin. Thromb Haemost Vol. 96, pp. 816–21

Niers, T.M.; Bruggemann, L.W.; Klerk, C.P.; et al. (2009). Differential effects of anticoagulants on tumor development of mouse cancer cell lines B16, K1735 and CT26 in lung. Clin Exp Metastasis Vol. 26, pp. 171–178

Lazennec, G. & Richmond, A. (2010). Chemokines and chemokine receptors: new insights into cancer-related inflammation. Trends in Mol. Med. Vol. 16, No.3, pp.133-144

Läubli, H. & Borsig, L. (2010). Selectins promote tumor metastasis. Semin. Cancer Biol. Vol. 20, No3, pp. 169-77

Kim, Y.J.; Borsig, L.; Varki, N.M. & Varki, A. (1998). P-selectin deficiency attenuates tumor growth and metastasis. Proc Natl Acad Sci U S A Vol. 95, pp.9325–9330.

Laubli, H.; Stevenson, J.L.; Varki, A.; Varki, N.N. & Borsig L. (2006). L-selectin facilitation of metastasis involves temporal induction of fut7-dependent ligands at sites of tumor cell arrest. Cancer Res. Vol. 66, pp. 1536–1542

Auguste, P.; Fallavollita, L.; Wang, N. et al (2007). The host inflammatory response promotes liver metastasis by increasing tumor cell arrest and extravasation. Am J Pathol Vol.170, pp. 1781–1792

Zacharski, L.R. & Lee, A.Y. (2008). Heparin as an anticancer therapeutic. Expert Opin. Investig. Drugs, Vol. 17, pp. 1029–1037

Borsig L. (2010) Antimetastatic activities of heparins and modified heparins. Experimental evidence. Thromb Res. Vol. 125 Suppl 2, pp. S66-71

Casu, B.; Vlodavsky, I. & Sanderson, R.D. (2008). Non-anticoagulant heparins and inhibition of cancer. Pathophysiol Haemost Thromb. Vol. 36, No. 3-4, pp. 195-203

Skinner, M. P.; Lucas, C. M.; Burns, G. F.; Chesterman, C. N. & Berndt, M. C. (1991) GMP-140 binding to neutrophils is inhibited by sulfated glycans. J. Biol. Chem. Vol. 266, pp. 5371-5374

Hostettler, N.; Naggi, A.; Torri, G.; et al. (2007). P-selectin- and heparanase-dependent antimetastatic activity of non-anticoagulant heparins. FASEB J. Vol. 21, pp. 3562–3572

Simonis, D.; Fritzsche, J.; Alban, S. & Bendas, G. (2007). Kinetic analysis of heparin and glucan sulfates binding to P-selectin and its impact on the general understanding of selectin inhibition. Biochemistry. Vol. 46, No. 20, pp. 6156-6164

Zhang, C.; Liu, Y. ; Gao, Y. et al. (2009). Modified heparins inhibit integrin alpha(IIb)beta(3) mediated adhesion of melanoma cells to platelets in vitro and in vivo. Int. J. Cancer Vol. 125, pp.2058–2065

Melnikova, V.O.; Villares, G.J. & Bar-Eli, M. (2008). Emerging roles of PAR-1 and PAFR in melanoma metastasis. Cancer Microenviron. Vol. 1, No. 1, pp. 103-111.

Okahara, H.; Yagita, H.; Miyake, K. & Okumura, K. (1994). Involvement of very late activation antigen 4 (VLA-4) and vascular cell adhesion molecule 1 (VCAM-1) in tumor necrosis factor alpha enhancement of experimental metastasis. Cancer Res. Vol. 54; pp. 3233-3236

Liang, S. & Dong, C. (2008) Integrin VLA-4 enhances sialyl-Lewisx/a-negative melanoma adhesion to and extravasation through the endothelium under low flow conditions. Am. J. Physiol. Cell Physiol. Vol. 295, pp. C701-707.

Garofalo, A.; Chirivi, R.G.; Foglieni, C.; Pigott, R.; Mortarini, R.; Martin-Padura, I.; et al. (1995) Involvement of the very late antigen 4 integrin on melanoma in interleukin 1-augmented experimental metastases. Cancer Res. Vol. 55, pp. 414-419

Schadendorf, D.; Heidel, J.; Gawlik, C.; Suter, L. & Czarnetzki, B.M. (1995). Association with clinical outcome of expression of VLA-4 in primary cutaneous malignant melanoma as well as P-selectin and E-selectin on intratumoral vessels. J. Natl. Cancer Inst. Vol. 87, pp. 366-371

Fritzsche, J.; Simonis, D. & Bendas, G. (2008). Melanoma cell adhesion can be blocked by heparin in vitro: suggestion of VLA-4 as a novel target for antimetastatic approaches. Thromb. Haemost. Vol.100, pp. 1166-1175

Schlesinger, M.; Simonis, D.; Schmitz, P.; Fritzsche, J. &, Bendas, G. (2009). Binding between heparin and the integrin VLA-4. Thromb. Haemost. Vol. 102, pp. 816-822.

Meier, F.; Busch, S.; Gast, D.; Goppert, A.; Altevogt, P.; Maczey, E. et al. (2006). The adhesion molecule L1 (CD171) promotes melanoma progression. Int J Cancer; Vol. 119, pp. 549–55.

Yamada, M.; Yanaba, K.; Hasegawa, M.; Matsushita, Y.; Horikawa, M.; Komura, K. et al. (2006). Regulation of local and metastatic host-mediated anti-tumour mechanisms by L-selectin and intercellular adhesion molecule-1. Clin Exp Immunol; Vol. 143 ; pp. 216–27.

Johnson, J. P.; Bar-Eli M.; Jansen, B. & Markhof, E. (1997). Melanoma progression-associated glycoprotein MUC18/MCAM mediates homotypic cell adhesion through interaction with a heterophilic ligand. Int J Cancer; Vol. 73, pp. 769–74.

Johnson, J. P. (1999). Cell adhesion molecules in the development and progression of malignant melanoma. Cancer Metastasis Rev; Vol 18 ; pp. 345–57.

Desgrosellier J. S. & Cheresh D. A. (2010). Integrins in cancer: biological implications and therapeutic opportunities. Nat Rev Cancer. Vol 1; pp 9-22

Shattil, S. J., Kim, C. & Ginsberg, M. H. (2010). The final steps of integrin activation: the end game. Nat Rev Mol Cell Biol. Vol 4 ; pp. 288-300.

Hsu, M. Y.; Wheelock, M. J.; Johnson, K. R. & Herlyn, M. (1996). Shifts in cadherin profiles between human normal melanocytes and melanomas. J Investig Dermatol Symp Proc; Vol. 1 ; pp. 188–94.

Hsu, M.; Andl, T.; Li, G.; Meinkoth, J. L. & Herlyn, M. (2000). Cadherin repertoire determines partner-specific gap junctional communication during melanoma progression. J Cell Sci. Vol. 113 ; pp. 1535–42.

Braeuer, R. R.; Zigler, M.; Villares, G.J.; Dobroff, A. S. & Bar-Eli, M. (2011). Transcriptional control of melanoma metastasis: the importance of the tumor microenvironment. Semin Cancer Biol. Vol. 2 ; pp. 83-8.

Schadendorf, D.; Heidel, J.; Gawlik, C.; Suter, L. & Czarnetzki, B. M. (1995). Association with clinical outcome of expression of VLA-4 in primary cutaneous malignantmelanoma as well as P-selectin and E-selectin on intratumoral vessels. J Natl Cancer Inst. Vol. 87 ; pp. 366–71.

Okahara, H.; Yagita, H.; Miyake, K. & Okumura, K. (1994). Involvement of very late activation antigen 4 (VLA-4) and vascular cell adhesion molecule 1 (VCAM-1) in tumor necrosis factor alpha enhancement of experimental metastasis. Cancer Res; Vol. 54 ; pp. 3233–6.

Morgan, M. R.; Humphries, M.J. & Bass, M. D. (2007). Synergistic control of cell adhesion by integrins and syndecans. Nat Rev Mol Cell Biol. Vol. 12 ; pp. 957-69.

Lau, T. L.; Kim, C.; Ginsberg, M. H. & Ulmer, T. S. (2009). The structure of the integrin alphaIIbbeta3 transmembrane complex explains integrin transmembrane signalling. EMBO J.; Vol. 9 ; pp. 1351-61.

Humphries, M. J. (2000). Integrin cell adhesion receptors and the concept of agonism. Trends Pharmacol Sci. Vol. 1 ; pp. 29-32.

Hynes, R. O. (2002). Integrins: bidirectional, allosteric signaling machines. Cell. Vol., 6. pp. 673-87.

Nermut, M. V.; Green, N. M.; Eason, P.; Yamada, S. S. & Yamada, K. M. (1988). Electron microscopy and structural model of human fibronectin receptor. EMBO J. Vol., 13. pp. 4093-9.

Assoian, R. K. & Klein, E. A. (2008). Growth control by intracellular tension and extracellular stiffness. Trends Cell Biol. ; Vol. 7. pp. 347-52.

Stupack, D. G. (2007). The biology of integrins. Oncology (Williston Park). Vol. 9. pp. 6-12.

Huveneers, S. & Danen, E. H. (2009). Adhesion signaling - crosstalk between integrins, Src and Rho. J Cell Sci. Vol. 122 ; pp. 1059-69.

Tybulewicz, V. L. & Henderson, R. B. (2009). Rho family GTPases and their regulators in lymphocytes. Nat Rev Immunol. Vol. 9 ; pp. 630-44.

Guo, W. & Giancotti, F. G. (2004). Integrin signalling during tumour progression. Nat Rev Mol Cell Biol. Vol. 10 ; pp. 816-26.

Parsons, J. T & Parsons, S. J. (1997). Src family protein tyrosine kinases: cooperating with growth factor and adhesion signaling pathways. Curr Opin Cell Biol. Vol. 2 ; pp.187-92.

Schlaepfer, D. D. & Hunter, T. (1998). Integrin signalling and tyrosine phosphorylation: just the FAKs? Trends Cell Biol. Vol. 4 ; pp. 151-7.

Cary, L. A.; Han, D. C. & Guan, J. L. (1999). Integrin-mediated signal transduction pathways. Histol Histopathol. Vol. 3; pp. 1001-9.

Wary, K. K.; Mariotti, A.; Zurzolo, C. & Giancotti, F. G. (1998). A requirement for caveolin-1 and associated kinase Fyn in integrin signaling and anchorage-dependent cell growth. Cell. Vol. 5 ; pp. 625-34.

Wary, K. K.; Mainiero, F.; Isakoff, S. J.; Marcantonio, E. E. & Giancotti, F. G. (1996). The adaptor protein Shc couples a class of integrins to the control of cell cycle progression. Cell. Vol. 4. ; pp. 733-43.

Arias-Salgado, E. G. et al. (2003). Src kinase activation by direct interaction with the integrin β cytoplasmic domain. Proc. Natl Acad. Sci. USA Vol. 100 ; pp. 13298–13302.

Gagnoux-Palacios, L.; Dans, M.; van't Hof, W.; Mariotti, A.; Pepe, A.; Meneguzzi, G.; Resh, M. D. & Giancotti, F. G. (2003). Compartmentalization of integrin α6β4 signaling in lipid rafts. J. Cell Biol. Vol. 162 ; pp. 1189–1196.

Mainiero, F. et al. (1995). Signal transduction by the α6β4 integrin: distinct β4 subunit sites mediate recruitment of Shc/Grb2 and association with the cytoskeleton of hemidesmosomes. EMBO J. Vol. 14 ; pp. 4470–4481.

Mainiero, F.; Murgia, C.; Wary, K. K.; Curatola, A. M.; Pepe, A.; Blumemberg, M.; Westwick, J. K.; Der, C. J. & Giancotti, F. G. (1997). The coupling of alpha6beta4 integrin to Ras-MAP kinase pathways mediated by Shc controls keratinocyte proliferation. EMBO J. Vol. 9 ; pp. 2365-75.

Shaw, L. M., Rabinovitz, I., Wang, H. H., Toker, A. & Mercurio, A. M. (1997). Activation of phosphoinositide 3-OH kinase by the α6β4 integrin promotes carcinoma invasion. Cell. Vol.7 ; pp. 949-60.

Shaw, L. M. (2001). Identification of insulin receptor substrate 1 (IRS-1) and IRS-2 as signaling intermediates in the α6β4 integrin-dependent activation of phosphoinositide 3-OH kinase and promotion of invasion. Mol. Cell Biol. Vol. 21 ; pp. 5082–5093.

Leitinger, B. & Hogg, N. (2002). The involvement of lipid rafts in the regulation of integrin function. J Cell Sci. Vol. 115 ; pp. 963-72.

Green, J. M.; Zhelesnyak, A.; Chung, J.; Lindberg, F. P.; Sarfati, M.; Frazier, W. A. & Brown, E. J. (1999). Role of cholesterol in formation and function of a signaling complex involving alphavbeta3, integrin-associated protein (CD47), and heterotrimeric G proteins. J Cell Biol. Vol. 3 ; pp. 673-82.

Meder, D. & Simons, K.(2005). Cell biology. Ras on the roundabout. Science. Vol. 307; pp. 1731-3.

Pechlivanis, M.; Ringel, R.; Popkirova, B.; Kuhlmann, J. (2007). Prenylation of Ras facilitates hSOS1-promoted nucleotide exchange, upon Ras binding to the regulatory site. Biochemistry. Vol. 18 ; pp. 5341-8.

Roy, S.; Wyse B.; Hancock, J. F. (2002). Mol. Cell. Biol. Vol. 22, pp. 5128

Chiu, V. K. et al. (2002). Nature Cell Biol. Vol. 4 pp. 343

Rocks, O.; Peyker, A.; Kahms, M.; Verveer, P. J.; Koerner, C.; Lumbierres, M.; Kuhlmann, J.; Waldmann, H.; Wittinghofer, A. & Bastiaens, P. I. (2005). An acylation cycle regulates localization and activity of palmitoylated Ras isoforms. Science. Vol. 307 ; pp. 1746-52.

Rocks, O.; Gerauer, M.; Vartak, N.; Koch, S.; Huang, Z. P.; Pechlivanis, M.; Kuhlmann, J.; Brunsveld, L.; Chandra, A.; Ellinger, B.; Waldmann, H. & Bastiaens, P. I. (2010). The palmitoylation machinery is a spatially organizing system for peripheral membrane proteins. Cell. Vol. 141 ; pp. 458-71.

Schadendorf, D.; Heidel, J.; Gawlik, C.; Suter, L. & Czarnetzki, B. M. (1995). Association with clinical outcome of expression of VLA-4 in primary cutaneous malignant melanoma as well as P-selectin and E-selectin on intratumoral vessels. J Natl Cancer Inst.Vol. 87 ; pp. :366-71.

Okahara, H.; Yagita, H.; Miyake, K. & Okumura, K. (1994). Involvement of very late activation antigen 4 (VLA-4) and vascular cell adhesion molecule 1 (VCAM-1) in tumor necrosis factor alpha enhancement of experimental metastasis. Cancer Res. Vol. 54 ; pp. 3233-6.

Jantscheff, P.; Schlesinger, M.; Fritzsche, J.; Taylor, L. A.; Graeser, R.; Kirfel, G.; Fürst, D. O.; Massing, U. & Bendas, G. (2011). Lysophosphatidylcholine pretreatment reduces VLA-4 and P-Selectin-mediated b16.f10 melanoma cell adhesion in vitro and inhibits metastasis-like lung invasion in vivo. Mol Cancer Ther. Vol. 10 ; pp. 186-97.

Graeser, R.; Bornmann, C.; Esser, N.; Ziroli, V.; Jantscheff, P.; Unger, C.; Hopt, U. T.; Schaechtele, C.; von Dobschuetz, E. & Massing, U. (2009) Antimetastatic effects of liposomal gemcitabine and empty liposomes in an orthotopic mouse model of pancreatic cancer. Pancreas. Vol. 38 ; pp. 330-7.

Mansilla, M. C., Banchio, C. E. & de Mendoza, D. (2008). Signalling pathways controlling fatty acid desaturation. Subcell Biochem, Vol. 49 ; pp. 71-99.

Stulnig, T. M., Huber, J., Leitinger, N., Imre, E. M., Angelisova, P., Nowotny, P. & Waldhausl, W. (2001). Polyunsaturated eicosapentaenoic acid displaces proteins from membrane rafts by altering raft lipid composition. J Biol Chem, Vol. 276 ; pp. 37335-37340.

Callaghan, R., Stafford, A. & Epand, R. M. (1993). Increased accumulation of drugs in a multidrug resistant cell line by alteration of membrane biophysical properties. Biochim Biophys Acta. Vol. 1175 ; pp. 277-282.

Hac-Wydro, K. & Wydro, P. (2007). The influence of fatty acids on model cholesterol/phospholipid membranes. Chem Phys Lipids, Vol. 150 ; pp. 66-81.

Hall, A. (1998). Rho GTPases and the actin cytoskeleton. Science. Vol. 279 ; pp. 509–514.

Hall A. (2009). The cytoskeleton and cancer. Cancer Metastasis Rev. Vol. 28 ; pp. 5-14.

Etienne-Manneville, S. & Hall, A. (2000). Rho GTPases in cell biology. Nature Vol. 420 ; pp. 629–635.

Etienne-Manneville, S. & Hall, A. (2001). Integrin-mediated activation of Ccd42 controls cell polarity in migrating astrocytes through PKCζ. Cell Vol. 106 ; pp. 489–498.

Etienne-Manneville, S. & Hall, A. (2002). Rho GTPases in cell biology. Nature Vol. 420 ; pp. 629–635.

Bishop, A. L. & Hall, A. (2000). Rho GTPases and their effector proteins. Biochemical Journal Vol. 348 ; pp. 241–255.

Burridge, K. & Wennerberg, K. (2004) Rho and Rac take center stage. Cell. Vol. 116 ; pp. 167-79.

Ausili, A.; Torrecillas, A.; Aranda, F. J.; Mollinedo, F.; Gajate, C.; Corbalán-García, S.; de Godos, A. & Gómez-Fernández, J. C. (2008). Edelfosine is incorporated into rafts and alters their organization. J Phys Chem B. Vol. 112 ; pp. 11643-54.

Gajate, C.; Gonzalez-Camacho, F. & Mollinedo, F. (2009). Involvement of raft aggregates enriched in Fas/CD95 death-inducing signaling complex in the antileukemic action of edelfosine in Jurkat cells. PLoS One. Vol. 4 ; pp. 5044.

Mollinedo, F. & Gajate, C. (2010). Lipid rafts and clusters of apoptotic signaling molecule-enriched rafts in cancer therapy. Future Oncol. Vol. 6 ; pp 811-21.

Mollinedo, F.; Fernandez-Luna, J. L.; Gajate, C.; Martin-Martin, B.; Benito, A.; Martinez-Dalmau, R. & Modolell, M. 1997. Cancer Res. Vol. 57 ; pp. 1320.

Gajate, C.; Fonteriz, R. I.; Cabaner, C. ; Alvarez-Noves, G.; Alvarez-Rodriguez, Y.; Modolell, M. & Mollinedo, F. (2000). Intracellular triggering of Fas, independently of FasL, as a new mechanism of antitumor ether lipid-induced apoptosis. Int J Cancer. Vol. 85 ; pp. 674-82.

Gajate, C.; Del Canto-Jañez, E.; Acuña, A. U.; Amat-Guerri, F.; Geijo, E.; Santos-Beneit, A. M.; Veldman, R. J. & Mollinedo, F. (2004). Intracellular triggering of Fas aggregation and recruitment of apoptotic molecules into Fas-enriched rafts in selective tumor cell apoptosis. J Exp Med. Vol. 200 ; pp 353-65.

Berdel, W. E.; Fink, U.; Egger, B.; Reichert, A.; Munder, P. G. & Rastetter, J. (1981). Alkyl-lysophospholipids inhibit the growth of hypernephroid carcinomas in vitro. J Cancer Res Clin Oncol. Vol. 101 ; pp. 325-30.

Berdel, W. E.; Greiner, E.; Fink, U.; Zänker, K. S.; Stavrou, D.; Trappe, A.; Fahlbusch, R.; Reichert, A. & Rastetter, J. (1984). Cytotoxic effects of alkyl-lysophospholipids in human brain tumor cells. Oncology. Vol. 41 ; pp. 140-5.

Denizot, Y.; Desplat, V.; Drouet, M.; Bertin, F. & Melloni, B. (2001). Is there a role of platelet-activating factor in human lung cancer? Lung Cancer. Vol. 33 ; pp. 195-202.

Haugland, H. K.; Nygaard, S. J. & Tysnes, O. B. (1999). Combined effect of alkyl-lysophospholipid and vincristine on proliferation, migration and invasion in human glioma cell lines in vitro. Anticancer Res. Vol. 19 ; pp. 149-56.

Houlihan, W. J.; Lee, M. L.; Munder, P. G.; Nemecek, G. M.; Handley, D. A.; Winslow, C. M.; Happy, J. & Jaeggi, C. (1987). Antitumor activity of SRI 62-834, a cyclic ether analog of ET-18-OCH3. Lipids. Vol. 22 ; pp. 884-90.

Kosano, H. & Takatani, O. (1988). Reduction of epidermal growth factor binding in human breast cancer cell lines by an alkyl-lysophospholipid. Cancer Res. Vol. 48 ; pp. 6033-6.

van der Luit, A. H.; Budde, M.; Ruurs, P.; Verheij, M. & van Blitterswijk, W. J. (2002). Alkyl-lysophospholipid accumulates in lipid rafts and induces apoptosis via raftdependent endocytosis and inhibition of phosphatidylcholine synthesis. J Biol Chem. Vol. 277 ; pp. 39541-7.

Gajate, C.; Del Canto-Jañez, E.; Acuña, A. U.; Amat-Guerri, F.; Geijo, E.; Santos-Beneit, A. M.; Veldman, R. J. & Mollinedo, F. (2004). Intracellular triggering of Fas aggregation and recruitment of apoptotic molecules into Fas-enriched rafts in selective tumor cell apoptosis. J Exp Med. Vol. 200 ; pp. 353-65.

Gajate, C. & Mollinedo, F. (2007). Edelfosine and perifosine induce selective apoptosis in multiple myeloma by recruitment of death receptors and downstream signaling molecules into lipid rafts. Blood. Vol. 109 ; pp. 711-9.

Mollinedo, F.; de la Iglesia-Vicente, J.; Gajate, C.; Estella-Hermoso de Mendoza, A.; Villa-Pulgarin, J. A.; Campanero, M. A. & Blanco-Prieto, M. J. (2010). Lipid raft-targeted therapy in multiple myeloma.

Zaremberg, V.; Gajate, C.; Cacharro, L. M.; Mollinedo, F. & McMaster, C. R. (2005). Cytotoxicity of an anti-cancer lysophospholipid through selective modification of lipid raft composition. J Biol Chem. Vol. 280 ; pp. 38047-58.

Santa-Rita, R. M., Henriques-Pons, A.; Barbosa, H. S. & de Castro, S. L. (2004). Effect of the lysophospholipid analogues edelfosine, ilmofosine and miltefosine against Leishmania amazonensis. J Antimicrob Chemother. Vol. 54 ; pp. 704-10.

Boggs, K.; Rock, C. O. & Jackowski, S. (1998). The antiproliferative effect of hexadecylphosphocholine toward HL60 cells is prevented by exogenous lysophosphatidylcholine. Biochim Biophys Acta Vol. 1389 ; pp 1-12.

Wieder, T.; Orfanos, C. E. & Geilen, C. C. (1998). Induction of ceramide-mediated apoptosis by the anticancer phospholipid analog, hexadecylphosphocholine. J Biol Chem Vol. 273 ; pp. 11025-31.

Rybczynska, M.; Spitaler, M.; Knebel, N. G.; Boeck, G.; Grunicke, H. & Hofmann, J. (2001). Effects of miltefosine on various biochemical parameters in a panel of tumor cell lines with different sensitivities. Biochem Pharmacol Vol. 62; pp. 765-772.

Jendrossek, V.; Hammersen, K.; Erdlenbruch, B.; Kugler, W.; Krugener, R.; Eibl, H. & Lakomek, M. (2002). Structure-activity relationships of alkylphosphocholine derivatives: antineoplastic action on brain tumor cell lines in vitro. Cancer Chemother Pharmacol. Vol. 50 ; pp. 71-79.

Jiménez-López, J. M.; Ríos-Marco, P.; Marco, C.; Segovia, J. L. & Carrasco, M. P. (2010). Alterations in the homeostasis of phospholipids and cholesterol by antitumor alkylphospholipids. Lipids Health Dis. Vol. 9 ; pp. 33.

Clive, S.; Gardiner, J. & Leonard, R. C. (1999). Miltefosine as a topical treatment for cutaneous metastases in breast carcinoma. Cancer Chemother Pharmacol Vol. 44 ; pp. 29-30.

Bermudez, O.; Pagès, G. & Gimond C. (2010). The Dual-Specificity MAP Kinase Phosphatases: critical roles in development and cancer. Am J Physiol Cell Physiol.

Calvisi, D.F., Pinna, F., Meloni, F., Ladu, S., Pellegrino, R., Sini, M., Daino, L., Simile, M.M., De Miglio, M.R., Virdis, P., Frau, M., Tomasi, M.L., Seddaiu, M.A., Muroni, M.R., Feo, F. & Pascale, R.M. (2008). Dual-specificity phosphatase 1 ubiquitination in extracellular signal-regulated kinase-mediated control of growth in human hepatocellular carcinoma. Cancer Res. Vol. 68 ; pp.:4192-200.

Liu, Y., Shepherd, E.G. & Nelin L.D. (2007). MAPK phosphatases--regulating the immune response. Nat Rev Immunol. Vol. 3 ; pp. 202-12.

Keyse, S.M. (2008). Dual-specificity MAP kinase phosphatases (MKPs) and cancer. Cancer Metastasis Rev. Vol. 2 ; pp. 253-61.

Britson, J.S., Barton, F., Balko, J.M. Black, E.P. (2009). Deregulation of DUSP activity in EGFR-mutant lung cancer cell lines contributes to sustained ERK1/2 signaling. Biochem Biophys Res Commun. Vol. 3 ; pp. 849-54